Laparoscopic Sleeve Gastrectomy

Salman Al-Sabah · Ali Aminian ·
Luigi Angrisani · Eliana Al Haddad ·
Lilian Kow

Editors

Laparoscopic Sleeve Gastrectomy

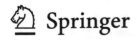 Springer

Editors
Salman Al-Sabah
Faculty of Medicine
Kuwait University
Safat, Kuwait

Luigi Angrisani
University of Naples Federico II
Napoli, Italy

Lilian Kow
Flinders University
Adelaide, Australia

Ali Aminian
Cleveland Clinic
Cleveland, OH, USA

Eliana Al Haddad
Columbia University Medical Center
New York, NY, USA

ISBN 978-3-030-57375-1   ISBN 978-3-030-57373-7   (eBook)
https://doi.org/10.1007/978-3-030-57373-7

This Springer imprint is published by the registered company Springer Nature Switzerland AG
The registered company address is: Gewerbestrasse 11, 6330 Cham, Switzerland

Foreword

Over the last century, we witnessed the obesity disease's rapid progression across all continents to become the pandemic that it now is in 2020. In parallel to this trend, bariatric surgeons have been trying to develop an ideal surgical approach that combines safety with durable weight loss and remission of associated comorbid illnesses. Bariatric surgery evolved from being initially hypoabsorptive (ileocolic bypass, biliopancreatic diversion, and jejunoileal bypass) to purely restrictive (vertical banded gastroplasty and gastric banding), and finally evolved further to combined hypoabsorptive and restrictive (gastric bypass).

Sleeve gastrectomy, first performed by Hess et al. as a restrictive component of the open biliopancreatic diversion and duodenal switch, has become an innovative and integral part of the bariatric surgery armamentarium. With the advent of laparoscopy, Gagner et al. introduced the concept of a step approach in super morbidly obese subjects and performed a laparoscopic sleeve gastrectomy (LSG), followed by a second step biliopancreatic diversion with duodenal switch (BPD-DS).

Not surprisingly, the initial excellent outcomes of LSG inclusive of patient-reported significant weight loss and remission of comorbidities at 6-month follow-up resulted in subjects foregoing the second stage BPD-DS.

The mechanism of action of LSG is still the subject of intense research and encompasses multiple mechanisms. LSG combines a restrictive element by significantly decreasing the gastric capacity to approximately 200 cc volume, and an anorectic component as it removes 80% of the ghrelin-producing cell mass. In addition, because the food transit is displaced toward the lesser curvature of the stomach or "Magenstrasse," a significant number of patients develop rapid emptying that results in stimulation of GLP1 hormones and dumping syndrome. Further characteristics are related to changes in the microbiome that seem to have an impact in the binding capacity of biliary acid with intestinal receptors.

Over the last decade, the indication of LSG as a final step continued to evolve until it has now become the most common stand-alone bariatric procedure performed worldwide. Its technical simplicity, in conjunction with excellent weight loss, remission of comorbid illnesses, and the best safety record ever in bariatric surgery, are the most important attributes responsible for this phenomenon.

As with any surgical approach, LSG is not exempt from short- and long-term complications and failures. In the short-term, and despite its technical simplicity, staple line disruptions can result in serious morbidity requiring a multidisciplinary treatment algorithm that might include a proximal gastrectomy and Roux-y reconstruction. Weight regain and the development of gastroesophageal reflux disease are the two most important long-term complications that result in disease recurrence and need for reoperative interventions.

This excellent monograph, put together by Dr. Salman Al-Sabah and co-authors, is a wonderful guide that will help surgeons navigate the different aspects of performing this procedure while managing the obesity disease. It thoroughly reviews all facets of a care path, including procedure indications, contraindications, technique, and reoperative strategies. It also provides the reader with a review of the most current nutritional and lifestyle interventions available to help our patients maintain their weight loss and have long-term success.

I congratulate Dr. Al-Sabah and the elite faculty he chose to author these chapters for this outstanding book and wish him and all readers continued health and success.

Raul J. Rosenthal MD FACS
Clinical Professor of Surgery
Lerner College of Medicine at CWRU
Chairman, Department of General Surgery
Director, Bariatric and Metabolic Institute
Co-editor in Chief
SOARD (Surgery for Obesity and Related Diseases)
Cleveland Clinic Weston
Weston, FL, USA

Preface

"المعدة بيت الداء"

"The Stomach is the home of disease"—Al-Harith ibn Kaladah (ancient Arab physician)

The prevalence of obesity is on a continuous rise worldwide, with an estimate of at least 1.9 billion adults (39%) considered as overweight and 600 million (13%) classified as obese in the year 2014. With it, this has brought a concomitant increase in the number of bariatric surgeries performed, with laparoscopic sleeve gastrectomy (LSG) becoming the most performed bariatric procedure as of 2014. This raise in the popularity of the LSG procedure has been attributed to its relative surgical simplicity, low complication rate, significant improvement in comorbidities, and evident weight loss.

"Laparoscopic Sleeve Gastrectomy is an easy, yet not a simple procedure." —Dr. Raul Rosenthal

Skill and expertise is required in the postoperative management of complications. Therefore, we decided to put this book together, to focus on all aspects related to the LSG, from how to choose the patient to long-term outcomes and options when the surgery fails.

Since the development of the LSG, many advances have been made in the field of bariatric surgery. The history of this procedure is more of an evolution of prior procedures than a discrete timeline of the development of a single procedure. The sleeve has its roots in the earliest gastroplasty procedures and as an observation from prior anti-reflux procedures in 1988. Since then, it has matured into its own technique and pioneered and refined over multiple meetings and summits by Dr. Michel Gagner. Bariatric surgeons have subsequently discussed its place in the field, comparing it to existing procedures and questioning its validity in the long-term. However, they are all in consensus that this procedure is an option for those seeking bariatric surgery.

I draw my inspiration from the highly readable and accessible works of my colleagues that have presented and published on this topic in world-renowned journals. It builds on the existing studies and literature that are in published journals regarding LSG, with its foundation concentrated around the Arab region, which has the highest levels of obesity prevalence worldwide.

It has been well established and accepted that the LSG is an effective bariatric procedure for those eligible for it. However, proper guidelines for choosing the proper bariatric procedure according to each individual patient has yet to be set. This book aims to lay out all aspects of the LSG, explaining and proposing guidelines for surgeons, the thought process and rationale behind choosing patients for this procedure, performing the procedure according to specific patient characteristics, the perioperative period, follow-up and postoperative requirements including exercise, nutrition, and supplementation, dealing with postoperative complications and morbidities, assessing success and knowing when the procedure has failed, discussing possible revision options for each patient according to their cause of failure. Additionally, this book discusses perspectives beyond the clinical, ranging from medicolegal aspects and medical tourism to recommended diet and exercise programs post-sleeve. The aim of this book is to consolidate all available information on LSG, putting it all in one place for bariatric surgeons and healthcare providers to refer to when needed.

Many papers and studies have been conducted covering multiple aspects of the LSG, looking at its effect on obesity, as well as comorbidities associated with obesity, short- and long-term outcomes, management of complications, the nutritional effect on the body, and so on. Surgeons have discussed it at length in conferences all around the world, speaking about its role in topics such as pediatric and adolescent obesity, debating future directions for its improvement and development.

The book is of interest to practicing surgeons working in the general and/or bariatric surgery field, as well as residents and trainees specializing in general surgery or have an interest in bariatric surgery. It involves a collaboration between multiple departments that deal with patients undergoing this procedure, providing insight from all those involved, and therefore, would also be beneficial to nutritionists working with bariatric patients, and researchers interested in metabolic medical issues and obesity. It also provides a highly accessible introduction to innovations in this topic, with a wide range of examples and areas covered being of interest to them, and concludes with the future directions in this field, thus making it "The Complete Book of Laparoscopic Sleeve Gastrectomy."

Safat, Kuwait   Salman Al-Sabah
Cleveland, USA   Ali Aminian
Napoli, Italy   Luigi Angrisani
New York, USA   Eliana Al Haddad
Adelaide, Australia   Lilian Kow

Acknowledgments by Salman Al-Sabah

If your actions inspire others to dream more, learn more, do more and become more, you are a leader—John Quincy Adams

I dedicate this book to my family for their constant support and also to all the mentors, colleagues, students over the past 20 years that have given the opportunity to learn and teach, الحمدلله. I believe as innovation increases, healthcare continues to evolve. It is important for surgeons to lead the way in the management of obesity and related chronic diseases. Mentorship and leadership are vital in our current environment and with more challenges come opportunities to innovate and lead. With the Arab region having a predominantly higher burden of obesity, I hope this book will be a success story from this region and inspire both surgeons and academics of this region to be great future leaders in surgery.

I would also like to acknowledge the contributions of my fellow editors and all the contributors of this book.

Acknowledgments by Dr. Eliana Al Haddad

I would firstly like to thank my colleague and friend, Dr. Salman Al-Sabah, who has been a guide and mentor to me throughout my medical journey. To my family and friends, who have unconditionally supported me every step of the way, I can never express the degree of my gratitude toward you all.

With enough hard work and dedication, we were able to put together this tremendous piece of literature, which will hopefully aid patients and surgeons alike in their weight loss journey.

"The purpose of life is not to be happy. It is to be useful, to be honorable, to be compassionate, to have it make some difference that you have lived and lived well."—Ralph Waldo Emerson

Acknowledgments by Lilian Kow

It is a big task when one sets out to write a "complete book" on a procedure. This is because like all bariatric surgery, it is not just about the surgery that determines the success of the procedure. For a successful outcome, one must understand the chronic multifactorial disease of obesity, the health burden to the individual and health stakeholders, and how to manage the patient in the long-term.

This book sets out to cover all aspects of the laparoscopic sleeve gastrectomy. It is appropriate to write this book just over 20 years since the first laparoscopic sleeve gastrectomy was performed by Professor Michel Gagner as a first stage laparoscopic BPD. Like most "good ideas", it was by serendipity that the sleeve gastrectomy was found to be as good as a stand-alone operation and because of its simplicity was adopted by bariatric surgeons all around the world overtaking both gastric banding and gastric bypass as the most commonly performed bariatric operation.

Despite its simplicity, it was not without risks and complications. Over the last 2 decades, this procedure has been extensively studied in clinical trials and RCTs, its mechanism on gut physiology systematically studied and refined. The production of this Complete Book of Laparoscopic Sleeve Gastrectomy is hence timely and appropriate as the book of resource systematically laid out from 2 decades of experiences for all bariatric surgeons.

June 2020

Lilian Kow
President IFSO

Contents

Potential Benefits of the LSG

LSG: Risks and Considerations

Editors and Contributors

About the Editors

Dr. Salman Al-Sabah is the Chairman of Surgery at Jaber Al-Ahmad Al-Sabah Hospital, Kuwait, and an associate professor at Kuwait University. He graduated from Kuwait Medical School and completed his residency in General Surgery and Master of Management and Health Leadership and Fellowship in Minimal Invasive and Bariatric Surgery at McGill University, Canada. He has contributed to several publications as well as presenting as a speaker and moderator in international conferences for the field of Minimally Invasive and Bariatric Surgery. His principal clinical foci are Metabolic/Bariatric Surgery, Minimally Invasive Surgery, Advanced Endoscopy, Health Policy, and research. Additionally, Dr. Al-Sabah is on the editorial board and reviewer of international peer-review journals. He is the founder and President of the Gulf Obesity Surgery Society, the Kuwait Association of Surgeons and Governor for Kuwait at the American College of Surgeons. Dr. Al-Sabah's research has been the foundation in the establishment of international guidelines in the fields of gastroenterology and metabolic and bariatric surgery. He is also the recipient of the prestigious 2018, Scientific Production Prize from the Kuwait Foundation for the Advancement of Sciences (KFAS) for his contributions in the field of Medical Health and Allied Sciences. Dr. Al-Sabah was instrumental in establishing the Kuwait National Bariatric Registry.

Ali Aminian, M.D. is Director of Bariatric and Metabolic Institute at the Cleveland Clinic. He is an Associate Professor of Surgery at the Cleveland Clinic Lerner College of Medicine. His clinical interests include gastrointestinal surgery, advanced laparoscopic surgery, and specifically surgery for severe obesity, diabetes, and metabolic disease. As an academic su^200), he has published high impact journals including New England Journal of Medicine, JAMA, Diabetes Care, and Annals of Surgery. His studies have been widely covered by the media such as New York Times, Wall Street Journal, TIME, Reuters, Forbes, and among the others.

Prof. Luigi Angrisani born in Naples. He received master's degree with honors in Medicine and Surgery at the University "Federico II" of Naples and postgraduate degree and medical practice in London, Pittsburgh, Lyon, Bombay, New York, Los Angeles, Birmingham, and Cambridge. He is Director of the Unit for General and Laparoscopic Surgery at San Giovanni Bosco Hospital in Naples; Professor of General Surgery at the Federico II University of Naples, Italy; and Past President of the Italian Society for Obesity and Metabolic Diseases (SICOB). He involved in editorial activity with several publications in the bariatric field worldwide. He is an Associate Editor of the scientific journal *Obesity Surgery* (Springer). He is Past President of IFSO, International Federation for the Surgery of Obesity and Metabolic Disorders; Chairman IFSO Board of Trustees; and President of IFSO World Congress Rome 2022.

Dr. Eliana Al Haddad obtained her bachelor's degree in biology from the American University of Beirut. She then graduated from Lebanese American University Gilbert and Rose-Mary Chagoury School of Medicine in 2016. After which, she completed a three-year postdoctoral research fellowship in congenital cardiac surgery at Columbia University Medical Center in New York. She has contributed to several international publications in the fields of bariatric and general surgery, as well as pediatric cardiothoracic surgery. She is currently working as a postdoctoral research fellow in the field of bariatric and general surgery with Dr. Salman Al- Sabah. Her principal foci are research in the fields previously mentioned. Additionally, Dr. Al Haddad is on the editorial board and a Reviewer of international peer-reviewed journals.

Lilian Kow is a Senior Consultant Surgeon at Flinders Medical Centre and Clinical Associate Professor at Flinders University of South Australia. She has been involved in training surgeons in bariatric surgery nationally and internationally. Lilian Kow was born in Malaysia. Her family migrated to Adelaide, Australia, where she completed her high school and qualified to study medicine at the Flinders University of South Australia. She went on to complete a Ph.D. in Neuroscience in the School of Medicine at the Flinders University of South Australia. Her thesis entitled "A systemic study of the regulation of intestinal motility in an organ culture system" was awarded by Flinders University of South Australia in 1996. After completing her advanced surgical training in general surgery, she became a Fellow of the Royal Australasian College of Surgeons FRACS in 1996. Lilian is a Co-Founder/Director of the Adelaide Bariatric Centre, which was established in 1995, as the first obesity surgical clinic in Adelaide. Over the years, Lilian has visited many bariatric clinics around the world and is of the firm belief that bariatric surgery works better with an effective support program. Lilian has been at the forefront along with her colleagues at the Adelaide Bariatric Centre in developing a very effective multidisciplinary program for supporting their patients in their weight loss journey. The program in Adelaide was one of the initial ones adopted in Australia and internationally and the first to be used in South Australia. Lilian and her colleagues have been firmly committed to providing this very important multidisciplinary support for our patients:

a program which clearly makes the Adelaide Bariatric Centre the leading centre for the management of weight loss in South Australia and one of the leading centres in Australia. She is the President of IFSO and the Past President of the IFSO-APC and the Obesity Surgical Society of Australia and New Zealand OSSANZ (ANZMOSS). She also runs the Education Portfolio as the executive member for Australian Chinese Medical Association (SA).

Contributors

Nadia Ahmad Obesity Medicine Institute, LLC, New Canaan, CT, United States; Eli Lilly & Company, Indianapolis, IN, USA

Mohammed Al Hadad MD, FRCS Glasg, FACS, Head of Bariatric Surgery Department, Healthpoint Hospital, Abu Dhabi, UAE

Eliana Al Haddad Columbia University Medical Center, New York, NY, USA; Amiri Hospital, Kuwait City, Kuwait

Salman Al Sabah Faculty of Medicine, Health Sciences Centre, Kuwait University, Jabriya, Kuwait

Sarah Al Youha Jaber Al Ahmad Al Sabah Hospital, Kuwait City, Kuwait

Naji Alamuddin Royal College of Surgeons in Ireland—Medical University of Bahrain, Busaiteen, Bahrain;
King Hamad University Hospital, Al Sayh, Bahrain;
Perelman School of Medicine at the University of Pennsylvania, Philadelphi, Pennsylvania, US

Abdullah Al-Darwish New You Medical Center, Riyadh, Saudi Arabia

Hanan M. Alghamdi HBP & Bariatric Surgeon, Imam Abdulrhman Bin Faisal University, Dammam, Saudi Arabia

Jasem Yousef AL-Hashel Faculty of Medicine, Department of Medicine, Kuwait University, Kuwait City, Kuwait;
Department of Neurology, Ibn Sina Hospital, Safat, Kuwait

Khawla F. Ali Department of Medicine, Royal College of Surgeons in Ireland-Medical University of Bahrain, Muharraq, Bahrain

Syed Mohamed Aljunid Department of Health Policy and Management, Faculty of Public Health, Kuwait University, Kuwait City, Kuwait

Ahmed Al-Khamis Jaber Al-Ahmed Al-Sabah Hospital, South Surra, Kuwait

Sulaiman Almazeedi Jaber Al-Ahmed Al-Sabah Hospital, South Surra, Kuwait

Meshari Almuhanna Bariatric & Metabolic Surgery Unit, Department of General Surgery, Jaber Al-Ahmad Al-Sabah Hospital, Kuwait, Kuwait;
Asia-Pacific Endoscopic Bariatric and Metabolic Surgical Center, Min-Sheng General Hospital, Taoyuan, Taiwan

Abdullah Al-Ozairi Department of Psychiatry, Faculty of Medicine, Kuwait University, Jabriya, Hawally, Kuwait

Aayed R. Alqahtani New You Medical Center, Riyadh, Saudi Arabia

Hanan Alsalem Department of Obstetrics and Gynecology, McMaster University, Gynecologic Minimally Invasive Clinical Fellow, Hamilton, ON, Canada

Abdulrahman Alserri Department of Obstetrics and Gynecology, Faculty of Medicine, Kuwait University, Kuwait City, Kuwait

Ahmad Al-Serri Unit of Human Genetics, Department of Pathology, Faculty of Medicine, Kuwait University, Jabriya, Kuwait

Husain Alshatti Neuropsychiatry Department, Al Amiri Hospital, Al-Asima, Kuwait

Dana AlTarrah Faculty of Public Health, Kuwait University, Kuwait City, Kuwait

Ali Aminian Department of General Surgery, Bariatric and Metabolic Institute, Clevland Clinic, Cleveland, OH, USA

Amin Andalib Center for Bariatric Surgery, Department of Surgery, McGill University, Montreal, QC, Canada

Meshka Kamal Anderson Surgery Residency Program, Department of Surgery, Carolinas Medical Center, Atrium Health, Charlotte, NC, USA

Luigi Angrisani Public Health Department, School of Medicine, "Federico II" University of Naples, Naples, Italy

Hutan Ashrafian Institute of Global Health Innovation at Imperial College London, London, UK

Moataz Bashah Bariatric and Metabolic Surgery Department, Hamad General Hospital, Doha, Qatar

Ahmad Bashir Gastrointestinal, Bariatric and Metabolic Center (GBMC), Jordan Hospital, Amman, Jordan

Mohammed A. Bawahab Upper GI, Laparoscopic, and Bariatric Surgeon, Department of Surgery, College of Medicine, King Khalid University, Abha, Saudi Arabia

Mohit Bhandari Head of Department At the Mohak Bariatric and Robotic Surgery Center, SAIMS University, Indore, India

Aparna Govil Bhasker Bariatric and Laparoscopic Surgeon, Gleneagles Global Hospital, Parel, Mumbai, India

Laurent Biertho IUCPQ—Laval University, Quebec, QC, Canada

Helmuth T. Billy Metabolic and Bariatric Surgery, St. John's Regional Medical Center, Oxnard, CA, USA;
Metabolic and Bariatric Surgery, Community Memorial Hospital, Ventura, CA, USA;
Bariatric Surgery, Hamad General Hospital, Doha, Qatar

Masoud S. Chopan Department of Surgical Education, Community Memorial Hospital, Ventura, CA, USA

Elie Chouillard Université Saint-Joseph, Chef de Service de Chirurgie Générale et Digestive Centre Hospitalier de Poissy/Saint-Germain-en-Laye, Saint-Germain-en-Laye, France

Michael Courtney Specialty Trainee in Upper GI/Bariatric Surgery, Sunderland Royal Hospital, Sunderland, UK

Jamil S. Dababneh American Pharmacists Association, American Marketing Association, Chicago, USA

Imane Ed dbali Emirates Specialty Hospital, Dubai, United Arab Emirates

Laura Divine High School Principal, Al-Bayan Bilingual School, Hawalli, Kuwait

Evangelos Efthimiou Chelsea and Westminster Hospital NHS Foundation Trust, Chelsea, London, UK

Maher El Chaar St Luke's University Hospital and Health Network, Fountain Hill, USA;
Lewis Katz School of Medicine, Temple University, Philadelphia, USA

Rawan El-Abd Faculty of Medicine, Health Sciences Centre, Kuwait University, Jabriya, Kuwait

Mohamed Elahmedi New You Medical Center, Riyadh, Saudi Arabia

Mohamad Hayssam Elfawal Clinical Assistant Professor of Surgery, CEO New You Center, Director Fellowship Program Bariatric and Metabolic Surgery at Beirut Arab University, Beirut, Lebanon

Waleed Gado Mansoura Faculty of Medicine, Mansoura, Egypt

Michel Gagner Department of Surgery, Sacré-Coeur Hospital, Montréal, QC, Canada

Ashraf Haddad Minimally Invasive, Advanced GI and Bariatric surgery, GBMC-Jordan Hospital, Amman, Jordan

Hidenori Haruta Weight Loss and Metabolic Surgery Center, Yotsuya Medical Cube, Tokyo, Japan

Jacques M. Himpens Delta CHIREC Hospitals, Brussels, Belgium; St Pierre University Hospital, Brussels, Belgium

Ismail Ibrahim Ismail Department of Neurology, Ibn Sina Hospital, Safat, Kuwait

Mohammad H. Jamal Department of Transplantation, Faculty of Medicine, Health Sciences Centre, Kuwait University, Kuwait City, Kuwait; Jaber Al-Ahmad Hospital, Kuwait City, Kuwait

François Julien IUCPQ—Laval University, Quebec, QC, Canada

Saleh Kanawati Department of Anesthesia, Chairman Department of Anesthesia, Makassed General Hospital, Beirut, Lebanon

Karin Karam Department of Surgery, Lebanese American University (LAU) Medical Center-Rizk Hospital, Beirut, Lebanon; Lebanese American University, Gilbert and Rose-Marie Chagoury School of Medicine, Beirut, Lebanon

Kazunori Kasama Weight Loss and Metabolic Surgery Center, Yotsuya Medical Cube, Tokyo, Japan

Shujhat Khan Milton Keynes University Hospital, London, UK

Nesreen Khidir Harvard T.H. Chan School of Public Health, PPCR, Boston, USA; Bariatric and Metabolic Surgery Department, Hamad General Hospital, Doha, Qatar

Carel W. le Roux Department of Experimental Pathology, University College Dublin, Dublin, Ireland

Stéfane Lebel Laval University, Quebec, QC, Canada

Wei-Jei Lee Asia-Pacific Endoscopic Bariatric and Metabolic Surgical Center, Min-Sheng General Hospital, Taoyuan, Taiwan

Alan Kawarai Lefor Division of Gastroenterological, General and Transplant Surgery, Jichi Medical University, Tochigi, Japan

Emanuele Lo Menzo Department of General Surgery and Director, Bariatric and Metabolic Institute, Cleveland Clinic Florida, Weston, FL, US

Kamal Mahawar Consultant General and Bariatric Surgeon, Sunderland Royal Hospital, Sunderland, UK

Tarek Mahdy Mansoura Faculty of Medicine, Mansoura, Egypt

Simon Marceau IUCPQ—Laval University, Quebec, QC, Canada

Andrés San Martin Médico Cirujano, Fellow Cirugía Bariátrica Clínica las Condes, Santiago, Chile

Thomas R. McCarty Brigham and Women's Hospital, Boston, USA

Karl A. Miller Diakonissen Private Hospital, Salzburg, Austria; Kings College Hospital London, Dubai, UAE

Diya Aldeen Mohammed Bariatric Surgeon, New You Center, Beirut, Lebanon

Mohanned-Al-Haddad Jaber Al-Ahmed Al-Sabah Hospital, Kuwait, Kuwait

Marius Nedelcu Bouchard Private Hospital, ELSAN, Clinique Saint Michel, ELSAN, MarseilleToulon, France

Abdelrahman Nimeri Atrium Health Weight Management, Section of Bariatric & Metabolic Surgery, Department of Surgery, Carolinas Medical Center, Atrium Health, Charlotte, NC, USA

Patrick Noel Emirates Specialty Hospital, Dubai, United Arab Emirates

Dimitri J. Pournaras Department of Upper GI Surgery, Southmead Hospital, Bristol, UK

Noe Rodriguez Department of General Surgery, Bariatric and Metabolic Institute, Clevland Clinic, Clevland, OH, USA

Raul J. Rosenthal Department of General Surgery and Director, Bariatric and Metabolic Institute, Cleveland Clinic Florida, Weston, FL, US

A. Ruano Department of Surgery, Complutense University of Madrid. Hospital Clinico San Carlos. IdISSC, Madrid, Spain

Kashif Saeed Department of General Surgery and Director, Bariatric and Metabolic Institute, Cleveland Clinic Florida, Weston, FL, US

Bassem Safadi Department of Surgery, Lebanese American University (LAU) Medical Center-Rizk Hospital, Beirut, Lebanon; Lebanese American University, Gilbert and Rose-Marie Chagoury School of Medicine, Beirut, Lebanon

Osama Samargandi Division of Plastic Surgery, Dalhousie University, Nova Scotia, Canada

C. Sanchez-del-Pueblo Department of Surgery, Complutense University of Madrid. Hospital Clinico San Carlos. IdISSC, Madrid, Spain

A. Sánchez-Pernaute Department of Surgery, Complutense University of Madrid. Hospital Clinico San Carlos. IdISSC, Madrid, Spain

Yosuke Seki Weight Loss and Metabolic Surgery Center, Yotsuya Medical Cube, Tokyo, Japan

Faiz Shariff Department of General Surgery, Wellspan Bariatric Surgery, York, Pennsylvania, USA

Iqbal Siddique Department of Medicine, Faculty of Medicine, Kuwait University, Jabriya, Kuwait

Terry L. Simpson Ventura Advanced Surgical Associates, Ventura, CA, USA

Samantha Stavola Nutrition for Celebrate Nutritional Supplements, Wadsworth, OH, USA

Christine Stier Sana Obesity Center Northrhine Westphalia, Hürth, Germany

Alexis C. Sudlow Department of Upper GI Surgery, Southmead Hospital, Bristol, UK

Samuel Szomstein Department of General Surgery and Director, Bariatric and Metabolic Institute, Cleveland Clinic Florida, Weston, FL, US

Safwan Taha Consultant Metabolic and Bariatric Surgeon, Mediclinic Airport Road Hospital, Abu Dhabi, UAE

André Tchernof IUCPQ—Laval University, Quebec, QC, Canada

Christopher C. Thompson Brigham and Women's Hospital, Boston, USA

A. Torres Department of Surgery, Complutense University of Madrid. Hospital Clinico San Carlos. IdISSC, Madrid, Spain

Peter K. H. Walton Dendrite Clinical Systems Ltd, Reading Bridge House, Reading, Berkshire RG1 8LS, UK

Rudolf Weiner Sana-Klinikum Offenbach, Frankfurt, Germany

Sylvia Weiner Krankenhaus Norwest, Frankfurt am Main, Germany

Jason G. Williams Division of Plastic Surgery, Dalhousie University, Nova Scotia, Canada

Camilo Boza Wilson Department of Digestive Surgery, Clinica Las Condes, Santiago, Chile

Rickesha L. Wilson Department of General Surgery, Bariatric and Metabolic Institute, Cleveland Clinic, Cleveland, OH, USA

Yuchen You Department of Surgical Education, Community Memorial Hospital, Ventura, CA, USA

Introduction

Learning About the Laparoscopic Sleeve Gastrectomy (lSG) The Birth and Evolution of Laparoscopic Sleeve Gastrectomy

Michel Gagner

Is sleeve gastrectomy the result of an omphaloskepsis? Omphaloskepsis or navel contemplation of one's self is known to be an aid to meditation. The word originates from the Greek omphalos, signifying "navel" and skepsis, meaning "viewing". In Hinduism, the navel is the site of a powerful chakra, focal point of mediation, the site of the universe, but it is also the exit of the sleeve gastrectomy specimen, transcending a powerful individual change.

The sleeve gastrectomy follows the duodenal switch evolution, but its originators did not create the concept of a stand alone or staged procedure called "sleeve gastrectomy". Doug Hess and Picard Marceau altered the open biliopancreatic diversion, modified it, and called it duodenal switch, generally called "DS", in 1988–90, with the needs for a major gastrectomy to diminish the acid load on the duodenal ileal anastomosis, causing dramatically less anastomotic ulcers [1, 2]. In Marceau's description, the BPD distal gastrectomy is replaced with a "65% parietal cell gastrectomy" along the greater curvature; note that this was not called "sleeve gastrectomy" at the time, leaving a stomach of at least 200 mL [3].

I initiated, as a principal investigator, a small animal swine pilot project in May 1999 at Mount Sinai School of Medicine where I had been an attending and professor of surgery, with the help of Dr. Gregg Jossart who was a clinical fellow in laparoscopic/bariatric surgery at Mount Sinai School of Medicine in New York under my directorship, has since served as the Director of Minimally Invasive Surgery at California Pacific Medical Center in San Francisco since 1999, assisted by Dr. John de Csepel, who was my research fellow and resident at the time from the same organization, who is now the Chief Medical Officer & Vice President of Medical Affairs for Medtronic's Minimally Invasive Therapy Group's for a

M. Gagner (✉)
Department of Surgery, Sacré-Coeur Hospital, Montréal, QC, Canada
e-mail: Gagner.Michel@cliniqueMichelGagner.com

© The Editor(s) (if applicable) and The Author(s), under exclusive license to Springer Nature Switzerland AG 2021
S. Al-Sabah et al. (eds.), *Laparoscopic Sleeve Gastrectomy*,
https://doi.org/10.1007/978-3-030-57373-7_1

diverse portfolio ($9 billion in annual revenues) in New York City, and Dr. Stephen Burpee, resident at the time who is now an attending bariatric surgeon in private practice in Tucson Arizona, Laparoscopic Duodenal Switch Feasibility study in 6 pigs was realised in the institution research centre, which was ultimately published later in 2001 [4].

This laboratory effort was to comprehend the complexities and technical impediments of performing such surgeries in real patients. After I initiated the first laparoscopic Roux-en-Y gastric bypass program at Mount Sinai in 1998, strong from my experience with the same surgery since 1995 at the Cleveland Clinic in Ohio, and preceding animal experiment on laparoscopic Roux-en-Y gastric bypass with our clinical fellow Dr. Mario Potvin at the Centre de Recherche de l'Hotel-Dieu de Montreal in 1993 [5], who is now an attending surgeon in the Marshfield Clinic Health System in Wisconsin, I embarked on July 2, 1999, 21 years ago, to perform the first Laparoscopic DS at Mount Sinai Hospital in New York. Dr. Christine Ren, our newest fellow of 1 day, following Dr. Jossart's fellowship year, a finishing general surgery resident from the NYU program, assisted me, NYU had no or minimal laparoscopic bariatric surgery experience at the time.

- This entailed a laparoscopic sleeve gastrectomy, using a bougie in place of 60Fr and multiple serial firings of laparoscopic linear staplers, followed with duodeno-ileostomy using a transabdominal circular stapler, end to side, antecolic, and a side-to-side ileo-ileostomy using a linear stapler and hand-sewn closure of the enterostomy. Initially, mesenteric defects were not closed, but later than a year afterwards, a 2.6% mesenteric internal hernia incidence was observed, mostly Petersen's, and routine closure of both mesenteric defects was initiated in 2000. It is amazing today, looking back at this era, that I had introduced this on patients with BMI >60 kg/m^2, as it was my conviction at the time, even today, that hypoabsorptive procedures should be completed in this class of super to super super obesity [7]. After her 1999–2000 fellowship with us, Dr. Christine Ren subsequently became Professor in the Department of Surgery at NYU Grossman School of Medicine and Division Chief of Bariatric Surgery.

We therefore initiated quite a series of patients such by December 1999, an abstract was submitted to the 2000 annual meeting of ASBS, not called ASMBS at the time, American Society of Bariatric Surgery, usually held in June, and accepted for an official podium presentation [8]. Dr. Gregg Jossart returned for an operating room visit to Mount Sinai NY in the fall of 1999, just before the annual meeting of the American College of Surgeons held in San Francisco, accompanied by Dr. Robert Rabkin, his new partner at the time in San Francisco, interested in learning and observing a live case of laparoscopic DS procedure, which they initiated afterwards with a hand assisted technique, not with complete laparoscopy. Dr. Jossart and Rabkin have displayed their preliminary experience at SAGES 2001, with 79 cases done, 27 lap assisted and 52 hand assisted which started in October 1999 until July 2000 [9]. At the Annual meeting of ASBS in June 2000, a short video presentation was produced from Dr. Jossart, Dr. R. Rabkin, and Dr. Donald Booth from Biloxi, and with an abstract revealing that they had started the complete laparoscopic technique in January of the same year [10].

By serendipity and providence, I could not perform a complete laparoscopic DS early in our experience, due to ventilator pressure problems, and tight pneumoperitoneum in spite of utmost muscular relaxation, and I decided to abandon after completion of the sleeve gastrectomy, which to this day, was constantly done first. My observation of weight loss, disappearance of co-morbidities, led me to believe that this group of high-risk patients, those with BMI >60 kg/m^2, it would be preferable to realize the long and tedious operation in 2 steps instead, with a 6 months interval as a minimum. As, a later review of our data had substantiated the higher mortality and morbidity rate of full laparoscopic DS in BMI >60 kg/m^2, much higher than a 2 stage procedure [11]. This led me to do the first presentation on laparoscopic sleeve gastrectomy "alone" at Dr. Phillip Schauer's meeting in Feb 20–25 2001, MISS Minimally Invasive Symposium in Snowbird, Utah, on sleeve gastrectomy as a 2 stages procedure. The reception was tepid, unenthusiastic, and because nobody was really doing laparoscopic duodenal switch at the time, as a large part of this crowd had been invited and paid by laparoscopic adjustable gastric band companies, it had generated no awareness from the audience, except for one individual in attendance. I suppose, it was either Dr. Peter Crookes or Dr. Gary Anthone who were working at USC Los Angeles at the time, who came forward during the coffee break, and confided to me that they had done a handful of patients with an open technique, as a salvage, but that they were not published and thought there was no interest in the subject at the time. They subsequently published this experience in 2004 and 2006, but I pondered if they would have published it, if it were not from my experience laparoscopically, and subsequent hype of the subject [12, 13].

Consequently, with Dr. Christine Chu, another clinical fellow, who is now working for Kaiser Permanente Northern California Bariatric Surgery Center, an abstract was sent for presentation at the annual meeting of SAGES in the spring of 2002. The abstract was published in Surgical Endoscopy, and this constitute the first official publication on the subject, entitled" Two-stage laparoscopic BPD/DS. An Alternative Approach to Super-Super Morbid Obesity", many co-authors represented my faculty partners and bariatric fellows at the time 2001–2002, at Mount Sinai hospital and School of Medicine in NY, NY [14]. From July 1999 until July 2001, 102 laparoscopic duodenal switches had been achieved, of which 7 were by two stages completed, and did not include also the sleeve alone that had not been converted for numerous motives, including patients who declined a second stage. On March 15th 2002, at the New York Hilton Hotel, the presentation of the first series, at an official societal meeting, on laparoscopic sleeve gastrectomy, took place.

I was part of the World Congress program in 2002, as it was combined for IFSES, the International Federation of Societies of Endoscopic Surgery, and this was a few months after the tragically September 11, 2001 events, which still attracted a large crowd in New York City, in spite of the fear of traveling and flying, they were even discussions to delay or cancelled the meeting. Fortunately, we had put an outstanding postgraduate laparoscopic bariatric course at Mount Sinai School of Medicine, with countless live surgeries, which encompassed laparoscopic Roux-en-y gastric bypasses, duodenal switch and sleeve gastrectomy as a stand-alone procedure. There was also an animal lab and a cadaver laboratory, where those techniques were tutored. Many participants remembered and reminisced, still exchange with me about this event as one of the turning point in their profession. During the same congress, Dr. Shoji Fukuyama, MD, Christine Chu, MD, Won Woo Kim, MD, and myself also presented a video of the two-stage procedure at the video session V02 on March 15th, 2002 [15]. Dr. Kim returned to Seoul Korea were he was an early adopter of sleeve gastrectomy in Asia, starting in 2003. Further, Dr. David Voellinger presented a poster, another clinical fellow that year, who did just before is residency at the University of Alabama in Birmingham, is now an attending bariatric surgeon and the Medical Director for the Novant Health Bariatric Center and Vice Chief of Staff at Presbyterian Medical Center in Charlotte, NC, entitled "Laparoscopic Sleeve Gastrectomy is a safe and effective Primary Procedure for Biliopancreatic Diversion With Duodenal Switch", because it had been turned down for a podium oral presentation, it was a poster abstract [16]. It included a series of 24 patients; initial mean weight was 414 lbs., with mean BMI of 65 (range 58–76 kgm^2). Mean operative time was 114 min with an average length of stay of 3 days (range 2–7) with a median of 3 days. Follow-up at 3 weeks, 3 months, and 6 months after sleeve resulted in an excess total body weight loss of 11, 23, and 32% and mean BMI of 60, 56 and 49 kgm^2. No major morbidity and no mortality ensued in this population. The conclusion was: Laparoscopic sleeve gastrectomy is feasible and can be performed with minimal morbidity as the primary stage of LBPDDS in the superobese. It also results in substantial short-term weight loss and should allow for a safer operation during second stages [16].

Dr. Bruce V. MacFadyen Jr. from the University of Texas-Houston Medical School, who was the main co-editor of Surgical Endoscopy at the time with Sir Alfred Cuschieri, turned down the manuscript submitted, for lack of long-term follow-up!! This infuriated me, as Surgical Endoscopy had an earlier tradition of publishing pioneering concepts a decade before. And this is why our second series has been published 1 year after, in 2003, in a distinct journal, more open minded to bariatric subjects, in Obesity Surgery, by our clinical fellow at the time Dr. Joseph Patrick Regan, and Barry Inabnet pushing for its publication on "Early experience with two-stage laparoscopic roux-en-Y gastric bypass as an alternative in the super-super obese patient" which is much quoted in the bariatric surgical literature [17]. As much commercial medical insurances were denying duodenal switches, although accepted by CMS, patients ended up, after their approval, with a second stage Roux-en-Y gastric bypass, which I considered an inferior operation for super-obeses. As I said, this was not my first cohort of patients, in this short paper in obesity Surgery, there were only 7 patients who had an initial sleeve followed several months later, with a mean of 11 months, a lap Roux-en-y gastric bypass, were the upper sleeve was transected, from a BMI of 63 to 50 kg/m^2

after a sleeve, and then to 44 kg/m^2, 2.5 months later. The very first sleeve gastrectomy series was published as a book chapter, with considerable delays, in 2005, which many referenced today, as the first series of laparoscopic sleeve gastrectomy [18] of note, Dr. Regan is now attending staff at Columbia St. Mary's Hospital Columbia, in Milwaukee, WI, as well as medical director and assistant Clinical Professor of Surgery of the Medical College of Wisconsin and member of the Milwaukee Institute of Minimally Invasive Surgery.

As I said earlier, Dr. Gregg Jossart who is now Director, Minimally Invasive Surgery, California Pacific Medical Center, San Francisco, California and Dr. Gary J. Anthone who as since left private bariatric surgery practice to be the chief medical officer and director of public health of Nebraska, have composed a short piece on the history of sleeve gastrectomy in the Bariatric Times in 2010 [19]. In 1997, Dr. Gary Anthone was performing an open duodenal switch on a 13-year-old girl with a history of common bile duct stones [12]. Intraoperatively, the common bile duct stones could not be completely cleared, and elected to just do an open sleeve gastrectomy in order to leave access for a postoperative endoscopic retrograde cholangiopancreatography (ERCP). From 1997 to 2001, he performed 21 open sleeve gastrectomies in high-risk patients with super-morbid obesity [12]. The lesser curve stomach left was approximately 100 mL in volume (presently the pouch volume is approximately 60 cm^3 or less) and the patients reached 40–50% excess weight loss (EWL). By October 2005, he had narrated on 118 open sleeve gastrectomies with similar outcomes [13].

Professor Michael J. McMahon, previously from the General Infirmary at Leeds, robust from the experience of Professor Johnston with Margenstrasse &Mill gastroplasty, had executed from January 2000 until December 2001, laparoscopic sleeve gastrectomy in 20 patients. Of note, Prof Michael J. McMahon had visited me at Mount Sinai School of Medicine during this time interval, where the laparoscopic sleeve gastrectomy had been performed 7 months earlier in duodenal switch patients. The technique described in their manuscript of 8-years results, is identical to the technique used at Mount Sinai, except for a smaller bougie of 32 Fr, the one that was currently used for M&M in Leeds. At 8 years, 55% of patients had more than 50% EWL [20].

In San Francisco, Dr. Gregg Jossart, our former fellow, was an early adopter of sleeve gastrectomy in the West coast, he had started to offer the stand-alone procedure with a 32 French calibre pouch (30–60 cm^3) to lower BMI patients, in November 2002 [21]. I had several conversations with him encouraging them to start the laparoscopic two stage procedure in San Francisco. The results of 216 patients compared successfully the other stapling procedures and certainly against adjustable gastric banding, with 75–85% EWL at two years of follow up [21].

Adjustable gastric banding has been almost abandoned, and performed less than 1% of the time in North America. Dr. Jacques Himpens from Brussels Belgium, an early adopter of the technique, has been convinced after video transmission of surgeries performed from Mount Sinai NY to Brussels and Europe, and had published some 6 years results in the Annals of Surgery, a landmark paper, where sleeves where performed between November 2001 and October 2002, in which the early technique was not fully understood, especially concerning the extent of fundus and crus dissections, giving its worst results [22].

Two additional posters at SAGES annual meeting in 2002 mentioned some aspects of early sleeve gastrectomy developments. Dr. Hazem Elariny from Virginia started in 2001 and had presented 30 patients of a laparoscopic non-banded vertical gastroplasty with sleeve gastrectomy [23]. Dr. Val Andrei from New Jersey, was our clinical fellow at Mount Sinai NY, at the same time as Dr. Jossart in 1998–1999, and described 3 cases of laparoscopic duodenal switches, one laparoscopic, one hand assisted and another converted from laparoscopic to open [24].

But this was antedated by one year, the SAGES annual meeting of 2001, where Dr. Theresa Quinn, who is working as a general surgeon in Wisconsin, our clinical fellow that year, presented on our updated experience "Laparoscopic Biliopancreatic Diversion with Duodenal switch: The early Experience" [25].

Since it had been clearly established that two stage procedures, with a laparoscopic sleeve gastrectomy performed first, had slashed impressively the mortality to zero, and gave an acceptably low morbidity rate in these high risk patients, I fully embraced the procedure from the very commencement [26].

I then embarked on the big task of educating a large population of bariatric, minimally invasive and gastro-intestinal surgeons worldwide in this new procedure. We started to display and teach this technique to visitors at Mount Sinai from 1999, and in official bariatric courses we had regularly. The very first international specific course on Laparoscopic Sleeve Gastrectomy was at Doral Golf Course in 2005, and Dr. Jacques Himpens was an invited foreign faculty. Afterwards, six International consensus conferences were established under my leadership and directorship, starting with the first one in New York City in October 25–27, 2007. The proceedings were published in obesity surgery in 2008 [27].

Following this great triumph, five more International Consensus conferences were held in New York City, Miami, Montreal and London, of which the first 5 ones have been published. Each of them had a sizeable component of live surgeries from countless expert surgeons demonstrating the easiness and convolutions of their operation, emanating form all continents. A didactic portion of the meeting had sessions on mechanisms, indications, and contraindications of that particular year, followed by management and detection of complications, conversions and revisions [28–31]. Worth stating, was also the Expert consensus meeting planned by Dr. Raul Rosenthal in Florida, sponsored by Ethicon Endosurgery, to establish consistency in the technical performance of sleeve gastrectomy, led to highly cited paper in 2012 [32].

The rest is history; ASMBS and IFSO have recognized Sleeve Gastrectomy as an acceptable option for a primary bariatric procedure or as a first-stage procedure in high-risk patients as part of a planned, staged approach. As with any bariatric procedure, long-term weight regain can occur after and may require one or more of reinterventions. Informed consent should be consistent with the other bariatric procedures and, as such, should include the risk of long-term weight regain and GERD.

I did organized the International Federation for the Surgery of Obesity and Metabolic Disorders (IFSO) annual meeting of 2014 and Fifth International Consensus Conference on Laparoscopic Sleeve Gastrectomy, in Montréal at the end of August 2014. An international expert panel was surveyed in 2014 and compared with the 2011 Sleeve Gastrectomy Consensus and with survey data taken from a general bariatric surgical group. The expert surgeons (based on having performed > 1000 cases) completed an online anonymous survey. The following indications were endorsed: as a stand-alone procedure (97.5%); in high-risk patients (92.4%); in kidney and liver transplant candidates (91.6%); in patients with metabolic syndrome (83.8%); body mass index 30–35 with associated co-morbidities (79.8%); in patients with inflammatory bowel disease (87.4%); and in the elderly (89.1%) [31]. Significant differences occurred between the expert and general surgeons groups in favouring several contraindications: Barrett's esophagus (80% versus 31% [P < 0.001]), gastroesophageal reflux disease (23% versus 53% [P < 0.001]), hiatal hernias (12% versus 54% [P < 0.001]), and body mass index > 60 kg/ m^2 (5% versus 28% [P < 0.001]). Mean reported weight loss outcomes 5 years postoperative were significantly greater for the expert surgeons group ($P = 0.005$), as were reported stricture (P = 0.001) and leakage (P = 0.005) rates. This conference emphasized areas of novel and enriched best practices on various aspects of laparoscopic sleeve gastrectomy performance among experts and bariatric surgeons [31].

In 2016, the numbers of bariatric procedures have been estimated to be 216,000 in USA alone [33]. Of these 58% have been sleeve gastrectomy, but if one looks at the number of primary laparoscopic procedures, sleeve gastrectomy has attained 73% of all, nearly 3 quarters of them, and still rising. But USA was unhurried to fully embrace it, because of private insurances slow processes. In countries where a national health system happens, like Chile, Kuwait or France, it has been the uppermost procedure before 2016.

Globally, the total bariatric surgical figures have approached 685,874; 634,897 (92.6%) of which were primary and 50,977 were revisional (7.4%) [34]. My estimate is that bariatric/metabolic surgeries are closer to 1 million procedures a year, as most nations do not have a countrywide registry of bariatric procedures. According to the latest IFSO assessment, the most performed primary procedure was sleeve gastrectomy (N = 340,550; 53.6%), followed by Roux-en-Y gastric bypass (N = 191,326; 30.1%), and single anastomosis gastric bypass (N = 30,563; 4.8%). In 2016, sleeve gastrectomy remains the most performed surgical procedure in the globe, with probably more than half a million cases done annually. It has the promise to grow to 5–10 times those numbers if they are being welcomed by national health care systems, and not restrained, due to biases and financial constraints, like in Canada or the UK for example.

References

1. Hess DS, Hess DW. Biliopancreatic Diversion with a duodenal switch. Obes Surg. 1998;8:267–82.
2. Lagace M, Marceau P, Marceau S, Hould FS, Potvin M, Bourque RA, Biron S. Biliopancreatic Diversion with a new type of gastrectomy: Some Previus conclusins revisited. Obes Surg. 1995;5:411–8.
3. Marceau P, Biron S, Bourque RA, et al. Biliopancreatic Diversion of a new type of gastrectomy. Obes Surg. 1993;3:2–36.
4. DeCsepel J, Burpee S, Jossart GJ, Gagner M. Laparoscopic biliopancreatic diversion with a duodenal switch for morbid obesity: a feasibility study in pigs. J Laparoendosc Adv Surg Tech A. 2001;11(2):79–83.
5. Potvin M, Gagner M, Pomp A. Laparoscopic Roux-en-Y gastric bypass for morbid obesity: a feasibility study in pigs. Surg Laparosc Endosc. 1997;7(4):294–7.
6. Ren CJ, Gagner M. Early results of laparoscopic Biliopancreatic diversion with duodenal switch for Morbid Obesity: A case series. Obes Surg. 2000;10:131.
7. Gagner M. Hypoabsorption Not Malabsorption, Hypoabsorptive Surgery and Not Malabsorptive Surgery. Obes Surg. 2016;26(11):2783–4.
8. Ren CJ, Patterson E, Gagner M. Early results of laparoscopic biliopancreatic diversion with duodenal switch: a case series of 40 consecutive patients. Obes Surg. 2000;10(6):514–23.
9. Jossart GH, Nuglozeh-Buck D, Rabkin RA. A laparoscopic technique for duodenal switch: Experience with 79 patients. Surg Endosc. 2001;15:S103.
10. Jossart G, Booth DJ, Rabkin R. A laparoscopic procedure for biliopancreatic BPD with Duodenal switch. Obes Surg. 2000;10:133.
11. Gagner M: The 2-stage Approach in Morbid Obesity: the benefits and rationale for a 2 stage approach in high risk patients and super Obesity. Symposium on Morbid Obesity 2006. XXIX International Meeting of Surgery, Doce de Octubre University Hospital. Madrid, Spain, May 24, 2006.
12. Almogy G, Crookes PF, Anthone GJ. Longitudinal gastrectomy as a treatment for the high-risk super-obese patient. Obes Surg. 2004;14:492–7.
13. Hamoui H, Anthone GJ, Kaufman HS, Crookes PF. Sleeve gastrectomy in the high-risk patient. Obes Surg. 2006;16:1445–9.
14. Chu C, Gagner M, Quinn T, Voellinger DC, Feng JJ, Inabnet WB, Herron D, Pomp A: Two-stage laparoscopic BPD/DS. An Alternative Approach To Super-Super Morbid Obesity. Surgical Endoscopy 2002; S187.
15. Fukuyama S, Chu C, Kim WW, Gagner M: The Second Stage of Laparoscopic biliopancreatic diversion BPD). SAGES 2002 annual meeting, NY, NY, manual proceedings, V047.
16. Voellinger D, Gagner M, Inabnet W, Chu C, Feng J, Mercado A, Quinn T, Pomp A: Laparoscopic Sleeve Gastrectomy is a safe and effective primary procedure for biliopancreatic diversion with duodenal Switch. Poster Abstract, SAGES 2002 manual proceedings, PF020. Surgical Endoscopy 2002; 16:S24.
17. Regan JP, Inabnet WB, Gagner M. Early experience with two-stage laparoscopic roux-en-Y gastric bypass as an alternative in the super-super obese patient. Obes Surg. 2003;13:861–4.
18. Gagner M, Inabnet W, Pomp A. Laparoscopic sleeve gastrectomy with second stage biliopancreatic diversion and duodenal switch in the superobese. In: Inabnet W, DeMaria E, Ikramuddin S, editors. Laparoscopic bariatric surgery. Philadelphia: Lippincott Williams & Wilkins; 2005. p. 143–50.
19. Jossart GH, Anthone G. The History of Sleeve Gastrectomy. Bariatric Times. 2010;7(2):9–10.
20. Sarela AI, Dexter SP, O'Kane M, Menon A, McMahon MJ. Long-term follow-up after laparoscopic sleeve gastrectomy: 8–9-year results. Surg Obes Relat Dis. 2012 Nov–Dec;8(6):679–84.

21. Lee CM, Cirangle PT, Jossart GH. Vertical gastrectomy for morbid obesity in 216 patients: report of two-year results. Surg Endosc. 2007;21(10):1810–6.
22. Himpens J, Dobbeleir J, Peeters G. Long-term results of laparoscopic sleeve gastrectomy for besity. Annals Surg. 2010;252:31–24.
23. Elariny H. Early results of laparoscopic non-banded vertical gastroplasty with sleeve gastrectomy –without duodenal switch in the treatment of morbid obesity. Surg Endosc. 2002;16:S241.
24. Andrei VE, Kortbawi P, Mehta V, Johnson BA, Villapaz A, Ramos C, Hancox W, Carey JC, Brolin RE. Laparoscopic Bariatric Surgery for the treatment of super-obesity: Biliopancreatic diversion with duodenal switch and Roux-en-Y Gastric bypass with a long limb: 24 month follow-up. Surg Endosc. 2002;16:S241.
25. Quinn T, Gagner M, Ren C, de Csepel J, Kini S, Gentileschi P, Herron D, Inabnet W, Pomp A. Laparoscopic biliopancreatic diversion with Duodenal switch: The early experience. Surg Endosc. 2001;15:S158.
26. Kim WW, Gagner M, Kini S, et al. Laparoscopic vs. open biliopancreatic diversion with a duodenal switch: a comparative study. J Gastrointest Surg. 2003;7(4):552–557.
27. Deitel M, Crosby RD, Gagner M. The first international consensus summit for sleeve gastrectomy (SG), New York City, October 25–27, 2007. Obes Surg. 2008;18(5):487–96.
28. Gagner M, Deitel M, Kalberer TL, Erickson AL, Crosby RD. The Second International Consensus Summit for Sleeve Gastrectomy, March 19-21, 2009. Surg Obes Relat Dis. 2009 Jul-Aug;5(4):476-85.
29. Deitel M, Gagner M, Erickson AL, Crosby RD. Third International Summit: Current status of sleeve gastrectomy. Surg Obes Relat Dis. 2011 Nov-Dec;7(6):749–59.
30. Gagner M, Deitel M, Erickson AL, Crosby RD. Survey on laparoscopic sleeve gastrectomy (LSG) at the Fourth International Consensus Summit on Sleeve Gastrectomy. Obes Surg. 2013;23(12):2013–7.
31. Gagner M, Hutchinson C, Rosenthal R. Fifth international consensus conference: current status of sleeve gastrectomy. Surg Obes Relat Dis. 2016;12(4):750–6.
32. Rosenthal RJ; International Sleeve Gastrectomy Expert Panel, Diaz AA, Arvidsson D, Baker RS, Basso N, Bellanger D, Boza C, El Mourad H, France M, Gagner M, Galvao-Neto M, Higa KD, Himpens J, Hutchinson CM, Jacobs M, Jorgensen JO, Jossart G, Lakdawala M, Nguyen NT, Nocca D, Prager G, Pomp A, Ramos AC, Rosenthal RJ, Shah S, Vix M, Wittgrove A, Zundel N. International Sleeve Gastrectomy Expert Panel Consensus Statement: best practice guidelines based on experience of >12,000 cases. Surg Obes Relat Dis. 2012 Jan-Feb;8(1):8–19.
33. English WJ, DeMaria EJ, Brethauer SA, Mattar SG, Rosenthal RJ, Morton JM. American Society for Metabolic and Bariatric Surgery estimation of metabolic and bariatric procedures performed in the United States in 2016. Surg Obes Relat Dis. 2018 Mar;14(3):259–263.
34. Angrisani L, Santonicola A, Iovino P, Vitiello A, Higa K, Himpens J, Buchwald H, Scopinaro N. IFSO Worldwide Survey 2016: Primary, Endoluminal, and Revisional Procedures. Obes Surg. 2018;28(12):3783–94.

Obesity, a Costly Epidemic

Syed Mohamed Aljunid

1 Introduction

Obesity is one of the major health problems affecting developed as well as developing countries. WHO defined Obesity and overweight as individual age 20 and above with Body Mass Index of 25 and above. Obesity itself is categorised into three groups: obesity class 1 (BMI 30 to <35), class II (BMI 35 to<39) and class III (BMI 40 and above). In this chapter we will focus on the cost and economic impact of both the overweight and obesity. WHO estimated in 2016, around 1.9 billion adult age 18 and above were overweight. Out of this 650 million were obese [25]. Generally, 39% of adult age 18 and above were overweight and 13% of them were obese in 2016.

Costing and economic burden studies were normally conducted for a number of reasons. Costing data is often use as a mechanism to inculcate cost consciousness among health stakeholders that include medical practitioners, their administrators and also consumers at large. All these three groups of stakeholders are highly relevant in prevention and management of obesity. Costing data can be used in comparing the cost of interventions over a period of time or in different health settings. These comparisons are important in order to understand the factors that lead to change in the cost and also to choose the most efficient setting in managing health conditions such as obesity. In some countries health services are contracted by the government to other players for various reasons. Costing information is very useful in ensuring that the government can purchase the services at the most efficient

S. M. Aljunid (✉)
Department of Health Policy and Management, Faculty of Public Health, Kuwait University, Kuwait City, Kuwait
e-mail: syed.junid@ku.edu.kw

price. Economic evaluation studies such as cost-effectiveness and cost-benefit analysis requires accurate costing data in order to impute the cost-outcome ratio. This is often used as the indicators to decide the most cost-effective intervention for a specific health problem such as obesity.

2   Costing Methods

There are at least three methods of costing in health care. The first method is called activity-based costing. The basic principle of this method is activities are the cost drivers. Each activity will consume resources in order to produce an output. Hence, each activity relates to specific health intervention should be identified. In management of obesity, all activities in the intervention should be recorded and costs are then assigned to each of each activity. The main advantage of activity-based costing is that it will produce a very detail and comprehensive costing information. However the main drawback of this method is that it will take too much time to complete and costly to execute since it is very labour intensive to conduct.

The second method is called step-down costing. In this method, the researchers will first need to know the total expenditure of the service unit involves in the interventions. This is followed by a series of drilling down the cost at various levels of subunits or cost-centres in the organisations until the lowest level, which is call the final cost-centres. The outcome of this costing is cost per day of stay for inpatient or cost per visit for outpatient care. The main strength of this costing method is that it can be carried out within a short period of time with low human resource need. However one of the limitations of this method is the requirement for researchers to establish the cost-centres and the need to use appropriate cost-allocation factors.

The third costing method is a combination of both activity-based costing and step-down costing. This is the most common method use by researchers in costing studies. In this method, the capital cost and some selected recurrent costs are distributed to the final cost centres using step-down costing while other recurrent cost such as drugs, investigations and selected surgical procedures are easily identified for each patients are allocated based on activity-based costing.

3   Costing Components

There are at least three major cost components in costing studies related to obesity from economics perspective, The first component is the direct cost. Direct cost refers to all costs due to resource use that are completely attributable to the use of a health care intervention or illness [26]. In this chapter, the direct cost of obesity will include cost of diseases related to obesity and overweight covering the inpatient cost, outpatient cost, cost of incurred by patients and their relatives and also cost of preventive services spend in the health system.

The second component of cost is the indirect cost. These are costs related to the loss of income due to the diseases or its intervention. In this chapter, the indirect cost covers the potential loss of income due to treatment of diseases related to obesity and overweight and premature deaths.

The third cost component is the intangible cost. This is the cost associated with pain and sufferings of diseases. Since this cost component is often difficult to quantify and not commonly covered in most costing studies, we will not include this component in our costing of obesity and overweight.

Another important aspect of costing study is the perspective of the costing. In this chapter, as far as possible we report the cost from societal perspective. This means that we will cover the direct and indirect cost of patients, their family members and also the cost incurred by health system on the whole. This will help us to provide a wider view in respect to the cost and economic burden of obesity and overweight.

4   Cost of Obesity and Overweight: The Evidence

In this chapter the evidence on the cost of obesity and overweight was obtained from literature search performed on the Medline (Pubmed) electronic database. Potentially relevant studies were published between 2000 and 2019 were identified through search of their title and abstract. The search terms used were: "Obesity OR Overweight and Cost OR Economic Burden". These were supplemented by hand search on key journals on obesity and reports from WHO and other relevant organisations.

The outcome is presented in two different parts: Overall cost of obesity in health system and cost of Non-communicable diseases related to obesity and overweight.

5   Overall Cost of Obesity

The estimation on the overall cost of obesity was done in the US health system. It was estimated that the direct cost of obesity is more than USD 92 billion per year. This is equivalent to 5% of adult health expenditure in the US [9]. The health care cost of obese individuals in US is 37% higher than non-obese persons, which amount to additional USD 732 per person per year. Another aspect of the impact of obesity is on the productivity of the workforce. Obese workers among a university employees loss a total of 376 productive working days per year. This is 27 times higher than those with healthy weight. The annual medical cost claims among these obese university employees is 13 times higher than those with healthy weight (USD 94,125 among the obese vs. USD 7,503 among those with healthy weight) [18].

A study conducted in North Carolina state in US estimated that the direct and indirect medical costs for eight unhealthy risk factors, including obesity were USD

57.8 billion. This is almost twice the annual budget of the state in 2010. The total cost of managing individuals with obesity and overweight was USD 17.60 billion or around 30% of the total health care cost. Hence, this position excessive weight as the most costly among the eight unhealthy risk factors [6]

Businesses and other commercial entities are also affected from having obese workforce. In another study, it was observed that obesity cost is as high as USD 12.7 billion per year to US businesses, of which USD 7.7 billion alone was on health care cost [22].

In United Kingdom, 66,000 deaths can be avoided in the year 2003–2004 if the population's BMI is 21 and below. Overweight and obesity is responsible for at least 7.3% of all morbidity and mortality in the UK. The total direct cost of obesity was estimated to be around £3.23 billion that is equivalent to 4.6% of the total NHS expenditure in 2002. However the indirect cost due to obesity is very much higher amounted to £11.23 billion. This amount is as high as 43% of the total NHS Budget [2].

In systematic reviews of articles on cost of obesity in Canada, Tran et al. [5] reported the outcome of ten published studies from 1990 to 2011. Annual cost of obesity in Canada range from CAD1.27 billion to CAD 11.08 billion, consuming between 2.2 and 12% of Canada's total health expenditures. One of the latest reviews on cost of obesity was by Anis et al. [4] using prevalence based approached covering 18 co-morbidities from societal perspective. Direct medical cost including hospital care, physicians' services, services by other health professionals and drugs were imputed in this study. The indirect cost was estimated from the morbidity cost due to short and long-term disability. The authors use human capital approach in estimating the indirect cost. It was found that the total direct cost was CD 5.96 billion and the indirect cost was CD 5.0 billion. The total cost of obesity is CD 10.6 billion, which is equivalent to 4.2% of total health expenditure of Canada.

The study conducted in Germany by Kannopka et al. (2011) reported a huge amount of resources are needed in managing obesity and overweight. The direct cost in their study covers inpatient, outpatient treatment, rehabilitation, and non-medical cost such an administration and research. As in the study in UK, the authors also used human capital approach in estimating the indirect cost. Output lost due to loss of income as the result of absence from work was imputed in this study. Most of the indirect costs are from loss of income due to early retirement and premature mortality related to obesity and overweight. The total cost of obesity was estimated at € 9.97 billion where 51% of the cost is indirect cost. The total cost is equivalent to 2.1% of total health expenditure of Germany.

Study on cost of obesity in low and middle-income countries is rare. Pitayatienanan et al. [19] conducted a study in Thailand that estimates the cost of obesity in the country. They used retrospective cost-of-illness approach in the study covering health care cost, cost of productivity loss due to premature death and hospital admissions. Twelve comorbidities related to obesity were included in this study. The cost of obesity was estimated to be Baht 12,142 million (USD PPP 725.3 million). This is equivalent to 0.13% of GDP. The healthcare cost account for 46% of the total cost or 1.5% of the total health expenditure of Thailand.

In South Korea, Kang et al. (2005) reported a study they conducted to estimate the socio-economic cost of obesity and overweight among adults age 20 and above. The direct cost included in the study is cost of inpatient care, outpatient care and medications. The indirect cost is loss of productivity due to premature deaths, inpatient care, transportation cost and nursing cost. The costing data for the study was sourced from National Health Insurance claims of eight co-morbid conditions associated with overweight and obesity. The total cost of obesity and overweight for Korea was found to be USD 1.78 billion per year. The direct cost was estimated to be USD 1.08 and the indirect cost was USD 0.7 billion. The costs represent 0.22% of GPD and 3.7% of total health expenditure of Korea.

6 Cost of Non-communicable Diseases Related to Obesity and Overweight

The chronic and communicable diseases that are most likely linked to obesity and overweight is given in Fig. 1.

6.1 Ischaemic Heart Disease and Stroke

Ischaemic heart diseases and stroke are among the top cardiovascular disases that has a strong link to obesity and overweight as riskfactors. Hansen et al. [15] in their study that followed-up 6,238 men and women in Denmark for a ten-year period showed that obese and overweight respondents had 2–3 times more likely to develop ischaemic hearth disease than the non-obese individuals. In another study done earlier, Thomsen and Nordestgaard [17] followed up a big chohort of 71,257 people for 3.6 years. They found that overweight and obese indiviuals with metabolic syndrome

Fig. 1 Chronic diseases linked to obesity and overweight

◆ Cardiovascular Diseases
  ▪ Ischemic Heart Disease
  ▪ Stroke
◆ Diabetes Mellitus
◆ Musculoskeletal Disorders
  ▪ Osteoarthritis
◆ Cancers
  ▪ Breast,
  ▪ Colorectal
  ▪ Uterine
  ▪ Ovary
  ▪ Prostate
  ▪ Liver
  ▪ Kidney

had higher risk of developing myocardial infarction by 1.7 and 2.3 times, respectively, than those with normal weights and without metabolic syndromes.

In term of stroke, Mitchell et al. [3] reported in their study involving 1,201 cases of obesity with 1,154 controls among young adults that obese subjects have nearly 60% higher risks of developing stroke. These findings re-confirmed the outcome of an earlier study among older adults, which covered more than 2 million subjects [12]. The cost of stroke attributable to obesity was estimated to be aroud CAD 106 million per year in Canada [13]. In the study in Canada, the population attributable fraction (PAF) of obesity for stroke was estimated to be vey low at only 4%. This is in mark contrast to study in UK where the PAF was estimated to be higher at 34%. The total cost of stroke attibutable to obesity was found to be £229 million per year.

Based on the Casemix Database in Malaysia and Indonesia for the year 2016, the direct cost from provider's perspective of managing both acute myocardial infarction and stroke were very high and may not be affordable by most sector of the population. In Malaysia, the cost of managing acute myocardial infaction per admission ranged from 5.5% for mild cases without any complications and comorbidity to 9.1% of percapita GDP for severe cases with major complications and comorbidity. For cases of stroke, the cost in Malaysia is higher than myocardial infaction ranging from 14% of percapita GDP for mild cases to 23.8% of GDP for severe cases (Table 1). The cost of mycoardial infarction and stroke in Indonesia

Table 1 Cost of inpatient care for myocardial infarction and stroke in Malaysia (2016)

	Severity	Cost per admission (RM)	USD (PPP)[a]	% GDP
Acute Myocardial Infarction	Mild	1,757	1,220	5.5
	Moderate	2,215	1,538	6.6
	Severe	2,925	2,031	9.1
Stroke	Mild	4,470	3,104	14.0
	Moderate	5,564	3,864	17.4
	Severe	7,602	5,279	23.8

[a]PPP Exchange Rate 2018: 1 USD PPP = 1.44 RM

Table 2 Cost of inpatient care for myocardial infarction and stroke in Indonesia (2016)

	Severity	Cost per Admission (Rupiah)	USD (PPP)[a]	% GDP
Acute Myocardial Infarction	Mild	4,810,699	1,135	12.0
	Moderate	8,589,900	2,027	21.5
	Severe	12,391,700	2,924	30.9
Stroke	Mild	8,763,300	2,068	21.8
	Moderate	11,715,800	2,764	29.2
	Severe	14,704,800	3,470	36.7

[a]PPP exchange rate 2018; PPP USD = 4,238 Rupiah

is much higher than Malaysia in term of percentage of percapita income. Overall, the cost for myocardial infarction in Indonesia ranged from 12 to 30% of percapita GDP. The cost of stroke in Indonesia is very much higher than myocardial infaction ranging from 21.8% to 36.7% of percapita GDP.

6.2   Diabetes Mellitus

Diabetes mellitus link with overweight and obesity is very clear and observed in most population in the world. The global prevalence of diabetes in 2019 is 9.3% affecting 463 million people. The prevalence is expected to raise to 10.2% by 2030 and 10.9% in 2045 [20]. International Diabetes Federation estimated that in 2019 the global expenditure on diabetes mellitus that accounts for the direct cost is USD 760 billion. This figure will raise to USD 825 billion in 2030 and USD 845 billion to 2045 [11]. Abdullah et al. [1] in a metaanalysis of 18 prospective cohort studies found that the relative risk of diabetes among the obese was 7.19 and the overweight was 2.99 compared to those with normal weight. Most of the studies that estimated the obesity and overweight cost of diabetes mellitus used the population attributable fraction (PAF) method. In UK, obesity and overweight contributes 79% of PAF of diabetes cost or 2.1% of the total annual DALYs lost. This is equivalent to £533 million in 2002 [2]. In an earlier study conducted by Birmingham et al. [13] in Canada the PAF for obesity in diabetes was estimated to be 50.7%. The total direct cost of diabetes mellitus attributable to obesity was CAD 423 million per year.

6.3   Osteoarthritis

Osteoarthritis is one of the major musculoskeletal conditions related to obesity. Study among women in UK found that highest tertile of BMI were six times more likely to develop osteoarthritis [21]. It was observed in another study that for every one standard deviation (SD) increase in BMI, the risk of developing osteoarthritis is increased by 40%. The PAF for obesity in osteoarthritis was estimated to be 21% in UK. The total cost of obesity in osteoarthritis was estimated to be around £229 million per year [2]. Chen et al. [8] in their reviews of series of literatures from North Americans, European and Asian regions reported that there are huge variation in the direct and indirect cost of managing osteoarthritis in these regions. The cost of topical and oral NSAID ranged from £19.2 to £26.65 million per year while the cost of knee and hip replacement exceeded £850 per year. The indirect cost of osteoarthritis due to loss of productivity was estimated to be £1.34 billion per year. In Spain, Loza et al. [16] estimated that the direct and indirect cost of osteoarthritis was £4.04 billion and £654 million per year, respectively. Based on PAF estimation from the study in UK, the cost of osteoarthritis due to obesity in Spain was £986 million per year. Le Pen et al. [14] conducted an economic burden study of osteoarthritis in France. They estimated that the total direct cost of osteoarthritis was £1.58 billion per year. Again if we use the same PAF of 21% as in the study in UK, the direct cost of osteoarthritis attributed to obesity is estimated to be £332 million per year. The cost is lower than Spain but slightly higher than the estimates in UK.

6.4   Cancers

Obesity and overweight are two known risk factors of cancers. In 2018, it was estimated there were 18.1 million cancer cases and 9.6 million deaths globally. Risks of 13 types of cancers increased with obesity and overweight that account for 3.6% new cancers among adults worldwide [7]. Cancers that are linked to obesity and overweight includes colon, endometrium, postmenopausal breast, kidney, esophagus, pancreas, gallbladder, liver, and hematological malignancy [23]. The overall cost of expenditure on cancers in US in 2017 was estimated to be USD 342 billion, which is equivalent to 1.8% of GDP. Loss of productivity and cost of premature deaths is 53% of the total cost. In the European Union the cost of cancer was estimated to be €141.8 billion or 1.07% of the total GDP.

Colorectal cancer is one of the commonest form of cancer associated with obesity and overweight. Around 10% of the total incidence of cancer in the world are colorectal cancers. In 2017, it was estimated that there were 1.8 million new cases of colorectal cancer with 896,000 deaths [10]. Obesity and overweight is attributed to 16% of the colorectal cancers that account for 2% of the total DALYs in UK. The cost of colorectal cancer due to obesity and overweight was estimated to be £61 million per annum [2]. Birmingham et al. [13] used a much lower value of PAF in estimating the obesity cost of colorectal cancers in Canada. Based on PAF of only 4.7%, they estimated that obesity and overweight contributed CAD 19.9 million per year of colorectal cancer cost.

Breast cancer is the most common cancer among women and accounted for 12% of all cancer cases globally. The cumulative risk of developing breast cancer among women age 75 years is 5%. The PAF for obesity and overweight in breast cancer was estimated to be around 12% in UK. Obesity and overweight is responsible for 1.8% of the total DALYs loss due to breast cancer. The total cost of breast cancer attributable to obesity and overweight in UK was £29 million per year [2]. A study in Canada reported that the obesity and overweight cause of breast cancer was CAD 19.8 million year. However, this study focussed on postmenopausal women and the PAF of 9.1% was used [13].

7   Conclusion

Overweight and obesity is a major public health problem in both developed and developing countries. Costing studies on these conditions can provide excellent insight to the policy makers on the scale of the problems that affect the health system. Outcome of such studies highlighted the significant amount of resources required in managing cases of overweight and obesity. The overall health expenditure to manage overweight and obesity ranged from 2% to as high 12% of the total national health expenditure. However, there are wide variations in the costing methods to estimate the direct and indirect cost as reported in the reviewed studies. Most of the studies employed the step-down approach in combination with PAF to estimate the total cost. Step-down costing was the preferred method in most of the studies because of lack of detail costing information required in activity-based costing. There is also wide range of PAF values depending on the countries where the study was conducted and the conditions linked to obesity and overweight. PAF values were as high as 79% for diabetes mellitus and was only 4.7% for colorectal cancers. One of the major future challenges for the researchers is to work towards standardization of the costing methods in order to increase the usability of the study outcome for policy decisions.

References

1. Abdullah A, Peeters A, de Courten M, Stoelwinder J. The magnitude of association between overweight and obesity and the risk of diabetes: a meta-analysis of prospective cohort studies. Diabetes Res Clin Pract. 2010;89(3):309–19.
2. Allender S, Rayner M. The burden of overweight and obesity related ill health in the UK. Obes Rev. 2007;8(5):467–73.
3. Mitchell AB, Cole JW, Patrick F, McArdle Y-C, Ryan KA, Sparks MJ, Mitchell BD, Kittner SJ. Obesity increases risk of ischemic stroke in young adults. Stroke. 2015;46:1690–2. https://doi.org/10.1161/STROKEAHA.115.008940.
4. Anis AH, Zhang W, Bansback N, Guh DP, Amarsi Z, Birmingham CL. Obesity and overweight in Canada: an updated cost-of-illness study. Obes Rev. 2010;11:31–40.
5. Tran BX, Nair AV, Kuhle S, Ohinma A, Veugelers PJ. Cost analyses of obesity in Canada: scope, quality, and implications. Cost Eff Resour Alloc. 2013;11(3):2–9. https://www.resource-allocation.com/content/11/1/3.
6. Be Active North Carolina. Tipping the scales: the high cost of unhealthy behaviour in North Carolina (2012). https://www.ncicdp.org/documents/Tipping-the-Scales-Final_2012.pdf.
7. Cancer Atlas (2029). https://canceratlas.cancer.org/content/uploads/2019/09/CA3_TheBurdenofCancer.pdf.
8. Chen A, Gupte C, Akhtar K, Smith P and Cobb J. The global economic cost of osteoarthritis: how the UK compares? Arthritis. 2012;2012, Article ID 698709, 6 pages https://doi.org/10.1155/2012/698709.
9. Finkelstein EA., Fiebelkorn IC, Wang G. National medical spending attributable to overweight and obesity: how much, and who's paying? Health Aff. 2003, Suppl Web Exclusives, W3-219–26.
10. GBD 2017 Colorectal Collaborators. The global, regional and national burden of colorectal cancer and its attributable risk factors in 195 countries and territories, 1990–2017: a systematic analysis for Global of Burden Disease Study 2017. Lancet Gasteroenterol Hepatol. 2019. https://doi.org/10.1016/S2468-1253(19)30345-0.
11. International Diabetes Federation. IDF Diabetes Atlas. 9th ed. 2019.
12. Meschia JF, Bushnell C, Boden-Albala B, Braun LT, Bravata DM, Chaturvedi S, Creager MA Eckel RH , Elkind MSV, Fornage M, Goldstein LB, Greenberg SM , Horvath SE, Iadecola C, Jauch EC, Moore WS and Wilson JA. Guidelines for the primary prevention of stroke a statement for healthcare professionals from the American heart association/American stroke association. Stroke. 2014;45:3754–832.

13. Laird Birmingham CL, Muller JL, Palepu A, Spinelli JJ and Anis AH. The cost of obesity in Canada. CMAJ. 1999;160:483–8.
14. Le Pen C, Reygrobellet C, Gerentes I. Financial cost of osteoarthritis in France: the "COART" France study. Joint Bone Spine. 2005;72(6):567–70.
15. Hansen L, Netterstrøm MK, Johansen NB, Rønn PF, Vistisen D, Husemoen LLN, Jørgensen ME, Faerch K. Metabolically Healthy Obesity and Ischemic HeartDisease: A 10-Year Follow-Up of the Inter99 Study. J Clin Endocrinol Metab. 2017;102:1934–42.
16. Loza E, Lopez-Gomez JM , Abasolo L, Maese J, Carmona L, Batlle-Gualdam E. Economic burden of knee and hip osteoarthritis in Spain. Arthritis Care Res. 2009;61(2):158–65.
17. Thomsen M, Nordestgaard BG. Myocardial Infarction and Ischemic Heart Disease in Overweight and Obesity with and Without Metabolic Syndrome. JAMA Intern Med. 2014;174(1):15–22.
18. Ostbye T, Dement JM, Krause KM. Obesity and workers' compensation: results from the duke health and safety surveillance system. Arch Intern Med. 2007;167:766–73.
19. Pitayatienanan P, Butchon R, Yothasamut J, Aekplakorn W, Teerawattananon Y, Suksomboon N and Thavorncharoensap M. Economic costs of obesity in Thailand: a retrospective cost-of-illness study. BMC Health Serv Res. 2014;14:146, 4–7. https://www.biomedcentral.com/1472-6963/14/146.
20. Saeedi P, Petersohn I, Salpea P, Malanda B,Karuranga S, Unwin N, Colagiuri S, Guariguata L, Motala A, Ogurtsova K, Shaw J, Bright D, Williams R. Global and regional diabetes prevalence estimates for 2019 and projections for 2030 and 2045: results from the international diabetes federation diabetes atlas, 9th edition. Diabetes Res Clin Pract. 2019;157(107843):1–9.
21. Sowers MFR and Karvonen-Gutierrez CA. The evolving role of obesity in knee osteoarthritis. Curr Opin Rheumatol. 22(5): 533–5. Curr Opin Rheumatol. 2010;22(5):533–7. https://doi.org/10.1097/BOR.0b013e32833b4682.
22. Thompson D, Edelsberg J, Kinsey KL, Oster G. Estimated economic costs of obesity to U.S. business. Am J Health Promot. 1998;13:120–7.
23. Vucenik V and Stains JP. Obesity and cancer risk: evidence, mechanisms, and recommendations. Ann NY Acad Sci. 2012;1271(2012):37–43 c 2012 New York Academy of Sciences. https://doi.org/10.1111/j.1749-6632.2012.06750.x
24. Wang F, Schultz AB, Musich S, McDonald T, Hirschland D, Edington DW. The relationship between National Heart, Lung, and Blood Institute Weight Guidelines and concurrent medical costs in a manufacturing population. Am J Health Promot. 2003;17(3):183–9.
25. WHO. 2020. https://www.who.int/en/news-room/fact-sheets/detail/obesity-and-overweight. Access 3rd March 2020.
26. Wilhelm K, editor. Encyclopedia of public health. 2008. https://link.springer.com/referencework entry/10.1007%2F978-1-4020-5614-7_799. https://doi.org/10.1007/978-1-4020-5614-7_799.

The Health Effects of Obesity

Nadia Ahmad

1 Obesity Reduces Life Expectancy

The effect of obesity on survival has been recognized for over 2500 years since Hippocrates first noted that "sudden death is more common in those who are naturally fat than lean." [1] Two centuries later, the physiologist Malcolm Flemyng described obesity as a disease "because it obstructs the free exercise of the animal functions and hath a tendency to shorten life" [1]. Indeed, obesity is associated with a striking reduction in life expectancy in both adult men and women and across racial and ethnic groups [2–4]. This observation has been confirmed in several large pooled analyses of prospective studies, including a meta-analysis of over 239 studies spanning 4 continents which found that every 5 kg/m^2 increase in body mass index (BMI) over 25 kg/m^2 is associated with a 29–39% increase in all-cause mortality [5–7]. The association of obesity and mortality even extends to individuals with so-called "metabolically healthy" obesity, who do not exhibit cardiometabolic abnormalities (e.g. high waist circumference, hypertension, hypertriglderidemia, low high-density lipoprotein, or abnormal glycemic parameters) [8]. The effect of obesity on survival is mediated by a broad range of conditions with the predominant mediators being cardiovascular diseases, respiratory diseases and cancer [7].

The direct relationship between BMI over 25 kg/m^2 and mortality has been challenged by some studies reporting a protective effect of overweight and/or Class I obesity in cardiovascular disease, cancer, respiratory disease, renal disease and the elderly. These observations have been termed "the obesity paradox" [9].

N. Ahmad (✉)
Obesity Medicine Institute, LLC, New Canaan, CT, United States
e-mail: nahmad1228@gmail.com

Eli Lilly & Company, Indianapolis, IN, USA

Table 1 Limitations of studies that observe an obesity paradox[a]

Methodological limitation	Example
Misclassification bias	BMI may inappropriately assign overweight status to individuals who are normal weight by body composition. This may underestimate mortality in the overweight group
Reverse causation	Weight loss in the normal weight group may be related to underlying illness and loss of fat free mass, leading to a higher relative mortality in that group compared to overweight groups
Collider stratification bias	Smoking may be a significant causal factor, and lower rates of smoking in the overweight group may present as improved survival

[a]Banack HR, Stokes A. The 'obesity paradox' may not be a paradox at all. *Int J Obes (Lond)*. 2017;41(8):1162–1163. https://doi.org/10.1038/ijo.2017.99

However, the obesity paradox is largely debunked when accounting for the methodological issues in these studies (Table 1).

2   Obesity and Cardiovascular Disease

Most cardiovascular disease is increased in the setting of obesity, including coronary heart disease, heart failure with reduced ejection fraction (HFrEF), heart failure with preserved ejection fraction (HFpEF), atrial fibrillation and stroke [10–11]. Obesity contributes to these diseases via both indirect and direct effects on the cardiovascular system. The indirect effects are well known and include hyperlipidemia, dyslipidemia, arterial hypertension, insulin resistance, hyperglycemia, and systemic inflammation [10]. These cardiometabolic risk factors correlate with fat mass in obesity, and particularly with visceral and ectopic fat depots that are known to have systemic metabolic effects [12].

The direct effects of obesity on cardiovascular health have received less attention in clinical care but are increasingly recognized in the literature. The epicardial fat depot, in particular, has been found to have direct lipotoxic effects on the underlying myocardium and coronary vasculature [13]. It releases inflammatory cytokines and reactive oxygen species that have paracrine and vasocrine effects creating a proatherogenic milieu. Epicardial fat may also contribute to structural and electrical remodeling leading to atrial fibrillation [3]. In addition, individuals with obesity not only have high levels of fat mass, but also have elevated fat-free mass (FFM), which is thought to be an adaptation to carrying an extra load or weight in their daily activities [10]. Increased FFM increases the circulating blood volume which, in turn, increases the left ventricular (LV) stroke volume and cardiac output, placing extra burden on the heart. This leads to altered cardiac structure and function including ventricular (both left and right) concentric hypertrophy and enlargement, left atrial enlargement, and systolic and diastolic dysfunction which can eventually manifest as obesity cardiomyopathy or congestive heart failure [10].

Both severity of obesity and duration of obesity are associated with cardiac performance and cardiovascular disease [10]. Increased cardiorespiratory fitness has been found to reverse much of the negative impact of obesity on cardiovascular health and mortality. However, only 20% of individuals with obesity are thought to have adequate cardiorespiratory fitness [10].

3   Obesity and Respiratory Disease

Respiratory function is adversely affected by obesity in a number of ways. Excess adiposity on the thoracic wall and in the abdomen limits chest wall movement and decreases lung compliance, heightening the demand on the diaphragm [14]. Although respiratory muscle strength is preserved, diaphragmatic endurance is reduced as much as 45%, which may explain the common occurrence of breathlessness and susceptibility to respiratory failure in patients with obesity in the setting of abdominal surgery, sepsis or metabolic derangements. Lung perfusion is impacted by obesity as well. Perfusion is greatest in the dependent portions of the lung. In obesity, however, shallow breathing leads to basal atelectasis and distributes ventilation to the upper lung zones leading to ventilation-perfusion mismatch and increased vulnerability to hypoxia.

Obesity also leads to reduced airway caliber and increased airway resistance. This may explain in part the relationship between obesity and asthma wherein a weight gain of >5 kg increases risk of asthma in a dose-dependent manner and obesity is associated with symptom severity and increased bronchodilator use [14].

Upper airway function is particularly impacted in obesity by both the mechanical load of excess adiposity on pharyngeal structures and obesity-related inflammatory cytokines that disrupt pharyngeal neuromuscular function [14]. These changes manifest in obstructive sleep apnea (OSA), which has a prevalence of over 70% in the bariatric surgical population. Despite its strong association with obesity, 80% of obstructive sleep apnea remains undiagnosed [14]. Hypopneas and apneas in OSA result in hypoxia, hypercapnia, increased sympathetic activity, increased respiratory effort, cortical arousal, and sleep fragmentation which in turn leads to functional and physiologic impairments [15]. Specifically, OSA causes neuropsychiatric disturbances, cardiac arrhythmias, pulmonary hypertension, corpulmonale, systemic hypertension, coronary artery disease, congestive heart failure, polycythemia, stroke and increased mortality [14–15]. These complications are worsened in obesity hypoventilation syndrome (OHS) which is characterized by non-apneic hypoxemia and CO_2 retention. Both mechanical and central mechanisms are thought to play a role in OHS [15].

Obesity is also associated with worse outcomes in respiratory infections, including community acquired pneumonia, H1N1 influenza and coronavirus disease 2019 (Covid-19) [15–17]. Higher rates of hospitalization, intubation and mortality in the setting of Covid -19 are possibly related to multiple mechanisms including the aforementioned alterations in respiratory function predisposing to respiratory failure and/or hypoxia, altered immune responses leading to weakened host defense and increased chances of cytokine storm, and increased quantities of angiotensin converting enzyme-2 (ACE-2), the transmembrane enzyme that SARS-CoV-2, the virus that causes Covid-19, uses for cell entry [17].

4   Obesity and Cancer

Obesity is associated with 13 types of cancer (Table 2) [18]. Among women in North America, Europe and the Middle East, the obesity-related cancer burden comprises 9% of the total cancer burden. There is increasing evidence of causal links between obesity and cancer that center on obesity-related metabolic and endocrine abnormalities. Specifically, alterations in sex hormone metabolism, insulin and insulin-like growth factor signaling, adipokines, and several inflammatory pathways have been implicated [18]. Despite the higher prevalence of various cancers in patients with obesity, rates of cancer screening have been shown to decrease with increasing BMI [19]. This disparity in care needs to be urgently addressed given the rising rates of both epidemics.

Although there is limited data to show the benefit of weight loss for cancer prevention or prognosis, it has been found that the mortality benefit of surgical weight loss is not only related to a reduction in cardiovascular mortality but also

Table 2 Obesity-related Cancers

Cancer site or type	Relative risk of highest BMI category evaluated versus normal BMI (95% CI)
Esophagus adenocarcinoma	4.8 (3.0–7.7)
Gastric cardia	1.8 (1.3–2.5)
Colon and rectum	1.3 (1.3–1.4)
Liver	1.8 (1.6–2.1)
Gallbladder	1.3 (1.2–1.4)
Pancreas	1.5 (1.2–1.8)
Breast (post-menopausal)	1.1 (1.1–1.2)[a]
Corpus uteri	7.1 (6.3–8.1)
Ovary	1.1 (1.1–1.2)
Kidney (renal cell)	1.8 (1.7–1.9)
Meningioma	1.5 (1.3–1.8)
Thyroid	1.1 (1.0–1.1)[a]
Multiple myeloma	1.5 (1.2–2.0)

Adapted from Lauby-Secretan B, Scoccianti C, Loomis D, et al. Body Fatness and Cancer–Viewpoint of the IARC Working Group. *N Engl J Med.* 2016;375(8):794–798. https://doi.org/10.1056/NEJMsr1606602
[a]Shown is the relative risk per 5 BMI units

a reduction in cancer mortality [20]. Weight loss has also been shown to improve prognosis in breast cancer treatment [18].

5 Other Obesity-Related Conditions

In clinical medicine, there has been a predominating focus on the impact of obesity on cardiovascular health, and more recently, an increased focus on the respiratory and oncologic diseases described thus far. This is due, in part, to the global burden of these specific co-morbidities, the high mortality associated with them and/or, in the case of cardiovascular disease, the well-established relationship between obesity and cardiovascular risk factors such as hypertension, dyslipidemia and type 2 diabetes.

The health effects of obesity, however, span every medical discipline and effect every organ system. Table 3 lists specific obesity-related diseases by system, which have not been discussed in the preceding sections. The range of obesity-related conditions, many of which are under-diagnosed or under-appreciated in routine clinical practice, points to the substantial morbidity and reduced quality of life that can be associated with excess adiposity.

6 Health Effects of Obesity in Special Populations

6.1 Transplant Recipients

Considering that obesity is a risk factor for end stage renal disease (ESRD), heart failure, and cirrhosis, it is not surprising that many transplant recipients have an elevated BMI. Unfortunately, obesity that has contributed to the end organ damage in these patients, also leads to worse post-transplant outcomes. The relationship between obesity and transplant has probably been most studied in the renal transplant field in which obesity has been associated with delayed graft function, graft failure, urine protein and acute rejection, independent of diabetes [29]. In lung transplant recipients, obesity affects short- and long-term survival above BMI ≥ 30 kg/m^2, whereas in liver transplant recipients it does not seem to confer added risk until much higher BMIs [30]. Obesity in heart transplant patients is associated with multiple complications related to the heart transplant, left ventricular assist devices, and cardiothoracic surgery more generally. These complications include infection, wound dehiscence, mediastinitis, prolonged mechanical ventilation and intensive care unit stays, thrombosis, premature device failure, cardiac arrythmias, and early and late mortality [31].

Due to the adverse effect of obesity on transplant outcomes, many transplant centers have implemented BMI thresholds resulting in an increased demand for more effective weight loss options in this population [30].

Table 3 Other obesity-associated conditions

System	Obesity-associated Condition
Gastrointestinal (21)	

Liver	• Non-alcoholic fatty liver disease (NAFLD)
	  ○ Increased cardiovascular mortality and hepatocellular carcinoma (HCC) risk
	• Non-alcoholic steatohepatitis (NASH)
	  ○ Increased mortality; 20% progress to cirrhosis
	• Cirrhosis

Gallbladder	• Gallstone disease
Pancreas	• Acute pancreatitis
Esophagus	• Esophageal dysmotility • Gastroesophageal reflux disease (GERD) • Erosive esophagitis • Barrett's esophagus
Stomach	• Erosive gastritis
Small intestine	• Diarrhea
Colon	• Diverticular disease • Colonic polyps • Clostridium difficile infection
Anorectum	• Dyssynergic defecation
Urogenital (22)	

Upper tract	• Chronic kidney disease (CKD)
	  ○ Related to hypertension and/or type 2 diabetes
	• End-stage renal disease (ESRD)
	  ○ Even when controlling for HTN and T2DM, obesity affects progression of CKD to ESRD
	• Obesity-related glomerulopathy
	• Kidneys stones
	  ○ Evidence strongest for uric acid stones but likely to increase calcium oxalate stones as well

Lower tract- women	• Urge incontinence • Stress incontinence
Lower tract- men	• Lower urinary tract symptoms (LUTS) • Benign prostatic hypertrophy
Neurologic (23)	
Central Nervous System	• Idiopathic intracranial hypertension • Alzheimer's dementia • Mild cognitive impairment ○ Attention deficits, poor executive function, impaired decision making, decreased verbal learning and memory
Peripheral Nervous System	
-Autonomic	• Autonomic dysfunction ○ Increased sympathetic outflow
-Somatosensory	• Peripheral polyneuropathy ○ Associated with obesity, prediabetes, and dyslipidemia; obesity also an independent risk factor
Psychiatric (24)	• Depression ○ Bidirectional relationship • Anxiety
Dermatologic (25)	
Physical effects	• Venous stasis, stasis pigmentation, stasis dermatitis • Venous ulcers

Table 3 (continued)

	• Lymphedema
	  o Lower limbs and abdominal wall
	• Recurrent cellulitis
	  o Lower limbs and abdominal wall; poor wound healing with prolonged hospitalizations
	• Hidradenitis suppurativa
	• Intertrigo and cutaneous infections (candida)

Inflammatory dermatoses	• Psoriasis o Increases both risk and severity
Cancer	• Melanoma • Non-melanoma skin cancer (excluding basal cell carcinoma)
Cosmetic	• Skin tags • Striae
Signs of metabolic disturbance	• Acanthosis nigricans (insulin resistance) • Acne, hirsutism, androgenetic alopecia (hyperandrogenism, polycystic ovarian syndrome)

Hematologic (15)	• Thromboembolic disease
	  o Higher in hospitalized patients and women
	  o May be related to immobility, endothelial dysfunction, and reduction in fibrinolysis

Rheumatologic/ Musculoskeletal (26, 27)	• Osteoarthritis
	• Degenerative joint disease
	• Plantar fasciitis
	• Low back pain
	• Carpal tunnel
	• Rheumatoid arthritis
	  o Associated with worse disease activity, increased odds of non-remission, worse functional ability and health-related quality of life
	• Psoriatic arthritis
	  o Recognized as a risk factor and associated with worse treatment efficiency
	• Ankylosing spondylitis
	  o Associated with adverse outcomes

Reproductive (28)	
Men	• Decreased testosterone • Erectile dysfunction
Women	• Polycystic ovarian syndrome • Reduced natural fecundity/ increased time to conception (even in ovulatory women) • Infertility • Anovulation / menstrual irregularities
Fertility treatment	• Increased gonadotropin requirement • Lower oocyte yield in severe obesity • Reduced implantation rates, clinical pregnancy rates and live birth rates • Increased pregnancy loss rate prior to 24 weeks gestation • If using egg donor, live birth rate per cycle is lower • Compromised pelvic ultrasound imaging for oocyte retrieval

6.2   Orthopedic Surgery Patients

Obesity is a risk factor for multiple musculoskeletal issues including knee osteoarthritis. There has been an increase in total knee arthroplasties in patients with elevated BMI [32]. In these patients, obesity is associated with a functional recovery
similar to those without obesity. However, there is a significant increase in mid- to
long-term revision rates in those with severe obesity. Obesity also poses a higher
risk of post-operative superficial wound infections and thromboembolism [32].
Many orthopedic surgeons recommend a BMI cut-off for knee replacements. As
is the case in transplant medicine, the BMI cut-offs lead to increased demands for
effective weight loss options in this population.

6.3   Pregnancy

Obesity impacts both maternal and neonatal health. Rates of miscarriage are
higher in women with obesity irrespective of spontaneous conception or in vitro
fertilization [28]. The rate of gestational diabetes doubles for BMI ≥ 30 kg/m^2 and
triples for BMI ≥ 40 kg/m^2. Risk of pre-eclampsia doubles with overweight and
triples with obesity. There is also a more than 30% chance of pre-term delivery
(before 37 weeks) in women with obesity. The peripartum risks include a prolonged first stage of labor, less success with vaginal birth after cesarean (VBAC),
and increased rates of cesarean section delivery. Other obstetrical risks include
increased fetal distress, instrumental deliveries, and shoulder dystocia. Wound
infection and dehiscence, perinatal hemorrhage, and deep venous thrombosis are
also more common in pregnant women with obesity. Neonatal effects of obesity
include macrosomia and congenital anomalies, such as neural tube defects, oral
clefts, hydrocephaly, anorectalatresia, limb reduction and cardiovascular anomalies [28].

6.4   Children and Adolescents

Much of the health effects of obesity in children and adolescents parallel those
in adults. The increasing prevalence of obesity in children is therefore accompanied by an increase in type 2 diabetes, dyslipidemia, hypertension, non-alcoholic
fatty liver disease (NAFLD), non-alcoholic steatohepatitis (NASH), and OSA [33].
There are, however, additional musculoskeletal and psychological considerations.
Obesity during periods of growth can exert biomechanical forces leading to flat-
foot, Blount's disease, and slipped capital femoral epiphysis. Children with obesity also experience significant psychosocial distress thought to be related to lower
self-esteem, social isolation, depressive symptoms, and body dissatisfaction [33].

7 Conclusion

Excess adiposity has widespread effects on health and well-being leading to significant morbidity and mortality. Obesity is not only a risk factor for numerous diseases, but it can also exacerbate underlying conditions leading to more severe symptoms, more rapid progression, and worse treatment prognosis. In some cases, obesity is even the primary cause of specific conditions such as obesity cardiomyopathy, NAFLD/NASH, and obesity-related glomerulopathy. The extensive endocrine and physical effects of excess and ectopic fat depots warrant a thoughtful and comprehensive assessment of the patient with obesity in clinical practice. The degree to which a therapy improves upon the many negative health effects of obesity also warrants evaluation, so the full risk–benefit of treatment is understood.

References

1. Rosen H. Is Obesity A Disease or A Behavior Abnormality? Did the AMA Get It Right? Mo Med. 2014;111(2):104–8.
2. Gu D, He J, Duan X, et al. Body weight and mortality among men and women in China. JAMA. 2006;295:776–83.
3. Fontaine KR, McCubrey R, Mehta T, et al. Body mass index and mortality rate among Hispanic adults: a pooled analysis of multiple epidemiologic data sets. International Journal of Obesity. 2012;36:1121.
4. Zheng W, McLerran DF, Rolland B, et al. Association between body-mass index and risk of death in more than 1 million Asians. N Engl J Med. 2011;364:719–29.
5. Whitlock G, Lewington S, Sherliker P, et al. Body-mass index and cause-specific mortality in 900 000 adults: collaborative analyses of 57 prospective studies. Lancet. 2009;373:1083–96.
6. Berrington de Gonzalez A, Hartge P, Cerhan JR, et al. Body-mass index and mortality among 1.46 million white adults. N Engl J Med. 2010;363:2211–9.
7. Global BMI Mortality Collaboration, Di Angelantonio E, Bhupathiraju ShN, et al. Body-mass index and all-cause mortality: individual-participant-data meta-analysis of 239 prospective studies in four continents. Lancet. 2016;388(10046):776–786. doi:https://doi.org/10.1016/S0140-6736(16)30175-1
8. Kramer CK, Zinman B, Retnakaran R. Are metabolically healthy overweight and obesity benign conditions?: A systematic review and meta-analysis. Ann Intern Med. 2013;159(11):758–69. https://doi.org/10.7326/0003-4819-159-11-201312030-00008.
9. Banack HR, Stokes A. The 'obesity paradox' may not be a paradox at all. Int J Obes (Lond). 2017;41(8):1162–3. https://doi.org/10.1038/ijo.2017.99.
10. Ortega FB, Lavie CJ, Blair SN. Obesity and Cardiovascular Disease. Circ Res. 2016;118(11):1752–70. https://doi.org/10.1161/CIRCRESAHA.115.306883.
11. Kernan WN, Inzucchi SE, Sawan C, Macko RF, Furie KL. Obesity: a stubbornly obvious target for stroke prevention. Stroke. 2013;44(1):278–86. https://doi.org/10.1161/STROKEAHA.111.639922.
12. Després JP. Body fat distribution and risk of cardiovascular disease: an update. Circulation. 2012;126(10):1301–13. https://doi.org/10.1161/CIRCULATIONAHA.111.067264.
13. Iacobellis G. Local and systemic effects of the multifaceted epicardial adipose tissue depot. Nat Rev Endocrinol. 2015;11(6):363–71. https://doi.org/10.1038/nrendo.2015.58.

14. Sebastian JC. Respiratory physiology and pulmonary complications in obesity. Best Pract Res Clin Endocrinol Metab. 2013;27(2):157–61. https://doi.org/10.1016/j.beem.2013.04.014.
15. Murugan AT, Sharma G. Obesity and respiratory diseases. Chron Respir Dis. 2008;5(4):233–42. https://doi.org/10.1177/1479972308096978.
16. Dietz W, Santos-Burgoa C. Obesity and its Implications for COVID-19 Mortality. Obesity (Silver Spring). 2020;28(6):1005. https://doi.org/10.1002/oby.22818.
17. Tan M, He FJ, MacGregor GA. Obesity and covid-19: the role of the food industry. BMJ. 2020;369:m2237. Published 2020 Jun 10. doi:https://doi.org/10.1136/bmj.m2237
18. Lauby-Secretan B, Scoccianti C, Loomis D, et al. Body fatness and cancer--viewpoint of the IARC Working Group. N Engl J Med. 2016;375(8):794-798. https://doi.org/10.1056/NEJMsr1606602.
19. Fagan HB, Wender R, Myers RE, Petrelli N. Obesity and Cancer Screening according to Race and Gender. J Obes. 2011;2011:218250. https://doi.org/10.1155/2011/218250.
20. Adams TD, Hunt SC. Cancer and Obesity: Effect of Bariatric Surgery. World J Surg. 2009;33:2028–33. https://doi.org/10.1007/s00268-009-0169-1.
21. Camilleri M, Malhi H, Acosta A. Gastrointestinal Complications of Obesity. Gastroenterology. 2017;152(7):1656–70. https://doi.org/10.1053/j.gastro.2016.12.052.
22. Morandi A, Maffeis C. Urogenital complications of obesity. Best Pract Res Clin Endocrinol Metab. 2013;27(2):209–18. https://doi.org/10.1016/j.beem.2013.04.002.
23. O'Brien PD, Hinder LM, Callaghan BC, Feldman EL. Neurological consequences of obesity. Lancet Neurol. 2017;16(6):465–77. https://doi.org/10.1016/S1474-4422(17)30084-4.
24. Rajan TM, Menon V. Psychiatric disorders and obesity: A review of association studies. J Postgrad Med. 2017;63(3):182–90. https://doi.org/10.4103/jpgm.JPGM_712_16.
25. Tobin AM, Ahern T, Rogers S, Collins P, O'Shea D, Kirby B. The dermatological consequences of obesity. Int J Dermatol. 2013;52(8):927–32. https://doi.org/10.1111/j.1365-4632.2012.05624.x.
26. Nikiphorou E, Fragoulis GE. Inflammation, obesity and rheumatic disease: common mechanistic links. A narrative review. Ther Adv Musculoskelet Dis. 2018;10(8):157–167. Published 2018 Jun 27. doi:https://doi.org/10.1177/1759720X18783894
27. Wearing SC, Hennig EM, Byrne NM, Steele JR, Hills AP. Musculoskeletal disorders associated with obesity: a biomechanical perspective. Obes Rev. 2006;7(3):239–50. https://doi.org/10.1111/j.1467-789X.2006.00251.x.
28. Mahutte N, Kamga-Ngande C, Sharma A, Sylvestre C. Obesity and Reproduction. J Obstet Gynaecol Can. 2018;40(7):950–66. https://doi.org/10.1016/j.jogc.2018.04.030.
29. Kwan JM, Hajjiri Z, Metwally A, Finn PW, Perkins DL. Effect of the obesity epidemic on kidney transplantation: obesity is independent of diabetes as a risk factor for adverse renal transplant outcomes. PLoS One. 2016;11(11):e0165712. Published 2016 Nov 16. https://doi.org/10.1371/journal.pone.0165712.
30. Hasse J. Pretransplant obesity: a weighty issue affecting transplant candidacy and outcomes. Nutr Clin Pract. 2007;22(5):494–504. https://doi.org/10.1177/0115426507022005494.
31. Wever-Pinzon J, Drakos SG, Fang JC. Con: The obese heart failure patient as a candidate for mechanical circulatory support: it's rarely appropriate. Am Coll Cardiol. June 29, 2015. Retrieved from https://www.acc.org/latest-in-cardiology/articles/2015/06/29/08/49/con-the-obese-heart-failure-patient-as-candidate-for-mechanical-circulatory-support-its-rarely-appropriate.
32. Boyce L, Prasad A, Barrett M, et al. The outcomes of total knee arthroplasty in morbidly obese patients: a systematic review of the literature. Arch Orthop Trauma Surg. 2019;139(4):553–60. https://doi.org/10.1007/s00402-019-03127-5.
33. Neef M, Weise S, Adler M, et al. Health impact in children and adolescents. Best Pract Res Clin Endocrinol Metab. 2013;27(2):229–38. https://doi.org/10.1016/j.beem.2013.02.007.

Obesity and Body Mass Index

Eliana Al Haddad

1 Definition of Obesity

Obesity is a complex health issue that results from a combination of causes and contributing factors that include behavior (dietary patterns, inactivity, medication use), environment (food and physical activity environment, education and skills, food marketing and promotion) and genetics (family history, variants of genes responsible for hunger and satiety). The intricate intertwining of these factors plays a major role in the existence of obesity and health at the individual and community level.

According to the Centre of Disease Control, in the year 2015–2016, obesity affected 93.3 million adults in the USA, making up 39.8% of the total population. This number has been showing a steady significant increase in the past decade, tripling since 1975, and demonstrating no sign of slowing down. This trend has been seen all over the world, with the estimated percentage of individuals aged 18 and above with a body mass index (BMI) of 30 and above in each of the Gulf countries as of 2014 proving to be 42.3% in Qatar, 39.7% in Kuwait, 37.2% in United Arab Emirates (UAE), 35.1% in Bahrain, 34.7 in Saudi Arabia, and 30.9% in Oman. When looking at he western counterparts, the USA showed 33.7%, New Zealand 29.2%, Australia 28.6%, the UK 28.1%, Mexico 28.1% and Canada showing obesity rates of 28% Obesity was also shown to affect people in the middle-aged group (40–59 years old) more than those considered to be in the young adult group (20–39 years old) with 42.8% of the former population proving to be defined as obese, versus 35.7% in the latter [1]. Due to the multiple comorbidities that have

E. Al Haddad (✉)
Columbia University Medical Centre, New York, USA
e-mail: Eliana.h91@gmail.com

Amiri Hospital, Kuwait City, Kuwait

been shown to be associated with obesity, alongside the burden of the disease itself, the estimated annual medical cost in the USA was shown to be $147 billion in 2008 alone. This corresponded to a medical cost of $1,429 higher for people with obesity than those of normal weight [2]. Furthermore, it was shown that Hispanics (47%) and non-Hispanic blacks (46.8%) had the highest age-adjusted prevalence of obesity compared to other race populations (Figs. 1, 2, 3) [1]. So how do we define this debilitating condition that has affected such a large population of the world, and what can be done about it?

2 Obesity and BMI

Obesity/overweight is defined as a weight that is higher than what is considered a healthy weight for a given height, causing an abnormal or excess fat accumulation that may impair health [3]. Currently, the most widely used tool to assess the degree of obesity is the body mass index (BMI), which divides a person's body weight in kilograms (kg) by their height in meters squared (m²).

$$BMI = weight\ (kg)/Height\ (m) * Height\ (m) = kg/m^2$$

The results of this calculation places people in specific weight categories as follows:

- If the BMI is lower than 18.5, it falls in the underweight range.
- If the BMI is between 18.5 and < 25, it is considered to be in the normal range.
- If the BMI is between 25.0 and < 30, it is in the overweight range.
- If the BMI is 30.0 and higher, it falls within the obese range.

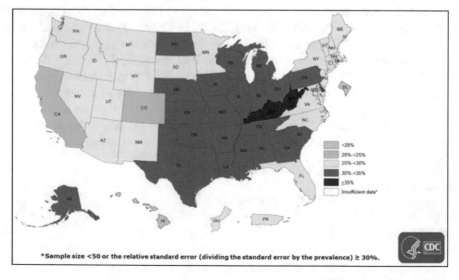

*Sample size <50 or the relative standard error (dividing the standard error by the prevalence) ≥ 30%.

Fig. 1 Prevalence of self-reported obesity among non-hispanic white adults, by State and Territory, BRFSS, 2016–2018

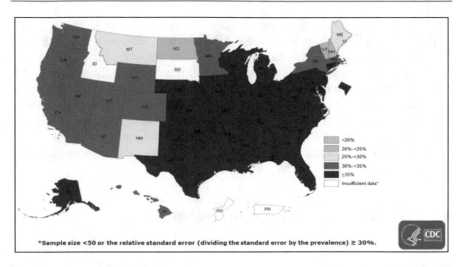

Fig. 2 Prevalence of self-reported obesity among non-hispanic black adults, by State and Territory, BRFSS, 2016–2018

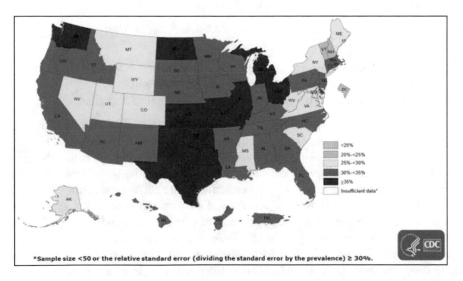

Fig. 3 Prevalence of self-reported obesity among hispanic adults, by State and Territory, BRFSS, 2016–2018

Obesity is also further subdivided into three class categories as follows:

- Class 1 obesity is defined as a BMI ranging between 30 to <35
- Class 2 obesity is defined as a BMI ranging between 35 to <40
- Class 3 obesity is defined as a BMI of 40 or higher, and is considered "severe" obesity.

BMI provides the most useful population-level measure of overweight and obesity as it is the same for both sexes and for all ages of adults. However, at an individual level, BMI is not diagnostic of body fatness or the health of the individual, but can be thought of as more of a useful screening tool. Research has shown that BMI is only moderately correlated with more direct measures of body fat obtained from skinfold thickness measurements, bioelectrical impedance, underwater weighing, dual energy x-ray absorptiometry (DXA) and other methods [4–6]. Furthermore, even though change in BMI can be used to assess weight loss and gain, other measures that employ the use of BMI have proven to provide more accurate depictions of weight change with time.

3   Percent Excess Weight Loss (%EWL)

Weight loss has been reported in many ways and by various methods according to the entity reporting it (for example dieticians vs bariatric surgeons); however, the best method should allow for the most accurate comparisons between the broadest ranges of patients' weight and population characteristics. One of the most widely used tools in the surgical community currently can be considered to be %EWL.

This is calculated using the following formula:

$$(\text{weight loss} / \text{baseline excess weight}) \times 100$$

where weight loss = preoperative weight−current weight;
baseline excess weight = preoperative weight − ideal weight,
and where ideal weight = weight corresponding to a BMI of 25 kg/m^2.

An advantage of %EWL is that it expresses weight loss that has been achieved relative to a defined goal. This goal is usually determined according to a BMI of 25 kg/m^2. However, a major concern when employing this method is that the definition of preoperative weight and ideal body weight can be ambiguous and vary between different studies and papers. Furthermore, the %EWL calculation can vary considerably if pre-operative weight is defined as the weight of the first visit, or the highest weight between first visit and the day of surgery. Ideal body weight (usually captured through the Metropolitan Life Tables) also varies depending upon which size body frame is used. As the Metropolitan Life Tables were originally created in the 1940s and have not been updated since 1983, many feel this method is outdated.

4   Percent Excess BMI loss (%EBMIL)

Due to the possible discrepancies previously discussed, experts from both the medical and surgical communities have proposed alternatives to %EWL. Percent excess BMI loss (%EBMIL) is one measure that is frequently used outside the United States and is favored by some experts.

This is calculated using the following formula:

$$\%EBMIL = [\Delta BMI/(Initial\ BMI - 25)]100$$

BMI is thought to be the easiest index of "fatness" when compared with hydro-densitometry studies [7, 8]. The accuracy of BMI continues to be challenged, however, particularly as it relates to individuals with normal weight obesity (defined as a combination of normal BMI and high body fat content) and muscular body types. Furthermore, when compared to dual-energy x-ray absorptiometry (DXA), a recent paper revealed that BMI misclassified 25% of men and 48% of women [9]. It is for this reason that many experts feel that the accuracy of BMI in diagnosing obesity is extremely limited.

5   Percent of Total Weight Loss (%TWL)

One of the key issues in this debate is determining what constitutes successful weight loss. Currently, the medical community prefers the calculation of percent total weight loss (%TWL).

The following formula can be used to calculate this:

$$\%TWL = [(Initial\ Weight) - (Postop\ Weight)]/[(Initial\ Weight)]100$$

Percent TWL is more accurate than kilograms of weight lost because it takes into account the fact that those with a high starting weight tend to lose more weight. Percent TWL can also be helpful to characterize reversal or prevention of obesity-related comorbidities. For example, in one diabetes prevention program, a seven-percent total weight loss prevented diabetes in 50% of the patients [10]. Also, a 10% total weight loss has been proven to produce improvements in a majority of metabolic and cardiac risk factors. One of the disadvantages of %TWL is that it does not take into account a therapeutic goal, nor does it express a patient's desire of how much weight he or she might wish to lose [11].

References

1. Hales CM, Carroll MD, Fryar CD, Ogden CL. Prevalence of Obesity Among Adults and Youth: United States, 2015–2016. NCHS Data Brief. 2017;288:1–8.
2. Finkelstein EA, Trogdon JG, Cohen JW, Dietz W. Annual medical spending attributable to obesity: payer-and service-specific estimates. Health Aff (Millwood). 2009;28(5):w822–31.
3. Organization WH. Obesity 2014 [Available from: https://www.who.int/topics/obesity/en/.
4. Freedman DS, Horlick M, Berenson GS. A comparison of the Slaughter skinfold-thickness equations and BMI in predicting body fatness and cardiovascular disease risk factor levels in children. Am J Clin Nutr. 2013;98(6):1417–24.
5. Garrow JS, Webster J. Quetelet's index (W/H2) as a measure of fatness. Int J Obes. 1985;9(2):147–53.
6. Wohlfahrt-Veje C, Tinggaard J, Winther K, Mouritsen A, Hagen CP, Mieritz MG, et al. Body fat throughout childhood in 2647 healthy Danish children: agreement of BMI, waist circumference, skinfolds with dual X-ray absorptiometry. Eur J Clin Nutr. 2014;68(6):664–70.

7. Deitel M. Comment on: reported excess weight loss after bariatric surgery could vary significantly depending on calculation method: a plea for standardization. Surg Obes Relat Dis. 2011;7(4):534–5.
8. Keys A, Fidanza F, Karvonen MJ, Kimura N, Taylor HL. Indices of relative weight and obesity. J Chronic Dis. 1972;25(6):329–43.
9. Shah NR, Braverman ER. Measuring adiposity in patients: the utility of body mass index (BMI), percent body fat, and leptin. PLoS ONE. 2012;7(4):e33308.
10. Knowler WC, Barrett-Connor E, Fowler SE, Hamman RF, Lachin JM, Walker EA, et al. Reduction in the incidence of type 2 diabetes with lifestyle intervention or metformin. N Engl J Med. 2002;346(6):393–403.
11. Bray GA, Bouchard C, Church TS, Cefalu WT, Greenway FL, Gupta AK, et al. Is it time to change the way we report and discuss weight loss? Obesity (Silver Spring). 2009;17(4):619–21.

Dealing with Obesity: Patient Perspective

Laura Divine

Stigma, bias, and condescension are something that people with obesity deal with on a daily basis and can cause an emotional and mental toll on those patients. They tend to feel like they stand out in any setting they are placed in, as well as struggle with physical movement, with finding clothing that fit, much less express their personal sense of style. Public transportation of any form pose a struggle - the seats are too small and they tend to feel self-conscience about taking space that belongs to someone else. From first hand experience, we know that we are constantly judged by others for the way we look and for the behaviors people assume we have. People generally assume that obese people have traits of laziness, gluttony, and unintelligence. As children we are bullied by other children and that unkindness from others often breaks into adulthood. Fat-shaming is commonplace globally and knows no age limit. It has been shown that obese people tend to be passed over for promotions at work, can find intimate relationships challenging, and often times find themselves trapped in a cycle of yo-yo dieting, weight loss, followed by weight gain repeated multiple times. Social situations can fill us with anxiety. Will I be the largest person in the room? Will I be stared at if I eat something? Is somebody going to make a comment about my weight? Some of us even struggle with body dysmorphia; as a person with obesity, at my heaviest, I failed to see how large I actually had gotten to, now at a much smaller size, I continue to struggle at times with photos, videos, and mirror images of myself, as I now see myself as much larger than I actually am. All of these experiences have a permanent negative effect our self-confidence and self-worth.

As a surgeon, you are frequently faced with patients presenting for the possibility of undergoing bariatric surgery. For most, the idea of bariatric surgery is

L. Divine (✉)
High School Principal, Al-Bayan Bilingual School, Hawalli, Kuwait
e-mail: laura.divine@bbs.edu.kw

S. Al-Sabah et al. (eds.), *Laparoscopic Sleeve Gastrectomy*,
https://doi.org/10.1007/978-3-030-57373-7_5

compelling due to its ease and simplicity as of recent years, and can be considered as an option at any point in their struggle to overcome obesity; maybe they've struggled with obesity but their visit to your office to inquire about bariatric surgery is the first time they have thought about dealing with it. Maybe they've tried multiple diet and exercise regimens, will drop weight only to gain it back and more as soon as they begin to experience some success. It could be possible that this isn't their first bariatric surgery and they are seeking a revision. Or they may even have been convinced or coerced to come to the consultation by a family member and are not ready to be there. But one thing remains certain. They are experiencing a range of emotions about this consultation: shame, vulnerability, hopefulness, hopelessness, and defensiveness being commonplace. This first consultation is critical to begin to foster the relationship between the doctor and the patient and to help establish the full extent of the education, preparation, and treatment the patient will need both pre- and post-operatively.

Patients with obesity have had a variety of interactions with doctors, many of them negative. Generally, the first thing they hear from any doctor is a statement about their weight and how it has affected their health negatively. Without going to a doctor who specializes in obesity treatment, patients will hear a variety of advice on how to lose weight, stemming from "eat less and exercise more" to recommendations for prescription drugs or surgical procedures; often these primary care physicians are not as well informed on the treatment of obesity and their advice has little follow-through attached to it.

The medical issue they are attempting to talk to the doctor about can be overshadowed by a focus on their weight. A patient relayed a story about a recent visit to an ob/gyn to discuss her issues with fibroid tumors. She had sought treatment for her fibroids before and was indicating that she had started to experience an ever-present feeling of fullness in her abdomen. The doctor, without further investigation, attributed the feeling she was describing as being related to her weight and his recommendation was for her to lose weight. Whether his assessment was or was not accurate, as the patient, she immediately felt dismissed, unheard, and uncared for. She ended up not following up with that doctor and has yet to get her fibroid tumor issues resolved.

It is essential that there is serious reflection and adjustment on how doctors' approach, talk to, relate to, and treat patients with obesity. The bias and stigma towards obesity and how the world and individuals treat those with obesity is a very real experience and it is a just as much a reality within the medical profession as anywhere else. If you ask most patients with obesity, there exists an obvious lack of empathy and understanding, and a condescension in how the medical community talks to and about them: a tendency to be talked AT and not TO, and an inconsistency of knowledge regarding the treatment of obesity within the medical community.

Medical professionals wield a powerful ability to influence, educate, and motivate their patients but implicit, intrinsic bias and stigmatization of obesity can have the opposite effect. There is often a lack of basic respect and humanity in the approach of doctors. There seems to be the opinion of "honesty" is best, a sense that people with obesity need to face reality, and if they simply controlled the amount and type of food they ate, and moved more, they would lose weight; the complexity of obesity is misunderstood and the blame for a person's obesity is placed solely on the behaviors of that person. The medical community has an obligation to openly discuss the bias and stigma that exists and collaborate on strategies and protocols that would embrace obesity as the chronic disease it is and work to make the treatment protocol for patients supportive, informative, and flexible.

1   Considering the Psychology of Obesity

I must make an absolute disclaimer. I am not a psychologist. I have no training in psychology and can only speak from my own experience. There is one thing that I know for sure—the psychology of obesity cannot be ignored. Though I may not be a psychologist, I am an educator. In my humble opinion, the key factor in creating a success story with weight loss, through bariatric surgery or not, is significant and consistent education. This cannot only be the education of the patient but also the education of the surgeon, any other advising healthcare professionals, and the public. If obesity is going to be classified as a chronic disease, then there has to be a more knowledgeable, overarching, and systematic approach to treatment. Bariatric surgery may give a physical advantage to prepare a person's body for weight loss, but the strength or weakness of a person's mental health is as much a part of that person's long-term success with their weight loss journey.

As a surgeon, how much time does your team spend assessing the mental and emotional state of your patients? How much time and consideration goes into your decision to operate on that patient? Are you only considering their physical readiness? How much time is spent considering if the patient sitting in front of you will be able to handle the psychological journey that is just as much a part of the weight loss journey as losing the weight itself? How do previous attempts with bariatric surgery help you gauge if a revision would be successful? Why did past attempts fail? Is there anything deeper than a pre-surgery psychological check? Was an initial pre-surgery psychological check even done?

If you are not considering if your patient will be able to handle the needed changes, both physical and psychological, are you ultimately failing your patients?

The less education, knowledge, preparedness, and self-awareness your patient has, the more likely their weight loss journey will not be successful.

I was not honest with my surgeon about the emotional triggers and adverse experiences that caused me to eat for comfort; in fact, I distinctly remember him asking if I was an emotional eater and I denied it. I'm sure he knew I was lying, but he showed no judgement. His gentle prodding into this area of my obesity may not have garnered the truth from me, but helped prompt the inner dialogue with myself about my eating habits and recognize them for what they were. I gradually was able to transform most of the habits I had and recognize them for what they were.

The more a patient is able to be honest with themselves and their doctors and feel secure enough to open up about their past experiences, their habits, their triggers, and are able to recognize and come to terms with some of their issues, the more successful their weight loss journey will be, especially post-operatively.

2   Education for Success

One of the most important aspects of preparing a patient to undergo bariatric surgery is to educate them as comprehensively as possible on the different types of procedures available. They need to be fully aware and informed of the decision they are about to make, as well as the advantages and disadvantages of each surgery, along with the pre-operative procedures and tests. They should have a full scope of understanding of the purpose of each test and what the results indicate. They should know what their post-operative physical condition will be and they should have planned how they will tackle each stage of the post-operative process, from how, what, and when to eat to how these changes in eating and habits will fit into their daily routine. The more information and support a patient has before, during, and after surgery, for this lifestyle change, the more likely they will begin to make the permanent changes they will need to make to be successful in the long-term.

How much guidance and instruction/support do they get from your office/clinic/hospital both pre- and post-operatively? Does the pre-operative care and post-operative care include psychological services and education on nutrition, meal planning, and tracking their progress? There should be an acknowledgment of the challenges of weight loss: the reality of dealing with stalls, nutritional deficiencies, relationship challenges, and psychological conditions such as body dysmorphia. Patients need to understand that much of their weight loss journey after surgery is going to be about finding out what works for them and how to make those adjustments in their habits permanent. They will need to accept that there will be a trial and error period in learning what they can and cannot eat, how frequently they need to eat, how to get the proper amount of water intake, and what exercise routines are going to work for them. Most of all, patients need to have an understanding of how their relationship with food and their emotions will impact their weight loss journey.

3   Understanding the Necessity of Mind Shift for Success

It was years later, after continuing to put on weight, that I considered having bariatric surgery again. After months of preparing myself for the removal of my lap band and learning about the VSG procedure, I ended up only having my lap band removed and no further surgery. When asked why I was ultimately successful in my weight loss, I could point to many factors: figuring out what diet restriction worked for me without making me feel deprived, tracking my food intake and watching my macros, regular use of a liraglutide, the incorporation of a regular exercise routine into my life and making sure that I made that exercise routine a priority over (almost) everything else, and for the first time working with doctors from whom I felt absolutely no judgement, only support.

I learned that it was vital to put myself first, that the world wouldn't fall apart if I wasn't available to everyone else all the time. I attempted to read everything I could about weight loss and bariatric surgery, joined online support groups, and educated myself as much as possible. I started to analyze how my relationship with food was tied to my emotions and life experiences.

But most significantly, what I could identify was that something in my mind completely shifted. I approached my weight loss on a day to day basis. Every day I made choices about what I ultimately wanted to achieve and made decisions that would bring me closer to that goal. I found balance in my lifestyle choices; I forgave myself when I didn't eat perfectly or missed a day of exercise, but made better choices the following days. I understood these were the choices I would be making for the rest of my life.

At a recent educational conference, we were tasked with connecting a group of hexagons in a way that would show how education could be individualized to ignite passion in learning. There was no correct arrangement. Working through the exercise, I couldn't help making connections between the hexagons and my own weight loss journey. Ideas such as personalizing the learning journey, learner agency & leadership, identity, culture, & values, and community wellness echoed my own beliefs that these are essential elements to create the paradigm shift necessary to alter the stigma and bias that currently exists in regards to obesity.

As a surgeon, I urge you to consider the full scope of a patient's obesity before operating on them. Start by assessing why a patient is choosing bariatric surgery, evaluating and supporting their psychological readiness, establish a system for making sure your patients receive the necessary education before the surgery: about the surgical procedure itself, the pre-op requirements, the nutritional information and support they will need to use post-operatively, and the support for the psychological issues they will need to continue to address and lifestyle changes they will need to continue to make. Above all, the incorporation of empathy, understanding, and education for everyone as The treatment of obesity continues to evolve.

The Future of Bariatric Surgery and Genetics

Ahmad Al-Serri

1   Heritability and Obesity

Both genetic and environmental factors contribute to the development of obesity. Heritability studies on twins and adoptees have estimated that about 40–70% of obesity is attributed to genetics [1–2]. Since the completion of the human genome project in 2003 hundreds of single nucleotide polymorphisms (SNPs) have been found to be associated with adiposity traits with pathway analysis showing these variants to play a role in the central nervous system involving lipid and energy metabolism, insulin secretion along with other pathways [3]. The most common SNP (rs9939609) associated with BMI to date is found in the *fat mass obesity* (*FTO*) gene [4]. Although the exact function of the *FTO* is unknow due to its ubiquitous expression however it is suggested to play a role in lipid metabolism and satiety, for a full review [5]. Moreover, monogenic mutations contribute to congenital obesity with the *MC4R* gene being the most commonly implicated monogenic form of obesity with a prevalence of 2–3% [6].

2   Weight Loss Interventions and Genetics

Differences in the amount of weight loss achieved between individuals from lifestyle interventions such as diet and physical activity can be attributed to the interactions between genetic variations and environmental factors [7]. Individuals on a high fat diet carrying the *FTO* risk allele were found to have higher BMI

A. Al-Serri (✉)
Unit of Human Genetics, Department of Pathology, Faculty of Medicine, Kuwait University, Jabriya, Kuwait
e-mail: ahmad.alserri@ku.edu.kw

© The Editor(s) (if applicable) and The Author(s), under exclusive license to Springer Nature Switzerland AG 2021
S. Al-Sabah et al. (eds.), *Laparoscopic Sleeve Gastrectomy*,
https://doi.org/10.1007/978-3-030-57373-7_6

and waist circumference (WC) compared to those carrying the protective allele, suggesting a gene-diet interaction [8]. Similarly, a study by Celis-Morales et al., showed an interaction between the *FTO* genotypes and physical activity levels [9]. The study found that individuals carrying the *FTO* risk allele had higher BMI and WC under low physical activity levels compared to those with the protective alleles, however, under high physical activity levels there were no differences in BMI and WC suggesting that the *FTO* is attenuated by physical activity [9].

3   Bariatric Surgery and Genetics

Individual differences between bariatric patients exists with about 20–30% appear to suffer from weight regain or insufficient weight loss [10]. In addition, differences in remission of comorbidities such as type 2 diabetes is also observed between patients [11].

A study by Rodrigues et al., on patients undergoing bariatric surgery (RYGB) showed that individuals carrying the *FTO* risk allele were more likely to have a lower %EWL and weight regain after 2-years of surgery compared to those with the protective allele [12]. Although differences were observed between the two *FTO* groups, however an EWL of above 50% was achieved independently of the existence of the risk allele indicating that the *FTO* alone has only a small effect on weight loss and regain [12]. In contrary, a study on 74 patients that have undergone SG showed no difference in %EWL between carriers of the *FTO* risk allele to those with the protective allele, however the study only evaluated the patients up to 6 months post-surgery [13]. Moreover, a recent study on a variant (rs1360780) in the *FK506 binding protein-5* (*FKBP5*) gene which is suggested to play a role in lipid accumulation has been found to be associated with weight loss after bariatric surgery [14]. The study which was conducted on both RYGB and SG patients found that carrying the risk allele was associated with higher BMI after 24 months in older males that have undergone SG [14]. In addition, a genome-wide association study (GWAS) found a variant (rs17702901) near the *solute carrier* (*SLC*) gene which plays a role in nutrient and metabolite transport to be associated with weight loss after 12 months post-surgery [15]. The study which was conducted on RYGB patients found that carriers of the risk allele only reached an average EWL of 33.5%, none of the patients carrying the risk allele exceeded an EWL of 50% after 12 months [15]. In addition, variants and mutations in the leptin-melanocortin pathway genes (*LEPR* and *MC4R*) have also been found to effect weight loss after bariatric surgery [16, 17]. A recent study by Cooiman et al., focused on monogenic mutations and investigated 52 obesity-associated genes in 1014 patients that have undergone bariatric surgery [17]. The study found that patients that have undergone SG with an *MC4R* mutation had a significant lower %TBWL compared to those without the mutation after 2-years of follow-up [17]. In contrast, patients that have undergone RYGB surgery with mutations in the *MC4R* showed no differences in %TBWL when compared to patients without a mutation. Such differences in findings may be attributed to the different physiological mechanisms between the two types of surgery and therefore may suggest that individuals with monogenic mutations in the *MC4R* gene are better off undergoing RYGB [18].

With the growing evidence of genetic variations impacting weight loss, this has facilitated the establishment of a Genetic Risk Score (GRS) to predict weight loss, regain, and remission of comorbidities such as type 2 diabetes prior to bariatric surgery [12, 19, 20]. Simply a GRS is the accumulation of genetic variations to estimate their cumulative effect on the phenotype being assessed. In 2014, Kakela et al., constructed a GRS from 33 SNPs associated with BMI and WHR [19]. Their findings on both SG and RYGB showed that the GRS did not predict %EWL or weight regain at 12 months nor did it predict it following that [19]. In contrast, a recent study by Katsareli et al., constructed a GRS from 108 SNPs also related to BMI and WHR [20]. Similarly, the study involved both SG and RYGB patients, however the GRS had a significant prediction on %EWL after 12 months and 24 months showing a positive correlation [20]. Such differences between the two studies may be attributed to the differences in SNP selection. Another recent study by Ciudin et al., found that a GRS of 57 SNPs was able to predict weight regain and diabetes remission after five years of follow-up [12].

In conclusion, it is clearly evident that genetic variations play a role in post-surgery outcomes and that the inconsistency observed between studies can be attributed to the differences in the study design of the current existing work. The type of surgery, the statistical methods to evaluate weight loss, the selection of genetic variations, sample size and longitudinal follow-ups of patients are critical factors that will need to be adjusted for. Once GRS are well established to predict the type of bariatric surgery along with predicting its success, we believe the term "surgenomics" will be used.

References

1. Stunkard AJ, Harris JR, Pedersen NL, McClearn GE. The body-mass index of twins who have been reared apart. N Engl J Med. 1990;322(21):1483–7.
2. Stunkard AJ, Sorensen TI, Hanis C, Teasdale TW, Chakraborty R, Schull WJ, et al. An adoption study of human obesity. N Engl J Med. 1986;314(4):193–8.
3. Locke AE, Kahali B, Berndt SI, Justice AE, Pers TH, Day FR, et al. Genetic studies of body mass index yield new insights for obesity biology. Nature. 2015;518(7538):197–206.
4. Frayling TM, Timpson NJ, Weedon MN, Zeggini E, Freathy RM, Lindgren CM, et al. A common variant in the FTO gene is associated with body mass index and predisposes to childhood and adult obesity. Science. 2007;316(5826):889–94.
5. Fawcett KA, Barroso I. The genetics of obesity: FTO leads the way. Trends Genet. 2010;26(6):266–274
6. Huvenne H, Dubern B, Clement K, Poitou C. Rare genetic forms of obesity: clinical approach and current treatments in 2016. Obes Facts. 2016;9(3):158–73.
7. Tan PY, Mitra SR, Amini F. Lifestyle interventions for weight control modified by genetic variation: a review of the evidence. Public Health Genomics. 2018;21(5–6):169–85.
8. Labayen I, Ruiz JR, Huybrechts I, Ortega FB, Arenaza L, Gonzalez-Gross M, et al. Dietary fat intake modifies the influence of the FTO rs9939609 polymorphism on adiposity in adolescents: the HELENA cross-sectional study. Nutr Metab Cardiovasc Dis. 2016;26(10):937–43.

9. Celis-Morales C, Marsaux CF, Livingstone KM, Navas-Carretero S, San-Cristobal R, O'Donovan CB, et al. Physical activity attenuates the effect of the FTO genotype on obesity traits in European adults: the Food4Me study. Obesity (Silver Spring). 2016;24(4):962–9.
10. Felsenreich DM, Langer FB, Kefurt R, Panhofer P, Schermann M, Beckerhinn P, et al. Weight loss, weight regain, and conversions to Roux-en-Y gastric bypass: 10-year results of laparoscopic sleeve gastrectomy. Surg Obes Relat Dis. 2016;12(9):1655–62.
11. Pucci A, Tymoszuk U, Cheung WH, Makaronidis JM, Scholes S, Tharakan G, et al. Type 2 diabetes remission 2 years post Roux-en-Y gastric bypass and sleeve gastrectomy: the role of the weight loss and comparison of DiaRem and DiaBetter scores. Diabet Med. 2018;35(3):360–7.
12. Ciudin A, Fidilio E, Ortiz A, Pich S, Salas E, Mesa J, et al. Genetic testing to predict weight loss and diabetes remission and long-term sustainability after bariatric surgery: a pilot study. J Clin Med. 2019;8(7).
13. Balasar O, Cakir T, Erkal O, Aslaner A, Cekic B, Uyar M, et al. The effect of rs9939609 FTO gene polymorphism on weight loss after laparoscopic sleeve gastrectomy. Surg Endosc. 2016;30(1):121–5.
14. Pena E, Caixas A, Arenas C, Rigla M, Crivilles S, Cardoner N, et al. Role of the FKBP5 polymorphism rs1360780, age, sex, and type of surgery in weight loss after bariatric surgery: a follow-up study. Surg Obes Relat Dis. 2020;16(4):581–9.
15. Hatoum IJ, Greenawalt DM, Cotsapas C, Daly MJ, Reitman ML, Kaplan LM. Weight loss after gastric bypass is associated with a variant at 15q26.1. Am J Hum Genet. 2013;92(5):827–34.
16. Kops NL, Vivan MA, Horvath JDC, de Castro MLD, Friedman R. FABP2, LEPR223, LEP656, and FTO polymorphisms: effect on weight loss 2 years after bariatric surgery. Obes Surg. 2018;28(9):2705–11.
17. Cooiman MI, Kleinendorst L, Aarts EO, Janssen IMC, van Amstel HKP, Blakemore AI, et al. Genetic obesity and bariatric surgery outcome in 1014 patients with morbid obesity. Obes Surg. 2020;30(2):470–7.
18. Pucci A, Batterham RL. Mechanisms underlying the weight loss effects of RYGB and SG: similar, yet different. J Endocrinol Invest. 2019;42(2):117–28.
19. Kakela P, Jaaskelainen T, Torpstrom J, Ilves I, Venesmaa S, Paakkonen M, et al. Genetic risk score does not predict the outcome of obesity surgery. Obes Surg. 2014;24(1):128–33.
20. Katsareli EA, Amerikanou C, Rouskas K, Dimopoulos A, Diamantis T, Alexandrou A, et al. A genetic risk score for the estimation of weight loss after bariatric surgery. Obes Surg. 2020;30(4):1482–90.
21. Stunkard AJ. Genetic contributions to human obesity. Res Publ Assoc Res Nerv Ment Dis. 1991;69:205–18.

Sleeve Gastrectomy Registries

Peter K. H. Walton

1 Introduction

The world is facing a frightening obesity epidemic and while randomized control trials (RCTs) and case series show very good evidence of improvement in diabetes control and reduction in obesity related diseases post-surgery, commissioners of care still need convincing that bariatric surgery should be funded on a much wider scale. Registries have the capability to provide this evidence on a global basis.

Tracking the results of sleeve gastrectomy surgery is part and parcel of capturing data on all patients undergoing bariatric and metabolic surgery. Indeed, there are distinct benefits in setting up registries that cover all procedures as they can provide comparative data on patient characteristics undergoing the different types of bariatric surgical approaches that are available. Even in those countries where sleeve gastrectomy operations represent some 80% of all procedures performed, as in Kuwait [1] the data are collected en masse via their national registry, rather than just for one operation type.

This chapter is therefore not designed to be a scientific review of sleeve gastrectomy surgery registries around the world, rather it is aimed at looking at the value of national bariatric surgery registries and to providing some practical perspectives on best practice when setting out to start a national registry and how to keep a good registry going.

P. K. H. Walton (✉)
Dendrite Clinical Systems Ltd, Reading Bridge House, George Street, Reading, Berkshire RG1 8LS, UK
e-mail: Peter.Walton@e-dendrite.com

S. Al-Sabah et al. (eds.), *Laparoscopic Sleeve Gastrectomy*,
https://doi.org/10.1007/978-3-030-57373-7_7

2   Definition of a Registry

"A Surgical Registry is a collection of observational data on consecutive patients undergoing a particular surgical procedure (or procedures) or for a given condition to enable systematic audit".

3   The Value of Registries

When looking at classical hierarchies in scientific evidence (Fig. 1) as first described by the Canadian Task Force on the Periodic Health Examination [2], typically registries would appear as a "cohort study" in terms of the value of evidence that they provide—hence with more observer bias than randomised control trials (RCTs).

Registries are very distinct from clinical trials which are designed to test hypotheses and require power calculations to determine the appropriate number of cases that need to be recruited in order to show statistical differences. Registries are not bound by power calculations and in the ideal world are never ending particularly because they can provide very useful trend data on patient demographics, surgical practice and outcomes which can change quite dramatically even over relatively short periods of time. This is well illustrated in the series of IFSO Global Registry Reports, the last of which—the Fifth Report [3] which shows a rapid uptake in sleeve gastrectomy worldwide in over just a few years, with a dip in the number of Roux-en-Y cases, and a new upsurge in One Anastomosis Gastric Bypass procedures especially in certain countries.

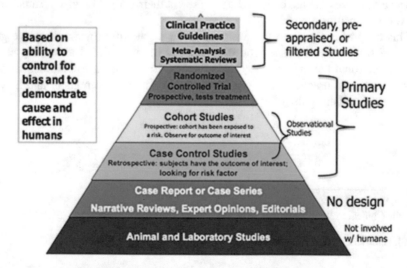

Fig. 1 Hierarchy of Research Designs and Levels of Scientific Evidence

It is probably a common mistake to simply think of clinical trials being more valuable or better than registries as trials and registries are really complementary and are not trying to compete with each other. It is better to think of registries being "Hypothesis Generators" and clinical trials as "Hypothesis Confirmers". This hypothesis generation component is very important and is well illustrated by the Swedish Obesity Surgery Registry [4], which has spawned an ever increasing number of scientific clinical papers over time, none of which could have been imagined at the starting point of the registry in the very first place.

Instead think of registries as helping to reset understanding about outcomes. They can report on real world practice instead of the best outcomes reported in the medical literature and can give surgeons confidence that they can compare their practice with others and share this information with patients.

Clinical Trials come to a natural end when the recruitment of patients and the collection of initial and follow up data has been completed and the data have been analysed, whereas registries can go on and probably should go on forever. Indeed, typically the functionality of high quality registries is that the inbuilt analysis capability can be extended and expanded over time. This is helped by the ever increasing speed of registry software development and innovation which leads to faster and more extensive reporting and analytic capability. The British National Bariatric and Metabolic Surgery Registry (NBSR) now offers instant dashboards and extensive one-button-push composite reports, neither of which could have been conceived of when the registry was first constructed. These reports have enhanced the functionality of the registry to provide surgeons with reports that can go straight into Appraisal files and can be created in seconds, whereas manually assembling the equivalent information even a year ago might have taken many days of effort for an individual surgeon to gather all the necessary data together. The real beauty is that registries can provide operational functionality that goes way beyond just addressing particular scientific questions, the real strength of registries is the capacity to provide a comprehensive suite of outputs:

- Ad hoc or automated analysis of:

  - Patient population demographics
  - BMI distributions and trends (by gender) prior to surgery
  - Levels of access-to-care on a geographical basis
  - Trends in comorbidities/obesity related diseases
  - Details of operative techniques
  - Interoperative complications
  - Post-operative and long-term complications
  - Volume/Outcome relationships
  - Long term outcomes by procedure type—weight loss, changes in the rates of obesity related diseases over time
  - Revision surgery outcomes

- Dashboard analyses

- Composite Reports
- Automated Patient Reports and automated generation of follow-up letters
- National and international benchmarking
- Links to Global Registries
- Outputs to public portals e.g. (https://nbsr.e-dendrite.com)

Therefore, working on the basis that registries are a good thing, how do you get one started and what are the secrets that makes a National Registry a success? There are ten key steps to building a successful registry, miss one or two out and a registry is at risk, miss three or more out and a registry will more than likely fail.

4 Key Step 1—Identify the Most Suitable Data Controller

Starting a National Registry is usually driven by either Specialist Societies wishing to provide a service to their surgical and patient community or by Ministries of Health and Governments wishing to monitor the performance of the bariatric service provision within a country.

The most successful registries are most often formed by specialist Surgical Societies. Why is this the case?

✓ Societies tend to have a long-lasting & uniform mission & "direction of travel", which can be independent of government policy which can change with each new administration
✓ Societies provide the safest legal haven for outcome data and offer exemption from Freedom of Information enquiries—again surgeons will often feel safer with a Society rather than an external body having ownership and oversight of their data
✓ Societies set standards of care and treatment protocols which are respected by their members
✓ Society Registry benchmarks can offer direct links with revalidation & re-accreditation processes
✓ Societies offer the strongest incentives for data submission (e.g. society membership requirements)
✓ Societies are the most "credible" location for registries
✓ and this concept *really* works and is very "*replicable*" and has been well tested over time

5 Key Step 2—Recruit a Respected Database Chairman with Long Tenure

Working on the basis that a Society is the most common Data Controller; the next challenge is to identify the best person to lead the development and implementation of a National Registry. Do not be tempted to appoint a surgeon for just a year or even two years for such a post. The development of a registry is a long process and it is vital that there is careful stewardship of the process over an extended period of time. Some would recommend a tenure for a Database Chairman of a minimum of 5 years with the option to extend between a further 3 and 5 years. The danger of rolling the position every one or two years is that by the time the individual has worked out how to do the job, it is being handed straight over to the next person who has to go through the same learning curve to get up to speed to manage the project—this roll-over process leads to too many "stops & starts" and can put a long term registry project at huge risk of failure.

When seeking to identify and recruit an individual to take on the role of Database Chairman there are a number of key attributes that are highly desirable. Namely the person should:

Be statesmanlike and a diplomat by nature
Be well respected and impartial
Be regarded as a "safe pair of hands"
Have a long term vision
Be a proven "deliverer"
Be able to demonstrate careful stewardship
Be an excellent communicator

6   Key Step 3—Define Clear Objectives for a Registry

Just in the same way that writing the objectives or mission statement for a surgical society or association is a necessary challenge, doing the same for a surgical registry is also an essential but not easy task. Indeed the two are often interlinked. Setting up a Surgical Society involves creating a constitution and key roles and responsibilities for both Executive Council members and for members of the Society. Setting up a registry also requires constitutional considerations, deciding who can sit on the Database Committee, how long the tenure should be, what determines quorate decisions and so on.

Writing down the objectives is so critically important as these then drive the dataset design and reporting requirements along with steering the required activities of the Committee and its chosen data management partner. The objectives may start off very simply indeed and may centre around feasibility of enrolling all centres within a country and demonstrating that basic data can be merged, analysed and reported. Down-the-road, second tier objectives are likely to be included, such as providing benchmarks of activity and performance. The objectives of a Registry should ideally be reviewed on an annual basis and should include sign-off from a Society Executive Board.

If the desire for a Society is to develop a Quality Improvement Programme, set up a mechanism to gain public trust, develop an education and training programme and provide a suitable regulatory background and public release of data.....it all starts with collecting and analysing data as seen in Fig. 2.

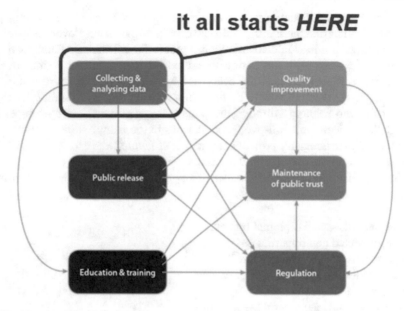

Fig. 2 Algorithm for the Development of a Quality Improvement Program

Along with defining objectives, the Database Committee should define roles and responsibilities for the major players in the Registry—for the Data Controller, the Data Processor & the Data Contributors.

7   Key Step 4—Contract with the Right Software Partner for You

The simple recommendation here is to choose an innovative and professional Data Management Company with long established experience in helping to set up and run national and international registries. Naturally they must have suitable security and information governance certification. In addition, ensure you choose a software company that has an established reputation for providing prompt support and fast turnaround telephone help whenever it is required.

There are three basic data flow "Models".

7.1   Direct-Data Entry Only

If the intention is to create a new registry with just Direct-Data-Entry then the web-database should be designed so that it is as easy to enter an operation record into a bariatric surgery registry as it is to book an airline ticket on-line—the software should be intuitive, navigation controls should simple and the process of data entry should be logical and easy with suitable onscreen prompts and/or hover tip messages available where additional user guidance is required. The SOReg Swedish National Bariatric Surgery Registry works on this model.

The simple rule of thumb is to ensure that it should take no more than 5 min per case to complete data entry into a national registry. Good database software design will ensure that there is on-line data validation to prevent inappropriate data entry e.g. to ensure there are date controls to prevent negative lengths of stay or to ensure that a balloon entry date cannot be subsequent to a definitive bariatric surgery procedure or to stop any dated data entry that is subsequent to the date of a patient's demise. Ideally a system will allow for detailed entry for complex cases but provide a very quick run through for simple cases. Limits should be set on integer or decimal answers to alert for an entry being an abnormal result and to stop the entry of answers that are physiologically impossible (i.e. normal ranges and absolute ranges). Good registry software will include rare event triggers to ensure that entry of such events (e.g. death) is not accidental and must be confirmed several times. A further step is to trigger an e-mail alert to a central administrator whenever such rare events are logged so that they can be checked and confirmed.

Inbuilt security measures must ensure that a given contributor can never see or access data that belongs to another surgeon or centre unless specific permissions have been granted.

7.2   Electronic Upload Only

It may be that when setting up a national registry, all the contributor hospitals already have local database systems in place, in which case a central database must have the capability of uploading data files, processing them to ensure they meet a defined upload specification and reporting back to contributors if there are any deficiencies in the upload files (e.g. fields that are out of range, incompatible data formats, missing desirable or mandatory fields) so that the uploader can constantly refine the source data file for re-upload of high quality data. The central registry must then have the capacity to merge all uploaded data so that is then available for data analysis and reporting. The Kuwait National Bariatric Surgery Registry works on this model.

7.3   Hybrid Model—Combined Direct-Data-Entry and Electronic Upload

The most common environment that is encountered when wishing to set up a new national registry is that are a mix of centres where the more established centres will already have a home grown or proprietary database system in place, whereas newer smaller centres may have not yet set up registry systems within their clinics/hospitals. In this scenario it is necessary to offer a hybrid system where data submissions can be en-bloc via electronic upload or by entering records on-line patient-by-patient. The UK National and IFSO Global Registries work in this fashion.

8 Key Step 5—Create a Suitable Minimum Dataset

With so many national bariatric and metabolic surgery registries already up and running around the world (there are examples from Australia/New Zealand to Austria, from Sweden to South Korea and from the USA to UK) it is now relatively easy to review minimum dataset that have been successfully used around the globe. Generally, these datasets are available in the public domain—as in the 2nd UK National Bariatric Surgery Registry Report [5], and these existing designs make a good starting point before adding in additional fields to suit local patient demographics, practice and both research and management or sponsor needs. The key is to make the dataset comprehensive enough to permit suitable analysis and reports but to avoid making the registry design too long and onerous for contributors to complete. As a rule, it is better to have a smaller but more complete registry than an extensively detailed dataset that nobody can ever complete on a consistent basis.

Datasets should include:

Demographics and medical/surgical history
Information on obesity related diseases (formerly described as comorbidities)
(Possibly laboratory tests e.g. HbA1C level)
Use of medical treatment or Balloons pre-operatively
Height and Weight on entry to the weight loss programme and weight at the time
    closest to the date of operation
Operative details
Peri/Post operative complications (if any)
Long term outcomes & details of any revision surgery
PROMS data

The International Federation for the Surgery of Obesity and Metabolic Disorders is proposing a full Delphi study to review existing datasets and to ensure that data collection is designed not just to track surgical outcomes, but also to consider patient perspectives and input from all stakeholders involved in bariatric and metabolic medicine and surgery. Likewise, there are attempts underway to develop a Patient Recorded Outcome Measure (PROM) that is very specific and tailored to obesity management.

9 Key Step 6—Layer in GDPR Compliance

In very recent years, Data Protection has become an important buzzword which has resulted in registries being required to comply with new legal standards, in particular the General Data Protection Regulation (GDPR) 2016/679 European

Union laws [6] on data protection and privacy. Every registry must now have in place not just a designated data controller but also the right documentation and processes around data management and patient confidentiality. For properly anonymised registries that are better described as "audit", consent is not a requirement, but it is nevertheless generally "advised" and indeed is mandatory if a national registry is collecting identifiable personal data.

Key documentation that needs to be in place for all registries:

1. **Data Processing Agreement (DPA)**—All "Data Controllers" are required to have a DPA with any and each organisation who will be processing their data (The Data Processors).
2. **Privacy Notice/Fair Processing Statement**—This document basically explains to the general public why you're collecting the data, what data you're collecting, what you intend doing with it, who it will be shared with etc. and also includes processes how to request what data the registry is holding and how patients can opt-out if they wish to remove their consent.
3. **Subject Access Request Page**—If a database is holding identifiable patient data of any kind, it is necessary to provide a means for the public to request what data may be held about them.... and also provide them with an opt-out mechanism. This should also be noted in the Privacy Notice/Fair Processing Statement which should describe the process that is followed/detailed in the Data Processing Agreement. Some databases also collect patient email addresses for PROMs—in this instance there needs to be TWO consent questions with an opt-out for both. The first for holding personal data on the registry, and another for holding their email address for PROMs.
4. **Data/Information Sharing Agreement**—Some Data Controllers implement Information/Data Sharing Agreements with the end-user data contributors so that they are aware of their own data collection responsibilities. This is not a mandatory requirement but it is best practice.

It is essential that any partnering data management company that is acting as the Registry "Data Processor" can demonstrate compliance with the highest levels of data security.

10   Key Step 7—Recognise that There are Multiple Stakeholders with an Interest in National Registries

It might be tempting to think that bariatric surgery registries are primarily for surgeons. In reality there are multiple other stakeholders who take a deep interest in the analyses and the reported outcomes coming from a registry including:

- Patients and Patient Advocacy Groups
- Governments because of focus on Cost & Quality and Healthcare Rationing
- Colleges of Surgeons

- Other National Specialist Medical & Surgical Societies
- Specialist Commissioners of Care
- Epidemiologists & Public Health
- Institutions/Hospitals (CEOs)
- Medical and Quality Assurance Directors
- Referring doctors—General Practitioners and other physicians
- Medical Device Companies
- Pharmaceutical Companies
- Health Observatories
- The Press
- International Audiences

With this long list in mind, it is wise to review datasets to ensure that all legitimate stakeholder interests are accounted for. Likewise when producing any reports the content, analyses and accompanying commentary should be carefully tailored to accommodate all pertinent audiences.

11   Key Step 8—Create a Suitable "Carrot and Stick" Environment to Recruit Contributors

As with the adoption of any new technology, registries are subject to the laws of Diffusion of Innovation (Fig. 3) as described by Everett Rogers, a Professor of Communication Studies which was first published in 1962, and is now in its fifth edition [7], which describes at what rate new ideas progress The important aspect to the observation is that the speed of take up of innovation determines the point of critical mass and/or success of a registry project.

There will always be a group of surgeons who are the innovators followed closely by early adopters. Fairly rapidly there will be an adoption swell of early majority and late majority users followed finally by the laggards who are reticent to adopt new technology unless they are forced to join, become too embarrassed by not taking part or just simply wait until they can see everybody else regards the project as a real success and being involved can no longer be avoided.

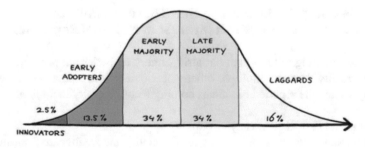

Fig. 3 An Illustration of the Laws of Diffusion and Innovation

There is constant discussion at surgical Scientific Congresses about who should shoulder the responsibility of Data Collection. Some will say that the data collector should be completely independent of the clinical team (in order to eliminate bias), often a North American viewpoint, whereas in other cultures e.g. the British environment there is a different mantra, namely: "The operation is not finished when you, or your assistant, puts the last stitch into the patient, the operation is finished when the data has been entered into a database". Professor Sir Bruce Keogh (former Medical Director of NHS England) in his introduction to the 1st UK National Bariatric Surgery Report [8] stated: "After all, in my view, if you can't describe what you're doing and define how well you're doing it, you have no right to be doing it at all".

12   Key Step 9. - Produce Regular Reports and Analytics and Other Outputs

It is an absolute imperative to ensure that registries do not become data cemeteries where data are never seen again. In order to encourage continued data collection and the success of any registry, regular outputs must be generated. These should span:

Individual patient reports—automated operation notes and discharge summaries
Individual surgeon/hospital dashboards
Ad hoc queries
Data output for research studies
National Reports [1, 3–5, 8]
On-line patient portals such as the UK Surgeon Specific Outcome Reports for NHS Bariatric Surgery [9]

Only by producing outputs to the benefit of surgeons can administrators of registries expect continued commitment to data entry.

13   Key Step 10—Recognise that Each Registry Has Its Own "Journey"

Developing a Registry is never a "single point action", it is never finished and will always be moving. The key is to remember that a registry is always "work in progress" and will evolve and mature over time. The great beauty of all registries is that as time passes, the historical data that has been entered increases in value, because, (a) trends appear and (b) long term follow up data evolves.

The very good news is that with any registry there is a possibility of a Hawthorne Effect [10], whereby the process of auditing itself helps drive improvements in the quality of care and brings reductions in all kinds of adverse outcomes: post-operative complication rates, long and short-term morbidity and mortality.

14　　Conclusion

Registries have the capacity to describe real-world data about patient populations, their characteristics along with patterns of practice and outcomes. These data help to inform a wide group of stakeholders as to the value of bariatric and metabolic surgery and enable surgeons to benchmark their performance against national and international standards. Starting a registry is not a trivial exercise as it is not only logistically complex but prone to failure unless all the necessary building blocks are in place. It is hoped that this chapter will encourage and guide both those that are about to embark on starting their own national registry or those who are determined to see an existing registry flourish.

The process of turning data into information to improve outcomes is ultimately to the benefit of patients who can be better informed about the risks and benefits of different procedures.

References

1. Al Sabah S, Walton P, Kinsman R. First Kuwait National Bariatric Surgery Database Report: April 2019. ISBN 978–0–9929942–9–7
2. Canadian Task Force on the Periodic Health Examination (3 November 1979). "Task Force Report: The periodic health examination". Can Med Assoc J. **121** (9): 1193–1254. PMC 1704686. PMID 115569.
3. Ramos A, Kow L, Brown W, Welbourn R, Kinsman R, Walton P. The 5th IFSO Global Registry Report September 2019. ISBN 978-1-9160207-3-3
4. Hedenbro JL, Naslund E, Boman L, et al. Formation of the Scandinavian obesity surgery registry SOReg. Obesity Surgery. 2015;25(10):1893–900.
5. Welbourn R, Small P, Finlay I, Walton P, Sareela A, Somers S, Mahawar K, Kinsman R. The United Kingdom National Bariatric Surgery Registry Second Registry Report: November 2014. ISBN 978-0-9568154-8-4
6. Regulation (EU) 2016/679 of the European Parliament and of the Council of 27 April 2016 on the protection of natural persons with regard to the processing of personal data and on the free movement of such data, and repealing Directive 95/46/EC (General Data Protection Regulation) (Text with EEA relevance) OJ L 119, 4.5.2016, p. 1–88 (BG, ES, CS, DA, DE, ET, EL, EN, FR, GA, HR, IT, LV, LT, HU, MT, NL, PL, PT, RO, SK, SL, FI, SV) ELI: https://data.europa. eu/eli/reg/2016/679/oj
7. Rogers, Everett (16 August 2003). Diffusion of Innovations, 5th Edition. Simon and Schuster. ISBN 978-0-7432-5823-4
8. Welbourn R, Fiennes A, Kinsman R, Walton P. The United Kingdom National Bariatric Surgery Registry First Registry Report: February 2011. ISBN 1-903968-27-5
9. Surgeon Specific Outcome Reports for NHS Bariatric Surgery updated April 2019. https://nbsr.e-dendrite.com
10. Landsberger HA. Hawthorne Revisited: management and the worker, its critics, and developments in human relations in industry. Ithaca: Cornell University; 1958.
11. Regulation (EU) 2016/679 of the European Parliament and of the Council of 27 April 2016 on the protection of natural persons with regard to the processing of personal data and on the free movement of such data, and repealing Directive 95/46/EC (General Data Protection Regulation) (Text with EEA relevance)

12. Regulation (EU) 2016/679 of the European Parliament and of the Council of 27 April 2016 on the protection of natural persons with regard to the processing of personal data and on the free movement of such data, and repealing Directive 95/46/EC (General Data Protection Regulation) (Text with EEA relevance)

Weight Loss: Diet Options

Khawla F. Ali

1   Introduction

The cornerstone therapy for obesity treatment is lifestyle modification. Adaption of a healthy lifestyle is founded by healthy dietary options, behavioral training and an increase in physical activity. In this chapter, we discuss the healthy dietary options available for weight loss, emphasizing on the behaviors that form the backbone of most dietary programs.

2   Principles in Dietary Therapies

Numerous dietary programs currently exist that are targeted to assist with the weight loss journey. A shared theme in most of these programs is the need for creating a caloric deficit that results in a negative energy balance [1]. A general approach to creating such a deficit is to reduce caloric intake by 500 kcal/day, or to restrict it by approximately 30% of total daily caloric need. The latter roughly translates to 1200–1500 kcal/day for women and 1500–1800 kcal/day for men [1].

The choice of a specific dietary program depends on several factors: degree of obesity, existence of comorbidities such as diabetes mellitus and patient preference. It is important to emphasize that no diet out there has been shown to consistently produce superior weight-loss results when compared to other diets. However, a strong predictive factor of success with any dietary program is patient adherence.

K. F. Ali (✉)
Department of Medicine, Royal College of Surgeons in Ireland-Medical University of Bahrain, Muharraq, Bahrain
e-mail: khawlafouad@hotmail.com

© The Editor(s) (if applicable) and The Author(s), under exclusive license to Springer Nature Switzerland AG 2021
S. Al-Sabah et al. (eds.), *Laparoscopic Sleeve Gastrectomy*,
https://doi.org/10.1007/978-3-030-57373-7_8

63

The programs that have shown to have the best weight-loss outcomes are those with the highest scores for patient adherence [2].

Most dietary programs produce mild-to-moderate weight loss of 5–15%. Additionally, most dietary interventions will reach their maximum efficacy 6-months post-initiation, with some patients re-gaining some or most of the weight in the months to follow. Therefore, it is essential for medical practitioners to discuss such figures with patients to ensure that their perceived weight goals and expectations align with the expected outcomes. It is also important to emphasize that weight loss and maintenance of as little as 5–7% still bears significant impact on health and wellbeing, and can lead to substantial improvements in medical comorbidities. The benefits of 5–7% weight loss were demonstrated in several landmark clinical trials. The Diabetes Prevention Program (DPP) is a good example. In the multicenter DPP trial, intensive lifestyle interventions aimed at weight loss of 7% showed significant reduction in the risk of progression from impaired glucose tolerance to diabetes by 58% [3]. Additionally, the landmark Look AHEAD study (Action for Health in Diabetes) for patients with type 2 diabetes mellitus and body mass index (BMI)>25 kg/m^2, showed that modest weight loss can lead to significant improvements in many comorbidities, such as, diabetes mellitus, sleep apnea, urinary incontinence, depression, physical function, mobility and overall quality of life [4, 5].

Several key principles should be emphasized in any dietary program. Increasing intake of fiber-rich foods such as fruits, vegetables, legumes and minimally processed whole grains is essential. Patients should also be advised to limit any processed or refined carbohydrates and meats, in addition to food items high in sodium and trans fats. The following are simple tips that can be provided to patients for improving their health and eating behaviors, regardless of whether a specific dietary program is being prescribed or not:

1. The plate method: patients should be encouraged to limit their plate size to a 9-inch plate. Half of the plate should contain non-starchy vegetables, such as lettuce, spinach, arugula, etc. A quarter of the plate should contain lean meats such as chicken, turkey or fish, and a quarter should contain whole grains such as brown rice, brown bread, etc.
2. Avoid sugar-sweetened beverages such as sodas, creamers, syrups and juices. Instead, patients should rely on water as a healthy liquid alternative.
3. Replace white carbohydrate options with whole grain ones. For instance, replace white bread with whole grain bread, replace white pasta with whole grain pasta, etc.
4. Avoid high-calorie, high-sugar snacks, such as cookies, chocolate and cakes. Instead, replace these with healthier snacks such as nuts, Greek yogurt and fruits.

Finally, dietary programs should always be combined with physical activity, particularly resistance anerobic training, for maximum preservations of muscle mass during the weight loss period.

3   Diet Options for Weight Loss

Several dietary interventions exist. Here, we outline a few of the most commonly prescribed diets in clinical practice.

- The Mediterranean Diet

The Mediterranean diet is typically rich in fruits, vegetables, nuts and whole grain sources of carbohydrate. The primary source of fat in this diet comes from the monounsaturated fatty acids of olive oil. Lean meat, such as chicken and fish are the primary sources of protein, with red meats being consumed as little as possible. Additionally, dairy sources should be low-fat or fat-free. The diet also allows low-to-moderate wine consumption.

The Mediterranean diet has been shown to have significant health benefits. In the large Primary Prevention of Cardiovascular Disease with a Mediterranean Diet Study (PREDIMED), the Mediterranean diet was associated with a 30% relative risk reduction in primary cardiovascular events, and a 40% relative risk reduction in the incidence of stroke [6]. Additionally, several observational studies have found a negative association between the Mediterranean diet and the incidence of cancers, such as colorectal, prostate and esophageal cancers [7].

The Mediterranean diet has also been shown to have significant impact on glycaemic measures in subjects with diabetes mellitus. In a recent meta-analysis examining its effects on type 2 diabetes patients, the Mediterranean diet resulted in significant reductions in haemoglobin A1c (HbA1c), fasting plasma glucose and fasting insulin levels compared to controls. Additionally, there were improvements in lipid profiles seen as reductions in total cholesterol and triglycerides, and increase in high-density lipoprotein (HDL) [8].

- Intermittent Fasting

Intermittent fasting refers to cyclic short periods of feeding followed by prolonged periods of fasting. An increased volume of literature supports the beneficial effects of intermittent fasting on disease modification and aging [9]. Additionally, recent studies have shown its beneficial effects on insulin resistance and glycemic control [10]. It has been theorized that the beneficial effects of intermittent fasting are not only due to its effects on weight reduction. Rather, it is thought to be due to adaptive cellular responses to fasting states. During prolonged periods of fasting, cells activate pathways that combat oxidative and metabolic stress, aiding in the process of cellular damage repair and reducing inflammation [9].

Several variations of intermittent fasting exist. Alternate-day fasting and daily time-restricted feeding are the most widely adapted variations. In the former, fasting is done on specific days of the week (one or more), when calories are reduced to less than 25% of the daily caloric requirements. The second form of intermittent fasting restricts caloric intake to certain hours of the day, typically ranging between 8 and 10 hours.

- Low-Carb and Very Low-Carb Diets

With the rise of diabetes mellitus prevalence worldwide, more specialists are advocating for low-carb and very-low carb diets as means of improving both glycemic measures and weight. Several short-term studies have demonstrated the efficacy of such diets on glycemic control, lipid profiles and weight in those with obesity and/or type 2 diabetes mellitus [11, 12].

Low-carbohydrate diets are usually composed of 60–130 g of carbohydrates per day. Very-low carbohydrate diets on the other hand, are usually composed of no more than 50 g of carbohydrates per day. The reduction in carbohydrate intake to less than 50 g per day typically depletes glycogen stores, and thus leads to the breakdown of fatty acids for the generation of ketone bodies and energy production. In both diets, the initial weight loss can be rapid, but is usually due to glycogen breakdown and water losses rather than true fat loss. The long-term superiority of low-carb and very-low carb diets versus other diets for weight loss has not been demonstrated [13]. Additionally, with lower carbohydrate intake, there is a higher likelihood for occurrence of adverse events, particularly with the very low-carb diets, such as constipation, headaches, generalized weakness and muscle cramps [14].

- Very-Low Calorie Diets

Very-low calorie diets (VLCD) refer to diets that provide less than 800 kcal per day. VLCD are effective at inducing rapid weight loss on the short-term. However, long-term outcomes of VLCD have not been demonstrated to be more superior compared to the more conventional diets. For instance, in a meta-analysis comparing the conventional low-calorie diets to VLCD, the short-term weight reduction was more pronounced in the VLCD (16% vs. 10% of initial body weight, for VLCD and conventional low-calorie diets, respectively). However, weight loss beyond one year did not differ (6.3% vs. 5%, for VLCD and conventional low-calorie diets, respectively) [15].

---

4   The Weight-Maintenance Diet

A major challenge post-weight loss via dietary methods is the maintenance of the weight loss achieved. The bodyweight is theorized to be set at a defined set point programmed at the level of the hypothalamus. Any attempt at lowering bodyweight via dieting and/or exercise would be met by internal resistance, in efforts to bring the body back to its original set point, no matter how pathological and disease-provoking this point may be. Resistance is typically seen in the form of increases in hunger signals such as ghrelin hormone, decreases in satiety signals such as glucagon-like peptide-1 and peptide YY, and decreases in basal metabolic rate [16].

Attempts at combatting weight regain have been investigated by several groups. Recent research has suggested a critical role of macronutrient composition on weight regain in the weight maintenance period. Diets composed of high-protein and low-glycemic index foods have been shown to be superior at maintaining weight loss, compared to low-protein and high-glycemic index diets [17].

5 Summary

Several dietary therapies exist. No single diet has been shown to be more superior or linked to more weight loss success. Rather, adherence is the key to weight loss success in any dietary program.

References

1. Garvey WT, Mechanick JI, Brett EM, et al. American association of clinical endocrinologists and american college of endocrinology comprehensive clinical practice guidelines for medical care of patients with obesity. Endocr Pract. 2016;22(Suppl 3):1.
2. Dansinger ML, Gleason JA, Griffith JL, et al. Comparison of the Atkins, Ornish, Weight Watchers, and Zone diets for weight loss and heart disease risk reduction: a randomized trial. JAMA. 2005;293:43.
3. Knowler WC, Barrett-Connor E, Fowler SE, et al. Reduction in the incidence of type 2 diabetes with lifestyle intervention or metformin. N Engl J Med. 2002;346:393.
4. Look AHEAD Research Group, Pi-Sunyer X, Blackburn G, et al. Reduction in weight and cardiovascular disease risk factors in individuals with type 2 diabetes: one-year results of the look AHEAD trial. Diabetes Care 2007; 30:1374.
5. Look AHEAD Research Group, Wing RR, Bolin P, et al. Cardiovascular effects of intensive lifestyle intervention in type 2 diabetes. N Engl J Med 2013; 369:145.
6. Estruch R, Ros E, Salas-Salvadó J, et al. Primary prevention of cardiovascular disease with a Mediterranean diet [retracted in: N Engl J Med. 2018 Jun 21;378(25):2441–2442]. N Engl J Med. 2013;368(14):1279–1290.
7. Schwingshackl L, Hoffmann G. Adherence to mediterranean diet and risk of cancer: a systematic review and meta-analysis of observational studies. Int J Cancer. 2014;135(8):1884–97.
8. Huo R, Du T, Xu Y, et al. Effects of Mediterranean-style diet on glycemic control, weight loss and cardiovascular risk factors among type 2 diabetes individuals: a meta-analysis. Eur J Clin Nutr. 2015;69(11):1200–8.
9. de Cabo R, Mattson MP. Effects of intermittent fasting on health, aging, and disease. N Engl J Med. 2019;381(26):2541–51.
10. Horne BD, Muhlestein JB, Anderson JL. Health effects of intermittent fasting: hormesis or harm? A systematic review. Am J Clin Nutr. 2015;102(2):464–70.
11. Boden G, Sargrad K, Homko C, et al. Effect of a low-carbohydrate diet on appetite, blood glucose levels, and insulin resistance in obese patients with type 2 diabetes. Ann Intern Med. 2005;142:403.
12. Gannon MC, Nuttall FQ. Effect of a high-protein, low-carbohydrate diet on blood glucose control in people with type 2 diabetes. Diabetes. 2004;53:2375.
13. Nordmann AJ, Nordmann A, Briel M, et al. Effects of low-carbohydrate vs. low-fat diets on weight loss and cardiovascular risk factors: a meta-analysis of randomized controlled trials. Arch Intern Med. 2006;166:285.

14. Yancy WS Jr, Olsen MK, Guyton JR, et al. A low-carbohydrate, ketogenic diet versus a low-fat diet to treat obesity and hyperlipidemia: a randomized, controlled trial. Ann Intern Med. 2004;140:769.
15. Tsai AG, Wadden TA. The evolution of very-low-calorie diets: an update and meta-analysis. Obesity (Silver Spring). 2006;14:1283.
16. Sumithran P, Prendergast LA, Delbridge E, et al. Long-term persistence of hormonal adaptations to weight loss. N Engl J Med. 2011;365:1597.
17. Larsen TM, Dalskov SM, van Baak M, et al. Diets with high or low protein content and glycemic index for weight-loss maintenance. N Engl J Med. 2010;363:2102.

Candidates for Sleeve Gastrectomy

Eligibility Criteria for Sleeve Gastrectomy

Faiz Shariff and Ali Aminian

1 Introduction

Global obesity is rising at an alarming rate, with estimates predicting that by 2030 nearly 1 in 2 adults will have obesity (BMI $\geq$ 30 kg/m^2), and 1 in 4 adults will have severe obesity (BMI $\geq$ 35 kg/m^2) [1]. It is well studied that obesity increases the risk of other chronic medical conditions, including type 2 diabetes mellitus, cardiovascular disease, cerebrovascular, chronic kidney disease, nonalcoholic fatty liver disease, metabolic syndrome, and many cancers. With an increasing number of patients with severe obesity and related comorbidities, there is an increasing role of bariatric surgery in managing these conditions, especially diabetes. Each year there is an increase in the number of bariatric procedures performed in the US as per the American Society for Metabolic and Bariatric Surgery (ASMBS) estimate of bariatric surgery numbers. The most significant upsurge seen in the number of sleeve gastrectomy (SG) performed rose from 17.8% of total procedures performed in 2011 to 61.4% of total procedures performed in 2018 [2, 3]. This increasing popularity of SG over the past decade has been due to its safety profile, technical ease, and excellent long-term efficacy. However, a blanket prescription of this procedure should be avoided, and an effort towards more personalized and evidence-based procedure selection should be adopted. In this chapter, we will first explore the current indications for metabolic and bariatric surgery, followed by a criterion that makes SG a better surgical option.

F. Shariff
Department of General Surgery, Wellspan Bariatric Surgery, Wellspan Hospital,
25 Monument Road, York, Pennsylvania, USA
e-mail: fshariff@wellspan.org

A. Aminian (✉)
Department of General Surgery, Bariatric and Metabolic Institute, Clevland Clinic,
Cleveland, Ohio, USA
e-mail: AMINIAA@ccf.org

S. Al-Sabah et al. (eds.), *Laparoscopic Sleeve Gastrectomy*,
https://doi.org/10.1007/978-3-030-57373-7_9

2   Current Eligibility Criteria for Bariatric Surgery

In 1991, National Institutes of Health (NIH) Consensus Development Panel first outlined the universally accepted guidelines for surgery for obesity and weight-related
disease [4]. Since then the guidelines have been repeatedly revised and expanded
over the years, most American and international societies have agreed on general
guidelines for the indication of bariatric and metabolic surgery as listed below.

- Adults with a BMI ≥ 40 kg/m² regardless of comorbid illness.
- Adults with a BMI 35.0–39.9 kg/m² with comorbidities, including:

  o   Type 2 diabetes (T2D)
  o   Hypertension
  o   Hyperlipidemia
  o   Obstructive sleep apnea (OSA)
  o   Nonalcoholic steatohepatitis (NASH)
  o   Pseudotumor cerebri
  o   Gastroesophageal reflux disease
  o   Asthma
  o   Venous stasis disease
  o   Severe urinary incontinence
  o   Debilitating arthritis
  o   Impaired quality of life

- Adults with a BMI 30.0–34.9 kg/m² with severe comorbidities listed above,
  especially T2D.
- Furthermore, potential surgical candidates must have the following conditions:
  - Inability to achieve a healthy weight loss for a while with prior weight loss
    efforts.
  - Absence of drug and alcohol problems
  - No uncontrolled psychological conditions
  - A capacity to understand the risks and commitment associated with the surgery.

3   Age

In their Consensus Statement of the NIH Consensus Development Conference
(1991) and the International Federation for the Surgery of Obesity and Metabolic
Disorders (IFSO) has age criterion—between the ages of 18 to 65 years [4, 5].
However, there is considerable flexibility in these recommendations [6]. In recent
years, there is a growing interest in the use of bariatric surgery at the extremes of
age. Bariatric surgery in the adolescent will be discussed in-depth in another section later in the chapter. Briefly, the ASMBS pediatric committee recommends an
adult BMI threshold selection criterion as it appears to be appropriate for adolescents, with some modification about associated comorbid disease thresholds [7]. A
significant concern when dealing with adolescents is their degree of maturity and

onset of puberty. These need to be taken into account when surgical treatment is recommended along with other psychological factors, metabolic issues, functional comorbidities, quality of life, and attention to long-term health risks in the absence of treatment in a patient who otherwise has a long life expectancy [6].

In the advanced age (>60 years), the higher perioperative risk due to anesthesia, complex medical comorbidities, and increased risk of mortality from complications have been cited as risk factors precluding bariatric surgery some series [8]. Besides, the elderly are less compliant with new dietary and lifestyle changes. However, more recent studies have shown not only low morbidity and mortality but a clinically significant weight loss and improvement in comorbidities in older patients [9–14]. In their comparison of patients >60 years who underwent bariatric surgery from 2009 to 2013, with those who underwent bariatric surgery from 1999 to 2005, Gebhart et al. found a significant decrease in mortality (0.3%) [15]. A systematic review by Giordano et al. of 26 articles with 8,149 patients showed a pooled mortality of 0.01%, and the overall complication rate was 15%. More recently, Nor Hanipah et al. suggested that bariatric surgery is safe and effective in patients aged ≥ 75 years older when carefully selected [14]. Similarly, Susmallian et al. analyzed the results of bariatric surgery in elderly patients (>65 years) for three years [12]. They noted a perioperative complication rate of 9%, with 1.3% needing re-operative intervention. These rates are slightly higher than those for the younger patient. However, most complications result from an increasing number of comorbidities seen in these patient populations. Often these complications do not need a major intervention. The authors believe that patients should not be denied bariatric surgery solely based on their age. It is vital to carefully counsel the elder patient about their slightly increased risks of morbidity and the possibility of less satisfactory outcomes.

4   BMI

From its inception, patient selection based on NIH Consensus statements for bariatric procedures has been based on BMI [4]. This selection criterion is inadequate as BMI is a poor indicator of adiposity, metabolic disease, and cardiovascular risk. It is a well known fact that a higher composition of visceral fat is associated with increased liver, muscle and pancreatic fat that results in a higher metabolic condition in individuals with same BMI [16–19]. BMI does not account for different body composition related to gender or age; that is, females and older patients have high body fat compared to males and younger patients, respectively. Also, there is an interracial difference in fat distribution; for example, an Asian has more body fat than a Caucasian with the same BMI [20]. The BMI criterion for bariatric procedures should be adjusted for ethnicity (e.g., 18.5–22.9 kg/m^2 is healthy range, 23–24.9 kg/m^2 overweight, and ≥25 kg/m^2 obesity for Asians). The recent ASMBS updated position statement on bariatric surgery in class I obesity recommends patients with a BMI of 30 to 35 kg/m^2 with obesity-related comorbidities be considered for surgical intervention after the failure of nonsurgical treatments [21]. This is particularly relevant for uncontrolled type 2 diabetes patients, as there are high-quality data that show significant benefit. Presently, patients in the 18 to 65 age group who have class I obesity along with severe comorbidities have the best evidence for bariatric and metabolic surgery.

5   Procedure Selection

A bariatric procedure should be selected based on individualized therapy goals, personalized risk stratification based on the patient's medical history, and available surgical expertise. Aminian et al. developed and validated an individualized metabolic surgery (IMS) score to aid the evidence-based procedure selection for T2D [22]. The IMS score uses four independent predictors of diabetes remission—preoperative duration of T2D, HbA1C level, number of diabetes medications, and insulin use before surgery. This was the largest reported cohort of patients with T2D (n = 900), which had a minimum 5-year glycemic data after RYGB and SG (median follow-up time of 7 years, range: 5–12 years). The IMS score categorizes T2D into three validated stages of severity to guide procedure selection—mild, moderate, and severe. In mild disease (IMS score 25 points or less), SG and RYGB are recommended as both are highly effective in the treatment of T2D. However, RYGB results in slightly higher long-term diabetes remission rates and a reduction in the number of diabetes medications. In severe T2D (IMS Score > 95) where there is a limited functional beta-cell reserve in the pancreas, both procedures have similarly low efficacy in achieving diabetes remission, reduction in HbA1C level, and use of diabetes medications. In the large intermediate disease group, RYGB is recommended over SG as it achieves better long-term diabetes remission, this is likely related to its more pronounced effect on the gut hormones and neuroendocrine milieu. In the original cohort with the intermediate diabetes severity, long term diabetes remission was observed in 60% of patients who underwent RYGB versus 25% of those who had SG. The IMS score calculator (smartphone application) computes a score when the patient's data are entered, and recommendation for an average surgical risk patient is provided. Given that the IMS cohort had patients with higher BMI and involved mostly patients from the US and Spain, it may not accurately apply to patients with class I obesity or Asian ethnicity. Another limitation of this model was that it did not include bariatric surgical procedures with more potent metabolic effects such as malabsorptive procedures (Duodenal Switch, SADI). Generally, RYGB and SG appear to be similarly effective in improving hypertension, dyslipidemia, and quality-of-life indices [23–26].

6   Other Considerations in Decision-Making

A procedure may be preferred over the other depending on the individual patient's condition [22, 25]. In patients with extremely high BMI and higher surgical risk, SG may be chosen because the limited working space makes a bypass procedure challenging and unsafe. After losing weight, these patients may be a candidate for diversionary procedures.

SG is favored in patients with multiple small bowel diseases like Crohn's disease [27], multiple small bowel resection, dense adhesions, large complex ventral hernias due to technical reasons [25].

Compared with GI bypass procedures, SG has minimal effect on the pharmacokinetics of medications as it does not alter gut absorption. This makes SG most suitable in patients with complex psychiatric and addiction history requiring psychotropic polypharmacy [22, 24, 28].

SG is a better choice for patients who smoke [29, 30] or are dependent on chronic nonsteroidal anti-inflammatory drugs as it circumvents the risk of marginal ulceration seen in RYGB patients [25].

Similarly, in patients with history of duodenal ulcer, increased risk of gastric cancer, or patient in whom access to distal stomach, duodenum, and biliary tree would be necessary in future, SG is a prudent choice, as RYGB precludes easy access to the remnant stomach and duodenum.

RYGB would be preferred over SG in patients with severe gastroesophageal reflux disorder (GERD) or Barrett's esophagus [28]. There are concerning reports of worsening or development of de novo GERD after SG, which may progress to Barrett's esophagus. Although its significance has yet to be determined, GERD after SG can be effectively treated with medical therapy in most cases. In 5% to 10% of patients with GERD after SG, medical management is ineffective controlling the symptoms. In these cases, a conversion to RYGB is warranted [25].

In patients with osteoporosis or decreased bone density, SG may be a better option compared with RYGB. Calcium and vitamin D deficiencies are commonly seen after bariatric surgery that is responsible for the accelerated bone loss. Multiple studies have shown more significant bone loss after RYGB than SG at the femoral neck [31, 32]. Comparative studies have noted a significantly increase in circulating bone turnover markers such as CTX, PINP, TRAcP5b in the RYGB compared with SG [33]. This could also be related to the different hormonal responses induced by these procedures [33–35].

A meta-analysis of 12 studies concluded that RYGB surgery is associated with a higher risk of renal stone and increased urine oxalate and calcium oxalate supersaturation [36]. In an another meta-analysis, SG was associated with reduced kidney stones formation (pooled risk ratio of 0.37, 95% CI 0.16–0.85) compared with RYGB that was associated with increased risk (pooled risk ratio of 1.73, 95% CI 1.30–2.30) [37]. The overall pooled risk ratio of kidney stones in patients undergoing bariatric surgery was 1.22 (95% CI 0.63–2.35). It has been postulated that the fat malabsorption induced enteric hyperoxaluria results in an increased risk of kidney stones in RYGB and other malabsorptive procedures.

Portomesenteric and splenic vein thrombosis (PMSVT) is a rare but potentially severe complication after bariatric surgery. A meta-analysis and systematic review of 41 studies reported that SG is associated with remarkably increased risk of PMSVT when compared with RYGB [38]. The estimated incidence was 0.4%, and 43% of patients had a history of the hypercoagulable disorder. Hence, in patients who have hypercoagulable disorders, an RYGB would be recommended.

Patients with increased risk of colon cancer need special consideration. In general, following bariatric surgery, the risk of hormone-related cancer like breast, endometrial, and prostate cancer reduces. However, an English study has shown that gastric bypass was also associated with a greater than two-fold increase risk of colorectal cancer (odd ratio 2·63, 95% CI 1·17 to 5·95) [39]. Similar results were seen in an earlier Swedish study [40] and a Nordic study, they also noted the increased risk is exaggerated with longer follow-ups [41]. There are some postulations to explain this anomaly to the protective effect of bariatric surgery on overall cancer incidence. The inflammatory environment stimulates hyperproliferation of the bowel mucosa after RYGB in a rat model [42]. Furthermore, similar results of increased proliferation of rectal mucosa along with elevated bio-marker levels were seen in patients who underwent RYGB [43]. The changes in the gut microbiome that partially mediates the metabolic changes could be responsible [44, 45]. In summary, the increased risk of colorectal cancer is that following RYGB, the local mucosal changes occur secondary to the malabsorptive effects and changes in the gut microbiome. The authors recommend that patients with an inherent increase risk of colorectal cancer undergo SG.

Management of blood sugar in some patients with type 1 diabetes after bariatric surgery can be extremely challenging. Particularly, some patients with type 1 diabetes may develop severe hypoglycemia after diversionary bariatric procedures. In patients with type 1 diabetes, SG, which is associated with more predictable absorption of carbohydrates and fat-soluble nutrients, would be a preferred procedure, unless there is a reason not to perform SG [46].

Outlined in Table 1 is the bariatric procedure selection (RYGB or SG) based on the patient's condition.

7 Summary

- In conclusion, for better outcomes, it is crucial to guide patients towards the most suitable bariatric procedure depending on their obesity-related comorbidities and overall medical conditions.
- BMI $\geq$ 40 kg/m^2 or BMI $\geq$ 35 kg/m^2 with obesity-related comorbidities are used as eligibility criteria for bariatric surgery selection. However, there are reliable data that support the positive impact of these operations in patients with lower BMI (30–35 kg/m^2) with uncontrolled metabolic conditions.
- The current review of the literature indicates that RYGB and SG have positive effects on improvement of T2D and that RYGB has a more substantial effect on remission. RYGB and SG appear to be similarly effective in improving hypertension, dyslipidemia, and quality-of-life indices.
- The IMS score is an evidence-based and validated prediction tool that can help in a personalized selection process of metabolic surgery in patients with T2D and obesity.
- The surgical risk, differential impact of each procedure on weight and other obesity-related diseases (e.g., GERD), presence of other medical and mental problems, patient's behavioral factors (e.g., postoperative compliance, active

Table 1 Bariatric procedure selection (RYGB or SG) based on patient's condition

Patient's condition	Suggested bariatric procedure
Average risk patient	RYGB or SG
High BMI	RYGB
Extremely high BMI (limiting working space)	SG
High-risk patient	SG
Complex large abdominal wall hernia	SG
Multiple small bowel resections	SG
Crohn's disease	SG
Transplant recipient/candidate	SG
Complex psychiatric history requiring polypharmacy	SG
Active smoker	SG
NSAID user	SG
Need for access to the duodenum and biliary tree	SG
Increased gastric cancer risk	SG
Increased colorectal cancer risk	SG
History of kidney stones	SG
Osteoporosis	SG
Severe GERD, Barrett's esophagus	RYGB
Hypercoagulable State	RYGB
Type 1 diabetes	SG
Type 2 Diabetes	
Mild (IMS score ≤ 25)	RYGB $\geq$ SG
Moderate ($25 <$ IMS score ≤ 95)	RYGB
Severe (IMS score > 95)	RYGB $=$ SG

BMI: body mass index; IMS score: individualized metabolic surgery score; GERD: gastroesophageal reflux disease; NSAID: nonsteroidal anti-inflammatory drug; RYGB: Roux-en-Y gastric bypass; SG: sleeve gastrectomy
Adapted and modified from Ref. [25]

smoking), medications (e.g., chronic nonsteroidal anti-inflammatory drugs, immunosuppressive medications, or psychotropic polypharmacy), and patient's values and goals should be considered when the patient and medical team make a shared decision about the most appropriate surgical procedure [25].

References

1. Ward ZJ, Bleich SN, Cradock AL, et al. Projected US state-level prevalence of adult obesity and severe obesity. N Engl J Med. 2019;381(25):2440–50. https://doi.org/10.1056/NEJMsa1909301.

2. Surgery AS for M and B. Estimate of Bariatric Surgery Numbers, 2011–2017. *WwwAsmbsOrg*. 2018.
3. English WJ, DeMaria EJ, Hutter MM, et al. American Society for Metabolic and Bariatric Surgery 2018 estimate of metabolic and bariatric procedures performed in the United States. Surg Obes Relat Dis. 2020;16(4):457–63. https://doi.org/10.1016/j.soard.2019.12.022.
4. Chair MG, Barondess JM, Bellegie NJ, et al. Gastrointestinal surgery for severe obesity: Consensus statement. Nutr Today. 1991;26(5):32–5. https://doi.org/10.1097/00017285-199109000-00007.
5. International Federation for the surgery of obesity. IFSO—Are you a candidate.
6. Luca M De, Angrisani L, Himpens J, et al. for the Surgery of Obesity and Metabolic Disorders (IFSO). 2018;26(8):1659–1696. doi:https://doi.org/10.1007/s11695-016-2271-4. Indications
7. Michalsky M, Reichard K, Inge T, Pratt J, Lenders C. ASMBS pediatric committee best practice guidelines. Surg Obes Relat Dis. 2012;8(1):1–7. https://doi.org/10.1016/j.soard.2011.09.009.
8. Livingston EH, Langert J. The impact of age and medicare status on bariatric surgical outcomes. Arch Surg. 2006;141(11):1115–20. https://doi.org/10.1001/archsurg.141.11.1115.
9. Aminian A, Brethauer SA, Sharafkhah M, Schauer PR. Development of a sleeve gastrectomy risk calculator. Surg Obes Relat Dis. 2015;11(4):758–64.
10. Sugerman HJ, DeMaria EJ, Kellum JM, Sugerman EL, Meador JG. Wolfe LG Effects of bariatric surgery in older patients. Ann Surg. 2004;240(2):243–7. https://doi.org/10.1097/01.sla.0000133361.68436.da.
11. Dunkle-Blatter SE, St. Jean MR, Whitehead C, et al. Outcomes among elderly bariatric patients at a high-volume center. *Surg Obes Relat Dis*. 2007;3(2):163–169. doi:https://doi.org/10.1016/j.soard.2006.12.004
12. Susmallian S, Raziel A, Barnea R, Paran H. Bariatric surgery in older adults. Medicine (Baltimore). 2019;98(3):e13824. https://doi.org/10.1097/md.0000000000013824.
13. Koh CY, Inaba CS, Sujatha-Bhaskar S, Nguyen NT. Outcomes of laparoscopic bariatric surgery in the elderly population. *Am Surg*. 2018.
14. Nor Hanipah Z, Punchai S, Karas LA, et al. The Outcome of Bariatric Surgery in Patients Aged 75 years and Older. Obes Surg. 2018. https://doi.org/10.1007/s11695-017-3020-z.
15. Gebhart A, Young MT, Nguyen NT. Bariatric surgery in the elderly: 2009–2013. Surg Obes Relat Dis. 2015;11(2):393–8. https://doi.org/10.1016/j.soard.2014.04.014.
16. Müller MJ, Lagerpusch M, Enderle J, Schautz B, Heller M, Bosy-Westphal A. Beyond the body mass index: Tracking body composition in the pathogenesis of obesity and the metabolic syndrome. *Obes Rev*. 2012;13(SUPPL.2):6–13. doi:https://doi.org/10.1111/j.1467-789X.2012.01033.x
17. Okorodudu DO, Jumean MF, Montori VM, et al. Diagnostic performance of body mass index to identify obesity as defined by body adiposity: A systematic review and meta-analysis. Int J Obes. 2010;34(5):791–9. https://doi.org/10.1038/ijo.2010.5.
18. Gómez-Ambrosi J, Silva C, Galofré JC, et al. Body mass index classification misses subjects with increased cardiometabolic risk factors related to elevated adiposity. Int J Obes. 2012;36(2):286–94. https://doi.org/10.1038/ijo.2011.100.
19. Gómez-Ambrosi J, Silva C, Galofré JC, et al. Body adiposity and type 2 diabetes: Increased risk with a high body fat percentage even having a normal BMI. Obesity. 2011;19(7):1439–44. https://doi.org/10.1038/oby.2011.36.
20. Corbel MJ, Tolari F, Yadava VK, WHO Expert Consultation. Appropriate body-mass index for Asian populations and its implications. *Lancet*. 2004;363(9403):157–163. doi:https://doi.org/10.1016/S0140-6736(03)15268-3
21. Aminian A, Chang J, Brethauer SA, Kim JJ. ASMBS updated position statement on bariatric surgery in class I obesity (BMI 30–35 kg/m 2). Surg Obes Relat Dis. 2018;14(8):1071–87. https://doi.org/10.1016/j.soard.2018.05.025.

22. Aminian A, Brethauer SA, Andalib A, et al. Individualized Metabolic Surgery Score: Procedure Selection Based on Diabetes Severity. In: *Annals of Surgery*. ; 2017. doi:https://doi.org/10.1097/SLA.0000000000002407

23. Schauer PR, Bhatt DL, Kirwan JP, et al. Bariatric surgery versus intensive medical therapy for diabetes—5-year outcomes. N Engl J Med. 2017. https://doi.org/10.1056/NEJMoa1600869.

24. Peterli R, Wolnerhanssen BK, Peters T, et al. Effect of laparoscopic sleeve gastrectomy vs laparoscopic roux-en-y gastric bypass onweight loss in patients with morbid obesity the sm-boss randomized clinical trial. JAMA—J Am Med Assoc. 2018. https://doi.org/10.1001/jama.2017.20897.

25. Aminian A. Bariatric procedure selection in patients with type 2 diabetes: choice between Roux-en-Y gastric bypass or sleeve gastrectomy. Surg Obes Relat Dis. 2020;16(2):332–9.

26. Salminen P, Helmio M, Ovaska J, et al. Effect of laparoscopic sleeve gastrectomy vs laparoscopic roux-en-y gastric bypass onweight loss at 5 years among patients with morbid obesity the SLEEVEPASS randomized clinical trial. JAMA—J Am Med Assoc. 2018. https://doi.org/10.1001/jama.2017.20313.

27. Aminian A, Andalib A, Ver MR, Corcelles R, Schauer PR, Brethauer SA. Outcomes of Bariatric Surgery in Patients with Inflammatory Bowel Disease. Obes Surg. 2016. https://doi.org/10.1007/s11695-015-1909-y.

28. Ames GE, Clark MM, Gothe KB, Collazo-Clavell ML, Elli EF. Which Bariatric Surgery is Best for My Patient: Guiding Patients Toward the Optimal Surgical Treatment for Obesity While Supporting Autonomy Bariatric Times. Bariatric Times. 2018;15(11):18–27.

29. Haskins IN, Nowacki AS, Khorgami Z, et al. Should recent smoking be a contraindication for sleeve gastrectomy? Surg Obes Relat Dis. 2017. https://doi.org/10.1016/j.soard.2017.02.028.

30. Inadomi M, Iyengar R, Fischer I, Chen X, Flagler E, Ghaferi AA. Effect of patient-reported smoking status on short-term bariatric surgery outcomes. Surg Endosc. 2018. https://doi.org/10.1007/s00464-017-5728-1.

31. Lupoli R, Lembo E, Saldalamacchia G, Avola CK, Angrisani L, Capaldo B. Bariatric surgery and long-term nutritional issues. World J Diabetes. 2017;8(11):464–74. https://doi.org/10.4239/wjd.v8.i11.464.

32. Bredella MA, Greenblatt LB, Eajazi A, Torriani M. Yu EW Effects of Roux-en-Y gastric bypass and sleeve gastrectomy on bone mineral density and marrow adipose tissue. Bone. 2017;95:85–90. https://doi.org/10.1016/j.bone.2016.11.014.

33. Ivaska KK, Huovinen V, Soinio M, et al. Changes in bone metabolism after bariatric surgery by gastric bypass or sleeve gastrectomy. Bone. 2017. https://doi.org/10.1016/j.bone.2016.11.001.

34. Hage MP, El-Hajj FG. Bone and mineral metabolism in patients undergoing Roux-en-Y gastric bypass. Osteoporos Int. 2014. https://doi.org/10.1007/s00198-013-2480-9.

35. Folli F, Sabowitz BN, Schwesinger W, Fanti P, Guardado-Mendoza R, Muscogiuri G. Bariatric surgery and bone disease: From clinical perspective to molecular insights. Int J Obes. 2012. https://doi.org/10.1038/ijo.2012.115.

36. Upala S, Jaruvongvanich V, Sanguankeo A. Risk of nephrolithiasis, hyperoxaluria, and calcium oxalate supersaturation increased after Roux-en-Y gastric bypass surgery: a systematic review and meta-analysis. Surg Obes Relat Dis. 2016. https://doi.org/10.1016/j.soard.2016.04.004.

37. Thongprayoon C, Cheungpasitporn W, Vijayvargiya P, Anthanont P, Erickson SB. The risk of kidney stones following bariatric surgery: A systematic review and meta-analysis. Ren Fail. 2016. https://doi.org/10.3109/0886022X.2015.1137186.

38. Shoar S, Saber AA, Rubenstein R, et al. Portomesentric and splenic vein thrombosis (PMSVT) after bariatric surgery: a systematic review of 110 patients. Surg Obes Relat Dis. 2018. https://doi.org/10.1016/j.soard.2017.09.512.

39. Mackenzie H, Markar SR, Askari A, et al. Obesity surgery and risk of cancer. Br J Surg. 2018;105(12):1650–7. https://doi.org/10.1002/bjs.10914.
40. Derogar M, Hull MA, Kant P, Östlund M, Lu Y, Lagergren J. Increased risk of colorectal cancer after obesity surgery. Ann Surg. 2013;258(6):983–8. https://doi.org/10.1097/SLA.0b013e318288463a.
41. Tao W, Artama M, von Euler-Chelpin M, et al. Colon and rectal cancer risk after bariatric surgery in a multicountry Nordic cohort study. *Int J Cancer*. 2019:1–8. doi:https://doi.org/10.1002/ijc.32770
42. Li JV, Reshat R, Wu Q, et al. Experimental bariatric surgery in rats generates a cytotoxic chemical environment in the gut contents. Front Microbiol. 2011. https://doi.org/10.3389/fmicb.2011.00183.
43. Kant P, Sainsbury A, Reed KR, et al. Rectal epithelial cell mitosis and expression of macrophage migration inhibitory factor are increased 3 years after Roux-en-Y gastric bypass (RYGB) for morbid obesity: Implications for long-term neoplastic risk following RYGB. Gut. 2011. https://doi.org/10.1136/gut.2010.230755.
44. Palleja A, Kashani A, Allin KH, et al. Roux-en-Y gastric bypass surgery of morbidly obese patients induces swift and persistent changes of the individual gut microbiota. Genome Med. 2016. https://doi.org/10.1186/s13073-016-0312-1.
45. Farin W, Oñate FP, Plassais J, et al. impact of laparoscopic Roux-en-Y gastric bypass and sleeve gastrectomy on gut microbiota: a metagenomic comparative analysis. Surg Obes Relat Dis. 2020. https://doi.org/10.1016/j.soard.2020.03.014.
46. Kirwan JP, Aminian A, Kashyap SR, Burguera B, Brethauer SA, Schauer PR. Bariatric Surgery in Obese Patients With Type 1 Diabetes. Diabetes Care. 2016;39(6):941–8. https://doi.org/10.2337/dc15-2732.

The Sleeve and Pregnancy

Hanan Alsalem

There is no doubt that obesity among women is on the rise world wide. According to World Health Organization (WHO) estimates, Kuwait is ranked amongst the top countries in the world in obesity prevalence. In a study published in 2014 by Weiderpass et al., they have concluded that eight out of 10 Kuwaitis were overweight or obese which is a great health concern [1].

Unfortunately, obesity have affected women in the reproductive age group on different levels. Pre-pregnancy challenges which were described by my colleague in the previous chapter as well as potential complications during pregnancy of which we will discuss in this chapter. We will pay a closer look into how weight management surgeries have affected this challenging group of patients.

1 Pre-pregnancy Weight Management

It's no doubt a crucial point of care to optimize weight prior to conception. This is agreed up on by various international guidelines. Advice on weight and lifestyle should be given during preconception counselling or contraceptive consultations. Weight and BMI should be measured to encourage women to optimise their weight before pregnancy. Women of childbearing age with a BMI 30 kg/m^2 or greater should receive information and advice about the risks of obesity during pregnancy as well as childbirth. They should be supported and encouraged to lose weight prior to conception and between pregnancies in line with National Institute for Health and Care Excellence (NICE) Clinical guideline (CG) 189. Women

H. Alsalem (✉)
Department of Obstetrics and Gynecology, McMaster University,
Gynecologic Minimally Invasive Clinical Fellow, Hamilton, ON, Canada
e-mail: dr.hananalsalem@yahoo.com

S. Al-Sabah et al. (eds.), *Laparoscopic Sleeve Gastrectomy*,
https://doi.org/10.1007/978-3-030-57373-7_10

should be informed that weight loss between pregnancies reduces the risk of still-birth, hypertensive complications and fetal macrosomia. Weight loss increases the chances of successful vaginal birth after caesarean (VBAC) section.

2 Pre-pregnancy Supplementation

Women with a BMI 30 kg/m^2 or greater wishing to become pregnant should be advised to take 5 mg folic acid supplementation daily, starting at least 1 month before conception and continuing during the first trimester of pregnancy. (RCOG). Metabolic and nutritional derangements can occur after bariatric surgery, particularly after malabsorptive procedures. Reduced oral intake and alterations in digestive physiology as well as anatomy can result in malabsorption of various micronutrients and minerals, particularly iron, folate, vitamin B12, calcium, and vitamin D. Absorption of iron and folate are reduced due to lower acid content in the gastric pouch and bypass of the duodenum, the main site of absorption. Calcium deficiency can also result from bypass of the duodenum, as well as reduced intake of both calcium and vitamin D. A reduction in the availability of both gastric acid and intrinsic factor may lead to B12 deficiency.

While women with prior malabsorptive procedures are at greatest risk for micronutrient deficiencies, women who undergo restrictive procedures may also develop iron, folate, and fat soluble vitamin deficiencies [2].

A number of adverse pregnancy outcomes have been linked to inadequate supplementation and resultant micronutrient deficiencies. Iron and B12 deficiencies have resulted in maternal anemia.

Specific supplementation regimens need to be tailored to the individual patient and the type of bariatric procedure performed [3]. Guidelines for optimum micronutrient supplementation during pregnancy have been extrapolated from data from the bariatric and obstetric literature. In general, during pregnancy, it is reasonable to continue the regimen recommended by the bariatric surgeon, but the multivitamin is generally advised and is replaced with a prenatal vitamin.

It is generally advised that the following tests are to be performed pre conception or at booking antenatal visit [4]:

- Complete blood count
- Ferritin
- Iron
- Vitamin B12
- Thiamine
- Folate
- Calcium
- Vitamin D

The previous tests will aid in identifying those who will require additional supplementation as well as ensure followup during the course of the pregnancy. Monthly repeat labs are also suggested to those with demonstrable deficiencies. At every trimester, the tests should be repeated to those with no documented deficiency.

Supplementation and screening should continue following delivery in women who breastfeed.

3 Acceptable Weight Changes in Pregnancy

There is a lack of consensus on optimal gestational weight gain in the obese population or post weight management surgery group. Until further evidence is achieved, the main advice by treating obstetrician is focus on a healthy diet that is more applicable than prescribed weight gain targets. None the less, a referral to a nutritionist could aid in managing both obese and post weight management surgery patients. Caloric restriction during pregnancy is not recommended, even if patients continue to be overweight after bariatric surgery, due to concerns that caloric restriction might impair fetal growth [5]. Anti-obesity medications are not recommended during pregnancy.

Optimal weight gain during pregnancy in women who have undergone bariatric surgery has not been studied. We suggest that women who are not achieving the minimum weight gain standards suggested by the IOM (0.5 lb [0.23 kg]/week for obese women in the second and third trimester) undergo ultrasound evaluation of fetal growth and dietary consultation. If adequate caloric intake is confirmed, we do not recommend encouraging the woman to consume significantly more calories.

4 Care During Pregnancy

Routine care and management for post weight management surgery patients is generally advise. Unless the starting (booking visit) BMI is elevated (>30 kg/m^2), then patient is to be followed up according to international guidelines for obese patients.

Once again, the main issue with post weight management surgery patients is attaining adequate nutrition. Nausea, vomiting might be more profound as the gestation advances. It is most importantly to ensure adequate supplementations in those patients. Needless to say, if symptoms persists, exclusion of acute causes is mandatory.

It is well known that obesity in pregnancy carries risks to both the mother as well as the fetus. Those risks can develop from early pregnancy till the post partum period. This includes early pregnancy loss, diabetes, hypertension, fetal macrosomia, failed induction of labor and ultimately undergoing a C-section. One potential issue during pregnancy is obstructive sleep apnea. Once again no solid evidence is found on the effect of wight management surgery specifically post sleeve gastrectomy is found. We will review some of the potential risks of wight management surgeries in the pregnant patient group.

Fetal growth—Given the plausible increased risk of intrauterine growth restriction and small for gestational age infants in post-bariatric surgery pregnancies, its been suggested to perform serial ultrasound examinations every four weeks to evaluate fetal growth in the third trimester, especially in women with poor weight gain and those who conceive within two years of surgery.

5 Gestational Diabetes

5.1 Screening

The glucose challenge test used to screen for gestational diabetes is typically not well tolerated in women with prior history of bariatric surgery due to dumping syndrome which is experienced in about 50% of patients following RYGB. It's been suggested that following fasting and postbreakfast blood sugars for one week as an alternative [6, 7]. Patients who regularly drink and tolerate sugared soft drinks are an exception; these women probably can tolerate a standard glucose challenge test. A third option is to measure glycated hemoglobin (A1C) and assume overt diabetes is present if it is elevated ($\geq 6.5\%$); women with a normal A1C should undergo screening as described.

Dumping syndrome typically does not occur in women who have undergone restrictive-type bariatric procedures such as gastric banding and those women can undergo standard testing for GDM.

5.2 Treatment

GDM conventional treatment involves nutritional therapy and insulin, some clinicians use oral anti-hyperglycemic agents, such as glyburide or metformin.

Monitoring for complications of bariatric surgery—The most common late sequelae of bariatric surgery are mild nutritional deficiencies, which are readily treated with replacement therapy.

5.3 Mode of Delivery

Cesarean delivery is performed for standard obstetric indications. Consultation with a bariatric surgeon is advisable if the patient had a complicated bariatric surgery [5]. Patients who have undergone uncomplicated bariatric surgery generally do not require changes in surgical technique. Some obstetricians may favor blunt entry into the peritoneum to minimize risk of iviscus injury that could be adherent to anterior abdominal wall.

5.4   Postpartum

Bariatric surgery should not adversely affect breast feeding and it should be encouraged.

As previously disclosed, micronutrient supplementation and screening should continue following delivery in women who breastfeed. Breastfed infants of women who have had gastric bypass procedures may develop nutritional deficiencies, especially those that are exclusively breastfed [7, 8].

References

1. Weiderpass E, Botteri E, Longenecker JC, Alkandari A, Al-Wotayan R, Al Duwairi Q, Tuomilehto J. The prevalence of overweight and obesity in an adult Kuwaiti population in 2014. Front Endocrinol. 2019. https://doi.org/10.3389/fendo.2019.00449.
2. Ledoux S, Msika S, Moussa F, Larger E, Boudou P, Salomon L, Roy C, Clerici C. Comparison of nutritional consequences of conventional therapy of obesity, adjustable gastric banding, and gastric bypass. Obes Surg. 2006;16(8):1041.
3. Guelinckx I, Devlieger R, Vansant G. Reproductive outcome after bariatric surgery: a critical review. Hum Reprod Update. 2009;15(2):189.
4. Poitou Bernert C, Ciangura C, Coupaye M, Czernichow S, Bouillot JL, Basdevant A. Nutritional deficiency after gastric bypass: diagnosis, prevention and treatment. Diabetes Metab. 2007;33(1):13.
5. American College of Obstetricians and Gynecologists. ACOG practice bulletin no. 105: bariatric surgery and pregnancy. Obstet Gynecol. 2009;113(6):1405. (The American College of Obstetricians and Gynecologists, Washington, DC 20090-6920)
6. American College of Obstetricians and Gynecologists. ACOG practice bulletin no. 105: bariatric surgery and pregnancy. Obstet Gynecol. 2009;113(6):1405. (The American College of Obstetricians and Gynecologists, Washington, DC 20090-6920, USA)
7. Wax JR, Pinette MG, Cartin A, Blackstone J. Female reproductive issues following bariatric surgery. Obstet Gynecol Surv. 2007;62(9):595.
8. Celiker MY, Chawla A. Congenital B12 deficiency following maternal gastric bypass. J Perinatol. 2009;29(9):640.
9. Grange DK, Finlay JL. Nutritional vitamin B12 deficiency in a breastfed infant following maternal gastric bypass. Pediatr Hematol Oncol. 1994;11(3):311.

The Sleeve and Reproductive Potential

Abdulrahman Alserri

1 Introduction

In this chapter we aim to cover the impact of obesity on both male and female fertility potential and to touch upon the effect of bariatric surgery on natural and assisted reproduction. The impact of obesity and bariatric surgery on pregnancy will be discussed in a separate chapter.

2 Obesity and Female Reproduction

Women who are obese are at increased risk of menstrual abnormalities. It is also noteworthy that menstrual irregularity is positively correlated with weight in obese women [1]. This in turn prolongs the time to conception in obese women as the spontaneous pregnancy rate decreases by about 4% for every kg/m^2 increase in BMI [2, 3].

A likely explanation for the lower spontaneous conception rate is the higher prevalence of ovulation dysfunction (oligoovulation/anovulation) in obese women [4]. Obese women with a BMI >27 kg/m^2 are three times more likely to suffer from anovulatory infertility compared to their lean counterparts [5]. The main mechanism explaining this is a decreased gonadotropin secretion secondary to negative feedback exerted from increased conversion of androgens to estrogens by adipose aromatase [6–8].

A. Alserri (✉)
Department of Obstetrics and Gynecology, Faculty of Medicine, Kuwait University, Kuwait City, Kuwait
e-mail: a.alserri@HSC.EDU.KW

© The Editor(s) (if applicable) and The Author(s), under exclusive license to Springer Nature Switzerland AG 2021
S. Al-Sabah et al. (eds.), *Laparoscopic Sleeve Gastrectomy*,
https://doi.org/10.1007/978-3-030-57373-7_11

Obese women also have more difficulty conceiving through assisted reproductive technologies (ART) compared to lean controls. A metanalysis of 33 In-Vitro-Fertilization (IVF) studies that included 47,967 IVF cycles concluded that obese women undergoing IVF have a lower chance of clinical pregnancy and live birth as compared with normal weight women [9].

The mechanisms that may explain the difference in ART success are as follows:

1. Reduced response to fertility medications: When inducing ovulation, Obese women require higher doses of medication and have a decreased chance of ovulation. In IVF, they require a higher total dose of gonadotropins to stimulate the ovaries, have fewer oocytes retrieved and have a higher cycle cancellation rate [8, 10–17].
2. Reduced oocyte quality: In IVF, when using autologous oocytes, obese women may experience altered oocyte morphology, lower fertilization, poorer embryo quality and therefore lower pregnancy rates [10, 18–21]. However, when using donor oocytes, obese women had better pregnancy rates [22, 23].
3. Altered endometrial function: Obesity appears to alter endometrial receptivity. This has been shown when third-party surrogate women with a BMI >35 kg/m^2 experienced a 50% lower live birth rate compared with those with a BMI <35 kg/m^2 [24, 25].
4. Technical issues: Obesity may also make procedures such as ultrasound, oocyte retrieval and embryo transfer, which are an essential part of ART success, more difficult [26, 27].

3   Obesity and Male Reproduction

Obese men may suffer from altered sexual function and are more likely to have erectile dysfunction [28–31]. They may also have poorer semen quality, where studies have shown an increased likelihood of oligospermia and asthenospermia [32–39]. However, the evidence is divided as to whether or not pregnancy outcomes are negatively impacted due to this [32, 39–45].

This is explained by increased androgen aromatization to estrogens by adipose tissue which in turn reduces gonadotropin secretion by the anterior pituitary gland and thereby reducing both the production of testosterone and hindering normal spermatogenesis [29, 43, 46–52]. Semen parameters may also be adversely affected by increased scrotal temperatures as the scrotum remains in closer contact with the surrounding adiposity in obese men [43, 53].

4   Female Reproduction Following Bariatric Surgery

Female reproductive potential improves following weight loss. Improvement is more pronounced in women with ovulation disorders specifically polycystic ovary syndrome (PCOS) [54, 55]. This is true for both nonsurgical and surgical weight loss [56–61].

Weight loss following bariatric surgery may restore menstrual regularity and promote ovulation [60, 62–64]. Furthermore, it has been shown to improve markers of PCOS specifically symptoms of hyperandrogenism like hirsutism, and Insulin resistance [56, 60, 63, 65–71]. Further, a study looking specifically at laparoscopic sleeve gastrectomy (LSG) found that PCOS patients who had LSG had a larger change in BMI at 1 year compared to controls without PCOS who had the same procedure [72].

Sexual function in females has also been shown to be enhanced following bariatric surgery with women reporting improvement in libido [67].

Both the improvement in ovulation regularity and sexual function has translated into better reproductive outcomes following bariatric surgery. It seems that the amount of weight lost and the BMI at the time of conception were both predictors of the chance of pregnancy following bariatric surgery but not the type of surgery itself [73–75].

However, even given this encouraging data, bariatric surgery should not be the primary treatment for infertility in obese women [76, 77].

5   Male Reproduction Following Bariatric Surgery

Weight loss following bariatric surgery may improve sexual function in some men as it increases gonadotropin secretion as a result of decreased adipose aromatization of androgens to estrogens. It is however not clear whether weight loss following bariatric surgery alters sperm parameters [78]. Some case reports have shown worsening semen parameters after bariatric surgery, possibly secondary to nutritional deficiencies affecting normal spermatogenesis [79, 80]. Other reports have shown that semen parameters remain stable after 1 year of follow up following bariatric surgery [81]. Therefore, in selected cases, men wishing to undergo bariatric surgery may want to consider semen cryopreservation before surgery as a back-up for future use [82].

6   Timing of Conception Following Bariatric Surgery

It is recommended that pregnancy be delayed until 1–2 years after bariatric surgery [36, 83–87]. This is to avoid the adverse effects of fetal exposure to nutritional deficiencies and rapid weight loss, and to optimize weight loss goals [57, 85]. If conception does occur before the recommended 1–2 years, there is limited data that suggests that surgery may not necessarily affect maternal and fetal health given proper pregnancy surveillance [75, 88, 89]. A study specifically looking at the time interval between laparoscopic sleeve gastrectomy and pregnancy found no difference in pregnancy outcome between women in the short interval group (within 18 months) versus those in the long interval group (after 18 months) [90]. In our opinion, time of conception should be individualized according to the patient's age, ovarian reserve and, if any, complications of surgery.

7 Assisted Reproductive Technologies (ART) Following Bariatric Surgery

According to a case series of five women who underwent in-vitro fertilization (IVF) 1–5 years after bariatric surgery, four out of the five women became pregnant and delivered at term without complications, suggesting that ART seems to be safe following bariatric surgery [91].

8 Conclusion

We conclude that obesity has a negative effect on both male and female fertility. In women, weight loss following surgery may be associated with improvement in reproductive potential and pregnancy rates. In men, weight loss following surgery may improve sexual function, but it is unclear if semen parameters are affected. That said, bariatric surgery should not be recommended as the primary treatment for male or female infertility.

References

1. Castillo-Martinez L, Lopez-Alvarenga JC, Villa AR, Gonzalez-Barranco J. Menstrual cycle length disorders in 18- to 40-y-old obese women. Nutrition. 2003;19(4):317–20.
2. Lake JK, Power C, Cole TJ. Women's reproductive health: the role of body mass index in early and adult life. Int J Obes Relat Metab Disord. 1997;21(6):432–8.
3. van der Steeg JW, Steures P, Eijkemans MJ, et al. Obesity affects spontaneous pregnancy chances in subfertile, ovulatory women. Hum Reprod. 2008;23(2):324–8.
4. Pathi A, Esen U, Hildreth A. A comparison of complications of pregnancy and delivery in morbidly obese and non-obese women. J Obstet Gynaecol. 2006;26(6):527–30.
5. Grodstein F, Goldman MB, Cramer DW. Body mass index and ovulatory infertility. Epidemiology. 1994;5(2):247–50.
6. McCartney CR, Blank SK, Prendergast KA, et al. Obesity and sex steroid changes across puberty: evidence for marked hyperandrogenemia in pre- and early pubertal obese girls. J Clin Endocrinol Metab. 2007;92(2):430–6.
7. Pasquali R, Casimirri F, Plate L, Capelli M. Characterization of obese women with reduced sex hormone-binding globulin concentrations. Horm Metab Res. 1990;22(5):303–6.
8. Pasquali R, Pelusi C, Genghini S, Cacciari M, Gambineri A. Obesity and reproductive disorders in women. Hum Reprod Update. 2003;9(4):359–72.
9. Rittenberg V, Seshadri S, Sunkara SK, Sobaleva S, Oteng-Ntim E, El-Toukhy T. Effect of body mass index on IVF treatment outcome: an updated systematic review and meta-analysis. Reprod Biomed Online. 2011;23(4):421–39.
10. Fedorcsak P, Dale PO, Storeng R, et al. Impact of overweight and underweight on assisted reproduction treatment. Hum Reprod. 2004;19(11):2523–8.
11. Imani B, Eijkemans MJ, te Velde ER, Habbema JD, Fauser BC. A nomogram to predict the probability of live birth after clomiphene citrate induction of ovulation in normogonadotropic oligoamenorrheic infertility. Fertil Steril. 2002;77(1):91–7.
12. Moragianni VA, Jones SM, Ryley DA. The effect of body mass index on the outcomes of first assisted reproductive technology cycles. Fertil Steril. 2012;98(1):102–8.

13. Mulders AG, Laven JS, Eijkemans MJ, Hughes EG, Fauser BC. Patient predictors for outcome of gonadotrophin ovulation induction in women with normogonadotrophic anovulatory infertility: a meta-analysis. Hum Reprod Update. 2003;9(5):429–49.
14. Pinborg A, Gaarslev C, Hougaard CO, et al. Influence of female bodyweight on IVF outcome: a longitudinal multicentre cohort study of 487 infertile couples. Reprod Biomed Online. 2011;23(4):490–9.
15. Shah DK, Missmer SA, Berry KF, Racowsky C, Ginsburg ES. Effect of obesity on oocyte and embryo quality in women undergoing in vitro fertilization. Obstet Gynecol. 2011;118(1):63–70.
16. Souter I, Baltagi LM, Kuleta D, Meeker JD, Petrozza JC. Women, weight, and fertility: the effect of body mass index on the outcome of superovulation/intrauterine insemination cycles. Fertil Steril. 2011;95(3):1042–7.
17. Wang JX, Davies M, Norman RJ. Body mass and probability of pregnancy during assisted reproduction treatment: retrospective study. BMJ. 2000;321(7272):1320–1.
18. Depalo R, Garruti G, Totaro I, et al. Oocyte morphological abnormalities in overweight women undergoing in vitro fertilization cycles. Gynecol Endocrinol. 2011;27(11):880–4.
19. Metwally M, Cutting R, Tipton A, Skull J, Ledger WL, Li TC. Effect of increased body mass index on oocyte and embryo quality in IVF patients. Reprod Biomed Online. 2007;15(5):532–8.
20. Orvieto R, Meltcer S, Nahum R, Rabinson J, Anteby EY, Ashkenazi J. The influence of body mass index on in vitro fertilization outcome. Int J Gynaecol Obstet. 2009;104(1):53–5.
21. Zhang D, Zhu Y, Gao H, et al. Overweight and obesity negatively affect the outcomes of ovarian stimulation and in vitro fertilisation: a cohort study of 2628 Chinese women. Gynecol Endocrinol. 2010;26(5):325–32.
22. Jungheim ES, Schoeller EL, Marquard KL, Louden ED, Schaffer JE, Moley KH. Diet-induced obesity model: abnormal oocytes and persistent growth abnormalities in the offspring. Endocrinology. 2010;151(8):4039–46.
23. Luke B, Brown MB, Stern JE, et al. Female obesity adversely affects assisted reproductive technology (ART) pregnancy and live birth rates. Hum Reprod. 2011;26(1):245–52.
24. Bellver J, Pellicer A, Garcia-Velasco JA, Ballesteros A, Remohi J, Meseguer M. Obesity reduces uterine receptivity: clinical experience from 9,587 first cycles of ovum donation with normal weight donors. Fertil Steril. 2013;100(4):1050–8.
25. DeUgarte DA, DeUgarte CM, Sahakian V. Surrogate obesity negatively impacts pregnancy rates in third-party reproduction. Fertil Steril. 2010;93(3):1008–10.
26. Beydoun HA, Stadtmauer L, Beydoun MA, Russell H, Zhao Y, Oehninger S. Polycystic ovary syndrome, body mass index and outcomes of assisted reproductive technologies. Reprod Biomed Online. 2009;18(6):856–63.
27. Wittemer C, Ohl J, Bailly M, Bettahar-Lebugle K, Nisand I. Does body mass index of infertile women have an impact on IVF procedure and outcome? J Assist Reprod Genet. 2000;17(10):547–52.
28. Cabler S, Agarwal A, Flint M, du Plessis SS. Obesity: modern man's fertility nemesis. Asian J Androl. 2010;12(4):480–9.
29. Pasquali R. Obesity and androgens: facts and perspectives. Fertil Steril. 2006;85(5):1319–40.
30. Ramlau-Hansen CH, Thulstrup AM, Nohr EA, Bonde JP, Sorensen TI, Olsen J. Subfecundity in overweight and obese couples. Hum Reprod. 2007;22(6):1634–7.
31. Sallmen M, Sandler DP, Hoppin JA, Blair A, Baird DD. Reduced fertility among overweight and obese men. Epidemiology. 2006;17(5):520–3.
32. Bakos HW, Henshaw RC, Mitchell M, Lane M. Paternal body mass index is associated with decreased blastocyst development and reduced live birth rates following assisted reproductive technology. Fertil Steril. 2011;95(5):1700–4.
33. Braga DP, Halpern G, Figueira Rde C, Setti AS, Iaconelli A Jr, Borges E Jr. Food intake and social habits in male patients and its relationship to intracytoplasmic sperm injection outcomes. Fertil Steril. 2012;97(1):53–9.

34. Hammiche F, Laven JS, Twigt JM, Boellaard WP, Steegers EA, Steegers-Theunissen RP. Body mass index and central adiposity are associated with sperm quality in men of subfertile couples. Hum Reprod. 2012;27(8):2365–72.
35. Hammoud AO, Wilde N, Gibson M, Parks A, Carrell DT, Meikle AW. Male obesity and alteration in sperm parameters. Fertil Steril. 2008;90(6):2222–5.
36. Kominiarek MA, Jungheim ES, Hoeger KM, Rogers AM, Kahan S, Kim JJ. American Society for Metabolic and Bariatric Surgery position statement on the impact of obesity and obesity treatment on fertility and fertility therapy Endorsed by the American College of Obstetricians and Gynecologists and the Obesity Society. Surg Obes Relat Dis. 2017;13(5):750–7.
37. Relwani R, Berger D, Santoro N, et al. Semen parameters are unrelated to BMI but vary with SSRI use and prior urological surgery. Reprod Sci. 2011;18(4):391–7.
38. Sermondade N, Faure C, Fezeu L, et al. BMI in relation to sperm count: an updated systematic review and collaborative meta-analysis. Hum Reprod Update. 2013;19(3):221–31.
39. Umul M, Kose SA, Bilen E, Altuncu AG, Oksay T, Guney M. Effect of increasing paternal body mass index on pregnancy and live birth rates in couples undergoing intracytoplasmic sperm injection. Andrologia. 2015;47(3):360–4.
40. Colaci DS, Afeiche M, Gaskins AJ, et al. Men's body mass index in relation to embryo quality and clinical outcomes in couples undergoing in vitro fertilization. Fertil Steril. 2012;98(5):1193–9 e1191.
41. Keltz J, Zapantis A, Jindal SK, Lieman HJ, Santoro N, Polotsky AJ. Overweight men: clinical pregnancy after ART is decreased in IVF but not in ICSI cycles. J Assist Reprod Genet. 2010;27(9–10):539–44.
42. Merhi ZO, Keltz J, Zapantis A, et al. Male adiposity impairs clinical pregnancy rate by in vitro fertilization without affecting day 3 embryo quality. Obesity (Silver Spring). 2013;21(8):1608–12.
43. Palmer NO, Bakos HW, Fullston T, Lane M. Impact of obesity on male fertility, sperm function and molecular composition. Spermatogenesis. 2012;2(4):253–63.
44. Ramasamy R, Bryson C, Reifsnyder JE, Neri Q, Palermo GD, Schlegel PN. Overweight men with nonobstructive azoospermia have worse pregnancy outcomes after microdissection testicular sperm extraction. Fertil Steril. 2013;99(2):372–6.
45. Thomsen L, Humaidan P, Bungum L, Bungum M. The impact of male overweight on semen quality and outcome of assisted reproduction. Asian J Androl. 2014;16(5):749–54.
46. Hakonsen LB, Thulstrup AM, Aggerholm AS, et al. Does weight loss improve semen quality and reproductive hormones? Results from a cohort of severely obese men. Reprod Health. 2011;8:24.
47. MacDonald AA, Herbison GP, Showell M, Farquhar CM. The impact of body mass index on semen parameters and reproductive hormones in human males: a systematic review with meta-analysis. Hum Reprod Update. 2010;16(3):293–311.
48. Pitteloud N, Hardin M, Dwyer AA, et al. Increasing insulin resistance is associated with a decrease in Leydig cell testosterone secretion in men. J Clin Endocrinol Metab. 2005;90(5):2636–41.
49. Teerds KJ, de Rooij DG, Keijer J. Functional relationship between obesity and male reproduction: from humans to animal models. Hum Reprod Update. 2011;17(5):667–83.
50. Tunc O, Bakos HW, Tremellen K. Impact of body mass index on seminal oxidative stress. Andrologia. 2011;43(2):121–8.
51. Vermeulen A, Kaufman JM, Deslypere JP, Thomas G. Attenuated luteinizing hormone (LH) pulse amplitude but normal LH pulse frequency, and its relation to plasma androgens in hypogonadism of obese men. J Clin Endocrinol Metab. 1993;76(5):1140–6.
52. Zumoff B, Strain GW, Miller LK, et al. Plasma free and non-sex-hormone-binding-globulin-bound testosterone are decreased in obese men in proportion to their degree of obesity. J Clin Endocrinol Metab. 1990;71(4):929–31.
53. Jung A, Schill WB. [Male infertility. Current life style could be responsible for infertility]. MMW Fortschr Med. 2000;142(37):31–3.

54. Clark AM, Ledger W, Galletly C, et al. Weight loss results in significant improvement in pregnancy and ovulation rates in anovulatory obese women. Hum Reprod. 1995;10(10):2705–12.
55. Clark AM, Thornley B, Tomlinson L, Galletley C, Norman RJ. Weight loss in obese infertile women results in improvement in reproductive outcome for all forms of fertility treatment. Hum Reprod. 1998;13(6):1502–5.
56. Eid GM, Cottam DR, Velcu LM, et al. Effective treatment of polycystic ovarian syndrome with Roux-en-Y gastric bypass. Surg Obes Relat Dis. 2005;1(2):77–80.
57. Marceau P, Kaufman D, Biron S, et al. Outcome of pregnancies after biliopancreatic diversion. Obes Surg. 2004;14(3):318–24.
58. Martin LF, Finigan KM, Nolan TE. Pregnancy after adjustable gastric banding. Obstet Gynecol. 2000;95(6 Pt 1):927–30.
59. Nelson SM, Fleming R. Obesity and reproduction: impact and interventions. Curr Opin Obstet Gynecol. 2007;19(4):384–9.
60. Teitelman M, Grotegut CA, Williams NN, Lewis JD. The impact of bariatric surgery on menstrual patterns. Obes Surg. 2006;16(11):1457–63.
61. Weiner R, Blanco-Engert R, Weiner S, Matkowitz R, Schaefer L, Pomhoff I. Outcome after laparoscopic adjustable gastric banding - 8 years experience. Obes Surg. 2003;13(3):427–34.
62. Maggard MA, Yermilov I, Li Z, et al. Pregnancy and fertility following bariatric surgery: a systematic review. JAMA. 2008;300(19):2286–96.
63. Tan O, Carr BR. The impact of bariatric surgery on obesity-related infertility and in vitro fertilization outcomes. Semin Reprod Med. 2012;30(6):517–28.
64. Zitsman JL, Digiorgi MF, Marr JR, Witt MA, Bessler M. Comparative outcomes of laparoscopic adjustable gastric banding in adolescents and adults. Surg Obes Relat Dis. 2011;7(6):720–6.
65. Escobar-Morreale HF, Botella-Carretero JI, Alvarez-Blasco F, Sancho J, San Millan JL. The polycystic ovary syndrome associated with morbid obesity may resolve after weight loss induced by bariatric surgery. J Clin Endocrinol Metab. 2005;90(12):6364–9.
66. Jamal M, Gunay Y, Capper A, Eid A, Heitshusen D, Samuel I. Roux-en-Y gastric bypass ameliorates polycystic ovary syndrome and dramatically improves conception rates: a 9-year analysis. Surg Obes Relat Dis. 2012;8(4):440–4.
67. Legro RS, Dodson WC, Gnatuk CL, et al. Effects of gastric bypass surgery on female reproductive function. J Clin Endocrinol Metab. 2012;97(12):4540–8.
68. Malik SM, Traub ML. Defining the role of bariatric surgery in polycystic ovarian syndrome patients. World J Diabetes. 2012;3(4):71–9.
69. Merhi ZO. Impact of bariatric surgery on female reproduction. Fertil Steril. 2009;92(5):1501–8.
70. Moran LJ, Norman RJ. The effect of bariatric surgery on female reproductive function. J Clin Endocrinol Metab. 2012;97(12):4352–4.
71. Rochester D, Jain A, Polotsky AJ, et al. Partial recovery of luteal function after bariatric surgery in obese women. Fertil Steril. 2009;92(4):1410–5.
72. Dilday J, Derickson M, Kuckelman J, et al. Sleeve gastrectomy for obesity in polycystic ovarian syndrome: a pilot study evaluating weight loss and fertility outcomes. Obes Surg. 2019;29(1):93–8.
73. Musella M, Milone M, Bellini M, Sosa Fernandez LM, Leongito M, Milone F. Effect of bariatric surgery on obesity-related infertility. Surg Obes Relat Dis. 2012;8(4):445–9.
74. Rinaldi AP, Kral JG. Comments on Sheiner et al.'s "Pregnancy outcome of patients who conceive during or after the first year following bariatric surgery". Am J Obstet Gynecol. 2011;205(4):e11; author reply e11–2.
75. Sheiner E, Edri A, Balaban E, Levi I, Aricha-Tamir B. Pregnancy outcome of patients who conceive during or after the first year following bariatric surgery. Am J Obstet Gynecol. 2011;204(1):50 e51–6.
76. Karmon A, Sheiner E. Pregnancy after bariatric surgery: a comprehensive review. Arch Gynecol Obstet. 2008;277(5):381–8.

77. Merhi ZO. Weight loss by bariatric surgery and subsequent fertility. Fertil Steril. 2007;87(2):430–2.
78. Reis LO, Zani EL, Saad RD, Chaim EA, de Oliveira LC, Fregonesi A. Bariatric surgery does not interfere with sperm quality—a preliminary long-term study. Reprod Sci. 2012;19(10):1057–62.
79. di Frega AS, Dale B, Di Matteo L, Wilding M. Secondary male factor infertility after Roux-en-Y gastric bypass for morbid obesity: case report. Hum Reprod. 2005;20(4):997–8.
80. Sermondade N, Massin N, Boitrelle F, et al. Sperm parameters and male fertility after bariatric surgery: three case series. Reprod Biomed Online. 2012;24(2):206–10.
81. Legro RS, Kunselman AR, Meadows JW, et al. Time-related increase in urinary testosterone levels and stable semen analysis parameters after bariatric surgery in men. Reprod Biomed Online. 2015;30(2):150–6.
82. Reis LO, Dias FG. Male fertility, obesity, and bariatric surgery. Reprod Sci. 2012;19(8):778–85.
83. American College of O, Gynecologists. ACOG practice bulletin no. 105: bariatric surgery and pregnancy. Obstet Gynecol. 2009;113(6):1405–13.
84. Apovian CM, Baker C, Ludwig DS, et al. Best practice guidelines in pediatric/adolescent weight loss surgery. Obes Res. 2005;13(2):274–82.
85. Beard JH, Bell RL, Duffy AJ. Reproductive considerations and pregnancy after bariatric surgery: current evidence and recommendations. Obes Surg. 2008;18(8):1023–7.
86. Guelinckx I, Devlieger R, Vansant G. Reproductive outcome after bariatric surgery: a critical review. Hum Reprod Update. 2009;15(2):189–201.
87. Mechanick JI, Youdim A, Jones DB, et al. Clinical practice guidelines for the perioperative nutritional, metabolic, and nonsurgical support of the bariatric surgery patient–2013 update: cosponsored by American Association of Clinical Endocrinologists, The Obesity Society, and American Society for Metabolic & Bariatric Surgery. Obesity (Silver Spring). 2013;21(Suppl 1):S1-27.
88. Dixon JB, Dixon ME, O'Brien PE. Birth outcomes in obese women after laparoscopic adjustable gastric banding. Obstet Gynecol. 2005;106(5 Pt 1):965–72.
89. Patel JA, Patel NA, Thomas RL, Nelms JK, Colella JJ. Pregnancy outcomes after laparoscopic Roux-en-Y gastric bypass. Surg Obes Relat Dis. 2008;4(1):39–45.
90. Rottenstreich A, Levin G, Kleinstern G, Rottenstreich M, Elchalal U, Elazary R. The effect of surgery-to-conception interval on pregnancy outcomes after sleeve gastrectomy. Surg Obes Relat Dis. 2018;14(12):1795–803.
91. Doblado MA, Lewkowksi BM, Odem RR, Jungheim ES. In vitro fertilization after bariatric surgery. Fertil Steril. 2010;94(7):2812–4.

The Sleeve as a Revisional Procedure

Camilo Boza Wilson and Andrés San Martin

1 Introduction

Bariatric surgery (BS) has widely shown its effectiveness in weight loss and improving comorbidities. According to ASMBC [1], in 2011 BS went from 158,000 to 252,000 cases in 2018. Revisional Surgery (RS) in the same period went from 6 to 15.4%. This increase also implies an increase in the number of failures and hence the need for RS. Long-term studies show that all primary techniques have a variable percentage of failures.

Sleeve gastrectomy (SG) is the most commonly performed primary bariatric procedure around the world. It is the technique that contributes with most of the cases in terms of weight regain, GERD and complications, and therefore that contributes the most to the number of RS. In 2016 it was the first time that RS numbers were shown worldwide, where 50,977 surgeries were reported. The percentages range from 1 to 11% of the total performed interventions, depending on the region (North America, Europe and Latin America respectively). Of the total numbers of RS 63% of these were due to insufficient weight loss or low response in comorbidities and 26% due to complications and 11% for both [2].

C. B. Wilson (✉)
Department of Digestive Surgery, Clinica Las Condes, Santiago, Chile
e-mail: bozauc@mac.com

A. S. Martin
Médico Cirujano, Fellow Cirugía Bariátrica Clínica las Condes, Santiago, Chile
e-mail: andresesanmartin@gmail.com

S. Al-Sabah et al. (eds.), *Laparoscopic Sleeve Gastrectomy*,
https://doi.org/10.1007/978-3-030-57373-7_12

2   General Considerations

As a general rule we should know that any RS is complex, technically demanding and associated with greater operating risks and complications than primary procedures [3–6]. When performed by experienced surgeons, the rate of complications is close to 13% [7]. When the team is assessing a RS should look at the causes of primary failure, presence of uncontrolled comorbidities, new symptoms that could have originated or worsen after the primary procedure (GERD, Dumping, anemia, micronutrient deficit) [8, 9], For this purpose all patients must be addressed by the multidisciplinary team.

The patient candidate for revision surgery must be carefully studied, in search of the causes of primary failure. Anatomy must be assessed with an endoscopy, radiologic studies, CT scan volumetry. Patients should also undergo laboratory analysis and in some cases Ph-impedance studies. For example, Re-Sleeve was generally proposed for patients with an excessively high residual gastric volume, as assessed by gastric CT volumetry) and/or with gastric pouch dilatation (as assessed by barium swallow) [10–12]. Keep in mind that GERD symptoms associated with Barret's esophagus are a contraindication for Re-Sleeve [13]. In addition to the above, patients must be assessed considering these procedures are technically complex in part due to the presence of adhesions, previous surgeries such, cholecystectomy or other bariatric procedures. Special attention should be noted in those with previous open surgery or abdominoplasty that increases difficulty.

3   Choice of Technique Based on Evidence

Evidence on RS is increasing, IFSO SURVEY presented RS as the current challenge of bariatric surgery. When BS fails, we have more than one RS alternative. In 2018 a survey was conducted with 460 bariatric surgeons from 27 countries about preferences in RS: For revision after LAGB, the RYGB (75.5%, n = 345) emerged as the most common option followed by SG (56.9%, n = 260) and one anastomosis gastric bypass (OAGB) (37.2%, n = 170). For the revision after SG, RYGB (77.7%, n = 355) was the preferred option followed by OAGB (42.45%, n = 194) and Re-Sleeve (22.32%, n = 102) [14].

Sleeve gastrectomy (SG) as RS has been described after multiple interventions, such as gastric band (LAGB), after Sleeve Gastrectomy; RYGB or endoscopic procedures.

4   Laparoscopic Adjustable Gastric Banding (LAGB)
         to Sleeve Gastrectomy (SG)

LAGB has been associated with high failure rates requiring RS [15–18]. Although band placement does not create a permanent anatomic alteration, it does not leave the stomach region undamaged. Erosion, scar tissue, pouch dilation, and adhesions make the area more complex and vulnerable during further interventions; this makes revisional surgery technically demanding [19, 20].

Recently SG has gained increased popularity as a revisional procedure after failed LAGB [21, 22]. In a systematic review and meta-analysis of Dimitrios E. Magouliotis et al. comparing RYGB versus SG after LAGB, they presented indications for conversion. The most frequent cause was insufficient weight loss (68%), band slippage/erosion (13.7%), gastric pouch dilation (3.6%) and intractable GE reflux (2.68%). Similar results are seen in other series. His team concluded that both techniques have no differences in clinical outcomes, hospital stay, complications, or excess weight loss (EWL) after a year. They found a better EWL at 2 years for RYGB [23]. Similarly, Jacobs et al. concludes that the SG has lower morbidity and mortality rates than converting to a RYGB with comparable weight loss. Average EWL was 60% at 26 months [24]. In his Sistematic review Alistair J. Sharples describes that the pooled morbidity and mortality rates for LAGB conversions are comparable to those reported for primary bariatric surgery. When comparing the EWL at 24 months, they showed 59.5% for conversion to RYGB and 61.8% after SG [7].

5   Sleeve Gastrectomy to Re-sleeve

Patients who have undergone SG but have experienced weight loss failure (insufficient weight loss or weight regain) or have developed certain complications can be treated surgically by a second intervention, such as Re-Sleeve. It is necessary to know the scope and causes of SG failures, as well as indications and results of revisions after SG. The most accepted indications for performing a Re-Sleeve are weight loss failure, if the barium swallow shows an upper gastric pouch dilation or a big, unresected fundus or if in the CT scan volumetry exceedes 250 cc. When deciding which RS to perform, the Re-Sleeve seems to be technically easier, than others, without anastomosis. With low conversion rates to open surgery and acceptable complication rates. Although it is still too early to conclude on its long-term efficacy [25, 26]. Al Sabah et al. presented a series with 24 patients undergoing Re-Sleeve compared to 12 patients undergoing RYGB after sleeve failure. Failure of SG was defined by a percentage of excessive weight loss (EWL%) of less than 50% after 1 year. All 24 patients underwent Re-Sleeve due to insufficient weight loss and dilation of gastric sleeve. Without intra-operative or postoperative complications, they achieved a mean EWL% of 57% after Re-Sleeve at 12 months vs 61% after revisional RYGB. They concluded that the results of re-sleeve and revisional RYGB for poor weight loss are feasible with good outcomes and comparable results after a 1-year follow-up [27]. Similar results were presented by Antonopulos C. et al. in 2019 comparing SG failure results, getting similar results in weight loss during the first year of follow-up in both techniques [28]. Kamal K. et al. review compared the results of the Re-Sleeve versus primary SG, where only 2 out of 7 studies showed a better weight loss in primary surgery, while in the rest it finds no differences [29]. Previously in 2015 Nedelcu et al., presented their series with 61 patients undergoing Re-Sleeve. All cases were completed by laparoscopy with no intraoperative complications. They found an EWL of 58.5% with 20 months of follow-up. Concluding that Re-Sleeve is a valid option for SG primary failure [30].

Compared with the malabsorptive procedures, Re-Sleeve offers several advantages, including increasing the restriction and decreasing the gastric output; lessening dumping syndrome by preserving the pylorus; decreasing risk of anemia, osteoporosis, and protein and vitamin deficiency (excepting B12 and thiamine level); and requiring shorter operative times. However, long term efficacy is still in debate specially in patients with higher BMI's [31].

6   RYGB to SG

The failure of a primary RYGB represents a great challenge for the multidisciplinary tema, due to the surgical difficulty and the few surgical options currently available. Himpens eta al presented a series with nine patients who presented poor weight loss (EWL < 10%) after primary RYGB. In these cases the bypass was reversed and converted to a SG, followed on a next stage to a duodenal switch in 3 patients. Two of them (28.6%) had a leak at the gastro-gastric anastomosis [10]. A few years before, the same group presented a small series with 4 patients converted from RYGB to SG, concluding that it is feasible and safe. The risk of gastric fistula is an important issue for this option (25% in this series). They reported a better weight loss, which leaves the patient in better condition to perform a second stage [32]. It could also be an option to consider when patients develops a sever malnutririon or the sleeve is as a first step for a planned biliopancreatic diversion with duodenal switch (BPD-DS) [33] or part of a conversion to Single-anastomosis duodeno-ileal bypass with sleeve gastrectomy (SADI-S) [34].

7   SG After Endoscopic Procedures

Currently, there are multiple endoscopic procedures to treat obesity. Some of which produce changes in the gastric anatomy and others only a temporary occupation of the stomach such as the intragastric balloon. These techniques are also not exempt from therapeutic failures or complications. The SG as revision surgery could be an alternative in these failures. Although at the moment there are few publications about its feasibility. Al Sabah et al. presented a case report of sleeve gastrectomy after primary obesity surgery endolumenal (POSE). The patient lost 20 kg after 6 months the revision [35]. Alqahtani et al. presented a series of 20 patients undergoing a conversion from Endoscopic Sleeve Gastrectomy (ESG) to LSG from a total of 1665 (1.2%) undergoing primary ESG. Patients who did not lose sufficient weight (defined as <5% of total weight) after at least three months from ESG, and those who experienced weight regain, were evaluated and considered for revisional options. They presented no mortality, reoperations or readmissions in any of the 20 patients after the conversion [36, 37].

8 Conclusion

All patients who are candidates for RS should be thoroughly evaluated. SG as RS is an efficient and reasonable option. It has improvements in comorbidities, weight loss and rate of complications similar to other techniques such as RYGB. The biggest drawback of this is the presence of GERD, hiatus hernia or barrett's esophagus where other options should be considered.

References

1. Estimate of Bariatric Surgery Numbers, 2011–2018. The American Society for Metabolic and Bariatric Surgery. https://asmbs.org/resources/estimate-of-bariatric-surgery-numbers (revisado el 13-05-2020).
2. Angrisani L, et al. IFSO worldwide survey 2016: primary, endoluminal, and revisional procedures. Obes Surg. https://doi.org/10.1007/s11695-018-3450-2.
3. Spyropoulos C, Kehagias I, Panagiotopoulos S, Mead N, Kalfarentzos F. Revisional bariatric surgery: 13-year experience from a tertiary institution. Arch Surg. 2010;145(2):173–7.
4. Sugerman HJ, Kellum JM Jr, DeMaria EJ, Reines HD. Conversion of failed or complicated vertical banded gastroplasty to gastric bypass in morbid obesity. Am J Surg. 1996;171(2):263–9.
5. Owens BM, Owens ML, Hill CW. Effect of revisional bariatric surgery on weight loss and frequency of complications. Obes Surg. 1996;6(6):479–84.
6. Schwartz RW, Strodel WE, Simpson WS, Griffen WO Jr. Gastric bypass revision: lessons learned from 920 cases. Surgery. 1988;104(4):806–12.
7. Sharples AJ et al. Systematic review and meta-analysis of outcomes after revisional bariatric surgery following a failed adjustable gastric band. Obes Surg. https://doi.org/10.1007/s11695-017-2677-7.
8. Daigle CR, Chaudhry R, Boules M, et al. Revisional bariatric surgery can improve refractory metabolic disease. Surg Obes Relat Dis. 2016;12(2):392–7.
9. McKenna D, Selzer D, Burchett M, Choi J, Mattar SG. Revisional bariatric surgery is more effective for improving obesity-related co-comorbidities than it is for reinducing major weight loss. Surg Obes Relat Dis. 2014;10(4):654–9.
10. Himpens J, Coromina L, Verbrugghe A, Cadiere GB. Outcomes of revisional procedures for insufficient weight loss or weight regain after Roux-en-Y gastric bypass. Obes Surg. https://doi.org/10.1007/s11695-012-0728-7.
11. van Rutte PW, Smulders JF, et al. Indications and short-term outcomes of revisional surgery after failed or complicated sleeve gastrectomy. Obes Surg. 2012;22(12):1903–8.
12. Rebibo L, Fuks D, Verhaeghe P, et al. Repeat sleeve gastrectomy compared with primary sleeve gastrectomy: a single-center, matched case study. Obes Surg. 2012;22:1909–15.
13. Gagner M. Is sleeve gastrectomy always an absolute contraindication in patients with Barrett's? Obes Surg. 2016;26:715–7.
14. Mahawar K, Nimeri A, Adamo M, Borg CM, Singhal R, Khan O, Small PK. Practices concerning revisional bariatric surgery: a survey of 460 surgeons. Obes Surg. 2018;28(9):2650–60. https://doi.org/10.1007/s11695-018-3226-8.
15. Chapman AE, Kiroff G, Game P, et al. Laparoscopic adjustable gastric banding in the treatment of obesity: a systematic literature review. Surgery. 2004;3:326–51.

16. Suter M, Calmes JM, Paroz A, et al. A 10-year experience with laparoscopic gastric banding for morbid obesity: high long-term complication and failure rates. Obes Surg. 2006;16:829–35.

17. Himpens J, Cadière GB, Bazi M, et al. Long-term outcomes of laparoscopic adjustable gastric banding. Arch Surg. 2011;7:802–7.

18. Jennings NA, Boyle M, Mahawar K, et al. Revisional laparoscopic Roux-en-Y gastric bypass following failed laparoscopic adjustable gastric banding. Obes Surg. 2013;23:947–52.

19. Moore R, Perugini R, Czerniach D, et al. Early results of conversion of laparoscopic adjustable gastric band to Roux-en-Y gastric bypass. Surg Obes Relat Dis. 2009;5(4):439–43.

20. Mognol P, Chosidow D, Marmuse JP. Laparoscopic conversion of laparoscopic gastric banding to Roux-en-Y gastric bypass: a review of 70 patients. Obes Surg. 2004;14(10):1349–53.

21. Patel S, Szomstein S, Rosenthal RJ. Reasons and outcomes of reoperative bariatric surgery for failed and complicated procedures (excluding adjustable gastric banding). Obes Surg. 2011;21:1209–19.

22. Patel S, Eckstein J, Acholonu E, et al. Reasons and outcomes of laparoscopic revisional surgery after laparoscopic adjustable gastric banding for morbid obesity. Surg Obes Relat Dis. 2010;6:391–8.

23. Magouliotis DE, Tasiopoulou VS, et al. Roux-En-Y gastric bypass versus sleeve gastrectomy as revisional procedure after adjustable gastric band: a systematic review and meta-analysis. Obes Surg. https://doi.org/10.1007/s11695-017-2644-3.

24. Jacobs M, et al. Failed restrictive surgery: is sleeve gastrectomy a good revisional procedure? Obes Surg. 2011;21:157–60. https://doi.org/10.1007/s11695-010-0315-8.

25. Gagner M, Rogula T. Laparoscopic reoperative sleeve gastrectomy for poor weight loss after bilio pancreatic diversion with duodenal switch. Obes Surg. 2003;13(4):649–54.

26. Baltasar A, Serra C, Pérez N, Bou R, Bengochea M. Re-sleeve gastrectomy. Obes Surg. 2006;16(11):1535–8.

27. AlSabah S, Alsharqawi N, Almulla A, Akrof S, Alenezi K, Buhaimed W, Al-Subaie S, Al Haddad M. Approach to poor weight loss after laparoscopic sleeve gastrectomy: re-sleeve vs. gastric bypass. Obes Surg. 2016;26(10):2302–7. https://doi.org/10.1007/s11695-016-2119-y.

28. Antonopulos C, Rebibo L, Calabrese D, et al. Comparison of repeat sleeve gastrectomy and Roux-en-Y gastric bypass in case of weight loss failure after sleeve gastrectomy. Obes Surg. 2019;29(12):3919–27. https://doi.org/10.1007/s11695-019-04123-9.

29. Mahawar KK, Graham Y, William R, et al. Revisional Roux-en-Y gastric bypass and sleeve gastrectomy: a systematic review of comparative outcomes with respective primary procedures. Obes Surg. https://doi.org/10.1007/s11695-015-1670-2.

30. Nedelcu M, Noel P, Iannelli A, Gagner M. Revised sleeve gastrectomy (re-sleeve). Surg Obes Relat Dis. 2015;11(6):1282–8. doi: https://doi.org/10.1016/j.soard.2015.02.009.

31. Mahawar KK, Himpens JM, Shikora SA, Ramos AC, Torres A, Somers S. The first consensus statement on revisional bariatric surgery using a modified Delphi approach. Surg Endosc. https://doi.org/10.1007/s00464-019-06937-1.

32. Dapri G, Cadière GB, Himpens J. Laparoscopic conversion of Roux-en-Y gastric bypass to sleeve gastrectomy as first step of duodenal switch: technique and preliminary outcomes. Obes Surg. 2011;21:517–23.

33. Nett PC, et al. Re-sleeve gastrectomy as revisional bariatric procedure after biliopancreatic diversion with duodenal switch. Surg Endosc. 2016;30:3511–5. https://doi.org/10.1007/s00464-015-4640-9.

34. Wu A, Tian J, Cao L, Gong F, Wu A, Dong G. Single-anastomosis duodeno-ileal bypass with sleeve gastrectomy (SADI-S) as a revisional surgery. Surg Obes Related Dis. 2018. https://doi.org/10.1016/j.soard.2018.08.008.

35. Al-Sabah S, Al Mulla A, Vaz JD. Revisional laparoscopic sleeve gastrectomy after primary obesity surgery endolumenal (POSE). https://doi.org/10.1016/j.soard.2016.12.027.

36. Alqahtani AR, Elahmedi M, Alqahtani YA, Al-Darwish A. Laparoscopic sleeve gastrectomy after endoscopic sleeve gastroplasty: technical aspects and short-term outcomes. Obes Surg. 2019. https://doi.org/10.1007/s11695-019-04024-x.
37. Alqahtani AR. Reply to letter to editor RE: laparoscopic sleeve gastrectomy after endoscopic sleeve gastroplasty: technical aspects and short-term outcomes. Obes Surg. 2019. https://doi.org/10.1007/s11695-019-04209-4.

Converting Endoscopic Bariatric Procedures to LSG: POSE, Endosleeve, and Balloon

Salman Al-Sabah and Eliana Al Haddad

1   Introduction

Bariatric surgery has now provided a new option for overweight patients that have attempted conventional weight loss methods and failed. With more studies being performed covering health and the detriments that come with increasing BMI's, the different emerging methods of weight loss have caught the attention of physicians, researchers, and patients alike, trying to provide the best option catered to each person individually. A systematic review and meta-analysis conducted by Gloy et al. [1] was able to demonstrate that bariatric surgery is a more effective method than non-surgical treatments for obesity, as well as the co-morbid conditions that come along with it. Therefore, more and more patients and physicians are starting to turn to bariatric surgeries, not only for the treatment of obesity, but also for the management of these co-morbid conditions.

Currently, multiple endoscopic procedures exist that are sought after due to the fact that they can be considered as 'less invasive' bariatric procedures. These include the Primary Obesity Surgery, Endolumenal (POSE) procedure, the endosleeve, and the balloon. However, long-term success rates of these procedures, especially in patients with higher BMI's, have shown to be lower than their surgical 'invasive' counterparts.

S. Al-Sabah (✉)
Faculty of Medicine, Kuwait University, Kuwait City, Kuwait
e-mail: salman.k.alsabah@gmail.com

E. Al Haddad
Columbia University Medical Center, New York, NY, USA
e-mail: Eliana.h91@gmail.com

E. Al Haddad
Amiri Hospital, Kuwait City, Kuwait

S. Al-Sabah et al. (eds.), *Laparoscopic Sleeve Gastrectomy*,
https://doi.org/10.1007/978-3-030-57373-7_13

103

Sleeve gastrectomy (SG) was initially conceived and first described in 1988 by Hess and Marceau as a restrictive component of the BPD-DS procedure at times when bariatric surgery was conducted via laparotomy. Nowadays, it has become the most performed bariatric procedure in the world (according to the numbers from the ASMBS), overtaking the Roux-en-Y gastric bypass. Therefore, it is understandable why it is considered a good option for revision following a failed endoscopic bariatric procedure.

2   The POSE Procedure

The POSE procedure was recently developed for patients with a BMI of 30–40; who have less than 100 lb (45 kg) of excess weight to lose. It currently has the advantage of being an incision-less weight loss option with fast recovery time over the popular bariatric surgeries, allowing patients to leave the hospital within 24 hours, as well as allowing for earlier intervention in obese patients for weight loss management.

2.1   How the POSE is Performed

The procedure is performed using an Incisionless Operating Platform (IOP) (USGI Medical, San Clemente, CA, USA) and endoscope, which is passed through the mouth and into the stomach. Once in the stomach, the IOP tools are used to grasp, fold, and fasten together full-thickness bites of stomach tissue. The POSE procedure involves making multiple stomach folds and securing them with expandable suture anchors. 14–18 stitches are placed in the fundus and antrum.

This procedure is still in its investigational stage in the USA, with limited data available currently on the short and long-term outcomes of it; however, its use outside the US has shown great positive results with one study from Spain showing patients losing up to 62% of their excess weight within a year [2]. Another study that followed patients who underwent this procedure for 1 year was able to demonstrate promising early results, with a 45% reduction in excess weight and an average of 50% reduction in hunger after that time [3]. A prospective observational study performed by Espinós et al. in Spain covering a period of 6 months post the POSE procedure was also able to demonstrate an EWL of 49.4%, as well as less hunger and early satiety in the patients [4]. Alhassani et al.'s study showed that all the patients that underwent the procedure reported less hunger following it, which was maintained with time, with a mean total body weight loss at 4 months of 13.21%. However, given that this procedure is still new, there isn't any significant evidence to support its effectiveness.

2.2 Converting a POSE to an LSG

Conversion from the POSE procedure after failed weight loss has been proven to be effective when necessary. The LSG is performed in a standard split-leg French position using four laparoscopic ports. Endoscopy would be used to visualize the stomach from the inside and to see the exact site of the stitches from the POSE procedure so that they can be avoided, as well as aid in the sleeve gastrectomy. Devascularization of the greater curvature of the stomach would then be carried out starting from 4 cm from the pylorus and up to the angle of His. The sleeve is then performed with a linear laparoscopic stapler using green cartridges for the antrum, body, and fundus, aiming for a final gastric pouch size of 100 ml. Endoscopy and laparoscopy are both used to ensure that the metal anchors of the POSE procedure are not incorporated or encountered when dividing the stomach. Endoscopy can also be utilized to assess for leak using air and inflation with water.

3 The Endosleeve

The Endoscopic sleeve gastroplasty, otherwise known as the endosleeve, has been showing increasing popularity around the world. It's aim is to mimic a sleeve gastrectomy by reducing the size of the gastric cavity to a tubular lumen with a line of clinched plications in the greater curvature [5]. It is indicated in patients with a BMI ranging from 30 to 49 kg/m^2 and requires an endoscopic suturing system (OverStitch; Apollo Endosurgery Inc., Austin, Texas) mounted onto a specific double- or single-channel endoscope, an esophageal overtube (US Endoscopy, Mentor, Ohio), and a tissue retraction screw (Helix; Apollo Endosurgery Inc., Austin, Texas).

3.1 How the Endosleeve is Performed

The procedure is performed under general anesthesia with orotracheal intubation. Full-thickness sutures (aiming at the muscularis propria) are delivered, starting distal (prepyloric antrum) to proximal (gastroesophageal junction), with a triangular stitch pattern (anterior wall—greater curvature—posterior wall). Each suture consists of around 3–6 full-thickness stitches. After all the sutures are clinched together, a plication is formed. To reduce the gastric lumen to the desired size, 6–8 plications are generally needed. A small fundus is, therefore, left in place (like a pouch) to delay gastric emptying.

Currently, the results are limited to short-term studies, however, showing promising results. For example, a multicentre analysis with 248 patients that were followed over 24 months demonstrated a %TBWL of 18.6% (15.7–21.5%); in an intention-to-treat analysis, 53% of these patients were able to achieve >10%TBWL [6].

It is important to note that this technique is not considered as competition to surgeries like sleeve gastrectomy or gastric bypass, but an alternative for less obese patients or those not willing to accept a surgical intervention [7, 8].

3.2   Converting Endosleeve to LSG

There is no robust literature about endosleeve failure and subsequent revisional surgery, with only a limited number of cases available [9, 10]. A recent study with 1000 patients that underwent endosleeve described the need for 8 revisions to sleeve gastrectomy in that population due to poor weight loss (%TBWL <5% after a 6-month period). However, there is no information about outcomes from that cohort [9].

A preoperative endoscopy is always mandatory to be performed before considering a revisional procedure. If none of the sutures are seen to be in place during the endoscopy, a typical SG can be offered without the need of a transoperative endoscopy. In that case, a stapler load of 4.1 mm or more is recommended along the sleeve line. The posterior wall should then be carefully dissected since anatomic modifications are typically present due to sutures and adhesions related to the inflammatory process that would have occurred post the initial endosleeve. On the other hand, if it is seen on endoscopy that some sutures have remained intact, a hybrid approach could be considered. The first part of the surgery would be to attempt to liberate the sutures during endoscopy. If this is not entirely possible, the endoscope will help to guide the correct placement of the stapler to avoid sutures and metal anchors. However, if during the procedure, a safe stapler position cannot be offered at the incisura, a gastric bypass should be considered instead. At the end of the procedure, an endoscopy is recommended to help identify any foreign body within the sleeved lumen.

4   The Balloon

The idea of using a gastric space-occupying device was first described by Nieben in 1982, based on the observation that a gastric bezoar can be well tolerated for an extended period of time and cause significant weight loss [11], however, had relatively high complication rate. The development of the saline-filled balloon revived interest in the method due to the fact that the balloon is a non-invasive restrictive bariatric procedure that is completely reversible and repeatable [12–14]. It is offered to morbidly obese patients who either refuse surgery or those who do not meet the International Federation of Surgical Obesity criteria for surgery and who had previously experienced poor results with conservative treatments [12–14]. It is also recommended for super-obese patients before undertaking elective or bariatric surgery to reduce surgical risk. However, it is essential to note that in the USA, the FDA have only approved it form patients with a BMI ranging from 30 to 40 [15, 16]. The balloon is generally designed to remain in the stomach for a maximum period of 6 months, after which there is an increased number of complications, mainly related to spontaneous deflation and intestinal obstruction [17]. It is also important to keep in mind that, given that it is a reversible short-term procedure, the maximum weight loss achieved with a balloon is significantly less than that of surgical options available.

In a published series of 19 patients with BMI 35–40 and 15 patients with BMI >40, mean %excess weight loss (%EWL) was 42.4% and 25.9% respectively on balloon extraction and 26.4% and 20.4% at 1-year post removal. In the morbidly obese patients, 7 remained with BMI >40, 4 had BMI 35–40, and only 4 patients had BMI 30–35 [18]. Although the number of patients is small, the results of this study confirm the recurrence of obesity after the removal of the balloon. The balloon, therefore, remains a good and safe method for temporary weight loss [12–14, 19–21], opening a path for other bariatric procedures afterward.

4.1   LSG Following Balloon Removal

Currently, no studies exist that examine whether there should be a delay between balloon removal and performance of a SG. While there is some debate on this subject, most authors [22–24] advocate performing a staged SG for the purpose of allowing gastric healing and hence reducing the incidence of perioperative complications; performing a staged SG a few weeks following balloon removal would ideally allow the gastric wall edema associated with the presence of an in-situ balloon to resolve. This may in turn, reduce the risk of the staple line leak and allow the fashioning of a narrower caliber sleeve.

5   Conclusion

Laparoscopic sleeve gastrectomy can be considered a safe and effective procedure to be undertaken after endoluminal procedures, given that a proper preoperative endoscopic examination is performed to ensure the viability of this surgery.

References

1. Gloy VL, Briel M, Bhatt DL, Kashyap SR, Schauer PR, Mingrone G, et al. Bariatric surgery versus non-surgical treatment for obesity: a systematic review and meta-analysis of randomised controlled trials. BMJ. 2013;347:f5934.
2. Espinos JC, Turro R, Moragas G, Bronstone A, Buchwald JN, Mearin F, et al. Gastrointestinal physiological changes and their relationship to weight loss following the POSE procedure. Obes Surg. 2016;26(5):1081–9.
3. Lopez-Nava G, Bautista-Castano I, Jimenez A, de Grado T, Fernandez-Corbelle JP. The Primary Obesity Surgery Endolumenal (POSE) procedure: one-year patient weight loss and safety outcomes. Surg Obes Relat Dis. 2015;11(4):861–5.
4. Espinos JC, Turro R, Mata A, Cruz M, da Costa M, Villa V, et al. Early experience with the Incisionless Operating Platform (IOP) for the treatment of obesity: the Primary Obesity Surgery Endolumenal (POSE) procedure. Obes Surg. 2013;23(9):1375–83.

5. Lopez-Nava G, Galvao MP, Bautista-Castano I, Jimenez-Banos A, Fernandez-Corbelle JP. Endoscopic sleeve gastroplasty: how I do it? Obes Surg. 2015;25(8):1534–8.
6. Lopez-Nava G, Sharaiha RZ, Vargas EJ, Bazerbachi F, Manoel GN, Bautista-Castano I, et al. Endoscopic sleeve gastroplasty for obesity: a multicenter study of 248 patients with 24 months follow-up. Obes Surg. 2017;27(10):2649–55.
7. Galvao-Neto MD, Grecco E, Souza TF, Quadros LG, Silva LB, Campos JM. Endoscopic sleeve gastroplasty—minimally invasive therapy for primary obesity treatment. Arq Bras Cir Dig. 2016;29(Suppl 1):95–7.
8. Kumar N, Abu Dayyeh BK, Lopez-Nava Breviere G, Galvao Neto MP, Sahdala NP, Shaikh SN, et al. Endoscopic sutured gastroplasty: procedure evolution from first-in-man cases through current technique. Surg Endosc. 2018;32(4):2159–64.
9. Alqahtani A, Al-Darwish A, Mahmoud AE, Alqahtani YA, Elahmedi M. Short-term outcomes of endoscopic sleeve gastroplasty in 1000 consecutive patients. Gastrointest Endosc. 2019;89(6):1132–8.
10. Ferrer-Marquez M, Ferrer-Ayza M, Rubio-Gil F, Torrente-Sanchez MJ, Martinez A-G. Revision bariatric surgery after endoscopic sleeve gastroplasty. Cir Cir. 2017;85(5):428–31.
11. Nieben OG, Harboe H. Intragastric balloon as an artificial bezoar for treatment of obesity. Lancet. 1982;1(8265):198–9.
12. Roman S, Napoleon B, Mion F, Bory RM, Guyot P, D'Orazio H, et al. Intragastric balloon for "non-morbid" obesity: a retrospective evaluation of tolerance and efficacy. Obes Surg. 2004;14(4):539–44.
13. Al-Momen A, El-Mogy I. Intragastric balloon for obesity: a retrospective evaluation of tolerance and efficacy. Obes Surg. 2005;15(1):101–5.
14. Genco A, Cipriano M, Bacci V, Cuzzolaro M, Materia A, Raparelli L, et al. BioEnterics Intragastric Balloon (BIB): a short-term, double-blind, randomised, controlled, crossover study on weight reduction in morbidly obese patients. Int J Obes (Lond). 2006;30(1):129–33.
15. Alfalah H, Philippe B, Ghazal F, Jany T, Arnalsteen L, Romon M, et al. Intragastric balloon for preoperative weight reduction in candidates for laparoscopic gastric bypass with massive obesity. Obes Surg. 2006;16(2):147–50.
16. De Waele B, Reynaert H, Urbain D, Willems G. Intragastric balloons for preoperative weight reduction. Obes Surg. 2000;10(1):58–60.
17. Mathus-Vliegen EM, Tytgat GN, Veldhuyzen-Offermans EA. Intragastric balloon in the treatment of super-morbid obesity. Double-blind, sham-controlled, crossover evaluation of 500-milliliter balloon. Gastroenterology. 1990;99(2):362–9.
18. Herve J, Wahlen CH, Schaeken A, Dallemagne B, Dewandre JM, Markiewicz S, et al. What becomes of patients one year after the intragastric balloon has been removed? Obes Surg. 2005;15(6):864–70.
19. Doldi SB, Micheletto G, Perrini MN, Librenti MC, Rella S. Treatment of morbid obesity with intragastric balloon in association with diet. Obes Surg. 2002;12(4):583–7.
20. Genco A, Bruni T, Doldi SB, Forestieri P, Marino M, Busetto L, et al. BioEnterics intragastric balloon: the Italian experience with 2,515 patients. Obes Surg. 2005;15(8):1161–4.
21. Sallet JA, Marchesini JB, Paiva DS, Komoto K, Pizani CE, Ribeiro ML, et al. Brazilian multicenter study of the intragastric balloon. Obes Surg. 2004;14(7):991–8.
22. Acholonu E, McBean E, Court I, Bellorin O, Szomstein S, Rosenthal RJ. Safety and short-term outcomes of laparoscopic sleeve gastrectomy as a revisional approach for failed laparoscopic adjustable gastric banding in the treatment of morbid obesity. Obes Surg. 2009;19(12):1612–6.
23. Foletto M, Prevedello L, Bernante P, Luca B, Vettor R, Francini-Pesenti F, et al. Sleeve gastrectomy as revisional procedure for failed gastric banding or gastroplasty. Surg Obes Relat Dis. 2010;6(2):146–51.
24. Goitein D, Feigin A, Segal-Lieberman G, Goitein O, Papa MZ, Zippel D. Laparoscopic sleeve gastrectomy as a revisional option after gastric band failure. Surg Endosc. 2011;25(8):2626–30.

The Sleeve Gastrectomy in Adolescents

Nesreen Khidir, Moataz Bashah and Luigi Angrisani

1 Introduction

The rapid development in science and technology has significantly impacted our lives. The lifestyle of the whole of society has changed, and people tend to adopt a sedentary way of living. Consequently, children nowadays prefer playing with technological equipment and electronic games to those that require physical activity. They tend to go for fast food and the unhealthy snacks which add to this harmful behaviour and results in them becoming overweight or obese.

The obesity in children and adolescent (2–19 years old) is measured by growth charts to determine age- and sex-specific body mass index (BMI), with a BMI $\geq$ 95th percentile being defined as obesity [1]. Approximately 18.5% of youth in the U.S. are obese, while 8.5% of those 12–19 are categorized as severely obese (BMI $\geq$ 120% of the 95th percentile); representing approximately 4.5 million children [2]. Children with obesity have a significantly higher risk of diabetes mellitus (DM), hypertension (HTN), and coronary artery disease (CAD) when they become obese adults. This risk decreases significantly if the child is non-obese by adulthood [3].

N. Khidir (✉)
Harvard T.H. Chan School of Public Health, PPCR, Boston, USA
e-mail: dr_sora4@hotmail.com

N. Khidir · M. Bashah
Bariatric and Metabolic Surgery Department, Hamad General Hospital, Doha, Qatar

L. Angrisani
Public Health Department, School of Medicine, "Federico II" University of Naples, Naples, Italy
e-mail: luigiangrisani@chirurgiaobesita.it

© The Editor(s) (if applicable) and The Author(s), under exclusive license to Springer Nature Switzerland AG 2021
S. Al-Sabah et al. (eds.), *Laparoscopic Sleeve Gastrectomy*,
https://doi.org/10.1007/978-3-030-57373-7_14

Bariatric surgery (BS), has proven its effectiveness in treating obese children [3, 4]. Recently, the American Society for Metabolic and Bariatric Surgery (ASMBS) has issued the paediatric metabolic and bariatric surgery guidelines which recommended sleeve gastrectomy (SG) as the best option for obese children alongside the roux en Y gastric bypass (RYGB) [2].

2   Eligibility

A broad range of moral issues is associated with BS for children and adolescents [3]. The adolescents' age group is very sensitive, and their lives are characterized by peaked physical, psychological and social development. Therefore, the decision of undergoing BS in children is multidisciplinary. The recent ASMBS guidelines consider BS as the standard of care for treatment of obese children and should be offered early to reverse the associated co-morbidities. However, the multidisciplinary approach for these patients is essential and of high importance. A team composed of paediatricians, bariatric physicians, psychotherapists and surgeons will be needed to offer the most appropriate care which will ultimately influence the patient's outcome.

The paediatricians and primary care physicians must be aware of the eligibility criteria and refer the paediatric patients to a specialized bariatric surgery centre to obtain the standard of care. There is an observed lack of enthusiasm to refer obese young patients to undergo bariatric surgery. However, all the published data as well as the recently issued guidelines encourage children to undergo bariatric surgery as early as possible.

2.1   Who is Eligible?

According to the ASMBS guidelines [2]: patients with a BMI >120% of the 95th percentile with a comorbidity or with a BMI >140% of the 95th percentile is eligible for bariatric surgery.

Adolescents are defined by the World Health Organization's (WHO) as persons between the ages of 10–19 years, however, younger children who meet the aforementioned criteria for bariatric surgery could be considered for the procedure, when benefit outweighs risk [2]. LSG has even proven its effectiveness in the pre-pubertal age group [5].

3   Which Procedure is Right for Adolescents

As mentioned above, the current guidelines recommend sleeve gastrectomy as the best surgical option for adolescents. LSG is known by its relative simplicity in comparison to the other bariatric procedures. However, it is the best option when it is chosen for the right patient.

An important controversial topic that needs to be considered is the link between LSG and gastroesophageal reflux disease (GERD) and its possible association with hiatal hernia (HH). Obese adolescents have a higher risk of GERD compared to their non-obese peers [6]. Data about the outcomes of GERD post LSG in adolescents is limited, nevertheless authors reported the incidence of new-onset GERD after LSG in 5.7–16.7% of adolescents [7].

The risks of long-standing GERD are well recognized; and those include the eventual development of reflux esophagitis, Barret's oesophagus and consequently oesophageal adenocarcinoma. Furthermore, the significant effect of GERD on patients' daily lives and dietary habits have been shown to severely impact the quality of life of patients suffering from it. Considering all the above factors and the early performance of LSG in youngsters, GERD symptoms should be evaluated cautiously during the pre-operative assessment. Pre-operative esophagogastroduodenoscopy is recommended routinely for all patients. Moreover, it is important to perform a meticulous intra-operative dissection and exploration of the hiatus for the presence of a hernia while undergoing BS. If present, it is crucial to combine hiatus repair alongside the sleeve. HH repair with LSG has been proven to relieve and improve GERD symptoms in LSG patients [8]. Another option for GERD patients would be RYGB, which has proven its effectiveness as the best option for obese patients with severe GERD.

Application of these principles to our clinical practice in the adolescent age group revealed that out of 696 adolescents; 667 patients (95.8%) had LSG, ten (1.4%) had RYGB, three (0.4%) had one anastomosis gastric bypass (OAGB) and sixteen had LSG with HH repair (2.3%). Laparoscopic adjustable gastric banding (LAGB) is still not FDA approved for patients less than 18-year-old [2]. However, some authors reported median BMI loss of 10 kg/m^2 at 4 years post-LSG [9]. Authors reported good results in term of weight loss and resolution of comorbidities in adolescents post (OAGB), with no incidence of growth disorders or malnutrition observed [10].

4   Pre- and Post-operative Nutritional Care

Assessment of the possible nutritional deficiencies post-LSG is crucial. Authors suggested that the existence of pre-operative nutritional deficiencies in adolescents (vitamin D, anemia, and hypoalbuminemia) persist or worsen post-operatively [11]. Hence, adolescents need vigorous pre-operative surveillance and appropriate post-operative monitoring. It is imperative to explain to the patient and his attendees the importance of post-operative compliance with vitamins and nutritional supplementation. A regular monthly follow-up after surgery for the first 3 months, then every 3 months for the first 2 years is highly recommended.

5   Psychological Concern

The current adolescents' guidelines have suggested that, except for active psychosis, suicidality, or substance abuse, mental health disorders are not a contraindication to metabolic and bariatric surgery in adolescents [2]. Nevertheless, these patients should be carefully monitored to promote positive mental health and reduce the potential risk of further mental health complications (i.e. new substance abuse or suicidality) [2].

Obese kids tend to suffer from bullying and insults by their peers. Weight loss could be the leading solution for this problem. Literature has proven that LSG has a positive psychosocial impact on paediatric patients and significant improvement of patients' quality of life [12]. The satisfactory weight loss results boost their self-esteem and perception of body image. Adolescent patients became more involved in social life and adopt a new lifestyle that is more constructive to their mental health.

6   The Outcomes of SG

Previous literature has been able to show satisfactory weight loss results in adolescents and children after undergoing sleeve gastrectomy [3, 5]. Patients had been able to maintain their weight loss in the long-term when compared to the older population. Authors relayed this to the easy implementation of life-style changes in the younger patients [3], as well as the age differences in physical activity and the basal metabolic rates that accompany the younger population.

The positive results of BS on obesity associated co-morbidities (DM, HTN, CAD, obstructive sleep apnoea) are well known. Having a child with an obesity associated co-morbidity has been shown to increase the risk of future morbidity and mortality. The impact of SG on obesity associated co-morbidities in the paediatric age group was very influential. Pre-diabetes was resolved completely in young populations [3]. DM was resolved in 63–100% of patients and no relapse was noticed at 5 years after SG [3, 13].

There is a worldwide lack of keenness to perform BS in children. However, it has been proven that there is well-established data that support and encourage the early intervention on this age group. Our previously published studies related to LSG on adolescents stressed on the importance of medical trials of weight loss before surgery. But the latest reviews and evidenced based clinical practice encourage interfering with the obesity problem in children as early as diagnosed. This will help the obese children to restart a new life and progress in their schools and social life easier and faster.

References

1. Centers for Disease Control and Prevention. Basics about childhood obesity. 2015. https://www.cdc.gov/obesity/childhood/basics.html. Accessed 20 Nov 2015.
2. Pratt JSA, Browne A, Browne NT, et al. ASMBS pediatric metabolic and bariatric surgery guidelines, 2018. Surg Obes Relat Dis. 2018;14(7):882–901. https://doi.org/10.1016/j.soard.2018.03.019.
3. Khidir N, El-Matbouly M, Sargsyan D, Al-Kuwari M, Bashah M, Gagner M. Five-year outcomes of laparoscopic sleeve gastrectomy: a comparison between adults and adolescents.

 4. Benedix F, Krause T, Adolf D, et al. Perioperative course, weight loss and resolution of comorbidities after primary sleeve gastrectomy for morbid obesity: are there differences between adolescents and adults? Obes Surg. 2017;27:1–10.
 5. Alqahtani A, Elahmedi M, Qahtani AR. Laparoscopic sleeve gastrectomy in children younger than 14 years: refuting the concerns. Ann Surg. 2016;263(2):312–9. https://doi.org/10.1097/SLA.0000000000001278.
 6. Koebnick C, Getahun D, Smith N, Porter AH, Der-Sarkissian JK, Jacobsen SJ. Extreme childhood obesity is associated with increased risk for gastroesophageal reflux disease in a large population-based study. Int J Pediatr Obes. 2011;6(2–2):e257–63. https://doi.org/10.3109/17477166.2010.491118.
 7. AboMostafa AI, El Attar AA, Mohamed AE, Shalaby MM, Atteyia MA. Pediatric and adolescent new-onset gastroesophageal reflux after laparoscopic sleeve gastrectomy. Tanta Med J. 2018;46:245–8.
 8. Soricelli E, Iossa A, Casella G, Abbatini F, Cali B, Basso N. Sleeve gastrectomy and crural repair in obese patients with gastroesophageal reflux disease and/or hiatal hernia. Surg Obes Relat Dis: Off J Am Soc Bariatr Surg. 2013;9(3):356–61.
 9. Pena AS, Delko T, Couper R, et al. Laparoscopic adjustable gastric banding in Australian adolescents: should it be done? Obes Surg. 2017.
10. Carbajo MA, Gonzalez-Ramirez G, Jimenez JM, et al. A 5-Year follow-up in children and adolescents undergoing One-Anastomosis Gastric Bypass (OAGB) at a European IFSO Excellence Center (EAC-BS). Obes Surg. 2019;29(9):2739–44.
11. Elhag W, El Ansari W, Abdulrazzaq S, et al. Evolution of 29 anthropometric, nutritional, and cardiometabolic parameters among morbidly obese adolescents 2 years post sleeve gastrectomy. Obes Surg. 2017. https://doi.org/10.1007/s11695-017-2868-2.
12. El-Matbouly MA, Khidir N, Touny HA, et al. A 5-year follow-up study of laparoscopic sleeve gastrectomy among morbidly obese adolescents: does it improve body image and prevent and treat diabetes? Obes Surg. 2017.
13. Stefater MA, Inge TH. Bariatric surgery for adolescents with type 2 diabetes: an emerging therapeutic strategy. Curr Diab Rep. 2017;17(8):62. https://doi.org/10.1007/s11892-017-0887-y.

Sleeve Gastrectomy in Non-alcoholic Steatohepatitis (NASH) and Liver Cirrhosis

Mohammad H. Jamal and Rawan El-Abd

1   Definition and Background

Non-Alcoholic Fatty Liver Disease (NAFLD) is a clinic-histopathological spectrum that results from fat accumulation in hepatocytes, that can be present without inflammatory changes (hepatic steatosis) or with concomitant inflammation (steatohepatitis), resulting in the condition called Non-Alcoholic Steatohepatitis (NASH). The histopathological finding of NASH is identical to that found in alcoholic steatohepatitis with the biopsy changes showing fat accumulation, lobular hepatitis, focal necrosis, inflammatory infiltrates, and Mallory bodies [1, 2].

2   Epidemiology

The prevalence of NAFLD is alarmingly increasing worldwide, not only in adults, where it is reported to be between 6 and 35% [3–5], but also in children and adolescents with the prevalence ranging from 0.7% for ages 2–4 and up to 17.3% for ages 15–19 years [6]. The highest prevalence of NAFLD is reported to be in the Middle East and South America [7]. The variable prevalence reported in the

M. H. Jamal (✉)
Department of Transplantation, Faculty of Medicine, Health Sciences Centre,
Kuwait University, Kuwait City, Kuwait
e-mail: mohammad.jamal@mail.mcgill.ca

Jaber Al-Ahmad Hospital, Kuwait City, Kuwait

R. El-Abd
Faculty of Medicine, Health Sciences Centre, Kuwait University, Kuwait City, Kuwait
e-mail: rawanela@gmail.com

S. Al-Sabah et al. (eds.), *Laparoscopic Sleeve Gastrectomy*,
https://doi.org/10.1007/978-3-030-57373-7_15

115

literature correlates with the coexistence of higher rates of obesity and other components of the metabolic syndrome in some countries but not others. Specifically, for NASH, literature review report it to affect 3–5% of the world's population [8]. The prevalence of NASH in NAFLD patients, however, is reported to be 60% [9]. Of those patients affected with NASH, 20% can progress to cirrhosis [10].

3 Risk Factors

Although the pathogenesis of NAFLD is not fully understood, the most accepted theory implicates insulin resistance as the cause, and this condition is said to be the hepatic manifestation of the metabolic syndrome [11]. Obesity has the strongest association with the development of NAFLD, and the risk of developing NAFLD increases the more obese the individual gets [12, 13]. Other risk factors include diabetes, hypertriglyceridemia, hypertension, disorders of lipid metabolism, total parental nutrition, severe weight loss, refeeding syndrome, and drugs [11].

4 Pathophysiology

There is strong evidence today that insulin resistance is the primary pathophysiological condition seen in patients with NAFLD/NASH who might or might not be obese. Insulin resistance in itself stimulates lipolysis, triglyceride synthesis, hepatic uptake of free fatty acids, and accumulation of hepatic triglyceride, which potentiates hepatic cell inflammation [14]. In addition, hormones such as adiponectin, leptin, and resistin, that regulate insulin sensitivity are found to exert important modulatory action through altered activation of numerous receptors and cytokines that eventually leads to hepatic cell dysregulation, inflammation, and apoptosis [15–17]. Several mechanisms are theorized to determine the extent and progression of necroinflammation in NASH. These include defects in mitochondrial function, impaired free oxygen radical scavenging, and increased hepatic iron [18–20]. The fibrosis seen in NASH is perisinusoidal (zone 3) and results due to activation of lobular stellate cells. Portal fibrosis, a feature of advanced disease, can also occur and is due to activation of a hepatic progenitor cells as a result of chronic hepatocyte injury. The degree of this fibrotic reaction correlates with the grade of NASH activity, which in turn correlated with insulin resistance [21].

5 Clinical Presentation

The clinical manifestations range from being asymptomatic with incidental discovery of the disease during imaging for unrelated conditions to biochemical finding of a persistently elevated liver enzymes and/or non-specific symptoms of fatigue, edema, pruritis, gastrointestinal bleeding, or ascites. Patients might have a normal physical examination (19–30%) or hepatomegaly (up to 53%), jaundice, splenomegaly, ascites, and/or stigmata of liver disease (5–16%).

6   Diagnosis

The diagnosis of NAFLD requires the presence of hepatic steatosis as identified by imaging or biopsy and exclusion of:

1. Significant alcohol consumption
2. Co-existing chronic liver disease
3. Other causes of hepatic steatosis (hepatitis C, medications, TPN, chronic liver diseases)

The amount of alcohol consumption considered to be significant defers according to different guidelines:

- EASL, NICE, and AISF Guidelines:

>30 g/d in men and >20 g/d in women.

a. AASLD guidance:
   >21 standard drink on average per week in men and >14 in women.
b. Asia–Pacific Guidelines:
   >7 standard alcoholic drinks/week (70 g ethanol) in women and >14 (140 g) in men.

The diagnosis of NASH, to date, relies on histologic examination showing hepatocyte ballooning degeneration, diffused lobular inflammation and fibrosis [11]. Fibrosis staging is an important factor to consider in all NAFLD patients as it was found to be the strongest predictor of all-cause and disease-specific mortality [22]. Actually, the severity of any chronic liver disease, in general, relies on the degree of fibrosis. By identifying patients with advanced fibrosis, physicians can plan more aggressive follow-up, investigations, and therapeutic measures. Although liver biopsy is the gold standard for evaluation of liver fibrosis, non-invasive investigations could substitute for invasive procedures in some patients. Table 1 presents a comprehensive list of the non-invasive methods used to detect fibrosis and assess the severity of liver disease listed by Trautwein et al. [23].

7   Non-invasive Tests

7.1   Laboratory Investigations

Laboratory abnormalities includes elevated AST and ALT (up to fivefold elevation), ALP (up to twofold), and AST:ALT ratio <1 unless cirrhosis develops. Bilirubin, albumin, and prothrombin time can be affected in late stages. However, normal liver function tests cannot exclude NAFLD and laboratory alterations may be due to a concomitant liver disease. Detection of laboratory abnormalities of elevated ferritin or low autoantibody titers (anti-nuclear antibodies and anti-smooth

Table 1 Non-invasive measures to assess liver fibrosis

Serum tests
• Enhanced Liver Fibrosis test
• FibroTest
• Fibrosis-4 test
• HepaScore
• FibroIndex
• Aspartate aminotransferase-to-platelet ratio
Liver Stiffness Measurement tests
• Transient Elastography
• Shear Wave Elastography
• Acoustic Radiation Force Impulse Imaging
• Magnetic Resonance Elastography
Magnetic Resonance-/Positron Emission Tomography-Based Imaging
• Liver inflammation score
• Proton density fat fraction
Functional Tests
• Cholate clearance test
• 13C-methacetin breath test
Clinical Scores
• Model for End-stage Liver Disease
• Child–Pugh
• Lille

muscle antibodies) may not be due to other liver disease but instead can be a sole manifestation of NALFD [24]. Kowdley et al. reported that serum ferritin >1.5 times the upper limit of normal was associated with advanced cirrhosis in 628 NAFLD patients [25]. For detecting and stages liver fibrosis, other investigations have been developed, including the Enhanced Liver Fibrosis (ELF) Panel, which tests for tissue inhibitor of metalloproteinases 1 (TIMP-1), amino-terminal propeptide of type III procollagen (PIIINP), and hyaluronic acid (HA) and was found to predict moderate fibrosis and cirrhosis in patients with chronic liver disease [26]. In fact, Kim et al. studied the use of ELF in the clinical setting on 170 patients chronic hepatitis B patients and reported it to predict liver related decompensation as good as TE with an AUROC of 0.8 [27].

7.2 Imaging

1. **Transient Elastography (TE)/Fibro scan**

Fibro scan is a sensitive imaging modality to measure hepatic steatosis and stiffness. This imaging modality incorporates ultrasonography and relies on the principle that velocity of a wave through a homogenous tissue is proportional to its elasticity/stiffness, expressed in kilopascals (kPa). It utilizes the use of a transducer probe, which emits low-frequency (50 Hz) vibrations into the liver. Those vibrations are then detected through pulse-echo acquisition, and by using an equation, the velocity of the wave is calculated. The stiffer the liver, the faster the velocity. TE is non-invasive, accessible for the outpatient setting, less expensive than a liver biopsy, free of side-effects, and requires 5–7 minutes to be performed. It also gives a more representable view of the hepatic parenchyma, as it evaluates a larger area compared to liver biopsy. In addition, the results are instantaneous enabling physicians to make quick decisions, all of which make TE useful for screening NAFLD patients and for follow-up of chronic liver diseases [28, 29].

Patients with an elastography value <6 kPa were repeatedly found to have no or minimal fibrosis and thus can be monitored with repeat TE instead of undergoing liver biopsy [30]. Eddowes et al. have studied 450 adults suspected to have NAFLD in a prospective analysis where they underwent both a diagnostic liver biopsy and Fibro scan, and they reported that Fibro scan was able to accurately identify patients with steatosis and fibrosis while using CAP and liver stiffness measurement (LSM) with an area under the receiver operating curve (AUROC) of 0.7–0.89 [31]. Also, a meta-analysis lead by Musso et al. on 32 articles evaluating the diagnostic accuracy of non-invasive tests against liver biopsy showed TE to have a sensitivity and specificity of $\geq 94\%$ and an AUROC of 0.94 when diagnosing NAFLD and differentiating its histological subtypes [32].

When used to detect significant fibrosis and severe fibrosis, TE was found to have an AUROC of 0.84 (0.82–0.86) and 0.89 (0.88–0.91), respectively [33]. Tamano et al. investigated the sensitivity of TE in detecting hepatic stiffness and fibrosis in 32 NAFLD compared to 32 chronic viral liver disease patients and found that TE is more sensitive in NAFLD than the later with its ability to differentiate between F 0 and F 1/F 2/F 3, F 1 and F 3/F 4, and F2 and F4 in NAFLD, while in chronic viral disease it differentiates F1/F2/F3 and F4 [34].

When it comes to its utility for diagnosing liver cirrhosis, a meta-analysis done by Shi et al. on 3644 patients reported TE to have a sensitivity and specificity of up to 90% in detecting portal hypertension for patients with cirrhosis [35], other meta-analysis also showed TE to be a sensitive method in detecting liver cirrhosis with an AUROC of 0.90 to 0.95 ranging from 0.90 to 0.95 [33, 36].

The main limitations of TE are faced when dealing with patients with ascites or those who are morbidly obese [29] but recent advances in creating XL probes is targeting this problem [37]. Garg et al. have tested the accuracy of Fibro scan in correctly diagnosing 76 morbidly obese individuals and found the imaging modality to have a success rate in diagnosing hepatic steatosis and fibrosis of 88% with AUROC for CAP and LSM ranging from 0.65 to 0.83 [38]. A Canadian study of 251 patients studied found that 14% had discordance between liver biopsy and TE results, with mild fibrosis, higher body mass index (BMI), alanine aminotransferase elevation, and variability in liver stiffness measurement being the main determinants of the discordant results [39]. Another study on 210 chronic liver disease patients with a BMI ≥ 28 kg/m^2 assessed the use of transient elastography XL probe and found that discordance in measurement of liver fibrosis by biopsy versus TE to be infrequent but a BMI greater than 40 led to a 4- to 5-fold increase in discordance [40].

2. Shear Wave Elastography (SWE)

This is an imaging modality that utilizes shear waves produced by ultrasound to detect liver stiffness. It was able to accurately stage fibrosis and differentiate fibrosis stages of F 0–1 from F 2–4 with high probability. It is reported to be as accurate or more accurate than TE [41]. Actually, Cassinotto et al. who have studied different imaging modalities for diagnosing 291 NAFLD patients found that both SWE and TE to have similar cutoff values for staging fibrosis: 6.3/6.2 kPa for ≥F2, 8.3/8.2 kPa for ≥F3, and 10.5/9.5 kPa for F4 [37].

3. Acoustic Radiation Force Impulse (ARFI)

ARFI performance is reported to be similar to transient elastography with the added benefits of the ability of using it on patients with ascites or those who are obese. Palmeri et al. conducted a study on 172 patients with NAFLD and found that ARFI imaging could differentiate between low (F0–2) and high (F3–4) stages of fibrosis with an AUROC, sensitivity, and specificity of 0.90. They also stated that a BMI greater than 40 did not affect results of this imaging technique [42]. Additionally, Freiedrich-Rust et al. published a meta-analysis of 518 patients supporting the diagnostic accuracy of ARFI imaging in diagnosing liver fibrosis, with AUROC curves of 0.87, 0.91, and 0.93 for significant fibrosis, severe fibrosis, and cirrhosis, respectively [43].

4. Magnetic Resonance Imaging (MRI)

MRI (proton density fat fraction or spectroscopy) is the most sensitive imaging modality to detect hepatic steatosis with a liver fat content as low as 5 – 10%. Its use, however, is limited to clinical studies due to its high cost, long time of execution, and limited availability [44]. **Magnetic Resonance Elastography (MRE)** combines MRI imaging with low-frequency vibrations to create visual images that reflect liver stiffness and can detect fibrosis, making it useful in the imaging of chronic liver disease. It is, however, costly, and labor intensive, making it a less favorable method over TE.

8 Scoring Systems

1. Fatty Liver Index (FLI)

The fatty liver index is an algorithm that predicts the presence of hepatic steatosis based on patient's waist circumference, body mass index (BMI, serum triglycerides, and gamma-glutamyl transferase (GGT). It's a score from 0 to 100, a FLI <30 rules out fatty liver, while a score ≥60 rules in the diagnosis [45].

2. NAFLD liver fat score

This score integrates hepatic transaminases and fasting insulin levels with the presence of the metabolic syndrome to predict the present or absence of hepatic steatosis. It is shown to be as effective as FLI [46].

3. Fibrosis Scoring systems

The scores used to date are the Fibrosis 4 calculator score [47] and NAFLD fibrosis score [48]. The former uses patient's age, AST, platelet count, and ALT to predict the presence of absence of fibrosis, while the later uses the same in addition to albumin, BMI, and the presence of absence of diabetes. By applying these scores, a significant proportion of NAFLD patients can avoid undergoing an invasive biopsy to diagnose their condition, with accurate prediction reaching up to 90%.

4. Biomarker Cytokeratin-18

Biomarkers of inflammation or fibrosis can predict prognosis of NAFLD patients although the presence of multiple co-morbidities is the most important predictor of progressing inflammation and fibrosis in NAFLD patients as per the AASLD guidelines. Cytokeratin-18 fragment is the most studied marker of inflammation and liver cell apoptosis and can be used to monitor NASH patients [49]. A meta-analysis found that the pooled AUROC, sensitivity, and specificity of cytokeratin-18 for diagnosing NASH to be 0.82 (0.78–0.88), 0.78 (0.64–0.92), and 0.87 (0.77–0.98), respectively [32].

8.1   Invasive Measure

8.1.1 Liver Biopsy

Biopsy remains the gold standard method to diagnose patients with the NAFLD spectrum. It can correctly differentiate Non- Alcoholic Fatty Liver (NAFL) from NASH and stage liver fibrosis, providing prognostic information regarding the risk of progression to cirrhosis [7]. NAFL is diagnosed when hepatic steatosis is >5% in liver biopsy in the absence of alcohol consumption [50]. Contrary to NASH, NAFL patients have <1% chance of developing cirrhosis or dying due to liver disease [30, 48].

Characteristically, NASH is defined by histologic examination showing zone 3, centrilobular macro vesicular steatosis with hepatocyte ballooning and inflammatory infiltrates [51]. It is important to detect these histological differences to guide management as the prognosis of NALF and NASH hugely differ. Although fibrosis tends to progress over the years in both NAFL and NASH patients as reported by a meta-analysis of 11 cohorts with a sample size of 411 biopsy-proven NAFLD patients, the progression is much faster for NASH [52].

For example, Matteoni et al., who have studied 137 NAFLD liver biop-sies found that the development of cirrhosis and later liver-related mortality is not the same across all patients with the NAFLD spectrum, and that poor outcomes are higher in patient's whom biopsy showed Mallory hyaline or fibrosis, as features of NASH [10]. This was also replicated by Ekstedt et al. who studied 229 biopsy-proven NAFLD patients for up to 33 years of follow up and found those with fibrosis stage of 3–4 had increased mortality with a Hazard Ratio (HR) of 3.3 (CI 2.27–4.76, P <0.001). In addition, a recent meta-analysis by Dulai et al. on 1,495 NAFLD patients with a person years follow-up of 17,452 showed that NAFLD patients who had fibrosis had an increased risk of all-cause and liver-related mortality with a dose response relationship. All-cause mortality of fibrosis stage 1 was Mortality Rate Ratio (MRR) = 1.58 (95% CI 1.19–2.11) while that of stage 4 was MRR = 6.40 (95% CI 4.11–9.95) and liver-related mortality was MRR = 1.41 (95% CI 0.17–11.95) for stage 1 and MRR = 42.30 (95% CI 3.51–510.34) for stage 4, concluding that the risk of mortality increases exponentially as fibrosis stage increases [53]. Even more, a study conducted by Angulo et al. included 619 multinational NAFLD patients with a median follow up of 13 years reported that fibrosis stage was independently associated with long-term overall mortal-ity and liver transplantation.

Performing a liver biopsy, however, has several limitations that include high cost, its invasive nature, pathologist variability, and sampling error [51, 54]. Thus, not all NAFLD patients should undergo liver biopsy [7, 55]. The AASLD guidelines advice to perform a liver biopsy for patients with the metabolic syn-drome, or when other non-invasive modalities classify the patient as high risk, as their disease status is more likely to be rapidly progressive, which necessi-ties accurate prognostic information. Actually, Bazick et al. have reported their results under the NASH Clinical Research Network assessing a new model to predict advanced fibrosis in diabetic patients with NAFLD on 435 patients, in which 69% were found to have NASH and 41% had advanced fibrosis, recon-firming that diabetes makes NAFLD patients a high-risk group instantly. Their model predicted fibrosis better than the NAFLD fibrosis score and can be used to assess the need for liver biopsy in diabetic patients [56]. Also, Simeone et al. have also studied the effect of diabetes on NAFLD progression in a cohort of 18,754 patients and found that diabetes was associated with 2 times the risk of disease progression and mortality [57].

The AASLD guidelines, in addition, advices a biopsy in the setting of high fer-ritin and high iron saturation levels or low titers of serum antinuclear antibody/ antismooth muscle antibody to rule out hemochromatosis, or autoimmune liver disease, respectively [7]. In addition, based on the EASL 2009 special conference, Ratziu et al. published that patients with thrombocytopenia, hypoalbuminemia and AST > ALT as signs of cirrhosis, or those undergoing bariatric surgery should be offered a liver biopsy for diagnosis and staging as NASH is highly prevalent in the bariatric patient population [55].

In summary of the above references, a liver biopsy is offered for patients who:

1. Have indicators of cirrhosis (stigmata of chronic liver disease, splenomegaly, or cytopenias)
2. Have a serum ferritin >1.5 times the upper limit of normal (NASH)
3. Are >45 years old or are obese + features of metabolic syndrome (high risk of fibrosis).
4. Have type 2 diabetes and elevated liver enzymes
5. Have low titers of serum antinuclear antibody/antismooth muscle antibody
6. Have an elevated value with a fibrosis scoring system
7. Have an elastography value >6 kPa or reliable value cannot be obtained due to obesity
8. Are undergoing bariatric surgery

Through biopsy, the NAFLD Activity Score (NAS) and Steatosis Activity Fibrosis scoring system (SAF) are used to assess disease activity.

1. **NAFLD Activity Score (NAS)**

The total NAS score (0–8) depends on 5 features on the biopsy specimens found to be independently associated with the diagnosis of NASH. These were steatosis (P = 0.009), lobular inflammation (P = 0.0001), hepatocellular ballooning (P = 0.0001), fibrosis (P = 0.0001), and absence of lipogranulomas (P = 0.001). The characteristic histologic feature of NAS found to be the most significant to diagnose NASH is ballooning. The score is the sum of steatosis, lobular inflammation, and hepatocellular ballooning scores and was found to have good reproducibility across pathologists. A score of ≥5 is diagnostic of NASH and a score of <3 excludes the condition [58]. A meta-analysis reported the pooled AUROC, sensitivity, and specificity of this score to be 0.85 (0.80–0.93), 0.90 (0.82–0.99), and 0.97 (0.94–0.99), respectively, in detecting NASH with advanced fibrosis [32].

2. **Steatosis Activity Fibrosis scoring system (SAF)**

SAF was developed in a study of a cohort of 679 obese patients undergoing bariatric surgery with intraoperative liver biopsy. This score also measures steatosis, lobular inflammation, and hepatocellular ballooning but reports a score for steatosis (S), activity (A), and fibrosis (F) to categorize patients as NASH, NALFD without NASH, and no NAFLD. The activity score (A) incorporates ballooning + lobular inflammation and can discriminate NASH if A >2 because all of the NASH patients in the study had A score ≥2 and no patients with A <2 had NASH [59].

9 Clinical Scores

1. Child–Pugh score:

This is a clinical score used to assess severity of liver disease to prioritize patients who would benefit from liver decompression or transplant allocation. It groups patients in to one of 3 categories:

- Child–Pugh A: 5 to 6 points - good hepatic function
- Child–Pugh B: 7 to 9 points - moderately impaired hepatic function
- Child–Pugh C: 10 to 15 points - advanced hepatic dysfunction

Five criterions are used to calculate the score:

1. Encephalopathy:

   - None = 1 point
   - Grade 1 and 2 = 2 points
   - Grade 3 and 4 = 3 points

2. Ascites:

   - None = 1 point
   - slight = 2 points
   - moderate = 3 points

3. Bilirubin:

   - <2 mg/ml = 1 point
   - 2 to 3 mg/ml = 2 points
   - >3 mg/ml = 3 points

4. Albumin:

   - >3.5 mg/ml = 1 point
   - 2.8 to 3.5 mg/ml = 2 points
   - <2.8 mg/ml = 3 points

5. INR:

   - <1.7 = 1 point
   - 1.7 to 2.2 = 2 points
   - >2.2 = 3 points

This score was found to help predict all-cause mortality and risk of development of liver-related complications, such as variceal bleeding. Infante-Rivard et al. studied the use of this score in 177 cirrhotic patients and found overall mortality for these patients to be 0% at one year for Child class A, 20% for Child class B, and 55% for Child class C [60]. Limitations of this score include the requirement of subjective assessment for grading ascites and encephalopathy and that it does not account for renal function.

2. MELD Score

MELD score stands for Model for end-stage liver disease (MELD) and was created to predict survival of patients undergoing transjugular intrahepatic portosystemic shunts (TIPS) [61]. This score incorporates: total bilirubin, creatinine, and INR, and it is used to prioritize patients for liver transplantation.

A comprehensive review and meta-analysis done by Peng et al. [62] to compare Child–Pugh versus MELD score for the assessment of prognosis in liver cirrhosis the concluded that both scores have similar prognostic significance in most of cases of liver disease and more studies are necessary to prioritize their use in specific patient populations.

10   Sleeve Gastrectomy in NAFLD and NASH

The hallmark of NAFLD and NASH is insulin resistance, therefore the comorbidities related to metabolic syndrome are usually present in these patients mainly, diabetes mellitus, hypertension, obstructive sleep apnea and hypercholesterolemia. Sleeve gastrectomy is therefore beneficial in treating morbid obesity in these patients and improve the control of their metabolic syndrome. The other advantage is the treatment of NASFLD and NASH in itself and the treatment of early stages of liver fibrosis halting the progress to late fibrosis and liver cirrhosis.

Souto et al., performed intraoperative liver biopsies in 521 patients while undergoing bariatric surgery and found that 95% of patients had NAFLD. NASH was common among the diabetic patients (59.4%) and prediabetic patients (49.2%) with higher rates of hepatic fibrosis in diabetic patients (56.4%) compared to prediabetic patients (29.2%) [63]. We therefore recommend performing routine liver biopsies in patients with diabetes mellitus, and the performance of preoperative fibroscan along with the addition of liver function tests and coagulation profile to routine labs in this group of patients.

Many studies reported resolution of NASH in liver biopsies post bariatric surgery [64–66]. A study evaluated 381 patients who underwent bariatric surgery and had liver biopsy taken at the time of surgery. They followed up the patients with liver biopsy at 1 and 5 years post bariatric surgery. The percentage of patients with probable or definite NASH decreased significantly over 5 years, from 27.4 to 14.2% [63].

11   Sleeve Gastrectomy in Liver Cirrhosis and Transplantation

In discussing liver disease and sleeve gastrectomy, we need to distinguish 7 group of patients:

1. Liver cirrhosis patients with low MELD score and low Child score without hepatic decompensation in the form of variceal haemorrhage, ascites, and hepatic encephalopathy who are recently diagnosed and not in the transplant list.

2. Liver cirrhosis patients with low MELD score and low Child score without hepatic decompensation in the form of variceal haemorrhage, ascites, and hepatic encephalopathy who are identified only at time of surgery.
3. Liver cirrhosis patients who need liver transplantation, but denied to be listed due to morbid obesity.
4. Liver cirrhosis patients who are morbidly obese and in the wait list for liver transplantation.
5. Liver cirrhosis patients who are morbidly obese and in the wait list for liver transplantation with a diagnosis of NASH as the cause of their cirrhosis.
6. Liver transplant recipients who had their transplant due to NASH and metabolic syndrome.
7. Liver transplant recipients who are morbidly obese, or with a diagnosis of metabolic syndrome.

The studies in the subject may be divided into studies on bariatric surgery in liver cirrhosis, studies on bariatric surgery in liver cirrhosis before transplant in patients listed for transplantation and studies on bariatric surgery during or after liver transplantation. Putting in mind these groups of patients will make us understand these studies better and allow for a future design of more robust studies to give evidence-based guidance to future recommendations.

Approximately 1–4% of bariatric patients are diagnosed with liver cirrhosis [67–69]. The dilemma in this case is which surgery to choose for these patients and how to work them up preoperatively to capture those patients and avoid a surprise diagnosis at time of surgery, which requires at times deviation from planned operative course. Another category of patients are those with known liver cirrhosis who are being worked up for liver transplant listing, who are generally presenting with more advanced disease. The timing of bariatric surgery in this category of patients is a matter of debate with scarce studies focusing on this question.

The challenges in performing sleeve gastrectomy in liver cirrhosis patients include the potential liver failure post operatively, bleeding due to low platelets and abnormal coagulation profile and increased chances of leak due to lower albumin and relative immunosuppression. Technical challenges also exist mainly due to the presence of varices in the abdominal wall and around the stomach especially gastroesophageal varices.

One of the earlier studies on the subject was by Mosko et al. [70], which evaluated patients who underwent bariatric surgery in the US, using the Nationwide Inpatient Sample (NIS) database. The outcomes of patients undergoing bariatric surgery were divided into three groups according to their liver disease: Patients with no cirrhosis, compensated cirrhosis and decompensated cirrhosis (mainly those with varices and ascites). They found that 3888 bariatric surgeries were performed in the US between 1998 and 2007 on compensated cirrhotic patients and 62 on decompensated cirrhotic patients. They reported that patients without cirrhosis had lower mortality rates than those with compensated and decompensated cirrhosis (0.3% vs. 0.9% and 16.3%, respectively). Patients with compensated cirrhosis had a more than twofold higher mortality rate (odds ratio, 2.17; 95% confidence interval, 1.03–4.55) than those without cirrhosis, while patients with decompensated cirrhosis had a greater than 20-fold higher mortality rate (odds ratio, 21.2; 95% confidence interval, 5.39–82.9), with a combined mortality rate of all cirrhotic patients at 1.2%. An important finding of this study is the relation between hospital bariatric volume and mortality in cirrhotic patients. In patients with decompensated cirrhosis, the mortality rate was 41% at low-volume centers (Performing less than 50 procedures per year), whereas there were no deaths among decompensated inpatients after bariatric surgery at high volume centers (Performing more than 100 procedures per year). In terms of the type of procedures performed, 85% of compensated cirrhotics underwent malabsorptive procedures and 57% of decompensated cirrhotics underwent the same [70].

A study on 23 patients with cirrhosis undergoing bariatric surgery revealed a complication rate of 35%. Most of the patients underwent laparoscopic Roux En Y Gastric Bypass (RYGB) and eight patients had sleeve gastrectomy with only one patient undergoing Laparoscopic adjustable gastric banding (LAGB). Only 12 of those patients were known cirrhotics and 11 patients were found to have cirrhosis at time of surgery, which changed the decision from the performance of RYGB to Sleeve gastrectomy in two of those eight patients. All the cohort were Child A except one Child B, and in two patients TIPS were performed before surgery in the form of sleeve gastrectomy. None of the patients developed hepatic decompensation and only one sudden death was reported 9 months after surgery due to unknown causes. Excess weight loss was adequate 67% ± 24.8% at 37 months follow-up [67].

Wolter et al. [71] identified 302 patients who underwent bariatric surgery and got a liver biopsy at time of surgery due to surgeon judging that the liver looked abnormal. Of the cohort 12 patients (4%), were found to have liver cirrhosis and 82.3% had an abnormal liver biopsy. Sleeve gastrectomy was performed in 49.7%, Roux-Y gastric bypass in 48.3%, and the rest were biliopancreatic diversions/duodenal switch as well as LAGB. All procedures were performed laparoscopically. Revisional bariatric surgery was performed in 11.6%. They reported a mortality rate of 0.3%, leak rate at 1%, and postoperative bleeding occurred in 3.3%. One patient developed portal vein thrombosis and one patient acute pancreatitis. They reported no postoperative hepatic decompensation and no association between histological findings and perioperative outcomes.

A Spanish multi-center study [72] included 41 patients with liver cirrhosis undergoing bariatric surgery, in which all but one were Child A patients. The majority of this cohort (68.3%) underwent sleeve gastrectomy. At one and five years of follow-up after surgery percentage of total weight loss (%TWL) was 26.33 ± 8.3% and 21.16 ± 15.32% respectively. They reported an early complication rate of 17% with one leak and no mortality. Hepatic decompensation was seen in the form of ascites in two patients only, less than 30 days post operatively. Type II DM went into remission in 53.6% of patients after one year of follow-up. What's interesting in this study is that only one patient is undergoing assessment for liver transplantation after 5 years of follow-up, with 20% of patients with child A progressing in their score and the one child B patient remaining without progressing. Six patients 14% found to have hepatocellular carcinoma in the follow-up period. We cannot deduct from this study that weight loss delays progression of liver disease, but it can be inferred and more studies are needed to confirm this hypothesis.

A study on 13 patients with Child A cirrhosis who underwent sleeve gastrectomy between March 2004 and January 2013 reported no mortality and a complication rate of 7.7%. Cirrhotic patients who underwent sleeve gastrectomy were matched to those without cirrhosis undergoing sleeve gastrectomy and found that complication rate and weight loss did not differ [73]. Therefore, we can see that benefits can outweigh risks in the absence of varices and especially in Child A patients. First of all, there is a possibility that sleeve gastrectomy causing weight loss and amelioration of metabolic syndrome can improve cirrhosis and reverse it in its early stages, thus saving the patient from undergoing a liver transplant. Secondly, there can be a delay in the progression of liver disease and a delay of the timing for transplantation, thirdly even if the patient progresses to requiring liver transplantation, weight loss post sleeve will improve the outcome of liver transplantation in terms of short and long term morbidity and mortality and fourthly many canters consider BMI >40 as a contraindication for liver transplantation and reducing the BMI by undergoing sleeve gastrectomy will qualify patients to be listed for liver transplantation. All these hypotheses require more extensive research to prove them, but there are reports utilizing Scientific Registry of Transplant Recipients (SRTR) data showing reduced post-transplant survival in obese liver transplant recipients [74]. A study by Conzen et al. [75] examined the effect of obesity in 785 patients undergoing orthotropic liver transplantation at a single institution. They found that a BMI of >35 kg/m^2 was associated with NASH cirrhosis, higher MELD score, and longer wait times for transplant. They found no difference in the operative time, intensive care unit or hospital length of stay, or perioperative complications. However, compared with non-obese recipients, recipients with a BMI of >40 kg/m^2 showed significantly reduced 5-year graft (49.0% versus 75.8%; P < 0.02) and patient (51.3% versus 78.8%; P < 0.01) survival.

Not all studies show that obesity carries a negative effect on liver transplantation, a study utilizing the Organ Procurement and Transplantation Network (OPTN) database included 48,226 patients who underwent liver transplantation between 2002 and 2013. They divided the cohort according to MELD score into 4 categories with MELD4 having those with a MELD of 25 and above. They found different outcomes according to the interaction between MELD and the BMI, where in MELD4 group the BMI did not affect the outcome and in MELD3 which contained patients with a MELD score between 19 and 24 the survival outcome actually increased with the increase in BMI [76]. Without stratifying patients for MELD score, the study found that the best survival was in those with a BMI of around 34. The study reported a relatively higher than expected mortality in the cohort at 25% with a mean of 1371 days follow-up. The issue is that at time of transplanting listing the MELD score differs than the time when a patient receives the transplant, therefore stratifying patients according to MELD may not influence the clinical decision of listing that is a controversy for morbidly obese patients. The same database (OPTN) were utilized in earlier studies showing worse outcome in obese patients [77, 78].

The cause of liver disease should be factored when examining studies looking at the relation of morbid obesity to liver transplant outcome. A metanalysis included studies from 1990 to 2013 looking at the impact of morbid obesity on liver transplant recipient survival. The authors examined thirteen studies that included 2275 obese and 72 212 non-obese patients, and found no difference in mortality between the two groups and no difference in mortality even when they performed a subgroup analysis looking at different BMI groups. However they found that obese patients had worse survival than non-obese when analysing the studies that had similar causes of liver disease [79].

In a single center study from Spain 11 obese liver transplant recipients (BMI >35) were identified out of 180 liver transplants performed between 2007 and 2013. The study found that the mortality of the obese group was clearly higher when compared to those with a BMI between 20–25 (72.7% vs. 38.9%; P = 0.032). They found no difference in postoperative morbidity or ICU and hospital stay between the groups, but obese patients were more likely to have portal vein thrombosis prior to transplants [80].

An important concept that should be taken into consideration, is that patients who are obese maybe less likely to be listed for liver transplant, therefore when examining studies looking at liver transplants in obese patients we should take into consideration that these are actually the patients who were discussed and approved for transplant listing, and they should be in theory the best group in terms of overall health conditions in comparison to the whole cohort of obese patients requiring liver transplant. A study using the 2003–2013 United Network for Organ Sharing (UNOS) data examined the association between obesity and DM and liver transplant wait list survival in hepatitis C patients. The study identified 43,478 chronic hepatitis C patients on the wait list for liver transplantation. Obesity was found to be associated with lower probability of receiving liver transplant (OR, 0.91; 95% CI, 0.85–0.97; P < 0.01), but lower probability of waitlist mortality (OR, 0.80; 95% CI, 0.72–0.89; P < 0.001) when compared to no obese patients. DM among HCV patients did not impact probability of waitlist survival or receiving liver transplant. When evaluating post liver transplant survival, compared to non-obese, non-DM patients, obese HCV patients had significantly lower post liver transplant mortality (HR 0.86; 95%CI, 0.81–0.92; P < 0.001); whereas, HCV patients with DM had significantly higher post-LT mortality (HR, 1.22; 95% CI, 1.12–1.33; P < 0.001). This highlight the complex interaction between metabolic syndrome and not obesity only on the outcome of liver transplantation and the need to evaluate the overall survival of obese patients with liver disease and not only those who will make it for transplantation [81].

12   Timing of Sleeve Gastrectomy in Liver Transplant Patients

The ideal timing for the performance of bariatric surgery in transplant candidates and recipients remain controversial. We need to distinguish between patients with early cirrhosis and patients who are declined to be listed for liver transplant and patients with cirrhosis who are already approved to be listed for transplantation. In this section we answer the question about the timing of liver transplantation in patients who are approved and listed for it.

13   Sleeve Gastrectomy Pre-transplant

The advantage of performing sleeve gastrectomy pre-transplant in patients who are listed for liver transplantation is that it may delay the need for transplantation and optimize patients' comorbidities such as DM II, hypertension, sleep apnoea and other obesity related comorbidities, thus improving liver transplant immediate postoperative outcomes and graft survival. The major disadvantage is increasing morbidity and mortality of sleeve gastrectomy due to hepatic decompensation, bleeding and leak. Optimizing the patient preoperatively is essential and identifying those with more advanced disease will allow better selection for those who will do well with sleeve gastrectomy pre liver transplantation. In general, patients with Child A cirrhosis without portal hypertension will be ideal to have their sleeve gastrectomy pre-liver transplant, but not all these patients will be listed for transplants. In the previous section we reviewed studies on this group of cirrhotic patients.

A study on patients listed for liver transplant and underwent sleeve gastrectomy included 32 patients with a median MELD score of 12 and a median BMI of 45. All of these patients had history of hepatic decompensation where 22% had a history of variceal haemorrhage, 44% had a history of ascites, and 38% had a history of hepatic encephalopathy. Hepatitis C virus was the most common primary etiology of liver disease (47%), followed by non-alcoholic fatty liver disease (31%), alcohol (9%), and hepatitis B virus (6%). Half of the patients were classified as Child–Pugh classification B and 5 of them underwent TIPS. They reported no liver related morbidity and no mortality but only one sleeve leak managed conservatively. Most patients 27/32 84% had either a stable or improved MELD score at 6 months postoperatively. In terms of liver transplant listing, 28 (88%) patients were considered eligible, with 7 patients considered too good to be listed due to their low MELD score post sleeve gastrectomy and 2 of those 7 patients were child B patients [82].

14   Simultaneous Liver Transplant and Sleeve Gastrectomy

Proponents of performing bariatric surgery at the time of liver transplantation, cite the avoidance of a second procedure, theoretical reduction of incidence of incisional hernia and the technical ease as most incisions for liver transplantation give good access to the left upper quadrant. More importantly performing sleeve gastrectomy at the time of liver transplantation with a new functioning liver will lead to the reduction of post-operative complications especially those related to liver decompensation that might occur when performing bariatric surgery pre liver transplantation. There are few reports published from groups performing the two operations simultaneously, but the largest experience comes from the Mayo Clinic in the USA, that published two studies on their outcomes [81, 83].

Heimbach et al. included 44 patients who are listed for LT with a BMI >35. All patients were enrolled in a pretransplant weight loss program, and 37 were able to reduce their weight with conservative measures and with ascites weight deducted. Seven patients underwent sleeve gastrectomy at time of LT in this cohort of patients. There were three deaths in patients who received LT without sleeve gastrectomy, and three patients lost their graft and needed retransplant. Weight regain to a BMI >35 was seen in 21/34 (60%) patients, DM post LT was seen in 12/34 (35%) patients and steatosis on ultrasound in 7/34 (20%) patients. No deaths or graft losses were seen in the combined sleeve and LT group but one patient had gastric leak and one patient had excessive weight loss. No patients in this group developed steatosis or post LT DM, and all patients had good weight loss with a mean BMI of 29, from a mean BMI of 48. All patients in the combined sleeve LT group had NASH, except one patient while 12/37 (32%) patients in the LT only group had NASH [83]. The same group published another report on their experience with longer follow-up [81]. In their updated report they included 49 patients with at least 3 years of post-transplant follow up, in which 13 patients underwent simultaneous LT and sleeve, while 36 patients managed to lower their BMI to below 35 and underwent LT alone. In the LT alone group, all regained their weight with a BMI more than 35 after 3 years of follow-up except 8/36 (22%) patients. In the simultaneous LT and sleeve group the %TBWL was (34.8 ± 17.3) compared to (3.9 ± 13.3) in the LT only group at three years follow-up. One patient from the LT and sleeve group died and four in the LT alone group at 3 years follow-up, however there were no statistically Signiant difference in survival between the groups.

15   Sleeve Gastrectomy After Liver Transplantation

The advantage of performing sleeve gastrectomy post transplantation is in mainly avoiding the complications resulting from hepatic decompensation, however surgical adhesions, including adhesions of the left lobe to the stomach as well as adhesions from incisional hernias can complicate these surgeries. Patients will be on immunosuppression, which can increase post-operative complications and will require special attention to monitor immunosuppression and avoid sub therapeutic levels due to inability to take medications or drug toxicity due to dehydration.

A single institution study reported 15 sleeve gastrectomies in patients post liver transplantation with median time from LT to sleeve at 2.2 years. They report no major complications, in particular no leak, no bleeding requiring reoperations or transfusion, no liver allograft rejection and no mortality. In the diabetic patients in their cohort, 60% stopped using insulin [84]. Another study evaluated 12 patients who underwent sleeve gastrectomy post LT and matched them to 36 patients who had sleeve gastrectomy without LT, reported three (25%) major complications in sleeve post LT group, where two patients required balloon dilatation due to poor oral intake and one patient requiring laparoscopic gastrostomy tube insertion due to poor oral intake. They report no mortality and no change in immunosuppression post sleeve and no liver related morbidity [85]. A study included six patients only who underwent sleeve gastrectomy post liver transplant. Three of these patients had their sleeve gastrectomy using an open approach due to incisional hernias. One patient had gastric fistula, requiring multiple interventions followed by death 19 months postoperatively and one patient developed chronic mesh infection requiring surgical removal [86].

Summary of Recommendations:

- Perform sleeve gastrectomy in Child A patients due to any cause of liver disease in morbidly obese patients with a BMI >35
- Perform sleeve gastrectomy in Child A patients due to NASH in patients with a BMI >32
- Perform sleeve gastrectomy in Child A patients due to NASH and Type II DM in patients with a BMI >30
- In patients with Child B, without varices or after TIPs and in case the patient is not approved for listing for liver transplantation due to morbid obesity a sleeve gastrectomy can be considered.
- In all other morbidly obese patients i.e. patients with Child B and C. We recommend performing sleeve gastrectomy at time of transplantation or post transplantation.
- In investigating diabetic patients preoperatively for sleeve, an abdominal ultrasound is highly recommended and a fibro scan is recommended.
- In investigating patients with Liver cirrhosis, referral to a cardiologist is highly recommended.

Better data is needed in the subject as most studies are case series. In particular a randomized controlled trial is required.

References

1. Ludwig J, Viggiano TR, McGill DB, Oh BJ. Nonalcoholic steatohepatitis: Mayo Clinic experiences with a hitherto unnamed disease. Mayo Clin Proc. 1980;55(7):434–8.
2. Sheth SG, Gordon FD, Chopra S. Nonalcoholic steatohepatitis. Ann Intern Med. 1997;126(2):137–45.
3. Williams CD, Stengel J, Asike MI, Torres DM, Shaw J, Contreras M, et al. Prevalence of nonalcoholic fatty liver disease and nonalcoholic steatohepatitis among a largely middle-aged population utilizing ultrasound and liver biopsy: a prospective study. Gastroenterology. 2011;140(1):124–31.
4. Browning JD, Szczepaniak LS, Dobbins R, Nuremberg P, Horton JD, Cohen JC, et al. Prevalence of hepatic steatosis in an urban population in the United States: impact of ethnicity. Hepatology. 2004;40(6):1387–95.

5. Amarapurkar DN, Hashimoto E, Lesmana LA, Sollano JD, Chen PJ, Goh KL. How common is non-alcoholic fatty liver disease in the Asia-Pacific region and are there local differences? J Gastroenterol Hepatol. 2007;22(6):788–93.

6. Schwimmer JB, Deutsch R, Kahen T, Lavine JE, Stanley C, Behling C. Prevalence of fatty liver in children and adolescents. Pediatrics. 2006;118(4):1388–93.

7. Chalasani N, Younossi Z, Lavine JE, Charlton M, Cusi K, Rinella M, et al. The diagnosis and management of nonalcoholic fatty liver disease: practice guidance from the American Association for the study of liver diseases. Hepatology. 2018;67(1):328–57.

8. Povsic M, Wong OY, Perry R, Bottomley J. A structured literature review of the epidemiology and disease burden of non-alcoholic steatohepatitis (NASH). Adv Ther. 2019;36(7):1574–94.

9. Younossi ZM, Koenig AB, Abdelatif D, Fazel Y, Henry L, Wymer M. Global epidemiology of nonalcoholic fatty liver disease—meta-analytic assessment of prevalence, incidence, and outcomes. Hepatology. 2016;64(1):73–84.

10. Matteoni CA, Younossi ZM, Gramlich T, Boparai N, Liu YC, McCullough AJ. Nonalcoholic fatty liver disease: a spectrum of clinical and pathological severity. Gastroenterology. 1999;116(6):1413–9.

11. Leoni S, Tovoli F, Napoli L, Serio I, Ferri S, Bolondi L. Current guidelines for the management of non-alcoholic fatty liver disease: a systematic review with comparative analysis. World J Gastroenterol. 2018;24(30):3361–73.

12. Luyckx FH, Desaive C, Thiry A, Dewe W, Scheen AJ, Gielen JE, et al. Liver abnormalities in severely obese subjects: effect of drastic weight loss after gastroplasty. Int J Obes Relat Metab Disord. 1998;22(3):222–6.

13. Andersen T, Gluud C. Liver morphology in morbid obesity: a literature study. Int J Obes. 1984;8(2):97–106.

14. Chitturi S, Abeygunasekera S, Farrell GC, Holmes-Walker J, Hui JM, Fung C, et al. NASH and insulin resistance: insulin hypersecretion and specific association with the insulin resistance syndrome. Hepatology. 2002;35(2):373–9.

15. Xu A, Wang Y, Keshaw H, Xu LY, Lam KS, Cooper GJ. The fat-derived hormone adiponectin alleviates alcoholic and nonalcoholic fatty liver diseases in mice. J Clin Invest. 2003;112(1):91–100.

16. Muse ED, Obici S, Bhanot S, Monia BP, McKay RA, Rajala MW, et al. Role of resistin in diet-induced hepatic insulin resistance. J Clin Invest. 2004;114(2):232–9.

17. Armstrong MJ, Gaunt P, Aithal GP, Barton D, Hull D, Parker R, et al. Liraglutide safety and efficacy in patients with non-alcoholic steatohepatitis (LEAN): a multicentre, double-blind, randomised, placebo-controlled phase 2 study. Lancet. 2016;387(10019):679–90.

18. Musso G, Gambino R, De Michieli F, Cassader M, Rizzetto M, Durazzo M, et al. Dietary habits and their relations to insulin resistance and postprandial lipemia in nonalcoholic steatohepatitis. Hepatology. 2003;37(4):909–16.

19. Valenti L, Fracanzani AL, Bugianesi E, Dongiovanni P, Galmozzi E, Vanni E, et al. HFE genotype, parenchymal iron accumulation, and liver fibrosis in patients with nonalcoholic fatty liver disease. Gastroenterology. 2010;138(3):905–12.

20. Wigg AJ, Roberts-Thomson IC, Dymock RB, McCarthy PJ, Grose RH, Cummins AG. The role of small intestinal bacterial overgrowth, intestinal permeability, endotoxaemia, and tumour necrosis factor alpha in the pathogenesis of non-alcoholic steatohepatitis. Gut. 2001;48(2):206–11.

21. Richardson MM, Jonsson JR, Powell EE, Brunt EM, Neuschwander-Tetri BA, Bhathal PS, et al. Progressive fibrosis in nonalcoholic steatohepatitis: association with altered regeneration and a ductular reaction. Gastroenterology. 2007;133(1):80–90.

22. Ekstedt M, Hagstrom H, Nasr P, Fredrikson M, Stal P, Kechagias S, et al. Fibrosis stage is the strongest predictor for disease-specific mortality in NAFLD after up to 33 years of follow-up. Hepatology. 2015;61(5):1547–54.

23. Trautwein C, Friedman SL, Schuppan D, Pinzani M. Hepatic fibrosis: Concept to treatment. J Hepatol. 2015;62(1 Suppl):S15-24.

24. Vuppalanchi R, Gould RJ, Wilson LA, Unalp-Arida A, Cummings OW, Chalasani N, et al. Clinical significance of serum autoantibodies in patients with NAFLD: results from the non-alcoholic steatohepatitis clinical research network. Hepatol Int. 2012;6(1):379–85.
25. Kowdley KV, Belt P, Wilson LA, Yeh MM, Neuschwander-Tetri BA, Chalasani N, et al. Serum ferritin is an independent predictor of histologic severity and advanced fibrosis in patients with nonalcoholic fatty liver disease. Hepatology. 2012;55(1):77–85.
26. Lichtinghagen R, Pietsch D, Bantel H, Manns MP, Brand K, Bahr MJ. The Enhanced Liver Fibrosis (ELF) score: normal values, influence factors and proposed cut-off values. J Hepatol. 2013;59(2):236–42.
27. Kim BK, Kim HS, Yoo EJ, Oh EJ, Park JY, Kim DY, et al. Risk assessment of clinical outcomes in Asian patients with chronic hepatitis B using enhanced liver fibrosis test. Hepatology. 2014;60(6):1911–9.
28. Wong VW, Chan WK, Chitturi S, Chawla Y, Dan YY, Duseja A, et al. Asia-Pacific working party on non-alcoholic fatty liver disease guidelines 2017-part 1: definition, risk factors and assessment. J Gastroenterol Hepatol. 2018;33(1):70–85.
29. Afdhal NH. Fibroscan (transient elastography) for the measurement of liver fibrosis. Gastroenterol Hepatol (N Y). 2012;8(9):605–7.
30. Gunn NT, Shiffman ML. The use of liver biopsy in nonalcoholic fatty liver disease: when to biopsy and in whom. Clin Liver Dis. 2018;22(1):109–19.
31. Eddowes PJ, Sasso M, Allison M, Tsochatzis E, Anstee QM, Sheridan D, et al. Accuracy of FibroScan controlled attenuation parameter and liver stiffness measurement in assessing steatosis and fibrosis in patients with nonalcoholic fatty liver disease. Gastroenterology. 2019;156(6):1717–30.
32. Musso G, Gambino R, Cassader M, Pagano G. Meta-analysis: natural history of non-alcoholic fatty liver disease (NAFLD) and diagnostic accuracy of non-invasive tests for liver disease severity. Ann Med. 2011;43(8):617–49.
33. Friedrich-Rust M, Ong MF, Martens S, Sarrazin C, Bojunga J, Zeuzem S, et al. Performance of transient elastography for the staging of liver fibrosis: a meta-analysis. Gastroenterology. 2008;134(4):960–74.
34. Tamano M, Kojima K, Akima T, Murohisa T, Hashimoto T, Uetake C, et al. The usefulness of measuring liver stiffness by transient elastography for assessing hepatic fibrosis in patients with various chronic liver diseases. Hepatogastroenterology. 2012;59(115):826–30.
35. Shi KQ, Fan YC, Pan ZZ, Lin XF, Liu WY, Chen YP, et al. Transient elastography: a meta-analysis of diagnostic accuracy in evaluation of portal hypertension in chronic liver disease. Liver Int. 2013;33(1):62–71.
36. Talwalkar JA, Kurtz DM, Schoenleber SJ, West CP, Montori VM. Ultrasound-based transient elastography for the detection of hepatic fibrosis: systematic review and meta-analysis. Clin Gastroenterol Hepatol. 2007;5(10):1214–20.
37. Cassinotto C, Boursier J, de Ledinghen V, Lebigot J, Lapuyade B, Cales P, et al. Liver stiffness in nonalcoholic fatty liver disease: a comparison of supersonic shear imaging, FibroScan, and ARFI with liver biopsy. Hepatology. 2016;63(6):1817–27.
38. Garg H, Aggarwal S, Shalimar, Yadav R, Datta Gupta S, Agarwal L, et al. Utility of transient elastography (fibroscan) and impact of bariatric surgery on nonalcoholic fatty liver disease (NAFLD) in morbidly obese patients. Surg Obes Relat Dis. 2018;14(1):81–91.
39. Myers RP, Crotty P, Pomier-Layrargues G, Ma M, Urbanski SJ, Elkashab M. Prevalence, risk factors and causes of discordance in fibrosis staging by transient elastography and liver biopsy. Liver Int. 2010;30(10):1471–80.
40. Myers RP, Pomier-Layrargues G, Kirsch R, Pollett A, Beaton M, Levstik M, et al. Discordance in fibrosis staging between liver biopsy and transient elastography using the FibroScan XL probe. J Hepatol. 2012;56(3):564–70.
41. Frulio N, Trillaud H. Ultrasound elastography in liver. Diagn Interv Imaging. 2013;94(5):515–34.

42. Palmeri ML, Wang MH, Rouze NC, Abdelmalek MF, Guy CD, Moser B, et al. Noninvasive evaluation of hepatic fibrosis using acoustic radiation force-based shear stiffness in patients with nonalcoholic fatty liver disease. J Hepatol. 2011;55(3):666–72.
43. Friedrich-Rust M, Nierhoff J, Lupsor M, Sporea I, Fierbinteanu-Braticevici C, Strobel D, et al. Performance of acoustic radiation force impulse imaging for the staging of liver fibrosis: a pooled meta-analysis. J Viral Hepat. 2012;19(2):e212–9.
44. Szczepaniak LS, Nurenberg P, Leonard D, Browning JD, Reingold JS, Grundy S, et al. Magnetic resonance spectroscopy to measure hepatic triglyceride content: prevalence of hepatic steatosis in the general population. Am J Physiol Endocrinol Metab. 2005;288(2):E462–8.
45. Bedogni G, Bellentani S, Miglioli L, Masutti F, Passalacqua M, Castiglione A, et al. The fatty liver index: a simple and accurate predictor of hepatic steatosis in the general population. BMC Gastroenterol. 2006;6:33.
46. Kotronen A, Peltonen M, Hakkarainen A, Sevastianova K, Bergholm R, Johansson LM, et al. Prediction of non-alcoholic fatty liver disease and liver fat using metabolic and genetic factors. Gastroenterology. 2009;137(3):865–72.
47. Sterling RK, Lissen E, Clumeck N, Sola R, Correa MC, Montaner J, et al. Development of a simple noninvasive index to predict significant fibrosis in patients with HIV/HCV coinfection. Hepatology. 2006;43(6):1317–25.
48. Angulo P, Hui JM, Marchesini G, Bugianesi E, George J, Farrell GC, et al. The NAFLD fibrosis score: a noninvasive system that identifies liver fibrosis in patients with NAFLD. Hepatology. 2007;45(4):846–54.
49. Feldstein AE, Wieckowska A, Lopez AR, Liu YC, Zein NN, McCullough AJ. Cytokeratin-18 fragment levels as noninvasive biomarkers for nonalcoholic steatohepatitis: a multicenter validation study. Hepatology. 2009;50(4):1072–8.
50. Kleiner DE, Makhlouf HR. Histology of nonalcoholic fatty liver disease and nonalcoholic steatohepatitis in adults and children. Clin Liver Dis. 2016;20(2):293–312.
51. Brunt EM, Janney CG, Di Bisceglie AM, Neuschwander-Tetri BA, Bacon BR. Nonalcoholic steatohepatitis: a proposal for grading and staging the histological lesions. Am J Gastroenterol. 1999;94(9):2467–74.
52. Singh S, Allen AM, Wang Z, Prokop LJ, Murad MH, Loomba R. Fibrosis progression in nonalcoholic fatty liver vs nonalcoholic steatohepatitis: a systematic review and meta-analysis of paired-biopsy studies. Clin Gastroenterol Hepatol. 2015;13(4):643–54.e1–9; quiz e39–40.
53. Dulai PS, Singh S, Patel J, Soni M, Prokop LJ, Younossi Z, et al. Increased risk of mortality by fibrosis stage in nonalcoholic fatty liver disease: systematic review and meta-analysis. Hepatology. 2017;65(5):1557–65.
54. Ratziu V, Charlotte F, Heurtier A, Gombert S, Giral P, Bruckert E, et al. Sampling variability of liver biopsy in nonalcoholic fatty liver disease. Gastroenterology. 2005;128(7):1898–906.
55. Ratziu V, Bellentani S, Cortez-Pinto H, Day C, Marchesini G. A position statement on NAFLD/NASH based on the EASL 2009 special conference. J Hepatol. 2010;53(2):372–84.
56. Bazick J, Donithan M, Neuschwander-Tetri BA, Kleiner D, Brunt EM, Wilson L, et al. Clinical model for NASH and advanced fibrosis in adult patients with diabetes and NAFLD: guidelines for referral in NAFLD. Diabetes Care. 2015;38(7):1347–55.
57. Simeone JC, Bae JP, Hoogwerf BJ, Li Q, Haupt A, Ali AK, et al. Clinical course of non-alcoholic fatty liver disease: an assessment of severity, progression, and outcomes. Clin Epidemiol. 2017;9:679–88.
58. Kleiner DE, Brunt EM, Van Natta M, Behling C, Contos MJ, Cummings OW, et al. Design and validation of a histological scoring system for nonalcoholic fatty liver disease. Hepatology. 2005;41(6):1313–21.
59. Bedossa P, Poitou C, Veyrie N, Bouillot JL, Basdevant A, Paradis V, et al. Histopathological algorithm and scoring system for evaluation of liver lesions in morbidly obese patients. Hepatology. 2012;56(5):1751–9.

60. Infante-Rivard C, Esnaola S, Villeneuve JP. Clinical and statistical validity of conventional prognostic factors in predicting short-term survival among cirrhotics. Hepatology. 1987;7(4):660–4.
61. Malinchoc M, Kamath PS, Gordon FD, Peine CJ, Rank J, ter Borg PC. A model to predict poor survival in patients undergoing transjugular intrahepatic portosystemic shunts. Hepatology. 2000;31(4):864–71.
62. Peng Y, Qi X, Guo X. Child-Pugh versus MELD score for the assessment of prognosis in liver cirrhosis: a systematic review and meta-analysis of observational studies. Medicine (Baltimore). 2016;95(8):e2877.
63. Souto KP, Meinhardt NG, Ramos MJ, Ulbrich-Kulkzynski JM, Stein AT, Damin DC. Nonalcoholic fatty liver disease in patients with different baseline glucose status undergoing bariatric surgery: analysis of intraoperative liver biopsies and literature review. Surg Obes Relat Dis. 2018;14(1):66–73.
64. Mathurin P, Hollebecque A, Arnalsteen L, Buob D, Leteurtre E, Caiazzo R, et al. Prospective study of the long-term effects of bariatric surgery on liver injury in patients without advanced disease. Gastroenterology. 2009;137(2):532–40.
65. Liu X, Lazenby AJ, Clements RH, Jhala N, Abrams GA. Resolution of nonalcoholic steatohepatits after gastric bypass surgery. Obes Surg. 2007;17(4):486–92.
66. Mattar SG, Velcu LM, Rabinovitz M, Demetris AJ, Krasinskas AM, Barinas-Mitchell E, et al. Surgically-induced weight loss significantly improves nonalcoholic fatty liver disease and the metabolic syndrome. Ann Surg. 2005;242(4):610–7; discussion 8–20.
67. Shimizu H, Phuong V, Maia M, Kroh M, Chand B, Schauer PR, et al. Bariatric surgery in patients with liver cirrhosis. Surg Obes Relat Dis. 2013;9(1):1–6.
68. Kral JG, Thung SN, Biron S, Hould FS, Lebel S, Marceau S, et al. Effects of surgical treatment of the metabolic syndrome on liver fibrosis and cirrhosis. Surgery. 2004;135(1):48–58.
69. Brolin RE, Bradley LJ, Taliwal RV. Unsuspected cirrhosis discovered during elective obesity operations. Arch Surg. 1998;133(1):84–8.
70. Mosko JD, Nguyen GC. Increased perioperative mortality following bariatric surgery among patients with cirrhosis. Clin Gastroenterol Hepatol. 2011;9(10):897–901.
71. Wolter S, Duprée A, Coelius C, El Gammal A, Kluwe J, Sauer N, et al. Influence of liver disease on perioperative outcome after bariatric surgery in a Northern German cohort. Obes Surg. 2017;27(1):90–5.
72. Miñambres I, Rubio MA, de Hollanda A, Breton I, Vilarrasa N, Pellitero S, et al. Outcomes of bariatric surgery in patients with cirrhosis. Obes Surg. 2019;29(2):585–92.
73. Rebibo L, Gerin O, Verhaeghe P, Dhahri A, Cosse C, Regimbeau JM. Laparoscopic sleeve gastrectomy in patients with NASH-related cirrhosis: a case-matched study. Surg Obes Relat Dis. 2014;10(3):405–10; quiz 565.
74. Perez-Protto SE, Quintini C, Reynolds LF, You J, Cywinski JB, Sessler DI, et al. Comparable graft and patient survival in lean and obese liver transplant recipients. Liver Transplant. 2013;19(8):907–15.
75. Conzen KD, Vachharajani N, Collins KM, Anderson CD, Lin Y, Wellen JR, et al. Morbid obesity in liver transplant recipients adversely affects longterm graft and patient survival in a single-institution analysis. HPB (Oxford). 2015;17(3):251–7.
76. Chang SH, Liu X, Carlsson NP, Park Y, Colditz GA, Garonzik-Wang JM, et al. Reexamining the association of body mass index with overall survival outcomes after liver transplantation. Transplant Direct. 2017;3(7):e172.
77. Nair S, Verma S, Thuluvath PJ. Obesity and its effect on survival in patients undergoing orthotopic liver transplantation in the United States. Hepatology. 2002;35(1):105–9.
78. Rustgi VK, Marino G, Rustgi S, Halpern MT, Johnson LB, Tolleris C, et al. Impact of body mass index on graft failure and overall survival following liver transplant. Clin Transplant. 2004;18(6):634–7.
79. Saab S, Lalezari D, Pruthi P, Alper T, Tong MJ. The impact of obesity on patient survival in liver transplant recipients: a meta-analysis. Liver Int. 2015;35(1):164–70.

80. Triguero J, García A, Molina A, San Miguel C, Notario P, Villegas T, et al. Complications associated with liver transplantation in recipients with body mass index >35 kg/m^2: would it be a poor prognosis predictive factor? Transplant Proc. 2015;47(9):2650–2.
81. Aguilar M, Liu B, Holt EW, Bhuket T, Wong RJ. Impact of obesity and diabetes on wait-list survival, probability of liver transplantation and post-transplant survival among chronic hepatitis C virus patients. Liver Int. 2016;36(8):1167–75.
82. Sharpton SR, Terrault NA, Posselt AM. Outcomes of sleeve gastrectomy in obese liver transplant candidates. Liver Transplant. 2019;25(4):538–44.
83. Heimbach JK, Watt KD, Poterucha JJ, Ziller NF, Cecco SD, Charlton MR, et al. Combined liver transplantation and gastric sleeve resection for patients with medically complicated obesity and end-stage liver disease. Am J Transplant. 2013;13(2):363–8.
84. Morris MC, Jung AD, Kim Y, Lee TC, Kaiser TE, Thompson JR, et al. Delayed sleeve gastrectomy following liver transplantation: a 5-year experience. Liver Transplant. 2019;25(11):1673–81.
85. Tsamalaidze L, Stauffer JA, Arasi LC, Villacreses DE, Franco JSS, Bowers S, et al. Laparoscopic sleeve gastrectomy for morbid obesity in patients after orthotopic liver transplant: a matched case-control study. Obes Surg. 2018;28(2):444–50.
86. Osseis M, Lazzati A, Salloum C, Gavara CG, Compagnon P, Feray C, et al. Sleeve gastrectomy after liver transplantation: feasibility and outcomes. Obes Surg. 2018;28(1):242–8.

Sleeve Gastrectomy in Immunocompromised Patients

Amin Andalib

1 Introduction

Over the course of the past decade and a half, sleeve gastrectomy (SG) has become the most frequently performed primary bariatric surgery worldwide [1, 2]. During this time period, the popularity of SG has mainly been driven by the inferior results after adjustable gastric banding coupled with SG procedure being technically easier to perform compared to bypass-type procedures [3, 4] as well as its safety profile and the satisfactory long-term outcomes [5–7]. Consequently, SG has turned into the procedure of choice in patients with complex medical histories including those suffering from advanced chronic kidney disease [8], renal transplant candidates [9] or patients suffering from inflammatory bowel disease (IBD) [10] and other conditions requiring chronic immunosuppressant therapy [11].

2 Safety and Postoperative Morbidity

In the general population and irrespective of comorbid conditions, laparoscopic SG is considered to be very safe with a thirty-day mortality and composite morbidity of 0.05% and 2.4%, respectively [12]. Two of the most troubling postoperative complications are postoperative staple-line leaks (0.6–1%) and hemorrhage (0.7–1.4%) [12–14].

In the current era of bariatric surgery, with the improved operative safety profiles and the established role for minimally invasive techniques, patients who

A. Andalib (✉)
Center for Bariatric Surgery, Department of Surgery, McGill University, Montreal, QC, Canada
e-mail: amin.andalib@mcgill.ca

undergo bariatric/metabolic procedures more frequently suffer from severe base-line chronic conditions including IBD, rheumatoid/autoimmune disorders, and solid organ transplantation. These conditions are routinely treated with immu-nosuppressive agents and other novel disease-modifying anti-rheumatic drugs (DMARDs). Consequently, the immunocompromised patients are considered a high-risk population for perioperative adverse events by the nature of their chronic use of immunosuppressants and other DMARDs that impact their wound healing and prone them to infectious postoperative complications [15, 16].

2.1 Postoperative Morbidity After SG in Immunocompromised Patients

For the immunocompromised patient population, SG is widely accepted as the bariatric/metabolic procedure of choice [17] and this is primarily due to its accept-able safety profile and low incidence of major postoperative complications.

In a large multicenter study using 2005–2013 data from the American College of Surgeons National Surgical Quality Improvement Program (ACS NSQIP), Andalib et al. evaluated the 30-day postoperative outcomes of primary SG and roux-en y gastric bypass (RYGB) in patients on chronic immunosuppressant medications within at least 30 days prior to surgery [11]. While 30-day postop-erative mortality and major morbidity were significantly higher among the patients dependent of chronic immunosuppression compared to those who were not (0.5% vs. 0.1% and 5.0% vs. 2.5%, respectively), the prevalence of such major complica-tions were acceptable. Furthermore, both SG and RYGB procedures were found to be equally safe in this patient population [11]. In another large study by Mazzei et al. using 2015–2016 Metabolic and Bariatric Surgery Accreditation and Quality Improvement Program (MBSAQIP) data, after a propensity-matched analysis, chronic preoperative use of corticosteroids was not found to be an independent predictor for worse outcomes except for a two-fold higher risk for leak (0.6% vs. 0.3%) along with slightly higher risk of readmission and reintervention after both SG and RYGB compared to patients who did not take steroids [18]. Despite the ele-vated risk, the overall incidence of such postoperative adverse events remains low. In addition, there is also data demonstrating the safety of continuing certain immu-nomodulators and biologic agents in the immediate perioperative period leading up to surgery such as cardiac, orthopedic and colorectal procedures [18–20].

2.2 Perioperative Timing of Immunosuppressive Therapy

Given that the use of immunosuppressant/modulators is often critical for mainte-nance and management of patients' chronic rheumatoid and autoimmune disor-ders, the consequences of withholding perioperative dosing should be carefully considered by bariatric surgeons and in consultation with the respective treating specialists. Moreover, due to the lack of high-quality studies on the perioperative use and management of these agents in patients undergoing bariatric surgery, there is great variability in clinical practice regarding holding or timing of perioperative dosing of immunosuppressive agents [21].

In a recent systematic review, Kassel et al. attempted to evaluate the impact and management of perioperative use of immunosuppressive agents in patients undergoing bariatric surgery [21]. However, given the limited literature available on the use of immunosuppressive therapies in patients undergoing bariatric surgery, data from non-bariatric procedures, specifically abdominal or other gastrointestinal operations were used to examine the risks associated with perioperative use of immunosuppressive agents and DMARDs. Also due to the small and heterogeneous nature of the available studies, the data could not be pooled to provide a meta-analysis [21]. Although immunosuppressants discussed in this review article were associated with an increased risk for infections, the limited data available suggest corticosteroids, methotrexate, and tumor necrosis factor-alpha (TNF-α) inhibitors may be safe to restart postoperatively provided there are no signs of infections [21]. Furthermore, if medically possible prior to elective bariatric surgery, one should aim to hold immunosuppressants 2–12 weeks preoperatively and until 2–4 weeks after surgery [22, 23]. For biologic immunomodulators and other DMARDs like TNF-α inhibitors, the timing of the surgery should ideally be planned according to the last dose since most agents are administered every 2–8 weeks (Table 1) and if needed only one dose may be skipped after surgery [24].

Therefore, management of each immunosuppressant agent must be handled individually and based on their respective routine interval dosing due to the

Table 1 Summary of preoperative dosing recommendations for selected TNF-α inhibitors. (Adapted from Ref. [21])

Generic name (Brand)	Route of administration	Dosing interval[a]	Half-life	Recommended administration of last dose (before surgery date)[b]
Adalimumab (Humira)	SC	1–2 weeks	14 days	2–3 weeks
Certolizumab (Cimzia)	SC	2–4 weeks	14 days	3–5 weeks
Etanercept (Enbrel)	SC	1–2 weeks	3 days	2–3 weeks
Golimumab (Simponi)	SC	4 weeks	14 days	5 weeks
	IV	8 weeks	–	9 weeks
Infliximab (Remicade)	SC	4–8 weeks	9 days	5–9 weeks

TNF-α = Tumor necrosis factor-alpha; SC = Subcutaneous; IV = Intravenous
[a]Dosing interval may vary based on the indication for the medication and the severity of the disease
[b]Administration of the last dose may vary depending on the dosing interval

varying disease-specific desired effects and the potential for undesired perioperative adverse events. Ideally, the decision and the timing to withhold the immuno-suppressant medications should be weighed against the benefits of their use for each case individually and in a multi-disciplinary fashion. Additional research is needed to determine, with more granularity, the timing recommendations to hold and restart these medications with respect to bariatric surgery.

3   Outcomes of SG in Immunocomromised Patients

3.1   Weight Loss and Improvements in Obesity-Related Conditions

As previously mentioned, the literature on the use of bariatric surgery especially SG in immunocompromised patients is scant. Therefore, the data on the beneficial outcomes of SG in this patient population is also mainly driven from case series [10, 25–27]. Furthermore, given the small sample size in reported studies, and an even smaller sample size for those who underwent SG, reported weight loss and comorbidity outcomes are pooled together and reported for all types of bariatric surgery included [10, 25–27].

In a systematic review, Shoar et al. discuss 7 studies that have reported outcomes of bariatric surgery in a total of 43 IBD patients of whom 58% suffered from Crohn's disease [27]. Crohn's patients more often underwent SG (72%), while those with ulcerative colitis underwent SG or RYGB in similar frequency (44%). Overall between 8 and 77 months after bariatric surgery, IBD patients had an average 71% excess weight loss (EWL) and a 14.3 kg/m^2 drop in body mass index (BMI) [27].

In a recent prospective cohort study, Xu et al. report on the 1-year outcomes of obese patients suffering from rheumatoid arthritis who underwent bariatric surgery ($n = 32$) and compared them to an obese non-surgical group ($n = 33$) [28]. In the surgical arm, 41% of patients underwent SG procedure and the rest had RYGB. At one-year, bariatric surgery yielded an average 33 kg weight loss equivalent to 11.3 kg/m^2 drop in BMI [28].

In terms of long-term weight loss after SG procedure in the general population, a 40–60% EWL or a mean BMI reduction of 8–10 kg/m^2 are realistic estimates to consider [29–31]. Moreover, long-term improvements in obesity-related conditions especially metabolic syndrome including type 2 diabetes mellitus after SG are impressive and occur in >60% of patient population [6, 30, 31]. When comparing long-term outcomes of SG to RYGB, a recent meta-analysis of 4 randomized control trials with reported 5-year outcomes of SG and RYGB procedures revealed that weight loss up to 5 years after surgery has been either comparable or favoring RYGB with only a modest difference in BMI (1–2 kg/m^2) and weight loss up to 5 kg [7]. Moreover, five years after surgery, the remission rate of type 2 diabetes mellitus was similar between SG and RYGB (55% vs. 60%, respectively; $p = 0.42$) [7]. Hence, SG procedure is highly effective for weight loss and improving obesity-related conditions. Finally, as demonstrated above the weight loss and related comorbidity outcomes after SG procedure appear to be similar among the immunocompromised patients and the general population.

3.2 Changes to Rheumatoid and Autoimmune Conditions

Obesity is common among patients with rheumatoid and autoimmune disorders such as rheumatoid arthritis and IBD [32, 33]. Moreover, obese patients with these conditions often have worse response to therapy after all types of DMARDs [34–36]. This association is not very surprising as obesity is linked to an increase in a pro-inflammatory state mediated by known cytokines such as interleukin-6, TNF-α, as well as adipokines such as leptin, adiponectin, and resistin, or neuro-peptides such as substance P, which are all molecules either produced within adipocytes or within macrophages and lymphocytes that infiltrate the mesenteric fat [37, 38]. Consequently, since both obesity and autoimmune disorders share a chronic inflammatory state, the advantage of bariatric/metabolic surgery in allevi-ating severity of such conditions is not surprising.

Various studies have demonstrated the improvement in many autoimmune dis-orders after bariatric surgery. In a study using 2004–2014 United States National Inpatient Sample database, Sharma et al. identified 15,319 morbidly obese patients who had a combined discharge diagnosis of IBD, of whom 3.2% (n=493) had prior bariatric surgeries (47% underwent SG; n=233) [39]. They found that a prior bariatric surgery was associated with lower incidence rate ratios for renal failure, malnutrition, and fistulae formation compared to obese non-surgical group [39]. The systematic review by Shoar et al. mentioned earlier evaluating out-comes of bariatric surgery in 43 IBD patients, of whom 58% had Crohn's disease mainly involving the small bowel, reported disease remission in 20 patients (48%), improvement in another two individuals (5%), but disease exacerbation was noted in 17% [27]. Interestingly, intestinal bacterial overgrowth that can develop due to bypass-type bariatric procedures like RYGB, may be associated with acute flare-ups of Crohn's disease [40, 41]. Also, there is a potential risk of flare-up cri-ses in patients with small bowel Crohn's disease, involving the operated segments of the small bowel after RYGB. Thus, one might argue that for obese patients with Crohn's disease especially those with small bowel involvement and previous bowel resections, SG should be the bariatric procedure of choice.

Similar association and improvements were shown after bariatric surgery for patients with other rheumatoid disorders including gout, psoriasis, systemic lupus erythematosus, multiple sclerosis, and rheumatoid arthritis [42–46]. As mentioned above, in a prospective cohort study, Xu et al. reported on 1-year outcomes of obese patients suffering from rheumatoid arthritis who underwent bariatric surgery (41% had SG surgery) compared to an obese non-surgical group [28]. At 1-year follow-up and compared to obese controls, patients who underwent bariatric sur-gery, showed significantly better American College of Rheumatology 20/50/70

(ACR 20/50/70) criteria and the weight loss after surgery was associated with lower disease activity [28].

Finally, although bariatric procedures are shown to improve outcomes of obese patients with rheumatoid disorders, bariatric surgery could also lead to some deleterious effects especially with respect to bone metabolism and is associated with an elevated risk of fractures [46]. SG is shown to have a less negative impact on bone metabolism compared to bypass-type procedures like RYGB or duodenal switch [47–49]. Thus, in the absence of any contraindication like severe gastroesophageal reflux disease, SG may once again be a better procedure choice in the immunocompromised patients due to rheumatoid disorders.

4   Summary

In summary, while studies on the perioperative use of immunosuppressive agents in patients undergoing bariatric surgery are lacking, the use of these medications in this population are not. The timing and the risk of withholding immunosuppressant medications should be weighed against the benefits of their use in each case and in a multi-disciplinary fashion. If medically possible prior to elective bariatric surgery, one should aim to hold immunosuppressants 2–12 weeks preoperatively and until 2–4 weeks after surgery. When applicable, for some DMARDs like TNF-α inhibitors, the timing of the surgery should be planned according to the last dose since most agents are administered every 2–8 weeks and if needed only one dose can be skipped after surgery. The beneficial outcomes of SG including weight loss and improvements in obesity-related conditions in the immunocompromised patients are comparable to those in immunocompetent individuals. Furthermore, given that both obesity and rheumatoid/autoimmune disorders share a chronic inflammatory state, it is not surprising that a reduction in obesity-induced inflammation after SG can lead to improvements in these conditions requiring immunosuppressive therapy.

References

1. Khorgami Z, Shoar S, Andalib A, Aminian A, Brethauer SA, Schauer PR. Trends in utilization of bariatric surgery, 2010–2014: sleeve gastrectomy dominates. Surg Obes Relat Dis. 2017;13:774–8.
2. Angrisani L, Santonicola A, Iovino P, Vitiello A, Zundel N, Buchwald H, Scopinaro N. Bariatric surgery and endoluminal procedures: IFSO worldwide survey 2014. Obes Surg. 2017;27:2279–89.
3. Aminian A, Chaudhry RM, Khorgami Z, Andalib A, Augustin T, Rodriguez J, Kroh M, Schauer PR, Brethauer SA. A challenge between trainee education and patient safety: does fellow participation impact postoperative outcomes following bariatric surgery? Obes Surg. 2016;26:1999–2005.
4. Bouchard P, Demyttenaere S, Court O, Franco EL, Andalib A. Surgeon and hospital volume outcomes in bariatric surgery: a population-level study. Surg Obes Relat Dis. 2020;16:674–81.

5. Aminian A, Brethauer SA, Andalib A, Punchai S, Mackey J, Rodriguez J, Rogula T, Kroh M, Schauer PR. Can sleeve gastrectomy "cure" diabetes? Long-term metabolic effects of sleeve gastrectomy in patients with type 2 diabetes. Ann Surg. 2016;264:674–81.

6. Schauer PR, Bhatt DL, Kirwan JP, Wolski K, Aminian A, Brethauer SA, Navaneethan SD, Singh RP, Pothier CE, Nissen SE, Kashyap SR. Bariatric surgery versus intensive medical therapy for diabetes—5-year outcomes. N Engl J Med. 2017;376:641–51.

7. Aminian A. Bariatric procedure selection in patients with type 2 diabetes: choice between Roux-en-Y gastric bypass or sleeve gastrectomy. Surg Obes Relat Dis. 2020;16:332–9.

8. Andalib A, Aminian A, Khorgami Z, Navaneethan SD, Schauer PR, Brethauer SA. Safety analysis of primary bariatric surgery in patients on chronic dialysis. Surg Endosc. 2016;30:2583–91.

9. Bouchard P, Tchervenkov J, Demyttenaere S, Court O, Andalib A. Safety and efficacy of the sleeve gastrectomy as a strategy towards kidney transplantation. Surg Endosc. 2020;34:2657–64.

10. Aminian A, Andalib A, Ver MR, Corcelles R, Schauer PR, Brethauer SA. Outcomes of bariatric surgery in patients with inflammatory bowel disease. Obes Surg. 2016;26:1186–90.

11. Andalib A, Aminian A, Khorgami Z, Jamal MH, Augustin T, Schauer PR, Brethauer SA. Early postoperative outcomes of primary bariatric surgery in patients on chronic steroid or immunosuppressive therapy. Obes Surg. 2016;26:1479–86.

12. Aminian A, Brethauer SA, Sharafkhah M, Schauer PR. Development of a sleeve gastrectomy risk calculator. Surg Obes Relat Dis. 2015;11:758–64.

13. Birkmeyer NJ, Dimick JB, Share D, Hawasli A, English WJ, Genaw J, Finks JF, Carlin AM, Birkmeyer JD, Michigan Bariatric Surgery C. Hospital complication rates with bariatric surgery in Michigan. JAMA. 2010;304:435–42.

14. Berger ER, Clements RH, Morton JM, Huffman KM, Wolfe BM, Nguyen NT, Ko CY, Hutter MM. The Impact of different surgical techniques on outcomes in laparoscopic sleeve gastrectomies: the first report from the Metabolic and Bariatric Surgery Accreditation and Quality Improvement Program (MBSAQIP). Ann Surg. 2016;264:464–73.

15. Ahmed Ali U, Martin ST, Rao AD, Kiran RP. Impact of preoperative immunosuppressive agents on postoperative outcomes in Crohn's disease. Dis Colon Rectum. 2014;57:663–74.

16. Abou Khalil M, Abou-Khalil J, Motter J, Vasilevsky CA, Morin N, Ghitulescu G, Boutros M. Immunosuppressed patients with Crohn's disease are at increased risk of postoperative complications: results from the ACS-NSQIP database. J Gastrointest Surg. 2019;23:1188–97.

17. Gagner M, Hutchinson C, Rosenthal R. Fifth international consensus conference: current status of sleeve gastrectomy. Surg Obes Relat Dis. 2016;12:750–6.

18. Mazzei M, Zhao H, Edwards MA. Perioperative outcomes of bariatric surgery in the setting of chronic steroid use: an MBSAQIP database analysis. Surg Obes Relat Dis. 2019;15:926–34.

19. Uchino M, Ikeuchi H, Bando T, Chohno T, Sasaki H, Horio Y, Kuwahara R, Minagawa T, Goto Y, Ichiki K, Nakajima K, Takahashi Y, Ueda T, Takesue Y. Associations between multiple immunosuppressive treatments before surgery and surgical morbidity in patients with ulcerative colitis during the era of biologics. Int J Colorectal Dis. 2019;34:699–710.

20. George MD, Baker JF, Winthrop KL, Goldstein SD, Alemao E, Chen L, Wu Q, Xie F, Curtis JR. Immunosuppression and the risk of readmission and mortality in patients with rheumatoid arthritis undergoing hip fracture, abdominopelvic and cardiac surgery. Ann Rheum Dis. 2020;79:573–80.

21. Kassel L, Hutton A, Zumach G, Rand J. Systematic review of perioperative use of immunosuppressive agents in patients undergoing bariatric surgery. Surg Obes Relat Dis. 2020;16:144–57.

22. Fleshner P. Expert commentary on perioperative management of biologic and immunosuppressive medications in Crohn's disease. Dis Colon Rectum. 2018;61:431–2.

23. Goodman SM, Springer B, Guyatt G, Abdel MP, Dasa V, George M, Gewurz-Singer O, Giles JT, Johnson B, Lee S, Mandl LA, Mont MA, Sculco P, Sporer S, Stryker L, Turgunbaev

M, Brause B, Chen AF, Gililland J, Goodman M, Hurley-Rosenblatt A, Kirou K, Losina E, MacKenzie R, Michaud K, Mikuls T, Russell L, Sah A, Miller AS, Singh JA, Yates A. 2017 American College of Rheumatology/American Association of Hip and Knee Surgeons guideline for the perioperative management of antirheumatic medication in patients with rheumatic diseases undergoing elective total hip or total knee arthroplasty. Arthritis Care Res (Hoboken). 2017;69:1111–24.

24. George MD, Baker JF. Perioperative management of immunosuppression in patients with rheumatoid arthritis. Curr Opin Rheumatol. 2019;31:300–6.

25. Keidar A, Hazan D, Sadot E, Kashtan H, Wasserberg N. The role of bariatric surgery in morbidly obese patients with inflammatory bowel disease. Surg Obes Relat Dis. 2015;11:132–6.

26. Sparks JA, Halperin F, Karlson JC, Karlson EW, Bermas BL. Impact of bariatric surgery on patients with rheumatoid arthritis. Arthritis Care Res (Hoboken). 2015;67:1619–26.

27. Shoar S, Shahabuddin Hoseini S, Naderan M, Mahmoodzadeh H, Ying Man F, Shoar N, Hosseini M, Bagheri-Hariri S. Bariatric surgery in morbidly obese patients with inflammatory bowel disease: a systematic review. Surg Obes Relat Dis. 2017;13:652–9.

28. Xu F, Yu C, Li DG, Yan Q, Zhang SX, Yang XD, Zhang Z. The outcomes of bariatric surgery on rheumatoid arthritis disease activity: a prospective cohort study. Sci Rep. 2020;10:3167.

29. Colquitt JL, Pickett K, Loveman E, Frampton GK. Surgery for weight loss in adults. Cochrane Database Syst Rev. 2014;Cd003641.

30. Salminen P, Helmio M, Ovaska J, Juuti A, Leivonen M, Peromaa-Haavisto P, Hurme S, Soinio M, Nuutila P, Victorzon M. Effect of laparoscopic sleeve gastrectomy vs laparoscopic Roux-en-Y gastric bypass on weight loss at 5 years among patients with morbid obesity: the SLEEVEPASS randomized clinical trial. JAMA. 2018;319:241–54.

31. Peterli R, Wolnerhanssen BK, Peters T, Vetter D, Kroll D, Borbely Y, Schultes B, Beglinger C, Drewe J, Schiesser M, Nett P, Bueter M. Effect of laparoscopic sleeve gastrectomy vs laparoscopic Roux-en-Y gastric bypass on weight loss in patients with morbid obesity: the SM-BOSS randomized clinical trial. JAMA. 2018;319:255–65.

32. Qin B, Yang M, Fu H, Ma N, Wei T, Tang Q, Hu Z, Liang Y, Yang Z, Zhong R. Body mass index and the risk of rheumatoid arthritis: a systematic review and dose-response meta-analysis. Arthritis Res Ther. 2015;17:86.

33. Long MD, Crandall WV, Leibowitz IH, Duffy L, del Rosario F, Kim SC, Integlia MJ, Berman J, Grunow J, Colletti RB, Schoen BT, Patel AS, Baron H, Israel E, Russell G, Ali S, Herfarth HH, Martin C, Kappelman MD, ImproveCareNow Collaborative for Pediatric IBD. Prevalence and epidemiology of overweight and obesity in children with inflammatory bowel disease. Inflamm Bowel Dis. 2011;17:2162–8.

34. Gonzalez-Gay MA, Gonzalez-Juanatey C. Rheumatoid arthritis: obesity impairs efficacy of anti-TNF therapy in patients with RA. Nat Rev Rheumatol. 2012;8:641–2.

35. Ottaviani S, Gardette A, Tubach F, Roy C, Palazzo E, Gill G, Meyer O, Dieude P. Body mass index and response to infliximab in rheumatoid arthritis. Clin Exp Rheumatol. 2015;33:478–83.

36. Moran GW, Dubeau MF, Kaplan GG, Panaccione R, Ghosh S. The increasing weight of Crohn's disease subjects in clinical trials: a hypothesis-generatings time-trend analysis. Inflamm Bowel Dis. 2013;19:2949–56.

37. Versini M, Jeandel PY, Rosenthal E, Shoenfeld Y. Obesity in autoimmune diseases: not a passive bystander. Autoimmun Rev. 2014;13:981–1000.

38. Karmiris K, Koutroubakis IE, Xidakis C, Polychronaki M, Voudouri T, Kouroumalis EA. Circulating levels of leptin, adiponectin, resistin, and ghrelin in inflammatory bowel disease. Inflamm Bowel Dis. 2006;12:100–5.

39. Sharma P, McCarty TR, Njei B. Impact of bariatric surgery on outcomes of patients with inflammatory bowel disease: a nationwide inpatient sample analysis, 2004–2014. Obes Surg. 2018;28:1015–24.

40. Woodard GA, Encarnacion B, Downey JR, Peraza J, Chong K, Hernandez-Boussard T, Morton JM. Probiotics improve outcomes after Roux-en-Y gastric bypass surgery: a prospective randomized trial. J Gastrointest Surg. 2009;13:1198–204.
41. Greco A, Caviglia GP, Brignolo P, Ribaldone DG, Reggiani S, Sguazzini C, Smedile A, Pellicano R, Resegotti A, Astegiano M, Bresso F. Glucose breath test and Crohn's disease: diagnosis of small intestinal bacterial overgrowth and evaluation of therapeutic response. Scand J Gastroenterol. 2015;50:1376–81.
42. Romero-Talamas H, Daigle CR, Aminian A, Corcelles R, Brethauer SA, Schauer PR. The effect of bariatric surgery on gout: a comparative study. Surg Obes Relat Dis. 2014;10:1161–5.
43. Romero-Talamas H, Aminian A, Corcelles R, Fernandez AP, Schauer PR, Brethauer S. Psoriasis improvement after bariatric surgery. Surg Obes Relat Dis. 2014;10:1155–9.
44. Corcelles R, Daigle CR, Talamas HR, Batayyah E, Brethauer SA, Schauer PR. Bariatric surgery outcomes in patients with systemic lupus erythematosus. Surg Obes Relat Dis. 2015;11:684–8.
45. Bencsath K, Jammoul A, Aminian A, Shimizu H, Fisher CJ, Schauer PR, Rae-Grant A, Brethauer SA. Outcomes of bariatric surgery in morbidly obese patients with multiple sclerosis. J Obes. 2017;2017:1935204.
46. Lespessailles E, Hammoud E, Toumi H, Ibrahim-Nasser N. Consequences of bariatric surgery on outcomes in rheumatic diseases. Arthritis Res Ther. 2019;21:83.
47. Cadart O, Degrandi O, Barnetche T, Mehsen-Cetre N, Monsaingeon-Henry M, Pupier E, Bosc L, Collet D, Gronnier C, Tremollieres F, Gatta-Cherifi B. Long-term effects of Roux-en-Y gastric bypass and sleeve gastrectomy on bone mineral density: a 4-year longitudinal study. Obes Surg. 2020
48. Bredella MA, Greenblatt LB, Eajazi A, Torriani M, Yu EW. Effects of Roux-en-Y gastric bypass and sleeve gastrectomy on bone mineral density and marrow adipose tissue. Bone. 2017;95:85–90.
49. Tian Z, Fan XT, Li SZ, Zhai T, Dong J. Changes in bone metabolism after sleeve gastrectomy versus gastric bypass: a meta-analysis. Obes Surg. 2020;30:77–86.

Sleeve Gastrectomy and Cancer

Sulaiman Almazeedi and Ahmed Al-Khamis

1   Obesity and Cancer

It is without question today that obesity is directly attributed to an increased risk of developing cancer. In the European Union alone, approximately 70,000 out of the 3.5 million (2.0%) new cases of cancer each year are linked to overweight or obesity, while in the United States, that number is around 85,000 out of 1.4 million (5.8%) [1, 2]. It was initially thought that obesity increased only hormone-dependent cancers, such as post-menopausal breast cancer, endometrial cancer, prostate and colon cancer, however evidence is proving day by day that the effect is much broader. As of the evidence available today, an elevated body mass index (BMI) has also been proven to be linked with pancreatic, gallbladder, esophageal, renal, and thyroid cancers, as well as leukemia and non-Hodgkin lymphoma [3–6]. Large population-based studies from Austria, Sweden and Denmark have proven this but showed variations in the effect's obesity had on individual cancer types in addition to differences in incidence across age groups and genders [3–5]. A meta-analysis by Renehen et al., which included 282,137 patients across four continents, showed that a 5 kg/m^2 increase in BMI was strongly associated with an increase in the incidence of the aforementioned cancers [6]. Obesity related cancer incidence was higher in men than in women for colon and rectal cancers ($p<0·0001$ and $p=0·003$ respectively), and were higher in women than in men for renal cancer ($p=0·004$). Interestingly, the incidence of two cancer types (lung and

S. Almazeedi (✉) · A. Al-Khamis
Jaber Al-Ahmed Al-Sabah Hospital, South Surra, Kuwait
e-mail: al_mazeedi@yahoo.com

A. Al-Khamis
e-mail: alkhamis.md@gmail.com

S. Al-Sabah et al. (eds.), *Laparoscopic Sleeve Gastrectomy*,
https://doi.org/10.1007/978-3-030-57373-7_17

esophageal squamous cell cancers) were found to be negatively associated with obesity.

Beyond the fact that obesity increases the incidence of certain cancers, it is also evident today that it is also linked to an increase in cancer mortality. In one of the largest studies of its kind, a collaborative analysis of 57 papers from Europe and North America of approximately 900,000 patients observed that for each 5 kg/m^2 increase in BMI, there was on average 10% increase in cancer mortality (HR 1.10 [1.06–1.15]) [7]. In addition, the authors found the BMI range 22.5–25 kg/m^2 to have the lowest all-cause mortality among both genders.

2 Pathogenesis of Cancer in the Obese

The underlying mechanism behind what predisposes obese patients to developing certain cancers remains a topic of much debate. Because of the wide range of cancer types and different physiology of each, it is difficult to group them together and draw conclusions of causality.

However, most studies on the subject have given rise to theories that mostly centered around diet, hormonal theories, and chronic inflammation.

The high-calorie "western diet" is infamous today for being a root cause behind many diseases. There are innumerable studies observing the detrimental health effects of such diet, with numerous meta-analyses proving a direct association with breast, colon and prostate cancer [8–10]. In addition, most of these studies also observed a reduction in cancer risk with a more prudent dietary pattern (i.e. high in fruits, vegetables, and low in fat, cholesterol and processed food).

The western diet is also related to an increase in insulin production, which is one of the culprits behind obesity and cancer in the hormonal theory [1]. Insulin and insulin-like growth factor 1 (IGF-1) both play a complex role in the initiation of cellular pathways that ultimately lead to promote cellular proliferation and possible tumor growth [11].

Sex hormones also play a role in linking obesity and cancer, with recent evidence showing that the excess estrogen produced from aromatization in the adipose tissue can lead to stimulation of cell division and subsequent carcinogenesis [1].

Finally, adipose tissue itself has been found to increase the overall state of chronic inflammation by the release of the so-called adipokine hormones, a group of pro-inflammatory cytokines. From the many adipokines identified to-date, leptin is one of the most widely studied in the literature, with research linking elevated levels to colon, breast, and even prostate cancer [12]. Although the underlying pathogenesis remains to be well-established, it is believed the long-standing overall state of inflammation in obese patients results in overwhelming oxidative stress and subsequent direct DNA damage.

3 Current Literature

Before the emergence of sleeve gastrectomy (SG) as one of the most common bariatric surgery procedures, the two most common procedures were Roux-en-Y gastric bypass (RYGB) and adjustable gastric banding (AGB). Despite the recent surge in SG popularity, it remains a relatively new standalone bariatric operation, and to this day RYGB remains the gold standard bariatric procedure. As a result, there is a lack of extensive data in the literature with appropriate sample size that specifically study SG and its association with cancer risk. Furthermore, many studies pool all bariatric procedures together in their analysis without differentiating patients who had SG from other procedures, or divide surgeries broadly into either restrictive or malabsorptive. Below, we provide a summary of the evidence regarding studies that specifically included patients undergoing SG in their cohort. Most of the available data observed the effects on colorectal cancer (CRC), and will therefore form the bulk of this section.

4 Bariatric Surgery and Cancer Risk

One of the more recent papers is by Schauer et al. who conducted a large retrospective study of 22,198 subjects undergoing bariatric surgery (61% RYGB, 27% SG, and 5.6% AGB) who were matched to 66,427 non-surgical obese subjects [13]. After a mean follow-up of 3.5 years, 2,543 cancer incidents were identified. They found patients who underwent bariatric surgery were 33% less likely to develop any cancer during follow-up (HR 0.67 [CI 0.60–0.74, p<0.001]) compared with matched patients with severe obesity who did not undergo bariatric surgery. These included postmenopausal breast cancer (HR 0.58 [CI 0.44–0.77, p<0.001]), colon cancer (HR 0.59 [CI 0.36–0.97, p=0.04]), endometrial cancer (HR 0.50 [CI 0.37–0.67, p<0.001]), and pancreatic cancer (HR 0.46 [CI 0.22–0.97, p=0.04]).

5 Colorectal Cancer (CRC)

CRC is one of the most common cancers all over the world and studying the relationship between SG and the risk of its development is of great importance. Interestingly, the data is at times controversial, especially with regard to RYGB versus SG as well as colon versus rectal cancer. A recently published systemic review and meta-analysis investigating the effect of bariatric surgery on the risk of developing CRC included seven large studies involving 1,213,727 individuals [14]. With a mean duration of follow-up of more than 7 years it was observed that patients who underwent bariatric surgery had a greater than 35% reduction in the risk of developing CRC compared with obese non-operated individuals (RR 0.64 [CI 0.42–0.98]).

Arvani et al. analyzed the data of over one million patients within the United Kingdom national health service (NHS), of whom 39,747 patients (3.9%) underwent bariatric surgery [15]. Overall, they reported almost half the surgeries were a purely restrictive procedures while the other half had a combined restrictive and malabsorptive procedure. Compared to the background general population, they found no significant increase in CRC in patients undergoing obesity surgery (SIR 1.26 [CI 0.92–1.71]), while obese patients who did not undergo bariatric surgery had a significant increase likelihood of developing CRC (SIR 1.12 [CI 1.08–1.16]). Breaking down the results according to type of surgery showed no significant difference between restrictive and combined restrictive and malabsorptive procedures and the risk of CRC.

6 CRC in RYGB Versus SG and AGB

Recent evidence has emerged regarding the increase in CRC risk among patients undergoing specific types of bariatric procedures. Mackenzie et al. performed a propensity match control study comparing 8,794 obese patients who had SG, RYGB, or AGB to obese patients who did not have obesity surgery [16]. Predominantly malabsorptive procedures (RYGB) but not predominantly restrictive procedures (SG and AGB) were associated with over two-fold increase in the risk of CRC (OR 2.63 [CI 1.17–5.95]). Their findings emulate the results reported by the two Swedish studies by Derogar et al. and Ostlund et al. who reported a two-fold increase in the risk of CRC after RYGB specifically [17, 18]. The reason RYGB, but not SG or AGB, was associated with increased risk of CRC was hypothesized to be related to significant changes in the gut microbiome and the increase in specific inflammatory markers promoting hyper-proliferation of bowel mucosa following RYGB. Kant et al. also observed that putative mucosal biomarkers of colorectal cancer risk and mucosal pro-inflammatory gene expression (pro-tumorigenic cytokine macrophage migratory inhibitory factor) were increased at least three years after RYGB compared with preoperative values [19]. These findings, contrary to previous assumptions, are likely secondary to malabsorptive effects of the procedure and appear to be increased more prominently in the rectal compared to colonic mucosa. This translates to potential higher risk of rectal cancer following the malabsorptive procedures such as RYGB but not necessary the predominantly restrictive procedures such as SG.

7 Breast and Endometrial Cancers

Studies looking at trends in reduction of breast and endometrial cancers after bariatric surgery seem to mimic those for CRC. In the United Kingdom NHS study, there was a reported lower risk of breast cancer in operated patients compared to non-operated ones across both restrictive and combined restrictive and malabsorptive procedures (SIR 0.76 [CI 0.62–0.92] and SIR 1.08 [CI 1.04–1.11] respectively) [15]. In addition, the Mackenzie et al. propensity score study found patients who had bariatric surgery (56.6% RYGB, 33.6% AGB, and 9.8% SG) exhibited a decreased risk of hormone-related cancers (OR 0·23 [CI 0.18–0.30]). This decrease was consistent for breast cancer (OR 0.25 [CI 0.19–0.33]) and endometrium cancer (OR 0.21 [CI 0.13–0.35]) [15]. In a study that included patients who underwent RYGB, SG, and AGB, Linkov et al. collected blood samples of 107 obese female patients before and 6 months postoperatively [20]. They studied several biomarkers associated with endometrial cancer including insulin, C-peptide, Leptin, adiponectin, C-reactive protein, and tumor necrosis factor alpha. Interestingly, they reported normalization of the cancer markers in the majority of their patients postoperatively.

8   SG and Gastro-esophageal Cancer

It has long been thought that the anatomical changes occurring around anastomotic sites in bariatric surgery predispose to neoplasia. This evidence came mostly from studies looking at long-term effects of partial gastrectomies after peptic ulcer surgeries [21]. The notion of whether or not this translates into bariatric surgery is still a topic of much debate, with the main issue being lack of evidence due to the scarcity of such cases. Most of the evidence is based solely on case reports, with the focus being on malabsorptive surgeries mostly due to the bile reflux in the gastric pouch [22]. This trend however, is changing, and a few gastro-esophageal cancers have been reported now in post SG cases. In a review from 2019, a total of 37 papers were found from 1991 to 2018 reporting post-bariatric gastro-esophageal cancers [23]. Of those, 19 cases occurred after gastric bypass procedures, 7 after vertical banded gastroplasty, 7 after AGB, and 7 after SG. Interestingly, the cancer cases reported after SG ranged in location from the distal esophagus to the antrum of the stomach, which questions whether or not they occurred de nova or were related to the actual surgery.

A recent finding that is gaining a lot of attention, however, is Barrett's esophagus (BE) after SG. Thought to be secondary to the increased gastro-esophageal reflux post-SG, a recent paper involving routine endoscopy post-SG observed an 18.8% prevalence of BE at least five years after SG [24]. Further research into the subject is of vital importance to set future follow-up guidelines and insure optimal and safe practice.

9   Conclusion

It is beyond any doubt that there exists a strong relationship between obesity and the pathophysiology of cancer development. This relationship appears to translate to an observed association between excess weight reduction and subsequent reduction in the risk of cancer. Bariatric surgery is today the most effective method of achieving sustainable weight loss, but the heterogeneity in the mechanism this is achieved across the different procedure types has yet to be explained in an optimal way. SG being one of the relatively novel procedures to be utilized in managing morbid obesity with increasing frequency, still lacks data differentiating it from other techniques with regard to its effect on cancer development in obese patients. More studies focusing on each surgical techniques' outcomes rather than the pooled analysis approach used by most studies is needed to explain the differences in results observed today.

References

1. Mcmillan DC, Sattar N, Lean M, et al. Obesity and cancer. BMJ. 2006;333(7578):1109–11.
2. Basen-Engquist K, Chang M. Obesity and cancer risk: recent review and evidence. Curr Oncol Rep. 2010;13(1):71–6.
3. Møller H, Mellemgaard A, Lindvig K, et al. Obesity and cancer risk: a danish record-linkage study. Eur J Cancer. 1994;30(3):344–50.
4. Wolk A, Gridley G, Svensson M, et al. A prospective study of obesity and cancer risk (Sweden). Cancer Causes Control. 2001;12(1):13–21.
5. Rapp K, Schroeder J, Klenk J, et al. Obesity and incidence of cancer: a large cohort study of over 145 000 adults in Austria. Br J Cancer. 2005;93(9):1062–7.
6. Renehan AG, Tyson M, Egger M, et al. Body-mass index and incidence of cancer: a systematic review and meta-analysis of prospective observational studies. The Lancet. 2008;371(9612):569–78.
7. MacMahon S, Baigent C, Duffy S, et al. Body-mass index and cause-specific mortality in 900 000 adults: collaborative analyses of 57 prospective studies. The Lancet. 2009;373(9669):1083–96.
8. Feng YL, Shu L, Zheng PF, et al. Dietary patterns and colorectal cancer risk: a meta-analysis. Eur J Cancer Prev. 2017;26(3):201–11.
9. Xiao Y, Xia J, Li L, et al. Associations between dietary patterns and the risk of breast cancer: a systematic review and meta-analysis of observational studies. Breast Cancer Res. 2019;21(1):1–22.
10. Fabiani R, Minelli L, Bertarelli G, et al. A western dietary pattern increases prostate cancer risk: a systematic review and meta-analysis. Nutrients. 2016;8(10):1–16.
11. Calle EE, Kaaks R. Overweight, obesity and cancer: epidemiological evidence and proposed mechanisms. Nat Rev Cancer. 2004;4(8):579–91.
12. Birmingham JM, Busik JV, Hansen-Smith FM, et al. Novel mechanism for obesity-induced colon cancer progression. Carcinogenesis. 2009;30(4):690–7.
13. Schauer DP, Feigelson HS, Koebnick C, et al. Bariatric surgery and the risk of cancer in a large multisite cohort. Ann Surg. 2019;269(1):95–101.
14. Almazeedi S, El-Abd R, Al-Khamis A, et al. Role of bariatric surgery in reducing the risk of colorectal cancer: a meta-analysis. Br J Surg. 2020;107(4):348–54.
15. Aravani A, Downing A, Thomas JD, et al. Obesity surgery and risk of colorectal and other obesity-related cancers: an English population-based cohort study. Cancer Epidemiol. 2018;53:99–104.
16. Mackenzie H, Markar SR, Askari A, et al. Obesity surgery and risk of cancer. Br J Surg. 2018;105(12):1650–7.
17. Derogar M, Hull MA, Kant P, et al. Increased risk of colorectal cancer after obesity surgery. Ann Surg. 2013;258(6):983–8.
18. Ostlund MP, Lu Y, Lagergren J. Risk of obesity-related cancer after obesity surgery in a population-based cohort study. Ann Surg. 2010;252(6):972–6.

19. Kant P, Perry SL, Dexter SP, et al. Mucosal biomarkers of colorectal cancer risk do not increase at 6 months following sleeve gastrectomy, unlike gastric bypass. Obesity (Silver Spring). 2014;22(1):202–10.
20. Linkov F, Goughnour SL, Ma T, et al. Changes in inflammatory endometrial cancer risk biomarkers in individuals undergoing surgical weight loss. Gynecol Oncol. 2017;147(1):133–8.
21. Safatle-Ribeiro AV, Ribeiro U, Reynolds JC. Gastric stump cancer: what is the risk? Dig Dis. 1998;16(3):159–68.
22. Orlando G, Pilone V, Vitiello A, et al. Gastric cancer following bariatric surgery. Surg Laparosc Endosc Percutaneous Tech. 2014;24(5):400–5.
23. Yamashita T, Tan J, Lim E, et al. A case of gastric cancer after sleeve gastrectomy. Asian J Endosc Surg. 2019; 1–6.
24. Sebastianelli L, Benois M, Vanbiervliet G, et al. Systematic endoscopy 5 years after sleeve gastrectomy results in a high rate of Barrett's esophagus: results of a multicenter study. Obes Surg. 2019;29(5):1462–9.

Multidisciplinary Care Before and After Sleeve Gastrectomy

Mohammed Al Hadad

1   Introduction

Obesity is defined as a chronic progressive relapsing multifactorial neurobehavioral disease which results in excessive accumulation of body fat sufficient to impair health and affect life expectancy [1]. The progressive relapsing and multifactorial nature of the disease needs a multimodal life-long treatment approach. Bariatric surgery is the only durable solution available at the time being with an acceptable success rate [2]. The success of bariatric surgery depends on many factors and would require intervention from different specialties to maintain it and prevent and manage possible complications.

Morbid obesity represents multiple challenges for medical, allied health, and ancillary health care providers. Bariatric surgery is a behavioral surgery in some aspects because of the fact that it helps the patients change their behavior by limiting the size of food portions, and more importantly, through the neuro-hormonal changes that help the patient to "change their lifestyle and relationship with food" which is more profound in the first year after surgery.

Management of the patient with obesity is a continuous process. It starts with educating the patient about the nature of the disease, followed by discussing the management plan, then providing guidance and motivational support that would lead to lifestyle modification. All that happens before undergoing bariatric surgery, which will need life-long follow up. Weight loss is not the sole indicator of success of bariatric surgery. Other factors like improvement or resolution of obesity related diseases and meeting the patient's expectations are important factors

M. Al Hadad (✉)
MD, FRCS Glasg, FACS, Head of Bariatric Surgery Department, Healthpoint Hospital, Abu Dhabi, UAE
e-mail: more991@hotmail.com

© The Editor(s) (if applicable) and The Author(s), under exclusive license to Springer   157
Nature Switzerland AG 2021
S. Al-Sabah et al. (eds.), *Laparoscopic Sleeve Gastrectomy*,
https://doi.org/10.1007/978-3-030-57373-7_18

in measuring the success. This continuous process needs a team of health care providers that can support the patient throughout the weight loss journey. The team consists of various specialties: Medical, allied health, and ancillary health practitioners.

Multidisciplinary bariatric surgery care is defined as the *integrated collaborative care between medical, allied health workers and ancillary practitioners to personalize the treatment plans for the patient with obesity*. The need for multidisciplinary care was first mentioned in the National Institute of Health criteria for bariatric surgery on March 1991, [3] candidates for bariatric surgery should be selected carefully after evaluation by a multidisciplinary care team with medical, surgical, psychiatry and nutritional expertise. Nowadays the core multidisciplinary bariatric team includes a bariatric/obesity specialist, bariatric psychologist, bariatric dietitian, bariatric coordinator, and bariatric surgeon. Many other specialties might be involved in the care team in certain cases, including but not limited to cardiology, pulmonology, gastroenterology, and plastic surgery.

Many studies evaluated the implementation of multidisciplinary care in bariatric surgery. Among those "The peri-operative bariatric surgery care in the Middle East region" [4]. The authors sent a questionnaire to bariatric surgeons in the Middle East region and they found that before surgery; 65% of bariatric surgeons referred their patients to a dietitian, 22.6% referred their patients to a psychologist, 78.3% referred their patients for smoking cessation clinic and 30% of surgeons screened for OSA. The authors of that study concluded that there is a wide variation in the preoperative care in the Middle East region. Similar findings were reported in Santry HP and his colleagues' study in which a survey about multidisciplinary care was sent to practicing bariatric surgeons in the USA [5]. Although 95% of respondent surgeons reported using a multidisciplinary team; only 53% had a general physician, nutritionist, and mental health specialist in their teams. Only 47% of the surgeons mandated primary care, nutrition, and mental health evaluations before the surgery (NIH-recommended evaluations).

This chapter will briefly discuss the role of the core members of the bariatric multidisciplinary team; including the bariatric/obesity specialist, bariatric dietitian, bariatric psychologist, and bariatric coordinator, before and after sleeve gastrectomy, which is the most commonly performed bariatric surgical operations at the time being.

2 Bariatric/Obesity Specialist

Bariatric/Obesity specialty is one of the relatively new specialties in the management of obesity. However, the bariatric/obesity specialist has one of the most essential and vital roles of the team. They are usually endocrinologists, internal medicine or family medicine specialists who are specialized in obesity medical management. In many countries around the world, obesity medical specialization is obtained through a fellowship that certifies physicians to work in the field of medical management of obesity.

Preoperatively: The bariatric specialist role is unique in many aspects of the management of obesity as they are the best source of health information for the patients. They work as a lynchpin for the multidisciplinary team members; their communication with the patient is usually patient-focused rather than procedure focused. They deliver weight-related information in a simple non-technical language. Their role starts with the education of the patients and a professionally directed lifestyle modification. It continues throughout the optimization of the medical problems like metabolic syndrome and type 2 diabetes, hypertension and hyperlipidemia and other weight-related diseases. Also, not to forget excluding secondary causes of obesity before considering bariatric surgery. They are in a better position than the bariatric surgeons in making a less biased decision of the risks versus benefits of bariatric surgery for each specific patient with obesity.

Postoperatively: The role of the bariatric/obesity specialist is significant postoperatively considering the chronicity and the progressive relapsing nature of the disease. Morbidly obese patients usually have multiple medical problems that require proper follow-up postoperatively. Their role is to maintain the success and prevent relapses and/or possible complications. This is done through, but not limited to, weight management and maintenance, management of weight-related diseases, monitoring nutritional and vitamin deficiencies, and detection of early cases of weight recidivism. In the latter case, they will work on putting patients on back on track programs by involving other team members like dietitian and psychologists and possibly considering pharmacotherapy to augment and maintain the weight loss.

3 Bariatric Dietitian

Preoperatively: The bariatric dietitian is a subspecialty for dietitians and nutritionists. The role of the bariatric dietitian is essential in many aspects of the management of obesity. It starts with education and assessment of the patients eating behaviors (frequency and type of meals per day, grazing, poor food choices, high-calorie food). It also includes detailed history about previous weight loss attempts, bariatric knowledge and food diaries. Their role continues with behavioral modifications like teaching the patient healthy habits, such as to eat when hungry, not to overeat, refrain from engaging in other activities while eating, and to avoid eating quickly. In addition, to practice mindfulness eating which is achieved through educating the patients about the satiety meter, as shown in Table 1. Before surgery, they teach the patient about the liver shrinkage diet, which might be a crucial step in preparing patients for surgery, especially in super and super super obese patients.

Table 2 shows an example of the bariatric dietitian assessment parameters before bariatric surgery.

Table 1 Mindful eating, satiety meter

Satiety meter	
0	Starving
1	1/4 Full
2	1/2 Full
3	3/4 Full
4	Full
5	Stuffed
6	Overstuffed
7	Sick

Table 2 Example for the bariatric dietitian assessment before bariatric surgery

Has realistic expectations for weight loss	Yes	No
Verbalized understanding of dietary changes post surgery	Yes	No
Verbalized understanding of supplements needs post surgery	Yes	No
Motivation to change	Yes	No
Verbalized understanding the plan of care and need for a major life style change	Yes	No
Predicted compliance on scale of 1–10		
Bariatric dietitian prediction of patient success		
Main factor predicting success		

Postoperatively: The role of the bariatric dietitian is very significant. It is life long, and it starts from the immediate post-operative period by guiding the patients throughout the stages of diet (fluid, pureed, soft, and then regular diet). Moreover, it continues to support the patient with dietary advice in all stages of weight loss and weight maintenance; and monitor for early signs of macro or micronutrional deficiencies.

4   Bariatric Clinical Psychologist

Preoperatively: Bariatric surgery is partly a behavioral surgery, as the outcomes are largely independent of the technical performance of the surgical operations. The long term maintenance of weight loss "one surrogate of success" is dependent on the patient's ability/willingness to make significant changes in their eating habits, exercise habits, and emotional relationships to food. The role of the bariatric clinical psychologists is not to decide which patient is fit for bariatric surgery and which patient is not. Rather it is guiding and providing psychological support for the patient throughout the journey of weight loss. All patients with obesity would need proper evaluation and support before undergoing bariatric surgery. This includes, but not limited to, the evaluation of their eating styles, relationship between mood and eating behavior, substance abuse, impulsive behavior, coping skills, motivation and expectations, mental health and current life situation and social support. The majority of patients would need minimal psychological support before the surgery. However, few patients may require extensive psychological support before bariatric surgery. That might be done throughout many sessions. Table 3 shows an example of an objective assessment for patients with obesity before undergoing bariatric surgery.

Postoperatively: A small percentage of patients would need psychological support as they realize that obesity was not the only problem in their lives and they were hiding their psychological/life problems behind obesity. Other psychological issues may appear as they get rid of the obesity; and start facing difficulties in dealing with life without obesity. This is seen in many people who previously found some sort of comfort in binge eating, which they can no longer do after the surgery. Proper evaluation before surgery and early identification and intervention after surgery for those patients is essential in preventing the progression into more severe psychological problems that would complicate their course of the obesity treatment.

5   Bariatric Coordinator

Morbidly obese patients have multiple unique challenges; one of those challenges is the coordination of their care between many medical/surgical specialties, allied health and ancillary care providers. All patients with morbid obesity who qualify for bariatric surgery would need evaluation from psychology, dietary, and a bariatric surgeon before surgery and some would need bariatric/obesity specialist. Many patients require evaluation of multiple other specialties like; cardiology, pulmonology, gastroenterology, etc. The bariatric coordinator has a vital role in coordinating the management plan and communicating properly with the patients. In addition to getting necessary insurance approval, maintaining proper follow up, coordinating the multidisciplinary team weekly meetings, participating in data collections and certification and audits. The bariatric coordinator is the real

Table 3 Example for the bariatric psychology assessment before bariatric surgery

Any psychological issues	Yes	No
Any eating disorders	Yes	No
Is the patient taking well informed consent (risk Versus benefit)?	Yes	No
Patient is putting things in perspectives	Yes	No
Patient is ready for the surgery and the big change	Yes	No
Patient has enough social and family support	Yes	No
Patient has realistic expectations	Yes	No
Patient can cope with stressors	Yes	No

link between all the specialties that manage obesity and also the link between the patient and the management team.

6 Conclusion

The multidisciplinary approach in managing obesity and its related diseases is essential for the success in the journey of managing the disease of obesity and maintaining the success. The characteristics of a properly functioning multidisciplinary team are: having a core team of bariatric/obesity specialist, bariatric clinical psychologist, bariatric dietitian, bariatric coordinator, and bariatric surgeon. All core members should have proper speciality training/certification in the field of management of obesity and its complications. Ideally, all team members should be in the same facility, where they meet regularly to discuss patients and they collect data and perform audits to identify problems and improve outcomes.

References

1. Bray GA, Kim KK, Wilding JPH on behalf of the World Obesity Federation. Position statement of the World Obesity Federation, 10 May 2017. https://doi.org/10.1111/obr.12551
2. O'Brien PE, Hindle A, Brennan L, Skinner S, Burton P, Smith A, Crosthwaite G, Brown W. Long-term outcomes after bariatric surgery: a systematic review and meta-analysis of weight loss at 10 or more years for all bariatric procedures and a single-centre review of 20-year outcomes after adjustable gastric banding, meta-analysis. Obes Surg. 2019;29(1):3–14. https://doi.org/10.1007/s11695-018-3525-0.
3. Consensus Statement, NIH Consensus Development Conference, 25–27 Mar 1991, Volume 9, Number 1. https://consensus.nih.gov/1991/1991GISurgeryObesity084PDF.pdf4.
4. Nimeri A, Al Hadad M, Khoursheed M, Maasher A, Al Qahtani A, Al Shaban T, Fawal H, Safadi B, Alderazi A, Abdalla E, Bashir A. The peri-operative bariatric surgery care in the Middle East region. Obes Surg. 2017;27(6):1543–7.
5. Santry HP, et al. The use of multidisciplinary teams to evaluate bariatric surgery patients: results from a national survey in the U.S.A. Obes Surg. 2006;16(1):59–66.

Psychiatric Evaluation: Pre and Post Sleeve

Abdullah Al-Ozairi and Husain Alshatti

1   Introduction

Mental health status of individuals should be considered prior any surgical procedure. Mental health does not only include all the psychiatric disorders but also the spiritual, the emotional and their general state of mind.

Lately, obesity became one of the significant health issues discussed worldwide. It became a global matter, especially since it's consideration as a disease by the American Medical Association (AMA) in 2013 [1]. It is associated with increased mortality and decreased quality of life [2] as well as psychiatric comorbidities, such as major depressive disorders, Anxiety disorders, eating, substance use disorder and self-harm [3–6]. Concerns about morbidity and mortality related to obesity are a significant concern especially in mental health populations, where obesity prevalence rates are as high as 60% in patients with severe mental illness.

Due to the increased demand of bariatric surgery and the high prevalence of psychiatric disorders, it is crucial to provide psychiatric evaluation to the candidates prior to the procedure and follow-up post-surgery. Such evaluation and follow-up should be done to support the candidates, prevent the onset of new psychiatric issue, or modify their medications if presented.

In this chapter will review the association between mental illness and bariatric surgery and how having mental illness might affect the outcome of the surgery. Having bariatric surgery may affect the mental health by triggering new

A. Al-Ozairi (✉)
Department of Psychiatry, Faculty of Medicine, Kuwait University, Jabriya, Hawally, Kuwait
e-mail: alozairi@gmail.com

H. Alshatti
Neuropsychiatry Department, Al Amiri Hospital, Sharq, Bin Misbah Street, Al-Asima, Kuwait

onset of a psychiatric disorder or suicidality. We will then review how the surgery affects psychotropic medications. We will also discuss the importance of psychiatric assessment prior the surgery, what aspects must be considered, and when it is contraindicated to do such surgery. Furthermore, we will review the tools to evaluate certain mental disorders (such as depression, psychosis, eating disorders, self-harm) as they have significant impact of the outcome of the surgery. Finally, it is important to talk about the post-surgery evaluation, management plan and follow-up from psychiatric point of view.

2   Preoperative Mental Health State of Bariatric Surgery Participants

Among the participants of bariatric surgery, the presence of psychiatric disorders is frequent. Around 25% of the participants reported that they are currently receiving pharmacological treatment from a mental health professional during the period of the surgery, and previously, up to 20% of the surgery candidates were excluded from the surgery due to the psychiatric complications that interfere with the surgery or their condition is contraindicated to undergo a surgery [7–9]. However, by incorporating psychiatric care into the multidisciplinary team, there have been centers which have successfully reduced this exclusion number to only 2%, especially in context of gastric sleeve surgery.

The most common conditions presented were mood disorders 23%, including major depressive disorders (19%) and dysthymia [7, 10, 11]. 12% of the participants had an anxiety disorder, mainly generalized anxiety disorder and social phobia [7, 10, 11]. The current estimation of eating disorders among candidates is 17%. Furthermore, 9% of the participants had a history of suicidal ideation and 3% suffered from substance use disorders [10].

In the following section, we will discuss the status of certain psychopathologies that are present among participants and may have an impact on the surgical outcome.

3   Depression

Major depressive disorder is considered the most prevalent psychopathology among the participants. It was also found that there are several associated factors between preoperative depression and the bariatric surgery. For instance, there is a positive relation between the severity of the depressive symptoms and obesity [12, 13].

It is well known that the relation between obesity and depression is bi-directional. Depression causes behavioural changes, such as social isolation, lower physical activity, increase in appetite or emotional eating, and feeling of guilt, which may facilitate further severity of obesity. On the other hand, obese individuals suffer from issues with body image, self-esteem, lower physical activity, and other behaviours that worsen the existence of depressive symptoms [12,

13]. The association between the two disorders goes further into polygenic genetic factors [14–16]. Such as the FTO (fat mass and obesity-associated) gene, which is linked with both depression and the severity of obesity [17, 18].

During the early stage after the surgery, there is significant improvement of depressive symptoms. The association between postoperative weight loss and improved depression symptoms, reduced severity, and lower prevalence can be explained by improvement in the body image and interpersonal relationships [19]. On the other hand, this improvement gradually decreases on a long-term basis [20].

4 Eating Disorders

As for eating disorder, the preoperative presentation of eating disorders among bariatric candidates usually is grouped as follows:

- **Binge Eating Disorders (BED)**: is experiencing binge eating without compensatory behavior such as induced vomiting, misuse of laxative, or excessive exercise, which is the main difference between BED and Bulimia nervosa. "Binge eating" is characterized as having two main points [21]:

  I. consumption of a relatively large amount of food in a discrete amount of time.
  II. the experience of loss of control.

It is considered the most common type of eating disorders among the candidates and is secondary only to depression. Several studies showed a wide range of prevalence of BED from 4–49%. This wide range can be explained by the fact that the diagnostic criteria of BED have only been formalized with the release of the Diagnostic and Statistical Manual of Mental Disorders (DSM-5) in 2013. Studies have produced mixed findings, with some studies linking BED with poorer postoperative weight loss while others suggesting no relation between BED and weight loss post-surgery. The tendency to eat in response to negative emotions is related to poorer postoperative weight loss.

- **Bulimia nervosa**: is characterized as experiencing recurrent binge eating with the compensatory behavior such as purging and misuse of laxative use, diuretics, enemas or other medications to prevent weight gain. Due to the inappropriate eating behavior of bulimia, it is considered contraindicated for a bariatric surgery. However, the prevalence among participants remains not well known, probably due to under-reporting by the candidates to avoid delaying or cancelling the surgery [22].
- **Anorexia nervosa**: is characterized by restriction of energy intake leading to a significant low body weight due to fear of gaining weight with the association of disturbed body image, despite the very low weight. The prevalence of

anorexia among the participants is not well known because of the insufficient data. However, there are reports of "Anorexia-like presentation" experienced postoperatively. Those behaviors include, dietary restriction, fear of weight gain and disturbances in body image [23].

- **Atypical Eating Disorders (AED)**: This is usually used for the two eating behaviors:
  I. "grazing" defined as continuous eating.
  II. "night eating syndrome"(NES) characterized by hyperphagia at night.

5   Anxiety

The prevalence of anxiety disorders among the candidates of the surgery vary from 12% and up to 24%. With a lifetime prevalence of up to 37% for a history of lifetime diagnosis of anxiety disorders [24]. Although the rate of anxiety disorders among the bariatric population is evident, there is no reported relation between anxiety and the post-surgical outcome [20]. This is supported by the prevalence of anxiety disorders after surgery, where the rates are the same as prior surgery [20].

6   Substance Use Disorders

Substance use disorder is prevalent among bariatric candidates, around 30% have a lifetime history prevalence of alcohol use disorder [25]. It is also found that the rate of alcohol use disorder and alcohol consumption increases even after the surgery, notably sleeve gastrectomy surgery. The reason for such increased rate was explained by multiple suggestions, such as changes in pharmacokinetics of alcohol from accelerated absorption and the long duration of elimination [10]. The effect of substance use disorder on the surgery outcome varies. The increased use of substances may contribute to further progression of the individual depression and may result in suicide [10]. Another possible effect is that individuals who are unable to change their substance use behavior are at risk of achieving only suboptimal weight change after the surgery, because they may fail to change their eating behavior to accommodate their new life style.

Toxicology screening is recommended by several studies for the preoperative evaluation, as the surgery should be delayed until the issue of substance use disorders is resolved, if present [26, 27].

7   Self-harm and Suicidal Ideation

Self-harm and suicidal ideation are important aspects to be assessed pre-surgery. The rate of suicidal behavior among individuals who had bariatric surgery is four times higher than the general population. In addition, during the first 3 years after the surgery showed an increased rate of reported self-harm behaviors among individuals after bariatric surgery [28]. Also, the prevalence of past suicidal attempts among the participants is 73 times higher than the normal population! This increased suicidal rate among this particular population could be affected by several circumstances, such as:

- difficulty adjusting to a new lifestyle which may lead to depression.
- not achieving the expected weight loss or experiencing weight regain, which may cause the feeling of disappointment.
- increased substance use, such as alcohol.

Screening for suicidal ideation preoperatively is as important as postoperatively. The presence of suicidal ideation can be a contraindication or a reason to delay the surgery [29].

8 Psychotropic Medications

As previously mentioned, up to 60% of the participants reported to have psychiatric disorder at the time of the preoperative evaluation, and around 25% receive psychotropic medication from a mental health provider [7–10]. By and large, the most common psychotropic medications used are antidepressants (87%), anxiolytics 9%, and 2% on mood stabilizers [30].

The change in drug absorption and pharmacokinetics of the psychotropics in bariatric surgery differs depending on the type of the procedure. Furthermore, this change affects the level of the medication in the body, thus, affecting its therapeutic effects and side effects. As an example, Hamad et al. in 2010 [31] measured the level of antidepressants in individuals immediately after bypass surgery. It was found that the level of antidepressants was reduced, and the reduction remained, in some individuals, up to 1 year after the surgery. The decreased level of antidepressant immediately after the surgery in those individuals can lead to discontinuation syndrome, which is causes discomfort to the patient and can be rarely fatal.

History of receiving psychotropic treatments is not contraindicated for bariatric surgery. However, it is highly recommended to be evaluated by a mental health provider, prior the surgery, and to follow up with a psychiatrist after the surgery on a regular basis. The post-operative follows up is essential to observe the course of the psychopathology and possibility of modification the treatment.

9 Psychological Predictors of Post-Surgical Weight Loss

Some studies found a relation between preoperative psychiatric history and reports of dietary noncompliance and medical complication postoperatively, these reports were not associated with weight loss [32, 33]. When analyzing this further, some studies that severity of the psychiatric disorders such as severe depression and anxiety, might have a negative effect on post-surgery weight loss but not mild-moderate in nature [34]. Recent studies have linked the effect of having multiple psychopathologies preoperatively on increasing the risk of having intermediate weight loss after the surgery [35–37].

It is believed that cognitive function has a direct effect on post-surgical weight loss, due to the influence of the cognitive function to develop an appropriate eating behavior and coping mechanisms later on.

Most studies have concluded that post-surgical eating behaviors influence the postoperative weight loss outcome. It is also believed that the impact of the preoperative mental status, cognitive function and personality of the participant on the total weight loss is linked to the postoperative eating behavior. Other psychiatric disorders may affect the weight loss outcome through the same previous principle, as seen in major depressive disorder among gastric sleeve participants [38].

In depression, there is a persistent depressed mood, loss of interest, feelings of guilt, and disturbed sleep and appetite [39]. Those symptoms may affect the eating behavior of the participant which includes dietary constrains and results in suboptimal weight loss. Also, depression affects the cognitive functions of the individual leading the participant focus on the negative sides of the circumstances [40]. This negative interpretation may interfere with participant's post-surgical adjustments and developing new cooking methods with weight loss and diet constrains.

10   Mental Health Preoperative Assessment

Psychiatric disorders and mental illness are prevalent among bariatric surgery participants, as was established earlier. Furthermore, the weight loss outcome relies not only on a successful procedure alone, but also on the behavioral, and the psychological status of the participant. Therefore, the psychological assessment prior the surgery is recommended. The goal of the assessment is not diagnostic, rather than screening. The screening must take place to reveal any contraindications such as current substance use disorder, recent suicidal attempt, or active psychosis [22]. The assessment should be done by mental health providers such as a psychologist, a psychiatrist.

It is important to emphasize that the psychiatrist role here is to enhance surgical outcomes and not just weight loss. For example, a patient with excellent weight loss post gastric sleeve, may still have psychosocial difficulties and challenges, ranging from disruptions in interpersonal relationships and body image dissatisfaction to concerns as serious as suicidal behaviour and substance abuse. The aim of the preoperative assessment is to improve all domains of surgical outcomes.

In this part, we will discuss the psychiatric evaluation of the bariatric surgery candidate, and the necessary tools should be used with considerations to certain psychopathologies, such as depression, and eating disorders.

11   Outline of Domains of the Evaluation

Guidelines published by the American Society for Metabolic and Bariatric Surgery (ASMBS 2016), show a systematic method to conduct a preoperative interview for bariatric surgery participants by psychiatrists. The interview contains four main elements to evaluate, including the current life, psychiatric, behavioral, and cognitive and emotional status.

Despite the previous published guideline, there are various protocols used across the globe tackling the issue of mental preoperative evaluation. Most of the protocols and guidelines agree on certain domains to be included in the evaluation, those are [22, 26, 41, 42]:

- history of weight loss and previous attempts
- physical activity
- medical history
- pathological eating behavior
- psychiatric history and screening of substance use
- patient's mental capacity (understanding the surgery, the outcome, possible complications, and expectations)
- support system

12   Psychiatric Contraindications for Bariatric Surgery

Having a psychiatric disorder, by itself, is not a contraindication per se, but there are psychiatric elements that prompt delay or cancellation of the surgery.

According to the American Psychaitric Association (APA), and the ASMBS, the most common elements considered as high risk, or contraindication, to undergo a bariatric surgery are:

- significant psychopathology such as active psychosis (including thought disorder symptoms),
- current substance dependence,
- untreated eating disorders (specifically anorexia nervosa or bulimia nervosa),
- untreated depression
- active suicidal ideation

Those mentioned contraindications, when present, the surgery either is canceled or delayed till the psychopathology is resolved, treated or reduced to a subclinical level.

Lastly, there are other elements considered as contraindications because they will interfere with the optimal weight loss after the surgery. Although they are not psychiatric in nature, they have to be evaluated by a mental health provider. Those elements are: unrealistic expectations for the goal weight, lack of knowledge of the surgery and the possible complications, and lack of social and family support [20, 29, 43, 44].

13   Conducting the Assessment

13.1   History of Weight Loss and Previous Attempts

During this part of the assessment, the examiner should review the pattern of weight changes of the participant, and the previous methods of weight loss was tried in a chronological manner, with the notion to the biological and environmental factors that may affect the weight change and the failed attempts. Knowing the age of onset and family history of obesity may reveal a genetic aspect in which helps the participant understand the factors affecting the obesity and what to expect after the surgery [42]. Asking about the effect of stressful events on weight changes may reveal inappropriate coping mechanism, such as emotional eating or loss of appetite. Such coping mechanisms may affect the post-surgical weight loss and may be erected later on.

13.2   Medical History

Asking about the medical history is an important part of any medical based interview. It is vital to know the medical diseases, and treatments the participant has to have an idea about the individual as a whole. Also, it will provide information that help the weight loss outcome. Certain medical conditions, or medications may intervene with the rate of post-surgical weight loss.

Furthermore, asking about the medical history reveals the level of adherence to the current medications, if present. This information will provide a prospective idea regarding future compliance to the postoperative management plan, such as respecting follow-ups, regular investigations, taking medications, and recommended behavioral changes [45].

13.3   Pathological Eating Behavior

This section involves two main aspects:

- eating and diet habits
- eating pathology

Eating habits of the participant should be known in detail or at least we should have an idea about this aspect. The eating habits include daily dietary preferences, number of main meals and snacks, meal portion sizes, and if there is a consistent timing of the meals. Understanding these habits may reveal inappropriate aspects of the participants eating behavior that were factors in the obesity or may cause weight to regain after surgery [46].

Eating pathology is another aspect to be considered in the assessment, besides eating habits. In this part we will discuss the types of eating disorders should be screened, and possible management plans prior undergoing with the surgery.

Understanding the eating patterns and detecting any related pathology is crucial for the after-surgery weight loss. As mentioned earlier, one of the factors that link the mental health status and not achieving optimal weight loss after the surgery is the inappropriate eating behavior. The most important eating disorders to screen for are (1) **anorexia nervosa** (2) **bulimia nervosa** (3) **binge eating disorder (BED)** (4) **night eating syndrome (NES)**. Other non-diagnostic eating disorders that are important to screen for are: overeating, grazing and emotional eating.

The use of scales and screening tools are useful to detect eating disorder. An example of those tools, eating disorder examination questionnaire (EDE-Q), which is a self-report instrument and it screens for symptoms of eating disorder in the last month [47, 48].

After screening for any pathological eating behavior, the next step is to determine the treatment and follow-up plan. The candidate should understand that the first few weeks after the surgery is a stressful period, mentally and physically. Furthermore, the participant should be educated that having this psychopathology may interfere with reaching the optimal weight [45].

The choice of therapy should depend on the psychopathology, e.g., cognitive behavioral therapy (CBT) and interpersonal therapy (IPT) are verified treatment options for BED [49]. The psychological approach found to be superior to the behavioral approach in treating BED [50]; however, the opposite is true in treating NES [51]. The basis of treating NES concentrates on the behavioral aspects [51].

As for the pharmacological aspects, the usual use of antidepressant has shown significant improvement of eating disorders symptoms and reducing the frequency of the episodes. As an example, Fluoxetine, a type of selective serotonin repute inhibitor (SSRI), is the only antidepressant approved by the food and drug administration (FDA) to treat bulimia nervosa with a therapeutic dose from 20 to 60 mg per day. For BED, antidepressants (SSRI and tricyclic antidepressants (TCA)) were superior to placebo in reducing the symptoms in a meta-analysis of 7 randomized control trails (RCT) [24]. As for NES, Sertraline (mean dose of 126.5 mg/day) [52], Escitalopram (mean dose of 20 mg/day) [53], and Agomelatine (mean dose of 50 mg/day) [54] showed superiority in treating NES when compared to placebo.

13.4   Psychiatric History and Screening of Substance Use

The psychiatric history should be brief and concentrate on screening the psychiatric disorders, rather than diagnosing. The screening should include past and current psychiatric history, mental state exam, substance abuse, psychiatric systemic review, active symptoms of psychosis, mood disorders, and suicidal ideation [43].

The main goal is to check if there are contraindications for the surgery, including suicide ideation, active psychosis, untreated substance use disorder, and untreated depression. Also, the screening should include other psychiatric disorders that may affect the cognitive functioning, such as schizophrenia, or bipolar disorder. Thus, affecting adherence and the behavior of the participant which causes achieving suboptimal weight loss. Furthermore, having surgical intervention is a stressful event, especially when it is affecting the lifestyle. The surgery may worsen the psychiatric symptoms and the patient may need further assessment and tailored management. In this section we will discuss further the screening of depression, substance use disorder, and suicide risk assessment.

Major depressive disorder in itself is not a contraindication for the surgery. However, if the depression is not treated, severe, or presented with active psychosis or suicidal ideation, then, postponing the surgery is considered. It is useful to use self-assessment tools, for example the patient health questionnaire-9 (PHQ-9), to screen and assess the severity of depression [55].

Suicide screening Active suicidal ideation is considered a contraindication to the bariatric surgery. To screen for suicide, ask the participant a clear direct question of intending of self-harm and having suicidal thoughts. If the participant had a positive answer, then continue with the suicide assessment. The American Psychiatric Association (APA) has approved a brief suicidal risk assessment named suicide assessment five-step evaluation and triage (SAFE-T) [56].

Substance use disorder is common among gastric sleeve candidates, especially alcohol use disorder, and the presence of this untreated pathology is contraindicated with the surgery. Thus, screening for substance use should be part of the psychiatric pre surgical evaluation. During this part of the assessment, the examiner should not rely solely on the self-report instruments. The screening instruments are complementary to the clinical assessment [57]. Accompanying the clinical interview, the change in biomarkers may give a hint to the degree of the substance use. As an example, in alcohol use, the liver enzymes are elevated such as alanine aminotransferase (ALT), serum aspartate aminotransferase (AST), and gamma glutamyl-transferase (GGT). However, these biomarkers are not sensitive, and they are affected by other medical issue, but they may support the clinical assessment [58].

Since alcohol use disorder is the most common type of substance abuse among the participants, there are brief methods to screen for the use of alcohol. The CAGE questionnaire is a self-administered questionnaire with high sensitivity around 91–93% for detecting heavy alcohol consumption [59] but is less sensitive for less severe alcohol misuse. The Alcohol Use Disorders Identification Test (AUDIT) is another widely used instrument to detect alcohol use disorders. It is a 10 items questionnaire that has two versions, the clinical administered and self-report. AUDIT is a validated and reliable instrument to detect different levels of alcohol use disorder. Furthermore, AUDIT uses a standardized levels of alcohol consumed regardless of the type of ingested drink [58].

Screening for substance use should also include screening of other addictive behaviors such as smoking cigarette, shoplifting, or food or any form of addiction. This addictive behavior is common among bariatric surgery participants and it might increase in frequency after the surgery. This can be explained by the concept of "addiction transfer". Addiction transfer is defined as individuals replacing one form of addiction with another one. In case of the bariatric population, it is the transfer from addiction to food to another form of addiction, such as consumption of alcohol, gambling, or other forms [57].

Educating the participants of the importance of this screening and the possible effect of the surgery. Also, participants should be educated about addiction transfer and how it affects the lifestyle. Individuals who suffer from untreated substance use disorders or addiction, should seek help prior the operation, or postponing the surgery is recommended till the issue is resolved.

The management plan may vary depending on the individual. Psychotherapy is widely used to treat addiction problems and substance use disorders, especially among the bariatric population undergoing bariatric surgery. Various methods are used depending on the patient, including motivational interviewing (MI), CBT, or 12- step programs [60, 61]. Pharmacological treatment is less evident among patients undergoing bariatric surgery; however, it may be useful for some patients more than others.

Adverse childhood experiences (ACE). In addition to the previous psychiatric history taken, asking about Adverse childhood experiences (ACE) might be useful to the evaluation. Childhood trauma, may be a factor in developing obesity or eating patterns that causes obesity. This could be explained that those individuals utilize the excess weight as a protective shield against stress or anxiety related issues triggered by intimate relationships. Those individuals may become more vulnerable when they lose significant weight via surgery, and the surgery may provoke new psychiatric issues [62].

13.5   Support System

Another aspect of the psychiatric preoperative assessment to explore, is the support system. Having a life changing surgery needs a good support system from family members and close relationships. The lack of support system may affect negatively the post surgical outcome. Some participants complain that their partners are feeling threatened after the significant weight loss after the surgery. It was elaborated that this feeling was due to the improved positive transformation after the weight loss, such as improved self-esteem and increased attractiveness of the participants [63].

13.6 Psychiatric Medication

The use of psychiatric medications is also common among the bariatric patients. Also, patients with mental illness are at higher risk of obesity and metabolic disturbances. The psychiatric medications may contribute to that risk. Screening for psychotropics should take place prior the surgery to look for any medication that might influence the weight the gain or affect the metabolism of the participant. Some antidepressants such as Amitriptyline and Mirtazapine may induce weight gain among the participants. Multips antipsychotics such as Olanzapine and Clozapine can cause metabolic disturbances that result in weight gain. Also, few of the mood-stabilizers such as Valproate and Lithium may increase appetite and induce weight gain [64].

14 Psychiatric Assessment Conclusion

Taking care of bariatric patients is done by a multidisciplinary team, and they must be informed about the readiness of the patient for the surgery from psychiatric point of view [43].

The majority of the candidates (96%) are cleared to have the surgery. The remaining 3–4% were absolutely contraindicated and were denied to have the surgery due to serious psychiatric issues, such as psychosis, thought disorder, suicidal ideation, active substance use, untreated eating disorder, and lack of decision making capacity. That small percentage was constant throughout several studies [29, 30, 65, 66].

A group of candidates are in a grey area. Those individuals have few psychiatric concerns, but they are cleared to have the surgery under certain conditions. The surgery is delayed for a short period of time till they start with the psychiatric treatment. Studies revealed that this issue could happen among 15–31% of participants [30, 67]. While delaying the surgery is beneficial to the participant, there is an undeniable rate who do not return for the surgery. Some studies found that up to 12% of the candidates never return for the surgery. Only 16% of participants return for the surgery after it was postponed due to an underlying eating disorder [17].

15 Special Populations

We will discuss the following three special populations due to the different nature of the problems they face. For example, adolescents and bariatric surgery is becoming more and more common, however, the preoperative assessment of pediatrics and adolescents requires a different approach with certain considerations, such as bullying and self-image issues. Another population are those with intellectual disability who, because of their deficit in their cognitive function, may find it difficult to adhere to the management plan or fathom the importance of having a strict diet for the first couple of weeks after the surgery, which affect the surgical outcome. Another population that may suffer from cognitive function limitation is the ageing adults.

In this section we will discuss populations (the adolescent and the intellectually disabled) and the difficulties we face and the solutions when assessing them.

15.1   The Adolescent Patient

The preoperative assessment of adolescents has a similar approach to adults. The evaluation should be comprehensive with a multidisciplinary team to assess if the participant is fit to have surgery. However, there are certain aspects should be considered when evaluating the adolescent candidate. Exploring those aspects will help a better surgical outcome.

The main issue of obesity troubling the adolescents is the social stigma. It is widely spread among individuals with obesity regardless of age, gender, and geographical distribution. However, the development of peer-focused social skills begins at adolescence when teens interact with their peers and develop sense of identity and being included in a social group as part of their social functioning. During this time, they are most vulnerable to the negative comments and social stigma about their weight or body shape. Bullying or weight related teasing has a great impact on adolescents and affect how they define themselves and their identity. This effect is noticeable among teenagers, the rate of depression has increased among teens with obesity and in particular among females [18].

Family environment is another major factor affecting the course of obesity in adolescences. During childhood, children are hugely affected by the behaviors and ideals of close family members. Some of those behaviors become tradition and some of those ideals become consolidated ideas shaping the individual's perception toward self and the community. Family support is a double sided weapon, the family may be a motivating factor for the adolescent to seek the sleeve gastrectomy procedure due to certain health concerns of the general well being of their child. One the other hand, within the same family environment there might be elements that contribute to weight gain. Those elements may be the family eating habits, unhealthy dietary choices, or the availability of unhealthy food. Since the family environment has a huge influence on the adolescents, they have difficulties change that environment without the help and support of their family members [68].

Another challenge is the adolescent client's adherence to management plans. During adolescence, a strong sense of independence and identity is developing. Lack of adherence to management plan among adolescent candidates is a well recognized issue [69] and that could be because of peer pressure and trying to fit in, as well as difficulty following dietary recommendations such as avoiding fast foods.

Adolescents seeking sleeve gastrectomy are motivated by many factors, such as health concerns, seeking better body image, the pressure of family members, or due to social concerns. This may lead to developing unrealistic expectations about the surgery, the post-surgical body shape, scars, optimal weight loss, the amount of excess skin, or life restrictive activities. The candidates may be unsatisfied with surgical results because they were not prepared from the beginning, and this may cause further discomfort in body image or even a new onset of psychiatric disorders like depression or body dysmorphic disorder. Experimentation with substance or sexuality is common during adolescence. The presented challenges after the surgery and the lack of preparation for the surgical outcome may raise an issue of substance use disorder.

It is crucial to explore the social and family environment domains of the adolescents with the addition to the other domains which are similarly evaluated in adults. Participants should be educated about the social stigma and its effect on understanding the consequences of the surgery. The participants should be asked about their expectations from the surgery, and any unrealistic ideas must be rectified to prepare them for the post surgical outcome. The psychological aspects of the rapid weight loss after the surgery should be addressed.

To avoid resisting the post surgical recommendations, clinicians and adolescents should be connecting. This can occur by understanding the values, goals, and cultural backgrounds of the adolescents. The young participants should be included in the management plan and their opinions should be considered. They must sense that their values are taken in consideration rather than ordering them around. These ways of communications with the adolescent candidates is helpful to improve the adherence to the management plan and better outcome. Motivating the participant to socially interact with other adolescents who share same goals to implement a strong social peers support.

15.2   Limited Cognitive Function

Cognitive function is one of the major factors affecting outcomes post sleeve gastrectomy. Thus, managing participants suffering from cognitive vulnerabilities is challenging. This group may include various populations, such as individuals with low IQ, learning disabilities, history of low educational achievement, or dementias. As previously mentioned, cognitive limitation affects the post-surgical weight loss through various aspects. Individuals who has difficulties in information consolidation may find it difficult to obtain and analyze vital information in respect to the procedure itself, possible complications, and lifestyle changes. Limited educational level could be an obstacle to the participants concerning the utility of self-monitoring methods and related educational materials. Participants with memory difficulties may not be able to recall crucial information or recommendations to optimize the weight loss, minimize complications, improve healing, taking medications, or diet plans after the surgery which may increase the risk of unpleasant events afterwards. A deficit in executive functions will have a great negative impact on the participant's capability of behavioral control, problem solving skills, analyzing current events and predicting the consequences. A dysfunction in such system is a predictor of reaching suboptimal weight loss or weight regain after the surgery [70].

Individuals suffering from limited cognitive function and seeking a sleeve gastrectomy should, at minimum, have the cognitive capacity to decision making in regards to the surgical procedure, understanding the possible consequences, and the importance of life changing behaviors. Further, it is important to assess their social supports and if they can cope with the changes post-sleeve gastrectomy.

16   The Impact of Bariatric Surgery on Mental Health

Individuals seek sleeve gastrectomy for multiples reasons. Some participants seek the surgery due to their unsatisfied body shape and image, to reduce their weight, or due to medical comorbidities. The surgery may improve general mental health, but also may trigger new onset of psychiatric disorders, like body dysmorphic disorder.

The literature is filled with studies indicating the significant improvement in health after sleeve gastrectomy [71, 72]. Major studies have explored this impact on the candidates for the short and long term. The main example of such studies is the Swedish obese subjects (SOS) study, which is a prospective study that followed participants for a long period of time for around two years. In this section we will discuss the impact of the sleeve gastrectomy on the mental health status, and the quality of life.

16.1   Quality of Life

It is evident in the literature that there is an improvement in health related quality of life after the surgery. This improvement might reach a peak and then slightly decline over time. This pattern is seen in the SOS study, it was found that patients reported significant improvements in health-related quality of life after a period of 6–12 months. However, these major improvements reached their peak at that period and a slight decline in such improvement is noticed after a period of two years after the surgery. Despite the slight decline two years after the surgery, the improvements in health-related quality of life were positively linked to the amount of weight lost [37].

The majority of the patients reported improvements in martial satisfaction and sexual activity [73]. Also, participants reported improvements in body image after the surgery [19].

16.2 Mental health status

16.2.1 Major Depressive Disorder, Anxiety Disorders and General Psychological Wellbeing

Several studies noted a major improvement in the mental health status among participants who suffer from current or previous psychiatric illness. Psychiatric patients who undergo sleeve gastrectomy showed improvement in their symptoms after 3–6 months from the surgery [74]. The SOS study, which followed 4047 bariatric surgery candidates for 2 years, found improvement in their general psychological symptoms. Further, they showed significant decrease in their depressive and anxiety symptoms after one year [37] and even after two or three years, there seems to be a mental health gain [74, 75].

A systemic review of 40 studies from 1982 till 2002 support the findings about the improvement in the psychiatric disorders among bariatric surgery participants who currently suffer from a psychiatric disorder or had a history of a psychiatric illness, particularly depression and anxiety disorders [76]. It was found that these significant improvements in mental health occurred mainly in patients who achieved their weight loss goal. Participants who suffered from postoperative weight regain were associated with increased depression. This reinforces the concept of the association between obesity and the psychiatric disorder, regardless of the underlying psychopathology [37].

Although the post-surgical weight loss may be associated with improvement in psychiatric symptoms, mental health gain after the surgery can be attributed to factors other than weight loss alone. This is said because the improvement of the psychiatric symptoms was not exclusive to those who achieved optimal weight loss after the surgery. There was mental health gain among individuals within the first few weeks after the surgery, where no significant weight loss achieved yet. Also, some participants who achieved only post-surgical suboptimal weight loss showed mental health gain [77]. This means there are other factors affect the improvement of the mental health post operatively, those include the type of the psychopathology and lifestyle changing, despite the fail to achieve the optimal weight loss.

Interestingly, Sleeve gastrectomy may have an independent effect on depression and anxiety reduction. The effect of Sleeve gastrectomy on depression and anxiety can be due to biological factors, such as the reduction of the inflammatory cytokines as a chronic effect from the surgery. It is known that inflammatory cytokines, like interleukin-6 and C-reactive protein, play major roles in depression and anxiety disorders, thus their reduction may actually improve the symptoms [74].

The baseline reduction in depression and anxiety symptoms happened among patients who either changed, stopped, or continued with the same medication. The change in medications or adjusting the dose is expected during the first 3 to 6 months. Approximately 90% of depression and anxiety patients who improved after the surgery, their medications were either reduced or discontinued. From 10 to 20% of patients needed to either increase the dose of their medication or switch to other class, which can be due to the disturbed absorption after the surgery [74].

Individuals who suffer from Anxiety benefit from the bariatric surgery as well. Improvement in Anxiety disorders showed similar improvements to depression after the surgery. Some studies showed around 50% improvement in anxiety after the Sleeve gastrectomy [74].

16.3   Suicide

The rate of suicide is noticed to be increasing post bariatric surgically on the long term, despite the general mental health gain. There is higher than expected suicide rate among participants after the surgery when candidates were followed-up for 8 years after the surgery [78]. It is difficult to explain why that is exactly and it is unclear if there is a difference between the types of surgeries.

16.4   Addiction

Substance use disorder and other addictive behaviors are very common among patients. Several studies showed an increased pattern in the addictive behaviors, including alcohol use, recreational drug use, smoking cigarette, gambling, sexual activity, shopping, that are present for at least the first 2 years among bariatric candidates after the surgery [79].

Alcohol use disorder (AUD) is one of the major substance use disorder suffered among the candidates and most of the studies explored this substance more than other addictive behaviors. The SOS study showed that AUD is still an issue even 15 years after the surgery [80]. The alcohol use might not just be a resistant problem but also the consumption might increase after a while. Longitudinal observational studies showed increase consumption of alcohol from the second year after the surgery when compared to 1 year before and after the surgery. Furthermore, a rate of 7.9% among the participants showed a new onset of AUD after the surgery [81].

There are several factors were noticed to be predicators of AUD after the surgery, those include males, family history of substance use disorder, history of AUD notably 1 year prior the surgery, and history of nicotine use prior the surgery [82]. The previous factors are also considered to increase the risk of developing substance use disorder after the surgery with the addition to history of food addiction and the consumption of high glycemic or high fat food before the surgery [83]. The relation of pre-surgery food addiction and the increased rate of substance use disorder after the surgery could be explained by the concept of "Addiction transfer", which is defined as the replacement of one addictive behavior with another. This patter is seen among bariatric patients who are addicted to food or suffer from a pathological eating behavior such as emotional eating, after the surgery they replace that pathological behavior into something else such as alcohol consumption, smoking cigarette, or gambling [84].

One of the common addictive behaviors is cigarette smoking. It is noticed that after the surgery, cigarette smoking is reduced more among older adults than a younger population. New-onset smoking can go up to 12% post-surgery [85].

16.5 Eating Disorders

Evaluating eating disorders after the surgery can be challenging. This is because they present in a different way than the classical presentation and they may not fulfil the criteria. For example, vomiting after surgery is common, but some patients vomit as a compensatory method for shape or weight concerns. After the surgery, eating huge amount of food at the same time uncontrollably, which is a criterion for binge eating, is difficult. Despite that, few months after the surgery participants reported feeling loss of control similar to that of binge eating disorder without the consumption of large amount of food [53]. Participants may suffer from marked fear of gaining weight or concerns about their shape after the surgery. This may lead to extreme diet restriction and causes anorexia. Although, many patients continue to have eaten disorders after the surgery, there are individuals reported improved symptoms. This could be due to following the recommended strict diet plan which may normalize the individual's eating pattern overtime [86].

16.6 Psychotropic Medication

Bariatric patients who use psychotropic medications may continue their medications after the surgery. The most common psychiatric treatment used among those patients are antidepressants. It is estimated that 35% of bariatric patients use at least one antidepressant on daily basis [87]. After the sleeve gastrectomy, the improvement in depression and mental gain noticed to occur among patients who either continued the same medication, switched their antidepressant into another class, or modified their dose [74]. Also, some patients experienced side effects of their usual medications that were not experienced before, or some found out that their usual treatment did not have a positive effect as before. This suggests that the procedure affects the current psychotropic medication by interfering with the pharmacokinetics of those medications. The effect of the bariatric surgery on the pharmacokinetics should be understood and considered when following up the participants after the surgery to optimize the positive effect and minimize the adverse effects.

All the bariatric surgeries affect the pharmacokinetics of the medications on various levels depending on the type of the surgery, but mainly they affect the absorption of the medications into the blood circulation since they make anatomical and functional alterations in the gastrointestinal (GI) track. The modification can be restrictive, malabsorptive, or a combination of both. The sleeve gastrectomy procedure has mainly a restrictive modification on the GI system since major part of the stomach is removed.

16.7 Postoperative Pharmacological Considerations

To avoid drug toxicity, major side effects, or having sub-therapeutic levels of the psychotropic medications after the sleeve gastrectomy, certain modifications should be considered depending on the clinical situation of the patient. It is not recommended to automatically change the doses or switch the treatment just because they are undergoing a gastric sleeve. Instead, close monitoring of the patient prior to the surgery and the use of baseline screening instruments, like the aforementioned PHQ-9 instrument for depression are highly recommended. If any early signs of reduced effectiveness of the medication, or signs of medication withdrawal, experiencing side effects, or signs of relapse occur then treatment modifications are considered.

The methods of treatment modifications are vary depending on the clinical situation and the type of the pharmacological treatment. One way is changing "controlled", "extended", and "sustained release" medications to "immediate release" drugs before or after the surgery to improve the rate of absorption. The goal of the controlled release drugs is to achieve the therapeutic effect and minimize dividing the doses throughout the day by prolongating the disintegration time of the drug. The extended release forms may have reduced absorption after the surgery [88]. With switching to the immediate release, it is recommended to divide the doses to several times per day to ensure achieving the therapeutic effect of the drugs.

Some psychotropics mediations come in liquid form or as orally disintegrated tablets. Those forms can be used instead of the tablet form in psychiatric patients undergoing a bariatric surgery, since they skip the process of disintegration and thus improving the absorption and metabolism of the active substance.

Unfortunately, not all psychiatric treatments are available in different forms. If the patient is on those medications and experienced early signs of relapse or sub therapeutic effectiveness, then other methods may be considered such as increasing the dose, dividing the dose throughout the day, or crushing the pills (if applicable).

Before taking the decision of modifying the pharmacological treatment of the psychiatric patient undergoing sleeve gastrectomy, assessing the mental health status of the patient and close monitoring should be done on regular basis. Some studies showed that the bioavailability of some psychotropic medications may normalize or even increase in some bariatric participants after a period of 6 month. This means that although those patients may experience signs of reduced effectiveness of their treatment, some of them might experience side effects of the drugs due to their increased blood level after 6 months after the surgery. This was noticed especially among patients who had increased doses of their antidepressants after a bariatric surgery due to signs of decreased absorption [89].

17   Conclusion

The Sleeve gastrectomy is one of the most successful methods of weight loss for obese individuals worldwide. The presence of psychiatric illness is common among this population and cannot be ignored. Also, a positive association exists between psychiatric illness and obesity, which means the bariatric surgery could also improve the mental health status of those individuals. The most common psychopathologies are mood disorders, anxiety, eating disorders, and substance use disorder. Having a mental illness is not a contraindication of the surgery in 97% of patients, but it can be challenging, and may interfere with the surgical outcome. Untreated or uncontrolled psychiatric illness may result in achieving only suboptimal weight loss, especially if the psychopathology affects the cognitive function of the patient. Those patients may not follow the postoperative recommendation and may not fully fathom the importance of lifestyle changes to this operation life changing operation. Thus, psychiatric evaluation prior making the decision of having the operation is crucial.

Sleeve gastrectomy benefits patients via quality of life, a noticeable mental health gain and patients with depression or anxiety show further improvement, while others are able to stop their medications. Despite the improvement in general mental health and in major psychiatric disorders, there are few setbacks. Patients with history of suicide, substance use, or addictive behavior may experience worsened symptoms or transfer their preoperative addictive behaviors to another.

Lastly, the psychiatric evaluation before the sleeve gastrectomy is necessary for all. It is important to avoid relapses of the present psychiatric issues, rectifying any false expectations, improving the mental health status, and implementing behavioral changes that help the participant reach the optimal weight loss and have the full care needed before and after the surgery.

References

1. Rosen H. Is obesity a disease or a behavior abnormality? Did the AMA get it right? Mo Med. 2014;111(2):104–8.
2. Adams KF, Schatzkin A, Harris TB, Kipnis V, Mouw T, Ballard-Barbash R, et al. Overweight, obesity, and mortality in a large prospective cohort of persons 50 to 71 years old. N Engl J Med. 2006;355:763–78.
3. Kalarchian MA, Marcus MD, Levine MD, Courcoulas AP, Pilkonis PA, Ringham RM, et al. Psychiatric disorders among bariatric surgery candidates: relationship to obesity and functional health status. Am J Psychiatry. 2007;164:328–34.
4. Luppino FS, de Wit LM, Bouvy PF, Stijnen T, Cuijpers P, Penninx BWJH, et al. Overweight, obesity, and depression: a systematic review and meta-analysis of longitudinal studies. Arch Gen Psychiatry. 2010;67:220–9.
5. Mühlhans B, Horbach T, de Zwaan M. Psychiatric disorders in bariatric surgery candidates: a review of the literature and results of a German prebariatric surgery sample. Gen Hosp Psychiatry. 2009;31:414–21.

6. Sarwer DB, Wadden TA, Fabricatore AN. Psychosocial and behavioral aspects of bariatric surgery. Obes Res. 2005;13:639–48.
7. Gertler R, Ramsey-Stewart G. Pre-operative psychiatric assessment of patients presenting for gastric bariatric surgery (surgical control of morbid obesity). Aust N Z J Surg. 1986;56:157–61.
8. Glinski J, Wetzler S, Goodman E. The psychology of gastric bypass surgery. Obes Surg. 2001;11:581–8.
9. Sarwer DB, Cohn NI, Magee L, et al. Psychiatric diagnoses and psychiatric treatment among bariatric surgery candidates. Obes Surg. 2004;9:148–56.
10. Dawes AJ, Maggard-Gibbons M, Maher AR, Booth MJ, Miake-Lye I, Beroes JM, et al. Mental health conditions among patients seeking and undergoing bariatric surgery: a meta-analysis. JAMA. 2016;315(2):150–63.
11. Black DW, Goldstein RB, Mason EE. Prevalence of mental disorder in 88 morbidly obese bariatric clinic patients. Am J Psychiatry. 1992;149:227–34.
12. Wadden TA, Sarwer DB, Womble LG, Foster GD, McGuckin BG, Schimmel A. Psychosocial aspects of obesity and obesity surgery. Surg Clin North Am. 2001;81:1001–24.
13. Wadden TA, Sarwer DB, Arnold ME, Gruen D, O'Neil PM. Psychosocial status of severely obese patients before and after bariatric surgery. Prob Gen Surg. 2000;17:13–22.
14. Afari N, Noonan C, Goldberg J, et al. Depression and obesity: do shared genes explain the relationship? Depress Anxiety. 2010;27(9):799–806.
15. Jokela M, Elovainio M, Keltikangas-Jarvinen L, et al. Body mass index and depressive symptoms: instrumental-variables regression with genetic risk score. Genes Brain Behav. 2012;11(8):942–8.
16. Samaan Z, Anand SS, Zhang X, et al. The protective effect of the obesity-associated rs9939609 A variant in fat mass- and obesity-associated gene on depression. Mol Psychiatry. 2013;18(12):1281–6.
17. Devlin MJ, Goldfein JA, Flancbaum L, Bessler M, Eisenstadt R. Surgical management of obese patients with eating disorders: a survey of current practice. Obes Surg. 2004;14(9):1252–7.
18. Needham BL, Crosnoe R. Overweight status and depressive symptoms during adolescence. J Adolesc Health. 2005;36(1):48–55.
19. Adami GF, Gandolfo P, Campostano A, Meneghelli A, Ravera G, Scopinaro N. Body image and body weight in obese patients. Int J Eat Disord. 1998;24:299–306.
20. Muller A, Mitchell JE, Sondag C, de Zwaan M. Psychiatric aspects of bariatric surgery. Curr Psychiatry Rep. 2013;15(10):397.
21. Spitzer RL, Devlin M, Walsh BT, et al. Binge-eating disorder: a multi site field trial of the diagnostic criteria. Int J Eat Disord. 1992;3:191–203.
22. Mechanick JI, Youdim A, Jones DB, Garvey WT, Hurley DL, McMahon MM, et al. Clinical practice guidelines for the perioperative nutritional, metabolic, and nonsurgical support of the bariatric surgery patient—2013 update: cosponsored by American Association of Clinical Endocrinologists, the Obesity Society, and American Society for Metabolic & Bariatric Surgery. Endocr Pract. 2013;19(2):337–72.
23. Marino JM, Ertelt TW, Lancaster K, Steffen K, Peterson L, de Zwaan M, et al. The emergence of eating pathology after bariatric surgery: a rare outcome with important clinical implications. Int J Eat Disord. 2012;45(2):179–84.
24. Stefano SC, Bacaltchuk J, Blay SL, Appolinário JC. Antidepressants in the short-term treatment of binge eating disorder: systematic review and meta-analysis. Eat Behav. 2008;9:129–36.
25. Marek RJ, Ben-Porath YS, Heinberg LJ. Understanding the role of psychopathology in bariatric surgery outcomes. Obes Rev. 2016;17(2):126–41.
26. Edwards-Hampton SA, Wedin S. Preoperative psychological assessment of patients seeking weight-loss surgery: identifying challenges and solutions. Psychol Res Behav Manag. 2015;8:263–72.

27. Heinberg LJ, Ashton K, Coughlin J. Alcohol and bariatric surgery: review and suggested recommendations for assessment and management. Surg Obes Relat Dis. 2012;8(3):357–63.
28. Bhatti JA, Nathens AB, Thiruchelvam D, Grantcharov T, Goldstein BI, Redelmeier DA. Self-harm emergencies after bariatric surgery: a population-based cohort study. JAMA Surg. 2016;151(3):226–32.
29. Bauchowitz AU, Gonder-Frederick LA, Olbrisch ME, Azarbad L, Ryee MY, Woodson M, et al. Psychosocial evaluation of bariatric surgery candidates: a survey of present practices. Psychosom Med. 2005;67(5):825–32.
30. Pawlow LA, O'Neil PM, White MA, Byrne TK. Findings and outcomes of psychological evaluations of gastric bypass applicants. Surg Obes Relat Dis. 2005;1(6):523–7. Discussion 8–9.
31. Hamad GG, Helsel JC, Perel JM, Kozak GM, McShea MC, Hughes C, et al. The effect of gastric bypass on the pharmacokinetics of serotonin reuptake inhibitors. Am J Psychiatry. 2012a;169(3):256–63.
32. Valley V, Grace M. Psychosocial risk factors in gastric surgery for obesity: identifying guidelines for screening. Int J Obes Relat Metab Disord. 1987;11:105–13.
33. Vallis MT, Ross MA. The role of psychological factors in bariatric surgery for morbid obesity: identification of psychological predictors of success. Obes Surg. 1993;3:346–59.
34. Herpertz S, Kielmann R, Wolf AM, Hebebrand J, Senf W. Do psychosocial variables predict weight loss or mentalhealth after obesity surgery? A systematic review. Obes Res. 2004;12(10):1554–69.
35. de Zwaan M, Enderle J, Wagner S, Mühlhans B, Ditzen B, Gefeller O, et al. Anxiety and depressionin bariatric surgery patients: a prospective, follow-upstudy using structured clinical interviews. J Affect Disord. 2011;133(1):61–8.
36. Lanyon RI, Maxwell BM. Predictors of outcome after gas-tric bypass surgery. Obes Surg. 2007;17(3):321–8.
37. Karlsson J, Sjöström L, Sullivan M. Swedish obese subjects (SOS)—an intervention study of obesity: two-year follow- up of health-related quality of life (HRQL) and eating behavior after gastric surgery for severe obesity. Int J Obes Relat Metab Disord. 1998;22:113–26.
38. Semanscin-Doerr DA, Windover A, Ashton K, Heinberg LJ. Mood disorders in laparoscopic sleeve gastrectomy patients: does it affect early weight loss? Surg Obes Relat Dis. 2010;6:191–6.
39. American Psychiatric Association. Diagnostic and Statistical Manual of Mental Disorders (DSM–IV). 4th ed. Washington, DC: American Psychiatric Publishing; 1994.
40. Beck AT. The evolution of the cognitive model of depression and its neurobiological correlates. Am J Psychiatry. 2008;165:969–77.
41. Greenberg I, Sogg S, Perna FM. Behavioral and psychological care in weight loss surgery: best practice update. Obesity (Silver Spring). 2009;17(5):880–4.
42. Wadden TA, Sarwer DB. Behavioral assessment of candidates for bariatric surgery: a patient-oriented approach. Surg Obes Relat Dis. 2006;2(2):171–9.
43. Fabricatore AN, Crerand CE, Wadden TA, Sarwer DB, Krasucki JL. How do mental health professionals evaluate candidates for bariatric surgery? Survey results. Obes Surg. 2006;16(5):567–73.
44. Walfish S, Vance D, Fabricatore AN. Psychological evaluation of bariatric surgery applicants: procedures and reasons for delay or denial of surgery. Obes Surg. 2007;17(12):1578–83.
45. Sogg S, Mori DL. Psychosocial evaluation for bariatric surgery: the Boston interview and opportunities for intervention. Obes Surg. 2009;19(3):369–77.
46. Sogg S, Mori DL. Revising the Boston interview: incorporating new knowledge and experience. Surg Obes Relat Dis. 2008;4(3):455–63.
47. Elder KA, Grilo CM. The Spanish language version of the Eating Disorder Examination Questionnaire: comparison with the Spanish language version of the eating disorder examination and test-retest reliability. Behav Res Ther. 2007;45(6):1369–77.

48. Kalarchian MA, Wilson GT, Brolin RE, Bradley L. Assessment of eating disorders in bariatric surgery candidates: self-report questionnaire versus interview. Int J Eat Disord. 2000;28:465–9.
49. Alfonsson S, Parling T, Ghaderi A. Group behavioral activation for patients with severe obesity and binge eating disorder: a randomized controlled trial. Behav Modif. 2015;39(2):270–94.
50. De Zwaan M, Hilbert A, Swan-Kremeier L, et al. Comprehensive interview assessment of eating behavior 18–35 months after gastric bypass surgery for morbid obesity. Surg Obes Relat Dis. 2010;6:79–87.
51. Berner LA, Allison KC. Behavioral management of night eating disorders. Psychol Res Behav Manag. 2013;6:1–8.
52. O'Reardon JP, Stunkard AJ, Allison KC. Clinical trial of sertraline in the treatment of night eating syndrome. Int J Eat Disord. 2004;35(1):16–26.
53. Kalarchian MA, Wilson GT, Brolin RE, Bradley L. Effects of bariatric surgery on binge eating and related psychopathology. Eat Weight Disord. 1999;4:1–5.
54. Milano W, De Rosa M, Milano L, Capasso A. Agomelatine efficacy in the night eating syndrome. Case Rep Med. 2013;2013:867650. https://doi.org/10.1155/2013/867650.
55. Kroenke K, Spitzer RL, Williams JB. The PHQ-9: validity of a brief depression severity measure. J Gen Intern Med. 2001;16(9):606–13. PubMed PMID: 11556941; PubMed Central PMCID: PMC1495268.
56. Practice parameter for the assessment and treatment of children and adolescents with suicidal behavior. J Am Acad Child Adolesc Psychiatry. 2001;40(7 Supplement):24s–51s.
57. Mitchell JE, Steffen K, Engel S, King WC, Chen JY, Winters K, et al. Addictive disorders after Roux-en-Y gastric bypass. Surg Obes Relat Dis. 2015;11(4):897–905.
58. Saunders JB, Aasland OG, Amundsen A, Grant M. Alcohol consumption and related problems among primary health care patients: WHO collaborative project on early detection of persons with harmful alcohol consumption—I. Addiction. 1993;88(3):349–62.
59. Bernadt MW, Mumford J, Taylor C, Smith B, Murray RM. Comparison of questionnaire and laboratory tests in the detection of excessive drinking and alcoholism. Lancet. 1982;1(8267):325–8.
60. Miller WR, Rollnick S. Talking oneself into change: motivational interviewing, stages of change, and therapeutic process. J Cogn Psychother. 2004;18(4):299–308.
61. Irvin JE, Bowers CA, Dunn ME, Wang MC. Efficacy of relapse prevention: a meta-analytic review. J Consult Clin Psychol. 1999;67(4):563–70.
62. Kalarchian MA, Marcus MD, Levine MD, Courcoulas AP, Pilkonis PA, Ringham RM, et al. Psychiatric disorders among bariatric surgery candidates: relationship to obesity and functional health status. Am J Psychiatry. 2007;164(2):328–34. Quiz 74.
63. Bocchieri LE, Meana M, Fisher BL. Perceived psychosocial outcomes of gastric bypass surgery: a qualitative study. Obes Surg. 2002;12(6):781–8.
64. Amodo G, Subramaniapillai M, Mansur R, McIntyre R. Choosing psychiatric medications for patients with severe obesity and pharmacological treatments for severe obesity in patients with psychiatric disorders: a case study. In: Psychiatric care in severe obesity—an interdisciplinary guide to integrated care. Springer International Publisher; 2017. p. 297–311.
65. Sarwer DB, Cohn NI, Gibbons LM, Magee L, Crerand CE, Raper SE, et al. Psychiatric diagnoses and psychiatric treatment among bariatric surgery candidates. Obes Surg. 2004;14(9):1148–56.
66. Sadhasivam S, Larson CJ, Lambert PJ, Mathiason MA, Kothari SN. Refusals, denials, and patient choice: reasons prospective patients do not undergo bariatric surgery. Surg Obes Relat Dis. 2007;3(5):531–5. Discussion 5–6.
67. Cunningham JL, Merrell CC, Sarr M, Somers KJ, McAlpine D, Reese M, et al. Investigation of antidepressant medication usage after bariatric surgery. Obes Surg. 2012;22(4):530–5.
68. Wansink B, van Ittersum K, Payne CR. Larger bowl size increases the amount of cereal children request, consume, and waste. J Pediatr. 2014;164(2):323–6.

69. Shaw RJ. Treatment adherence in adolescents: development and psychopathology. Clin Child Psychol Psychiatry. 2001;6(1):137–50.
70. Rieber N, Giel KE, Meile T, Enck P, Zipfel S, Teufel M. Psychological dimensions after laparoscopic sleeve gastrectomy: reduced mental burden, improved eating behavior, and ongoing need for cognitive eating control. Surg Obes Relat Dis. 2013;9(4):569–73.
71. Choban PS, Onyejekwe J, Burge JC, Flancbaum L. A health status assessment of the impact of weight loss following Roux-en-Y gastric bypass for clinically severe obesity. J Am Coll Surg. 1999;188:491–7.
72. Schok M, Greenen R, van Antwerpen T, de Wit P, Brand N, van Ramshorst B. Quality of life after laparoscopic Psychosocial and Behavior Aspects of Bariatric Surgery, Sarwer, Wadden, and Fabricatore adjustable gastric banding for severe obesity: postoperative and retrospective preoperative evaluations. Obes Surg. 2000; 10:502–8. 75. Dixon JB.
73. Camps MA, Zervos E, Goode S, Rosemurgy AS. Impact of bariatric surgery on body image perception and sexuality in morbidly obese patients and their partners. Obes Surg. 1996;6:356–60.
74. Scott M, Kristen R, Esra M, Joseph C. Impact of sleeve gastrectomy on psychiatric medication use and symptoms. J Obes. 2018;2018.
75. Frigg A, Peterli R, Peters T, Ackermann C, Tondelli P. Reduction in co-morbidities 4 years after laparoscopic adjustable gastric banding. Obes Surg. 2004;14(2):216–23.
76. Herpertz S, Kielmann R, Wolf AM, Langkafel M, Senf W, Hebebrand J. Does obesity surgery improve psychosocial functioning? A systematic review. Int J Obes. 2003;27(11):1300–14.
77. Dymek MP, le Grange D, Neven K, Alverdy J. Quality of life and psychosocial adjustment in patients after Roux-en-Y gastric Bypass: a brief report. Obes Surg. 2001;11(1):32–9.
78. Pories WJ, Swanson MS, MacDonald KG, et al. Who would have thought it? An operation proves to be the most effective therapy for adult-onset diabetes mellitus. Ann Surg. 1995;222:339–52.
79. Conason A, Teixeira J, Hsu CH, Puma L, Knafo D, Geliebter A. Substance use following bariatric weight loss surgery. JAMA Surg. 2013;148(2):145–50.
80. Svensson PA, Anveden A, Romeo S, Peltonen M, Ahlin S, Burza MA, et al. Alcohol consumption and alcohol problems after bariatric surgery in the Swedish obese subjects study. Obesity (Silver Spring). 2013;21(12):2444–51.
81. King WC, Chen JY, Mitchell JE, Kalarchian MA, Steffen KJ, Engel SG, et al. Prevalence of alcohol use disorders before and after bariatric surgery. JAMA. 2012;307(23):2516–25.
82. Substance Abuse and Mental Health Services Administration. Results from the 2013 national survey on drug use and health: summary of national findings. Rockville, MD: Mental Health Services Administration (SAMHSA); 2014. NSDUH Series H-48, HHS Publication No. (SMA) 14-4863.
83. Fowler L, Ivezaj V, Saules KK. Problematic intake of high-sugar/low-fat and high glycemic index foods by bariatric patients is associated with development of post-surgical new onset substance use disorders. Eat Behav. 2014;15(3):505–8.
84. Engel SG, Kahler KA, Lystad CM, Crosby RD, Simonich HK, Wonderlich SA, et al. Eating behavior in obese BED, obese non-BED, and non-obese control participants: a naturalistic study. Behav Res Ther. 2009;47(10):897–900.
85. Lent MR, Hayes SM, Wood GC, Napolitano MA, Argyropoulos G, Gerhard GS, et al. Smoking and alcohol use in gastric bypass patients. Eat Behav. 2013;14(4):460–3.
86. van Hout GCM, Boekestein P, Fortuin FAM, Pelle AJM, vanHeck GL. Psychosocial functioning following bariatric surgery. Obes Surg. 2006;16(6):787–94.
87. Mitchell JE, King WC, Chen J-Y, Devlin MJ, Flum D, Garcia L, et al. Course of depressive symptoms and treatment in the longitudinal assessment of bariatric surgery (LABS-2) study. Obesity (Silver Spring). 2014;22:1799–806. https://doi.org/10.1002/oby.20738.

88. Padwal R, Brocks D, Sharma AM. A systematic review of drug absorption following bariatric surgery and its theoretical implications. Obes Rev. 2010;11:41–50. https://doi.org/10.1111/j.1467-789X.2009.00614.x.
89. Hamad GG, Helsel JC, Perel JM, Kozak GM, McShea MC, Hughes C, et al. The effect of gastric bypass on the pharmacokinetics of serotonin reuptake inhibitors. Am J Psychiatry. 2012;169:256–63. https://doi.org/10.1176/appi.ajp.2011.11050719.

Insurance, Self-Pay and Medical Tourism

How Much Does the Sleeve Cost

Eliana Al Haddad

The popularity of Sleeve gastrectomy's is on a continues rise, with the sums performed outnumbering those of other bariatric procedures in many countries around the world [1]. In the USA alone, the percentage of sleeve's went up from 38 to 63% from the years 2012 to 2015, corresponding to a decrease in the number of Roux-en-Y gastric bypass from 44 to 30%, while the laparoscopic adjustable gastric band has shown a significant decrease from 13 to 2% in that time period. This brings into question the importance of analyzing the cost-effectiveness of these procedures in order to provide each individual patient with the most appropriate plan of action according to their needs. This information, however, has been sparse, with only the By-Band-Sleeve (BBS) trial currently being conducted to fill these gaps [2]. In comparison to other bariatric surgery trials, the BBS study will assess both clinical and economic outcomes for the three most common approaches to bariatric surgery, in the largest sample size studied in a comparative trial to date (expected to randomize 447 patients per group), over a substantial follow-up period (36 months). However, an important first step in estimating the economic outcomes in the BBS study will be to obtain detailed and 'accurate' costs of the three types of bariatric surgery.

E. Al Haddad (✉)
Columbia University Medical Center, New York, NY, USA
e-mail: Eliana.h91@gmail.com

E. Al Haddad
Amiri Hospital, Kuwait City, Kuwait

S. Al-Sabah et al. (eds.), *Laparoscopic Sleeve Gastrectomy*,
https://doi.org/10.1007/978-3-030-57373-7_20

1   A Cost Evaluation Methodology for Surgical Technologies

Until recently, the cost of new surgical procedures in developed countries was a secondary consideration to all parties involved: patients who were well covered by state or private insurance, hospitals, with healthy profit margins and surgeons, who were concerned with improving patient care (or marketing their services) no matter the cost. However, with recent global financial constraints, a shift in thinking of payers and regulatory services, as well as hospitals had to be adopted, especially for procedures that are considered elective and non-emergency such as bariatric surgery. With no consistent metrics to measure costs, comparative analysis becomes impossible.

To be fair, the economics of surgical interventions are extremely complex and not straightforward. Hospitals are complex economic environments that deal with a multitude of vendors, different levels of staff, administration and policy, and so on. In most systems, there is no simple way to determine the "cost" of something.

More socialized systems have global budget funding, and granular details of expenditures are often poorly documented. Other systems, based on billing for services, have a multitude of customers and use complex cost-shifting strategies to maintain an operating profit. Ismail et al. [3] was able to create an effective classification for surgical procedures which includes the following.

1.1   Economic Methodologies

An important first step is to create definitions for the different elements. The cost is the price paid by the producer (hospital) for resources consumed during the production process (surgery). Charge is the price paid by the consumer (patient) needed for the institution to break even and to be solvent.

Furthermore, a distinction must be made between fixed versus variable and direct versus indirect costs. A cost is considered fixed if it does not vary according to the level of activity, and variable if it does. A direct cost reflects the price of resources that are directly attributable to the project, whereas indirect costs are not directly attributable to the completion of the studied activity and have to be estimated using an allocation formula].

They chose to follow a micro-costing approach for direct costs separated into two categories: fixed and variable. This choice is meant to provide hospitals with detailed information on when, where, how and if they can optimize surgery cost.

The elements taken into account in each category include medical devices and personnel as fixed costs, whereas the variable costs encompass re-usable instruments and disposables. Note that if the personnel's salaries were based on hourly remunerations, the personnel cost would then be considered as variable.

1.2   Fixed Costs: Medical Devices

In today's technology leveraged surgical practice, the initial purchase price of surgical equipment needed to perform the procedure is only part of the financial investment required. Most advanced technologies need some type of routine maintenance or upkeep which is usually covered by "maintenance/service contracts" with the company or third-party vendors.

For mechanical and software based technologies, accounting principles dictate a "life expectancy" for the device. This is based on the average replacement cycle for the technology based on mechanical failure and obsolescence. It is an indication that allows projected amortization of the purchase price and maintenance cost.

1.3   Fixed Costs: Personnel

Even though most bariatric surgeries are now performed laparoscopically, the number of personnel involved is still as high as open surgeries, with similar operating times. These surgical operations translate into an increase in surgery cost with respect to the personnel cost.

1.4   Variable Costs: Reusable Instruments

Hospitals today are faced with many management choices that affect operating costs. The choice of reusable versus disposable operating room supplies used to be clear-cut: reusable supplies were less expensive but disposable supplies were more convenient. Today, with patient safety concerns, increasing regulations, labor costs and increasing disposable costs, this simplified view no longer holds. Both reprocessing expenses and disposable costs must be taken into account when evaluating the cost of a procedure.

1.5   Variable Costs: Disposables

Depending on the procedure, number of complications and other factors, various consumables (anaesthetic agent, implants, units of blood, etc.) will add to the operation cost. Integrating this element into our equation is an easy task. The challenge, however, lies in the time-consuming process of collecting such detailed data.

2   Bariatric Surgery Costs

When it comes to looking at the costs associated with bariatric surgery, they can be classified into either resources consumed, and the unit costs associated with those resources. To identify these parameters, a number of different approaches can be utilized.

2.1   Methods for Identifying Cost Components

Gross-costing: Involve identifying cost components at a highly aggregated level (e.g. costing an intervention based only on the associated inpatient days) [4].

Micro-costing: A precise method, where an attempt is made to identify every input consumed in the treatment of a particular patient [4].

2.2   Methods for Valuing Cost Components

Top-down costing: An approach where relative value units such as hospital days or some other metric are used to separate out relevant costs from comprehensive sources (e.g. the finance department's annual accounts) and apportion them to individual services or procedures [5]. For example, the sum of the annual budget of an intensive care unit and hospital overhead may be divided by the number of patient days to estimate an average cost per patient per day [6].

Bottom-up costing: An approach where cost components are valued by identifying resource use directly employed for a patient, resulting in patient-specific unit costs [7].

The seven 'important' cost components included:

- Cost, not charge data used in the analysis;
- Operating room costs reported separate from hospital admission costs;
- Medical device costs reported (e.g. endoscopy column, laparoscopic tower);
- Personnel costs reported (e.g. surgeon, nurse, anaesthesiologist time);
- Re-usable instrument costs reported (e.g. bowel graspers, surgical scissors);
- Disposable instrument/consumables costs reported (e.g. needles, disposable staplers); and
- Overhead costs reported.

3   The Cost of the Sleeve Around the World

We conducted a survey that was sent to bariatric surgeons around the world to attempt to obtain an average cost of bariatric procedures from the countries they represent. Table 1 summarizes these findings. The prices have all been converted into united states dollars for comparison purposes.

Table 1 Cost of bariatric procedures from around the world

	Procedure cost in USD			
	Balloon	LSG	Bypass	Band
Argentina	1322	3439	3439	2116
Australia	3612	14,446	15,891	5778
Colombia	2200	8000	6000	NA
Egypt	1116	1116	2512	2233
France	4753	17,147	18,290	4000
Iraq	1380	4350	4950	2500
Jordan	1990	4615	5742	2713
Kuwait	3365	6858	7641	5490
Lebanon	1962	5143	5619	2833
Libya	5358	11,073	14,288	1071
Oman	3117	6495	7793	
KSA	2665	6444	9098	3650
Syria	1,029	2,330	3,106	1,747
United Arab Emirates	3,412	11,000	9,348	3,921
United Kingdom	6,231	16,202	18,694	8,724
United States of America	15,000	21,000	20,000	9,000
Yemen	2000	3000	5000	2500

The cost of Gastric Sleeve surgery in Turkey varies from one clinic to the other. The amount you are expected to pay will cover things like the surgeon's fee, anesthesia used during the surgery, the meds you will use after the surgery, etc. All-in-all, you can expect to pay something like $7,700 on average. India is one of the countries that perform Gastric Sleeve surgery at a low cost. In India, you can five times less to what you are expected to pay in the US. Similarly, the cost of Gastric Sleeve in the UK is three times the cost in India, with an average of $5,500. Just like Turkey, Poland is now regarded as a medical tourism destination. Over the years, this European country has made notable strides in improving its medical infrastructure. Although there are a handful of reputable hospitals in Warsaw, the cost of the Gastric Sleeve procedure is relatively cheap as compared to what it costs in the UK, coming in at around $7,700. Based on the data gathered by the National Statistics Institute, 75% of medical facilities in Romania are privately-owned. Statistics show that the number of private Hospitals in Romania increased from 2 to 161, between 1997 and 2014. So, if you are to have a Gastric Sleeve surgery in Romania, there is a 75% probability that you are going to have the surgery at a private hospital. The cost of the procedure range between $7,500 to $9,000.

However, it is important to note that these methods look specifically at the cost of the procedure, and do not take into account the costs of nutritional and psychological evaluations, 6–12 months of medical weight management, re-admissions, postoperative complications, routine vitamin supplements and laboratory testing for the life of the patient after surgery.

References

1. Kizy S, Jahansouz C, Downey MC, Hevelone N, Ikramuddin S, Leslie D. National trends in bariatric surgery 2012–2015: demographics, procedure selection, readmissions, and cost. Obes Surg. 2017;27(11):2933–9.
2. Rogers CA, Welbourn R, Byrne J, Donovan JL, Reeves BC, Wordsworth S, et al. The By-Band study: gastric bypass or adjustable gastric band surgery to treat morbid obesity: study protocol for a multi-centre randomised controlled trial with an internal pilot phase. Trials. 2014;15:53.
3. Ismail I, Wolff S, Gronfier A, Mutter D, Swanstrom LL. A cost evaluation methodology for surgical technologies. Surg Endosc. 2015;29(8):2423–32.
4. Gold M. Panel on cost-effectiveness in health and medicine. Med Care. 1996;34(12 Suppl):DS197–9.
5. Chapko MK, Liu CF, Perkins M, Li YF, Fortney JC, Maciejewski ML. Equivalence of two healthcare costing methods: bottom-up and top-down. Health Econ. 2009;18(10):1188–201.
6. Edbrooke D, Hibbert C, Ridley S, Long T, Dickie H. The development of a method for comparative costing of individual intensive care units. The Intensive Care Working Group on Costing. Anaesthesia. 1999;54(2):110–20.
7. Tan SS, Rutten FF, van Ineveld BM, Redekop WK, Hakkaart-van RL. Comparing methodologies for the cost estimation of hospital services. Eur J Health Econ. 2009;10(1):39–45.

Analysis of LSG Competitors

Jamil S. Dababneh

Here, we are going to take Porter's five forces model as a tool to identify and analyze the five competitive forces that come into play when considering competitors in the bariatric world and to analyze the weight reduction tools and market.

1 Competition in the Industry

Weight loss surgery, or as it is commonly referred to as the bariatric surgery umbrella includes several procedures:

- Laparoscopic Sleeve Gastrectomy (LSG): The most commonly performed procedure in the United States as of recent years is the gastric sleeve procedure.
- Gastric bypass: the second most commonly performed bariatric surgery
- Gastric bypass surgery has been proven to be clinically useful for long-term weight loss. However, without the proper guidance before and after surgery, it may still fail.
- Lap Band surgery: the third most popular procedure in the United States.
- Duodenal Switch is another very effective, although less frequently performed, procedure.
- Newly FDA approved procedures such as gastric balloons.

J. S. Dababneh (✉)
American Pharmacists Association, American Marketing Association, Chicago, USA
e-mail: jamil.dababneh@hotmail.com

© The Editor(s) (if applicable) and The Author(s), under exclusive license to Springer
Nature Switzerland AG 2021
S. Al-Sabah et al. (eds.), *Laparoscopic Sleeve Gastrectomy*,
https://doi.org/10.1007/978-3-030-57373-7_21

2   Potential of New Entrants into the Industry

Until recently, the only options for combating obesity were lifestyle modification, medications and, if those methods proved ineffective, bariatric surgery.

The entry barrier to this domain is relatively medium with new techniques and developments introduced to this market. Also, it is imperative to take into consideration the expertise needed to master the surgical procedures once they are introduced into the market niche.

The exit barrier is also considered medium because of the average capital investment in hospitals for these procedures.

3   Threat of Substitute Products

There are numerous products that can be considered as substitutes for LSG, unlike the direct competitors, the substitutes are non-surgical. Many patients don't meet surgical requirements or are unwilling to undergo operations because of anxiety or fear and therefore, these products can come in handy for such patients.

The Substitutes that currently exist are:

3.1   Anti-obesity Medications

These are strong substitutes, (e.g. Orlistat (Alli®, Xenical®), Lorcaserin (Belviq®), Phentermine and topiramate (Qsymia®), Bupropion and naltrexone (Contrave®), Liraglutide (Saxenda®, Victoza®). However, it is important to note that LSG has outperformed them in terms of efficacy and endurance.

3.2   Herbal and Alternative Medicine

These are substances or procedures that are usually marketed with the goal of suppressing hunger or increasing metabolism and lean body mass.

Many products such as botanical weight loss supplements actually contain unapproved stimulants including analogues of amphetamine, methamphetamine and ephedra.

Some botanical supplements include high dosages of compounds found in plants with stimulant effects including Yohimbine and Higenamine.

Still, LSG has proven to outrank them in terms of outcomes and immediate response.

3.3   Diet Program

Dietitians have numerous roles to fill, one of which is to treat overweight patients, however, their results, when taken individually, are considered inferior compared to LSG in terms of results and time needed to achieve them.

3.4   Exercise

As with anything to demonstrate effective results, a lot of time, effort and dedication are needed in order for exercise to reduce the weight effectively. Therefore, LSG has become an easier tool to achieve better result in a shorter period of time.

3.5   Acupuncture and Acupressure for Weight Loss

Acupuncture is the traditional Chinese medical practice of stimulating specific points on the body, primarily with the insertion of very thin needles through the skin.

Advocates of acupuncture for weight loss believe that acupuncture can stimulate the body's energy flow (chi) to impact factors that can reverse obesity, such as increasing metabolism, reducing appetite, lowering stress, as well as affecting the part of the brain that feels hunger.

Weight gain, according to traditional Chinese medicine, is caused by internal body imbalance.

There have been studies suggesting that acupuncture is likely effective for weight loss. Those studies suggested that these results weren't completely convincing because of problems with the way the studies had been carried out.

Therefore, these traditional techniques do not form any significant threat to LSG.

4   Power of Customers

Customers could be considered as the insurance companies or third-party payers, or even the patients themselves.

The strongest bargaining power comes from the insurance companies.

While most of the major insurance carriers offer coverage for bariatric surgery, not all policies include coverage.

5   Power of Suppliers

Not all bariatric surgeons perform every procedure; Not all hospitals provide these surgeries.

Therefore, suppliers exert low to medium bargaining power in this domain.

What about the SWOT (Strengths, Weaknesses, Opportunities and Threats) analysis?

5.1   Strengths

Gastric Bypass Surgery: has a long history of success and clinical studies to validate its effectiveness [1, 2].

- Average Excess Weight Loss: 60–80%
- Serious Complication Rate: 1.25%
- Average 30 Day Mortality Rate (Death Rate): 0.14%
- May reduce hunger.
- Excellent rate of diabetes cessation after surgery.
- May relieve heartburn and acid reflux.

Gastric Sleeve Surgery [3, 4]:

- Average Excess Weight Loss: 57–70%
- Serious Complication Rate: 0.96%
- Average 30 Day Mortality Rate (Death Rate): 0.08%
- An average hospital stay of 2 nights, but in some cases, can be performed as an outpatient procedure.
- May reduce hunger.
- No foreign objects like that with Lap Bands.
- No re-routing of the intestines as seen with gastric bypass.
- A straightforward procedure that is relatively easy to replicate.

Duodenal Switch Surgery [5]:

- Average Excess Weight Loss: 80–90%
- Serious Complication Rate: 2–3%
- Average Mortality Rate (Death Rate): 0.29–2.7%
- The best weight loss profile, up to 85% excess weight loss.
- The best long-term weight loss success rate (better than 50% excess weight loss) of 95%.
- Best rate of comorbidity reduction.

5.2   Weaknesses

There are trade-offs. Bariatric surgery carries some long-term risks for patients, including: Dumping syndrome, a condition that can lead to symptoms like nausea and dizziness. Low blood sugar and malnutrition.

Bypass is more effective for weight loss, but has a greater risk of short-term complications.

It is a technically challenging procedure and typically requires longer time under anesthesia compared to other popular bariatric surgeries.

There is a risk of long-term nutritional deficiencies. Vitamins and minerals are required for life. However, the risk of vitamin and mineral deficiencies is lower than the duodenal switch and gastric bypass.

5.3   Weaknesses of Duodenal Switch Surgery

Duodenal Switch surgery is not a new surgery, many surgeons avoid it and prefer LSG to it, due to the following complexities:

- The highest risk for malnutrition.
- Strictest dietary guidelines.
- The longest and most complex procedure of the three primary bariatric procedures (bypass, sleeve, and duodenal switch).
- Highest 30-day serious complication rate.
- Strict adherence to vitamins and minerals and post-operative diet are required for success and to prevent malnutrition.

However, it is important to keep in mind that these complexities are not permanent. Lifestyle changes are paramount for lasting weight loss for any procedure and must be made clear to all patients before undergoing bariatric surgery. When considering gastric balloons, patients can expect 10 to 30% excess weight loss.

5.4   Opportunities

According to data from the Centers for Disease Control and Prevention (CDC), over a third of adults in the United States live with obesity.

Obesity is the next major epidemiologic challenge facing today's doctors, with the annual allocation of healthcare resources for this disease and related comorbidities projected to exceed $150 billion in the United States.

Furthermore, the incidence of obesity has risen in the United States over the past 30 years; it has been shown that 60% of adults are currently either obese or overweight.

Obesity is associated with a higher incidence of a number of diseases, including diabetes, cardiovascular disease, and cancer.

Consumption of fast food, trans fatty acids (TFAs), and fructose—combined with increasing portion sizes and decreased physical activity—has been implicated as a potential contributing factor in the obesity crisis.

5.5   Threats

New procedures are entering this market e.g. Gastric Balloons are a new tool for patients with a Body Mass Index (BMI) of 30–40 that want to lose weight but do not want to have surgery.

This new option now offers the patient a pill to swallow, and a balloon is then inflated and left in the stomach for six months. This results in reduced hunger and an increase in the feeling of satiety.

References

1. Phillips E, Ponce J, Cunneen SA, et al. Safety and effectiveness of REALIZE adjustable gastric band: 3-year prospective study in the United States. Surg Obes Relat Dis. 2009;5:588–97.
2. Tice, et al. Gastric banding or bypass? A systematic review comparing the two popular procedures. Am J Med. 2008;121:885–93.
3. O'Brian P, et al. Systematic review of medium-term weight loss after bariatric surgery. Obes Surg. 2006;16:1031–40.
4. Tice JA, Karliner L, Walsh J, et al. gastric banding or bypass? A systematic review comparing the two most popular procedures. Am J Med. 2008;121:885–93.
5. Cottam et al. A case-controlled match-paired cohort study of lap. RNY gastric bypass and lap band patient in a single US center with three year follow up. Obes. Surg. 2006;16: 534–40.

Medical Tourism: Global Bariatric Healthcare

Ahmad Bashir

1   Introduction

With the increase in world connectivity and ease of travel, ASMBS issued its position statement on medical tourism in bariatric surgery calling it 'Global Bariatric Healthcare' [1]. They feared the term 'Medical Tourism' would not accurately describe all the issues or concerns associated with bariatric surgery. They defined global bariatric healthcare as "travel to undergo bariatric surgery across any distance that precludes routine follow-up and continuity of care with the surgeon or program". Any distance associated with such conditions, was seen to fulfill this definition, even if within the same country, across cities, regions or states.

Based on commercial estimates, in 2018, the medical tourism market size was valued at 36.9 billion USD [2]. It is projected to be 179.6 billion USD by 2026, not including all potential countries, suggesting that physicians, societies and medical industry should put more emphasis on studying this sector, along with working to decrease the risks, concerns and burdens associated with it.

The number of publications addressing medical tourism has been increasing exponentially since 2004 (Fig. 1), in line with the increase in value mentioned above. However, there are plethora of areas for potential research to understand the realities of this sector. In this chapter, we will try to review the available literature to understand the impact of global bariatric healthcare on bariatric surgery outcomes worldwide, while identifying the areas of deficiency to promote more research to address them.

A. Bashir (✉)
Gastrointestinal, Bariatric and Metabolic Center (GBMC), Jordan Hospital, Amman, Jordan
e-mail: ahmad.bashir.md@gmail.com

S. Al-Sabah et al. (eds.), *Laparoscopic Sleeve Gastrectomy*,
https://doi.org/10.1007/978-3-030-57373-7_22

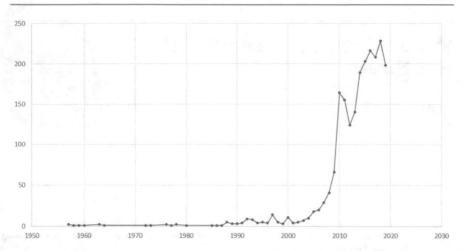

Fig. 1 Pubmed publications 1957–2019 on 'Medical Tourism'—CSV file obtained from pumed. com

---

2   The Impetus Behind Global Healthcare

The incentives behind the global healthcare growing vary according to different perspectives. From the eyes of surgeons accepting medical tourism; patients travel seeking bariatric surgery due to higher cost of care in the private sector of their own country, with long waiting lists within their national health system, lack of insurance coverage for bariatric surgery or lack of service providers able to perform bariatric surgery [3]. In a survey by Kowalewski et al. in which 93 bariatric surgeons from thirty-three countries responded to, bariatric surgery costs ranged from 2,300 to 35,000 USD with a mean of 7760 USD (±4035). The cost of treatment correlated weakly with gross domestic product GDP, influencing the flux of patients to nearby countries with lower cost of care as mentioned in several patterns within the survey (Fig. 2). This phenomenon is not unique to bariatric surgery, as it is noted in cosmetic surgery, fertility medicine, dental care, transplant, orthopedic surgery among several others [4].

The patients' view is similar, however with more barriers. Snyder et al. [5] interviewed patients who pursued care outside Canada (9% undergoing bariatric surgery). Long wait times for necessary procedures were seen as unethical and the primary driver for patients to seek treatment abroad. Having the ability to travel for treatment heightened the patients sense of control, as they felt justified to do so. Patients perceived the health system, in their study, as stifling to surgeons' ability to innovate, as it lacks the proper incentives to do so. Canada provided coverage for patients to undergo bariatric surgery in the United States in the recent past [6]. As the need for regional and local ability to provide these services was recognized, the country invested in building these services. However, the long

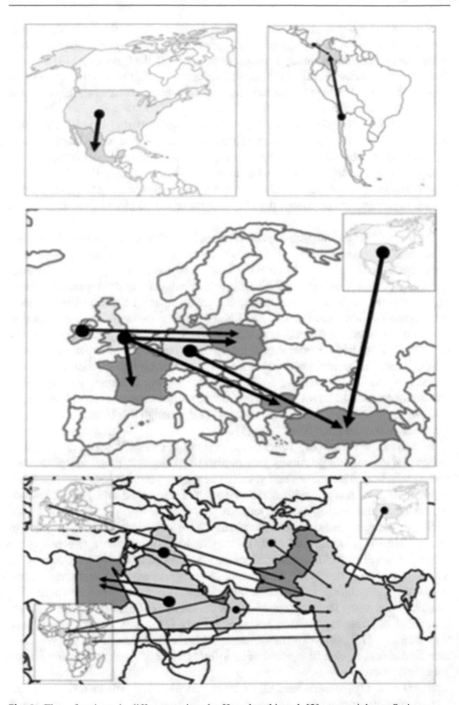

Fig. 2 Flux of patients in different regions by Kowalewski et al. [3]—copyrights to Springer

wait times of 5 years at times, with 1% out of 20% suffering from obesity getting access to care seems to drive patients to travel outside despite the patients having to pay out of pocket to undergo bariatric surgery [7]. Jackson et al. [8] showed that patients experienced all of the above barriers: long wait time, strict criteria for surgery, on top of limited options in certain areas, which incentivized them to seek different treatment abroad.

In the United Kingdom (UK), Hanefeld et al. [9] reported besides all of the mentioned above, the patients' lack of trust towards the National Health System (NHS) while on the waiting list for bariatric surgery. Informal networks, support groups and patient referrals seemed to boost the process of traveling abroad once trust is established with a physician accepting medical tourism. Providers abroad tended to have networks within the UK, and some would offer follow up even in the UK.

As for the effect of the industry, Sa Dang et al. [10] recently showed the impact of economy and competition in the medical tourism industry among six south-east Asian countries. In addition to excellent innovative and relatively cheaper medical services, additional tourism activities are a factor in driving more patients to that region. Healthcare facilities and infrastructure, together with the quality of medical tourism providers are the first conditions to any traveler, prior to considering lower costs of care. Governments in those countries play a major role in reducing other burdens: providing educational information on the travel experience, lower air fare costs, tax returns, and travel insurances. Among many reports, Thailand seemed to perform best among countries in that region. Cosmetic surgery is the number one reason to travel to Thailand, but bariatric surgery is second on the list and gaining momentum as a reason to travel [2], although this differs according to the different sources (Fig. 3 and Table 1).

In a systemic review of 'Patient care without borders', Foley et al. [11] also recognized the cultural proximity as a motive for patients to travel to destinations with similar language, culture and values. The positive economic impact has influenced more job creation, with additional sectors developed and geared towards promoting and facilitating medical tourism.

Sleeve gastrectomy, as a procedure, may have contributed to the increase in medical tourism. Kowalewski et al. [3] reported that the number one procedure offered to patients seeking bariatric surgery abroad, was sleeve gastrectomy in 89.1% of surgeons surveyed. Worldwide, sleeve gastrectomy is the number one procedure done among all bariatric procedures [12]. The procedure's relative simplicity and steep learning curve (easier to learn) [13] also led to an increase in number of surgeons offering bariatric surgery [14], with many being sleeve only surgeons [15]. One can only include with these factors, that the procedure increased access to care along with increasing number of bariatric tourists undergoing this procedure.

Rokni et al. [16] summarized all of these into push and pull factors: push factors pushing patients away from their current national health system, while pull factors pulling them into another medical tourism healthcare system or provider (Table 2).

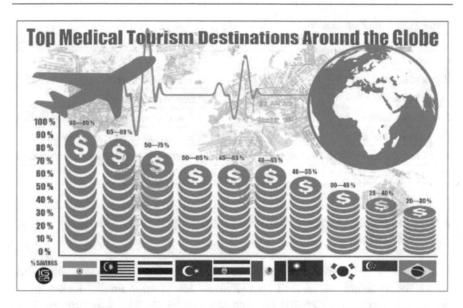

Fig. 3 Top 10 worldwide destinations according to (*AJN* ▼ July 2017 ▼ Vol. 117, No. 7): From left to right: India, Malaysia, Thailand, Turkey, Costa Rica, Mexico, Taiwan, South Korea, Singapore and Brazil. The percentage ranges above each bar indicate cost saving range of receiving medical treatment in each country compared to receiving it in USA. Image courtesy in the report was given to IgeaHub.com (no longer active). If displaying this image is not feasible, then the second option below

Table 1 Top ten medical tourism destinations, based on value and numbers

Top ten medical tourism destinations by value	US $m	Top ten medical tourism destinations by numbers	000K
USA	3,500	Malaysia	900
South Korea	655	USA	500
Turkey	600	South Korea	365
Thailand	600	Thailand	350
Germany	575	Dubal	350
India	450	South Africa	300
UK	350	Taiwan	300
Malaysia	350	Germany	255
Mexico	350	Mexico	250
Iran	315	Turkey	200

Source [16] Rokni et al. adopted from medical tourism and travel market briefing 2018

Table 2 Pull and Push factors

Pull factors	Push factors
Low-cost	High cost of private treatment
High-quality healthcare	Inefficient healthcare system
Expert physicians	Limited access to care
Cultural similarities	Lack of several professional treatments
Geographical proximity	Lack of trust in the national system
Touristic attractions with tourism support	Geographical, political or safety concerns
Level of trust	

3 The Deficiencies, Downside and Upside of Medical Tourism

Unfortunately, the countries with national health systems with long waiting lists, are on the receiving end of their own residents returning at times with complications, after undergoing bariatric or other procedures elsewhere. Before we delve into such reports, it is important to note that patients doing well otherwise are possibly not well represented in the medical literature, as they either follow up with their primary care only, or are just not following up with any physician. Eventually patients tend to seek medical advice if they are vigilant on maintaining their good health, or are experiencing a health problem. Those who only see physicians due to a health problem, will never do so if they are well in their own opinion. This raises the possible matter of medical tourism being impacted with a larger number of negative publications, especially among the countries on the receiving end of complications.

Foley et al. [11] in their systemic review recognized the challenges of having a current well-defined denominator of the number of patients inflowing or outflowing. Several survey studies are limited to specific number of medical tourism providers, without the ability to extrapolate the entire number. Noree et al. [17], showed conflicting numbers between the origin (UK) and recipient (Thailand) countries on the number of patients and types of procedures performed. This confusing conflict in the literature, has led to difficulty in estimating accurate costs, revenue and health outcomes. Commercial reports are also said to overestimate the industry, but without any alternative, several studies quoted these numbers and possibly misrepresented the reality.

Sheppard et al. [18] estimated that the complication rate of medical tourism within Alberta, Canada ranged between 42.2 and 56.1%, a leak rate alone of 12.8–17%, an estimate that far exceeds the complication rate of bariatric surgery performed of 16.6% in Alberta. Venous thromboembolic events (VTE) occurred 4–6 times higher in tourist patients. They estimated that the cost of these complications to exceed performing 250 bariatric procedures within Alberta and managing their potential complications. Their group showed similar results again in 2016 [7]. Unfortunately, bariatric tourists returning home with acute complications, may end up in non-specialized hospitals without proper knowledge of bariatric complications, which may worsen their outcome. This has led some to educate general surgeons on various bariatric procedures, their complications and how to effectively deal with them [19].

Unique bacterial infections have been reported away from bariatric surgery [20]. Usually the ones reported are either rare otherwise or multidrug resistant. Among transplant tourism utilizing commercial organs, this was highest.

In patients from relatively poorer countries seeking treatment when local expertise is not present, a good portion would end up paying catastrophic amount of money leading to a huge financial burden on the individual, family and even the society where patients reside [20].

Other social difficulties were reported by Awano et al. [21] in Japan. Language barriers, inadequate or inaccurate referral information, difference in cultural habits led to more confusion in some patients, with a few going elsewhere for treatment. Caregiver-companions; family or friends traveling with medical tourists, also face a great burden while abroad [22]. They have a heightened sense of responsibility, with most feeling vulnerable emotionally and strained financially if complications occur while abroad.

Perhaps one of the major criticisms of the ethical side of the tourism industry, is the lack of proper informed consent on potential risks of medical tourism [11]. Only 11.7% of a Canadian broker sites reported in Foley et al. review, mentioned the risks properly. Although the risks in the literature may be overstated, they felt the current status had to be mentioned and the tourism sites have to be encouraged to share their outcomes.

Still, several gaps exist that need to be addressed in research. This has led some as Peters et al. [23] to call for national bariatric tourism registry to define the actual cohort of patients seeking bariatric tourism. Till then, together with ASMBS position statement [1], they suggested increasing patients awareness on risks, identifying good providers within a Joint Commission International (JCI) accredited healthcare facility, while enforcing payers to maintain continuity of care with maintaining access to complications.

With all negatives mentioned above, there is still an upside to medical tourism. The economic upside as mentioned above, with expected growth to countries investing in health tourism [2, 10, 23]. This may aid in decreasing costs to healthcare for locals. It also may improve the level of overall care provided.

The overall access to care with decrease in the burden of overall wait time can be achieved at a lower cost, if complication rates were low or minimized. A standard enforced by societies together with a unified global registry may aid in identifying profile of patients seeking bariatric tourism with their true outcomes. Established registries, such as American College of Surgeons (ACS) National Surgery Quality Improvement Project (NSQIP) or Metabolic & Bariatric Surgery

Accreditation & Quality Improvement Project (MBSAQIP), Global Registry of International Federation for Surgery of Obesity (IFSO) and Bariatric Outcomes Longitudinal Database (BOLD), should consider adding a variable to define if a patient is a medical tourist or not, as all other parameters of follow up are otherwise well defined. This may be the beginning to answer the deficits present in the research today, to help us understand the true outcomes of bariatric tourism.

4 Conclusion

Medical tourism is growing globally. It stemmed from inefficiencies and higher costs within certain healthcare systems, with patients seeking care mainly at lower cost, but with excellent healthcare facilities with trusted providers. Sleeve gastrectomy contributed to the increase in bariatric tourism.

Risks with medical tourism are reportedly high, however, the outcomes of the overall tourism cohort are lacking with additional research needed. A call for national and unified shared global registry within the different bariatric societies may aid in the complete understanding of the true outcomes of bariatric tourism. A bridge between scientific bodies and the commercial providers of medical tourism has to be established to initiate the complete understanding of this phenomenon.

References

1. American Society for, M., C. Bariatric Surgery Clinical Issues. American Society for Metabolic and Bariatric Surgery position statement on global bariatric healthcare. Surg Obes Relat Dis. 2011;7(6): 669–71.
2. Grand view research. Medical Tourism Market Size, Share & Trends Analysis Report By Country (Turkey, Costa Rica, Thailand, India, Mexico, Singapore, Brazil, Malaysia, Taiwan, Colombia, South Korea), and Segment Forecasts, 2019–2026. https://www.grandviewresearch.com/press-release/global-medical-tourism-market.
3. Kowalewski PK, et al. Current practice of global bariatric tourism-survey-based study. Obes Surg. 2019;29(11):3553–9.
4. Leggat P. Medical tourism. Aust Fam Phys. 2015;44(1–2):16–21.
5. Snyder J, Crooks VA, Johnston R. Perceptions of the ethics of medical tourism: comparing patient and academic perspectives. Public Health Ethics. 2012;5(1):38–46. https://doi.org/10.1093/phe/phr034.
6. Gagner M. Bariatric surgery tourism hidden costs? How Canada is not doing its part in covering bariatric surgery under the Canada Health Act. Can J Surg. 2017;60(4):222–3.
7. Kim DH, et al. Financial costs and patients' perceptions of medical tourism in bariatric surgery. Can J Surg. 2016;59(1):59–61.
8. Jackson C, et al. I didn't have to prove to anybody that I was a good candidate": a case study framing international bariatric tourism by Canadians as circumvention tourism. BMC Health Serv Res. 2018;18(1):573.
9. Hanefeld J, et al. Why do medical tourists travel to where they do? The role of networks in determining medical travel. Soc Sci Med. 2015;124:356–63.
10. Dang HS et al. Grey system theory in the study of medical tourism industry and its economic impact. Int J Environ Res Public Health. 2020;17(3).

11. Foley BM et al. Patient care without borders: a systematic review of medical and surgical tourism. J Travel Med. 2019;26(6).
12. Angrisani L, et al. IFSO Worldwide Survey 2016: primary, endoluminal, and revisional procedures. Obes Surg. 2018;28(12):3783–94.
13. Carandina S, et al. Laparoscopic sleeve gastrectomy learning curve: clinical and economical impact. Obes Surg. 2019;29(1):143–8.
14. Janik MR, Stanowski E, Pasnik K. Present status of bariatric surgery in Poland. Wideochir Inne Tech Maloinwazyjne. 2016;11(1):22–5.
15. Udelsman BV, et al. Surgeon factors are strongly correlated with who receives a sleeve gastrectomy versus a Roux-en-Y gastric bypass. Surg Obes Relat Dis. 2019;15(6):856–63.
16. Rokni L, Park SH. Medical tourism in Iran, reevaluation on the new trends: a narrative review. Iran J Public Health. 2019;48(7):1191–202.
17. Noree T, Hanefeld J, Smith R. UK medical tourists in Thailand: they are not who you think they are. Global Health. 2014;10:29.
18. Sheppard CE, et al. Medical tourism and bariatric surgery: who pays? Surg Endosc. 2014;28(12):3329–36.
19. Healy P, et al. Complications of bariatric surgery–what the general surgeon needs to know. Surgeon. 2016;14(2):91–8.
20. Lunt N, Horsfall D, Hanefeld J. Medical tourism: a snapshot of evidence on treatment abroad. Maturitas. 2016;88:37–44.
21. Awano N, et al. Issues associated with medical tourism for cancer care in Japan. Jpn J Clin Oncol. 2019;49(8):708–13.
22. Whitmore R, Crooks VA, Snyder J. Ethics of care in medical tourism: Informal caregivers' narratives of responsibility, vulnerability and mutuality. Health Place. 2015;35:113–8.
23. Peters X, Gangemi A. An update on bariatric tourism: time for a national registry? Surg Obes Relat Dis. 2018;14(4):528–32.

Sleeve Gastrectomy: Medicolegal Aspects

Evangelos Efthimiou

Laparoscopic stapling bariatric procedures such laparoscopy gastric bypass started gaining popularity in UK and Europe the last 15–20 years and superseded the laparoscopic adjustable gastric band in numbers and popularity. In the last 10 years laparoscopic sleeve gastrectomy has become the most commonly performed bariatric procedure superseding the laparoscopic R-en-Y gastric bypass which many bariatric surgeons consider the gold standard [1]. For the last 5 years the one anastomosis gastric bypass has increasingly gaining ground as an alternative to the R-en-Y gastric bypass. These three procedures appear to dominate the bariatric domain, with the ideal bariatric procedure remaining illusive.

The rapid acceptance of laparoscopic sleeve gastrectomy in the bariatric domain as a stand-alone procedure was fuelled by its technical simplicity and the continuous improvement of modern stapling guns providing a reliable, secure, and haemostatic long staple line. The simplicity of sleeve gastrectomy appealed to prospective patients as an easier procedure to understand, avoiding the technicalities of bypassing the bowel and its restoration of continuity either in an "Y" or loop configuration. As the general public's appeal for sleeve gastrectomy increased many Upper GI surgeons without formal bariatric training undertook these operations leading to bad outcomes and fuelling litigation. Insurance premiums for surgeons performing bariatric surgery are generally higher than general surgery.

The lack of private insurance coverage for bariatric procedures in many countries, including UK, necessitated many patients self-funding their operation, providing a rather low threshold for litigation in cases of unexpected or adverse outcomes which escalate cost of treatment and lead to loss of income.

E. Efthimiou (✉)
Chelsea and Westminster Hospital NHS Foundation Trust, Chelsea, London, UK
e-mail: e.efthimiou@doctors.org.uk

S. Al-Sabah et al. (eds.), *Laparoscopic Sleeve Gastrectomy*,
https://doi.org/10.1007/978-3-030-57373-7_23

As obesity affects mostly lower socioeconomic classes in developed countries the ability of patients to absorb loss of income is limited and can lead to devastating effects for them and their families. The "no win no fee" option from personal injury lawyers provides a relative straightforward road for patients to pursue compensation and lowers the threshold to commence the litigation process.

International health tourism with many patients travelling abroad for bariatric operations in search for lower costs of surgery further complicates matters, as the route to pursue financial claims related to potential malpractice varies from country to country leaving many patients potentially vulnerable and uncertain on how to proceed.

The best strategy for a surgeon to deal with litigation is its avoidance. From the author's experience in medicolegal cases involving bariatric surgery and specifically sleeve gastrectomy the commonest causes for patients to initiate litigation procedures fall in three categories.

a. claims of incompetence in performing the operation (with leaks from sleeve gastrectomy as the commonest)
b. claims of delay in diagnosis and treatment of complications
c. claims of substandard information given about the operation and its potential complications during the consent process.

Gastric sleeve leaks heal much slower than leaks from gastric bypass with a higher incidence of chronic leak and need for repetitive procedures and prolonged hospitalisation. In UK, surgeons are bound to abide with the Montgomery ruling [2] when they obtain consent for a surgical procedure. In practical terms simply mentioning the generally quoted 0.5–1% leak rate following sleeve gastrectomy is not enough. Many patients will be unaware of what a leak is and what the treatment of the leak entails and assume that the low risk of leak makes the complication insignificant. The consent process should inform and record that in case of a leak hospitalisation will be prolonged even for weeks and further procedures or even operations will be required to deal with the leak as well as the potential for chronicity of the leak and need for major future surgery. The level of information should be tailored to the individual patient.

A freelance oil trader launched a litigation process following a leak from a sleeve gastrectomy that required significant time in hospital, increased hospital fees and led to loss of income. In his argument he claimed he had not been fully informed prior to his sleeve gastrectomy about the exact consequences of a leak. If he had known these he would not have gone ahead with the operation as even the risk was small the effects in his work would have been significant. The low 1% risk of leak rate made him feel safe and he assumed that the treatment of the leak would not have been as complicated as it proved to be. Naming a list of complications and their associate incidence is not considered acceptable practice and will leave the surgeon exposed to potentially successful litigation. The surgeon should explain and record the required treatment and consequences of such a serious complication in the context of a fully informed patient. The Montgomery rule applies retrospectively. A retired builder launched litigation procedures against a surgeon who quoted a 1% leak rate and wrote in his letter to the patient he had never experienced a leak in over 1,500 procedures. A staple line leak occurred a few days after surgery and was successfully treated but resulted in prolonged hospitalisation and loss of income. The patient claimed he understood from his discussion with the surgeon that the particular surgeon never gets leaks and felt reassured it would not happen to him. The surgeon was asked to provide evidence for both of his claims of number of cases and 0% leak rate. The publicly available record of cases the surgeon had recorded in the national bariatric data base was significantly smaller than the number he claimed. Frank discussion backed by facts and provision of written visual or audio material to enhance patient information prior to the operation is crucial to avoid and defend litigation suits. Providing a direct line of communication with the surgeon for the first few days after surgery until the leak risk lessens avoids the problems with the patient seeking advice out of hours from those unfamiliar with the procedure medical services that can delay access to the appropriate level of care for investigation and treatment.

In hospital setting delays in recognising leaks and delays in providing definitive treatment has the potential to cause seriously unfavourable outcomes with subsequent legal suits. The faster the leak is recognised and the sooner a bariatric surgeon is involved the higher the chances of a successful outcome which will lessen the risk of litigation.

Robust adherence to DVT prophylaxis protocols which are regularly reviewed and updated according to the emerging evidence will bolster the bariatric practice from the risk of successful litigation.

Assessing all potential candidates for stapling procedures within the auspices of a multidisciplinary team, irrespective the payor (state, self-funding, private insurer) is a pre-requisite of a successful and safe bariatric practice.

Meticulous data collection including case mix, volume and complications for every surgeon, collected independently and available for the public to view in an understandable format provided by National Bariatric Registers should be a requirement before any surgeon is granted privileges for bariatric surgery either in private or state funded hospitals.

The most devastating for the patient is the development of Wernicke's encephalopathy following bariatric surgery. A machinery operator underwent sleeve gastrectomy and experienced significant nausea and vomiting the following three months following and multiple admissions for dehydration in the bariatric unit he was operated. The radiological investigation revealed a normal looking sleeve, but the patient remained unable to proceed to the expected stages of diet and remained nauseous and vomiting sporadically. Alternative routes of temporary alimentation were not explored and during the last admission the patient experienced loss of vision and ability to walk unaided. His dehydration had been treated with intravenous Dextrose 5%. The neurological opinion was of Wernicke's encephalopathy and was backed by the results of low thiamine levels performed a few days prior to the development of neurological signs. Thiamine replacement was not considered until the development of neurological signs. The patient despite commencement of intravenous thiamine replacement lost most of his vision and his ability to walk became wheelchair bound and required significant levels of assistance with his daily activities of life. Negligence and liability were admitted, and the final claim was settled for a seven-figure number. Wernicke's encephalopathy is a serious and mostly irreversible condition which is fully preventable with high level of suspicion when there has been a history of continuous vomiting for more than two weeks or chronic persisting vomiting. High level of suspicion and early and adequate thiamine orally or intravenously supplementation with avoidance of Dextrose intravenous fluid until thiamine has been intravenously administered is paramount.

There are published reports of Barrett's oesophagus developing in patients following sleeve gastrectomy [3]. These reports raise the issue of patient awareness about the possibility of Barrett's development with the need for regular endoscopic surveillance to detect development of Barrett's and monitor for development of dysplasia according to the established protocols of surveillance. If all the patients after a sleeve gastrectomy should have regular endoscopic monitoring and how frequently is a matter that will need addressing by the bariatric surgical societies to avoid future lawsuits.

Complications are inherent in surgical practice and will continue to occur no matter how advanced surgery becomes. Litigation process is a tedious and long process both for the patient and the surgeon involved. The way surgeons inform patients about these complications requires to evolve and embrace modern technology and formats patients understand easily, avoiding medical jargon.

Accreditation of bariatric surgeons via dedicated fellowship programmes, restriction of bariatric procedures in dedicated bariatric programs with a multidisciplinary patient assessment, protocol based treatment of complications in bariatric patients and availability of direct lines of communication between the patients and bariatric surgeon and service will prevent late presentations of serious complications with potentially unfavourable outcomes and litigation procedures, ensuring data, patient, and surgeon confidentiality is some of the strategies health care systems will require to adopt.

References

1. https://www.ifso.com/pdf/5th-ifso-global-registry-report-september-2019.pdf.
2. https://www.supremecourt.uk/cases/docs/uksc-2013-0136-judgment.pdf.
3. Systematic Endoscopy 5 Years After Sleeve Gastrectomy Results in a High Rate of Barrett's Esophagus: Results of a Multicenter Study Lionel Sebastianelli1,2 & Marine Benois1,2 & Geoffroy Vanbiervliet1,2 & Laurent Bailly1,3 & Maud Robert4 & Nicolas Turrin5 & Emmanuel Gizard5 & Mirto Foletto6 & Marco Bisello6 & Alice Albanese6 & Antonella Santonicola7 & Paola Iovino7 & Thierry Piche1,2 & Luigi Angrisani8 & Laurent Turchi9 & Luigi Schiavo10 & Antonio Iannelli1,2,11 Published online: 21 January 2019 # Springer Science+Business Media, LLC, part of Springer Nature; 2019.

Laparoscopic Sleeve Gastrectomy 101

How the LSG is Performed: A Step-By-Step Procedure

Bassem Safadi and Karin Karam

There are multiple technical approaches to performing a laparoscopic sleeve gastrectomy (LSG) with countless variations [1–4]. I put together a description of my approach after 2500 consecutive procedures. I modified this approach over the past 10 years and standardized it 5 years ago with the intent of balancing the weight loss aspect of the procedure along with reduction in complication potential. Now that we understand LSG not only as a restrictive but also satiety-reducing procedure, we put more emphasis on complete excision of the fundus and do not necessarily make the gastric tube too tight [5, 6]. We are also cognizant of the deleterious effect of reflux esophagitis on patients long-term so we emphasize the need to detect and repair hiatal hernias intra-operatively with tight crural repair [2, 7]. Reflux esophagitis results not only from hiatal hernias but more likely from any anatomic or functional gastric obstruction. That is why it is important to avoid twists or narrowing particularly at the Angularis Incisura [1, 8]. Bleeding and staple line leak remain the two most common short-term complications of LSG. Choosing the appropriate staple line height, over sewing or re-enforcing the staple line and avoiding gastric tube narrowing are all key technical elements that reduce these risks [9]. Lastly, we routinely fix the gastric tube to the transverse colon mesentery at the inferior border of the pancreas to minimize the risk of axial torsion and perhaps provide a form of fixation of the stomach in the abdomen to reduce of risk of intra-thoracic migration [10].

B. Safadi (✉) · K. Karam
Department of Surgery, Lebanese American University (LAU) Medical Center-Rizk Hospital, Beirut, Lebanon
e-mail: bassem.safadi@lau.edu.lb

K. Karam
e-mail: karin.karam@lau.edu
B. Safadi · K. Karam Lebanese American University, Gilbert and Rose-Marie Chagoury School of Medicine, Beirut, Lebanon

S. Al-Sabah et al. (eds.), *Laparoscopic Sleeve Gastrectomy*,
https://doi.org/10.1007/978-3-030-57373-7_24

219

The following describes how I do the LSG step by step:

A. Patient positioning and port placement

The patient is placed in the supine position with arms comfortably placed on lateral arm boards. Mechanical venous compression apparatus is placed on the lower extremities (Foot pumps, sequential compression device, etc.) (Fig. 1). The table is placed in mild reverse Trendelenburg (around 15–20 degrees) with slight downward tilt to the right side. For most patients I start by placing a 12–15 mm port in the infra-umbilical position under direct vision. In super-obese patients were the umbilical skin in displaced far caudally I choose a point around 35-cm below the Xyphoid process slightly to the right

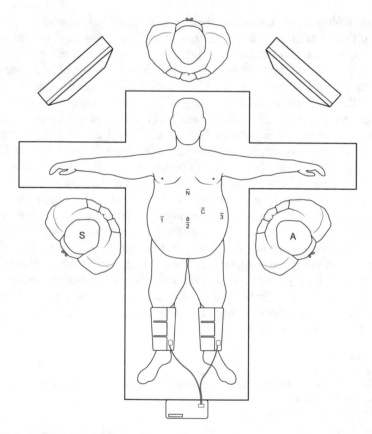

Fig. 1 Patient positioning and port placement: Surgeon (S) stands on the right side of the patient working with ports 1 and 2. In the majority of patients, port 2 is at the umbilicus. The assistant (A) holds the scope with the left hand through the Camera (C) port and assists with port 3. The sub-xyphoid incision allows the introduction of the "Nathanson" liver blade. The LSG can be performed without the N and Port 3 in cases where the liver is small, exposure is easy and the surgeon is sufficiently experienced

of midline. This port will serve as a working port for dissection, stapling and suturing. Then, in sequence, I place two lateral ports along the anterior axillary lines few cms above the level of the umbilicus. The camera port is placed 25-cm below the xyphoid process at the left mid-clavicular level. It is crucial that the camera port is placed high enough to provide clear view of the hiatus and in particular the left crus of the diaphragm. Finally, a "Nathanson" liver blade is used to retract the left lateral segment of the liver and is fixed to a table-mounted retractor arm.

The surgeon stands to the right side of the patient using the right lateral and umbilical port. The assistant stands on the left holding the camera with the left hand and assisting with the right hand using the left sided port. The scope is angled (typically 30-degrees) for better visualization.

There is a rationale for using the umbilical level to work and in particular to staple and I will try to use Fig. 2 to explain it. The stapler shaft and tip should ideally placed parallel to the orogastric tube as the surgeons advances it toward to Angle of His. This will reduce the risks of kinks and twists in gastric tube and will align the staples in sequence to avoid staple crossover. If the stapler is introduced via a high lying port, it will come at an angle and the surgeon will have to compensate by torqueing and angulating the stapler which increases the risk of twist in the gastric tube. The main disadvantage in using relatively low ports is working at a long distance and for that one would need long instruments to work with. The instruments including staplers are long (at least 43-cm long).

B. Freeing up the stomach

There are numerous vessel sealing devices that are available in the market with different sealing technology. I prefer using a long instrument (43-cm) and one that generates the least fumes or vapor. I sometimes use a smoke evacuator system and that seems to cut down on operative time, clears the view and minimizes the number of times the scope has to be removed for cleaning. The

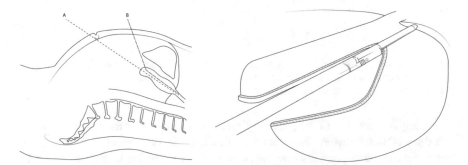

Fig. 2 This figure illustrates the importance of placing the stapling port low enough to ensure that the staple line is perfectly aligned from the Angularis Incisura to the EG junction. The sagittal representation of the abdomen on the left shows an appropriate placement of the stapling port in the infra-umbilical location (A) which allows formation of a consecutive rows of staples parallel to the shaft of the stapling device. When the port is placed high (B) the staple device would come at an angle with the staple line and that may lead to spiral twists in the sleeved stomach

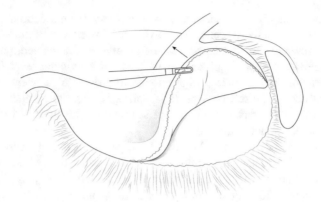

Fig. 3 Sealing and dividing the gastro-epiploic vessels starts at the mid greater curvature and continues toward the short gastric vessels at the upper pole of the spleen

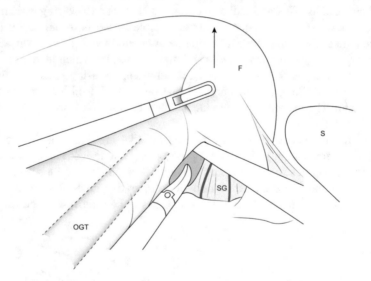

Fig. 4 After reaching the superior pole of the spleen (S), it is easier to lift the fundus anteriorly, develop the avascular plane along the oro-gastric tube (OGT) and then divide the posterior short gastric vessels (SG) from medial to lateral

sealing and division of the gastro-epiploic vessels starts at the mid greater curvature of the stomach since that part has little to no posterior attachment to the pancreas and provides easy and efficient access to the lesser sac. Once the lesser sac is opened and the posterior aspect of the stomach is visualized sealing and dividing branches of the gastro-epiploic vessels along the greater curvature of the stomach and the posterior short gastric ensues all the way to the Angle of His (Fig. 3). It is easier and safer to expose the short gastric vessels by lifting the fundus upward and sealing/dividing them posteriorly starting medially and then heading laterally toward the spleen. This is particularly helpful when the fundus is stuck close to the spleen. The dissection stops when the left crus of the diaphragm is reached (Fig. 4).

Sealing and division of the vessels continues distally separating the greater omentum from the stomach reaching 2 to 4 cms proximal to the pylorus. All posterior attachments between the stomach and the pancreas are released by cautery or sharp dissection until the greater curvature of the stomach is completely free and mobile.

C. Delineating the presence of a hiatal hernia

We perform routine gastroscopy on all patients pre-operatively so we know ahead of time who has a hiatus hernia or a wide hiatus by the Hill classification and those patients deserve a thorough intra-operative examination to determine if there is a hiatal hernia. Hiatal hernias are sometimes easily seen on initial exploration when there is a frank dimple sign or when the esophageal fat pad is seen herniating into the mediastinum. More often, small hiatal hernias are not easily seen upon initial exploration. When we get to the left crus of the diaphragm, we incise the peritoneal layer overlying the inferior border of the left crus and at that stage we should see clearly the longitudinal fibers of the esophagus. If not, then we continue dissection of the phreno-esophageal membrane anteriorly until we are sure the esophagus is seen. We routinely dissect the esophageal fat pad and divide it at the level of the Angle of His. Sometimes we see a large posterior fat pad herniating into the mediastinum and in that case would reduce it and excise it and that will expose the defect in the hiatus. Once we identify or highly suspect a hiatal hernia, we divide the gastro-hepatic ligament. Any dominant left accessory or replaced hepatic artery is preserved. The peritoneum at the inferior border of the right crus is incised to expose the esophagus. The rest of the dissection is done bluntly. A plane is developed behind the esophagus and posterior vagus nerve and the distal esophagus is encircled with a Penrose drain and retracted. The rest of the peritoneal attachments between the esophagus-crura and mediastinal attachments including distal perforators are sealed and divided to mobilize the esophagus and ensure at least 2–4 cm of esophagus in the abdomen without tension. Approximation of the crura is accomplished with non-absorbable sutures posteriorly and sometimes anteriorly taking care not to kink the esophagus anteriorly with excessive posterior approximation. The closure of the hiatus is calibrated using the 40-Fr. Oro-gastric tube. I usually perform the cruroplasty after stapling.

D. Stapling step by step

The stapling of the stomach should mirror the lesser curvature of the stomach to get a symmetrical gastric tube at the end. I now use a 40-Fr. Oro-gastric tube as a guide and no longer use the 32-Fr and 36-Fr tubes because of few cases of gastric tube stenosis that developed while using these tubes. The association between narrower oro-gastric tubes and higher complication rates has been reported in numerous studies [11]. Stomachs come in different sizes and shapes and some situations can create a challenge when it comes to stapling. A J-shaped stomach with an acute angle at the Incisura is such an example. I always start stapling from the right lateral port at 4-cm proximal to the Pylorus and reticulate the stapler so that it is aligned parallel to the lesser curvature (Fig. 5). The gastric wall here is thick and abundant with muscle and

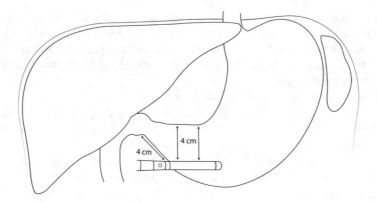

Fig. 5 The first stapler is introduced via the right sided lateral port (Port 1, Fig. 1) and is placed parallel to the lesser curvature at a point around 4 cm proximal to the pylorus. The distance between the lesser curvature and the stapler is no less than 4 cm

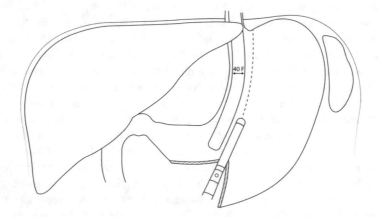

Fig. 6 The second stapler is probably the most critical one during the LSG. It is introduced via the umbilical port in most patients and is reticulated to an angle with the first staple to mimic the lesser curvature bend at the Angularis Incisura. The 40-Fr. Orogastric tube is advanced into the antrum after the stapler has been placed and before it is "fired" to ensure that the newly formed gastric tube is not tight or twisted

therefore the stapler should be 60 mm long and at least 3.0 mm in height. The gastric mucosa and submucosa gets displaced inward several millimeters so it is important not to tighten the tube here and I try to keep it around 4 cm wide. At this stage, I keep the 40-Fr. oro-gastric tube in the proximal aspect of the stomach and do not advance it. The second 60-mm stapler is introduced from the umbilical port with slight reticulation to the right (Fig. 6). This is probably the most important staple application and it is crucial to avoid narrowing the Angularis Incisura or torqueing/twisting the stomach here. Again, the orogastric tube is advanced only after the stapler is positioned to guarantee that the tube can be advanced without difficulty. The stapler is applied and the stomach is stapled and divided. There is a potential risk when the orogastric tube is advanced early to the antrum and stapling is done with the tube in place distally because the tube can distort the shape of the stomach and deceivingly "straighten" the stomach. This can result in narrowing and kinking at the Angularis Incisura especially in J-shaped stomachs and that can only become apparent once the tube in withdrawn.

The remaining staple applications past the Angularis Incisura are placed snug alongside the tube with 3 applications of the 60-mm staplers on average (total 4–7 staplers with a median of 5) (Fig. 7). It is important to check the crotch of the staple line and remove any loose staples as these might lead to subsequent staple malfunction. I toss the stomach back and forth anterior to posterior to make sure I am not leaving any redundant stomach posteriorly, especially the fundus that has to be completely excised. The last stapler is placed around 5 mm on the gastric side of the Angle of His. I try my best to avoid leaving any significant fundic "dog ear" and in case that is present in excess I advocate resection with another stapler [6] (Fig. 8).

E. Extraction of the resected stomach

Once stapling is completed, I remove the resected stomach from the umbilical incision. I do it at this stage since the patient would still be paralyzed and it is easier to remove it with adequate muscle relaxation. I do not place the stomach in a bag but do make sure that the abdominal wall opening is lax enough to allow easy retrieval and avoid excessive traction. Gastric dehiscence while retrieving the stomach could result in significant intra-abdominal and wound complications and should be avoided at all cost. If there is any concern, I would re-introduce the stomach back in, placed it in a bag and repeat the process of extraction.

F. Staple line re-enforcement/gastropexy

Several studies have shown that staple line re-enforcement reduces the risk of bleeding and may reduce the risk of leak and I am a big proponent of staple

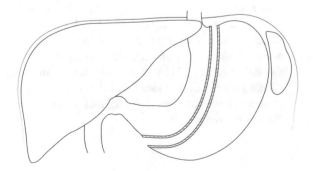

Fig. 7 Stapling is completed with sequential 60-mm staplers introduced via the umbilical port alongside a 40-Fr. Orogastric tube. A small (5-mm) rim of fundus is left just below the EG junction

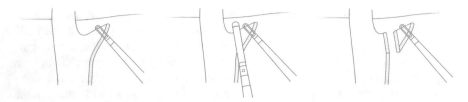

Fig. 8 Residual fundic tissue can enlarge and develop a "neo-fundus. It is better to excise such "dog ears" by re-stapling parallel to the oro-gastric tube to prevent the formation of a "neo-fundus"

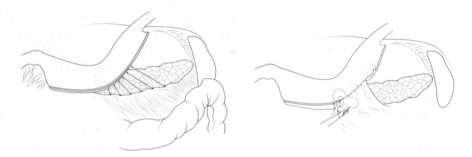

Fig. 9 The newly formed gastric tube is fixed with sutures to the transverse mesocolon at the inferior border of the pancreas. This may help reduce the risk of axial twist and possibly mediastinal migration

line re-enforcement with serosa-to-serosa plication over the staple line [4, 9–11]. I use an absorbable suture such as 3-O or 2-O polydioxanone PDS suture (Johnson & Johnson Medical N.V.). Once we get proximal to the Angularis Incisura, we use the same suture to attach the gastric tube to the transverse mesocolon at the inferior edge of the pancreas to provide a form of gastropexy that might help reduce axial rotation of the gastric tube and perhaps fix the stomach intra-abdominally to reduce the risk of intra-thoracic migration [10] (Fig. 9).

G. Closing

I do not routinely test the staple line with provocative tests such as Methylene blue or air insufflation. The risk of leak or staple line bleeding using this technique is under 1%, and reserve testing for difficult cases or when there is any doubt of a technical mishap. Endoscopy is probably the best method in testing the safety of the LSG and that has shown in some studies [12]. I use 12-mm dilating trocars on the sides so I don't close these. The fascia in the umbilicus is closed with interrupted absorbable sutures and the skin with skin staples or absorbable sutures.

References

1. Bhandari M, Fobi MAL, Buchwald JN. Bariatric Metabolic Surgery Standardization (BMSS) working group: standardization of bariatric metabolic procedures: world consensus meeting statement. Obes Surg. 2019;29(Suppl 4):309–45.
2. Dakour Aridi H, Alami R, Tamim H, Shamseddine G, Fouani T, Safadi B. Long-term outcomes of laparoscopic sleeve gastrectomy: a Lebanese center experience. Surg Obes Relat Dis. 2016;12(9):1689–96.
3. Varban OA, Thumma JR, Finks JF, Carlin AM, Kemmeter PR, Ghaferi AA, Dimick JB. Assessing variation in technique for sleeve gastrectomy based on outcomes of surgeons ranked by safety and efficacy: a video-based study. Surg Endosc. 2019;33(3):895–903.
4. Taha O, Abdelaal M, Talaat M, Abozeid M. A randomized comparison between staple-line oversewing versus no reinforcement during laparoscopic vertical sleeve gastrectomy. Obes Surg. 2018;28(1):218–25.
5. Goitein D, Lederfein D, Tzioni R, Berkenstadt H, Venturero M, Rubin M. Mapping of ghrelin gene expression and cell distribution in the stomach of morbidly obese patients—a possible guide for efficient sleeve gastrectomy construction. Obes Surg. 2012;22(4):617–22.
6. Silecchia G, De Angelis F, Rizzello M, Albanese A, Longo F, Foletto M. Residual fundus or neofundus after laparoscopic sleeve gastrectomy: is fundectomy safe and effective as revision surgery? Surg Endosc. 2015;29(10):2899–903.
7. Dakour Aridi H, Asali M, Fouani T, Alami RS, Safadi BY. Gastroesophageal reflux disease after laparoscopic sleeve gastrectomy with concomitant hiatal hernia repair: an unresolved question. Obes Surg. 2017;27(11):2898–904.
8. Nedelcu M, Manos T, Cotirlet A, Noel P, Gagner M. Outcome of leaks after sleeve gastrectomy based on a new algorithm adressing leak size and gastric stenosis. Obes Surg. 2015;25(3):559–63.
9. Debs T, Petrucciani N, Kassir R, Sejor E, Karam S, Ben Amor I, Gugenheim J. Complications after laparoscopic sleeve gastrectomy: can we approach a 0% rate using the largest staple height with reinforcement all along the staple line? Short-term results and technical considerations. Surg Obes Relat Dis. 2018;14(12):1804–10.
10. Abdallah E, Fikry M, Rady O, Elfeki H. Plicated Sleeve Gastrectomy with Combined Mesocolon and Greater Omentum Fixation After T-Shaped Omentoplasty: How to Do it? Obes Surg. 2020;30(3):1173–4.
11. Parikh M, Issa R, McCrillis A, Saunders JK, Ude-Welcome A, Gagner M. Surgical strategies that may decrease leak after laparoscopic sleeve gastrectomy: a systematic review and meta-analysis of 9991 cases. Ann Surg. 2013;257(2):231–7.'
12. Minhem MA, Safadi BY, Tamim H, Mailhac A, Alami RS. Does intraoperative endoscopy decrease complications after bariatric surgery? Analysis of American College of surgeons national surgical quality improvement program database. Surg Endosc. 2019;33(11):3629–34.

Robotic Sleeve Gastrectomy

Maher El Chaar

1   Introduction

Innovation and technology have become an integral part of the rapid evolution of bariatric surgery. Since the first laparoscopic Roux-en-Y gastric bypass was performed by Wittgrove et al. in 1993, laparoscopy has become the standard approach to bariatric surgery and the advantages of the minimally invasive approach have been well validated [1, 2]. Despite its widespread use and acceptance, there remains limitations to the laparoscopic approach to bariatric surgery which include limitations of movement due to thick abdominal walls and hepatomegaly, limited workspace secondary to increased intra-abdominal fat, limited surgical dexterity, and poor ergonomics. Because of these limitations and in light of recent evidence from the gynecologic literature indicating certain advantages when operating on morbidly obese patients [3, 4], we witnessed an increased interest in the use of robotic platforms in bariatric surgery. However, the use of robotics in bariatric surgery remains controversial because of concerns related to the increased health care costs associated with this new technology and the lack of level I evidence to support its widespread use [5, 6].

In addition to the widely popular Intuitive da Vinci platform, new platforms are increasingly being implemented to improve on the capabilities of previously established systems. A number of new FDA approved robotic surgical platforms with the potential to be used in bariatric surgery have entered the market. These

M. El Chaar (✉)
St Luke's University Hospital and Health Network, Fountain Hill, USA
e-mail: maher.elchaar@gmail.com

M. El Chaar
Lewis Katz School of Medicine, Temple University, Philadelphia, USA

© The Editor(s) (if applicable) and The Author(s), under exclusive license to Springer Nature Switzerland AG 2021
S. Al-Sabah et al. (eds.), *Laparoscopic Sleeve Gastrectomy*,
https://doi.org/10.1007/978-3-030-57373-7_25

include Senhance™ Surgical System (TransEnterix), Versius (CMR Surgical), Verb Surgical (Google, Johnson & Johnson), and Medrobotics Flex® Robotic System. Future studies are needed to further evaluate the advantages and disadvantages of each robotic surgical device and platform as well as their role in bariatric surgery.

Currently, the sleeve gastrectomy (SG) is the most commonly performed procedure in the United States according to the most recent estimates by the American Society for Metabolic and Bariatric Surgery (ASMBS) and its world-wide prevalence has significantly increased in the last years as well [7]. Multiple reports have been published to evaluate the safety and feasibility of robotic-assisted sleeve gastrectomy (RSG) in addition to the cost associated with this new innovative approach. This chapter will evaluate the available literature on robotic assisted sleeve gastrectomy and explore the steps necessary for the establishment of a robotic bariatric program.

2   Robotic-Assisted Sleeve Gastrectomy

According to the most recent estimates by the ASMBS, the SG   is now the most commonly performed bariatric surgery in the United States [7]. Its popularity is a reflection of its relative ease, low complication rate, and excellent short- and intermediate-term outcomes. Most SG procedures are performed using conventional laparoscopy in a largely standardized fashion, though some variation exists, such as in the management of the staple line after transection of the greater curvature. However, the growing popularity of the da Vinci robotic platform (Intuitive Surgical, Atlanta, GA, USA) in other surgical specialties has prompted its limited but growing use in bariatric surgery, presently accounting for 7% of all SG performed in the Metabolic and Bariatric Surgery Accreditation and Quality Improvement Program (MBSAQIP) database [8].

There are a number of potential advantages of robotic technology in bariatric procedures. These advantages are accentuated in the super morbid obese population (BMI>50). Sleeve gastrectomy performed in this population can be technically challenging due to the increased liver size, excess omental fat, and difficulty obtaining adequate pneumoperitoneum, all of which decrease the working space in the upper abdomen [9]. Additionally, the increased abdominal wall thickness of these patients requires additional torque, making fine movements more technically challenging with laparoscopic instruments. Robotic bariatric surgery overcomes some of the limitations of laparoscopic techniques by allowing for 3-dimensional visualization, improved surgeon dexterity, and increased degrees of motion [10–13]. Another proposed benefit of robotic surgery in the super morbid obese population is decreased port site trauma due to a decrease in abdominal wall torque with the remote-center technology [14]. The robotic arms provide the mechanical power to overcome the increased torque required to manipulate instruments in patients with thick abdominal walls thus allowing for finer movements and decreasing surgeon fatigue.

The primary arguments against RSG are the higher costs and longer operating times and the lack of outcome data to support its superiority [5, 6]. These obstacles have resulted in the lack of widespread acceptance and adoption of this technology in bariatric surgery.

3   Cost of Robotic-Assisted Sleeve Gastrectomy

Although use of the da Vinci robotic platform in bariatric surgery is gaining momentum, there are many financial concerns. The issue of cost is a critically important issue for hospital administrators and third-party payers. Increased health care cost associated with this technology is one of the main obstacles preventing its widespread adoption in bariatric surgery.

In a recent meta-analysis, Li et al. was able to show that robotic surgery results in increased health care costs [6]. However, other single institution studies have shown that robotic surgery can be cost effective. In a retrospective study evaluating the cost of robotically assisted sleeve gastrectomy (R-SG) versus conventional laparoscopic sleeve gastrectomy (L-SG), El Chaar et al. reported that the overall cost for RSG and LSG was not statistically different (mean total cost for RSG and LSG was $5308.99 and $4918.88, respectively) with a trend toward shorter length of stay for R-SG over time (1.4 versus 1.5 d, respectively) [15] (see Table 3). These findings, however, cannot be generalized given that cost data is institution specific. More cost data should be collected in light of the new cheaper robotic platforms and extended uses of robotic equipment in order to make meaningful conclusions on whether robotic surgery is cost effective or not.

4   Adoption and Evolution of a Bariatric Robotic Program

Clinical outcomes, training, cost, efficiency, and available local resources and expertise are all critical components to consider when creating a robotic bariatric program. Having a validated training curriculum is very important for patient safety and to avoid issues with credentialing and associated liability. Proficiency-based training curricula that comprehensively address the skills necessary to perform robotic operations have shown construct and content validity as well as feasibility [16–19].

In the development of our robotic surgery program at St Luke's University Hospital and Health Network, we have observed the importance of a systematic approach through the establishment of training programs for both surgeons and the operating room nursing staff, as well as creation of a dedicated robotic OR team. Every new robotic surgeon is required to go through a strict and regimented robotic training pathway involving many hours of on-robot training in a dry lab setting, simulation, live case observations at robotic epicenters around the country, and then a 1 to 2-day intensive training at the da Vinci accredited lab in Atlanta,

GA, USA. The staff also goes through a similar process where they receive hours of online and hands on training prior to being allowed in the robot room with a patient. A specialized OR efficiency team called Genesis was used to help assemble robotic trays, organize equipment, and decrease turnover times. At the initiation of our robotic program, we started with a core robotic team of 5–6 surgical technologists and nurses. Since that time, we have evolved into a much larger robotic team and trained additional staff members due to the increased volume of robotic cases. It is also very important for robotic programs to collect its data and analyze it on a regular basis to improve efficiency, patient outcomes, and safety.

5   Operative Technique

For a RSG, the robotic team generally consists of a console surgeon and a bedside surgeon or assistant. It is best performed in a dedicated robotic operating room with dedicated robotically trained staff. Depending on what robotic platform is available, the room layout and docking techniques may vary. Additionally, depending on the type and availability of robotic stapling devices, a fully robotic or hybrid laparoscopic and robotic approach may be employed. In this chapter, the authors describe a robotic sleeve gastrectomy technique using the Da Vinci Xi platform. For

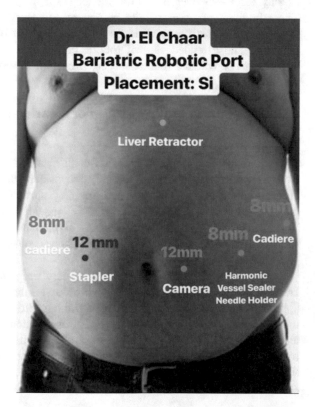

Fig. 1 Trocar placement for robotic sleeve gastrectomy using the da Vinci Si platform. Using the Si system requires stapling through the 12 mm assistant port using a laparoscopic stapler in hybrid-type technique

information on docking and approach to robotic sleeve gastrectomy using the Da Vinci Si system, please refer to Fig. 1.

After induction of general anesthesia, the patient is placed in the supine position with both arms extended and secured to arm boards. A foot board is used to allow for steep reverse Trendelenburg position during the surgery. The patient's abdominal wall is prepped and draped, and the robotic arms are draped in a sterile fashion. The anesthesia drape barrier should be positioned low enough to allow for sufficient working space for the robotic arms.

The procedure is then begun by obtaining access to the abdominal cavity using a Veress needle technique. Once adequate insufflation is obtained, a 0 degree 5-mm laparoscope inside a robotic 8-mm Optiview trocar is used for optical entry at the same site of Veress needle insertion. After inspection of the abdominal cavity, we routinely perform a transverse abdominis plane (TAP) block using a mixture of Exparel, Marcaine, and saline. Additional trocars are then placed under direct visualization with an 8-mm trocar and a 12-mm trocar on the right side of the abdominal wall, and an additional 8-mm trocar and 12-mm assistant port on the left side of the abdominal wall (Fig. 2). It is critical to place all robotic trocar sites at least 8 cm apart (10 cm with Si platform) to avoid collisions of the arms.

Fig. 2 Trocar placement for robotic sleeve gastrectomy using the da Vinci Xi platform

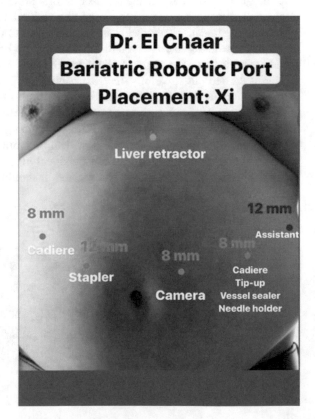

The patient is then placed in steep reverse Trendelenburg position at a minimum of 20°. A Nathanson liver retractor is placed through a small stab incision below the xiphoid process and is used to retract the left lobe of the liver in a medial fashion. When securing the Nathanson liver retractor to the bed rail, it is important to place the post low enough to allow for sufficient clearance for the robotic arms.

Once the trocars and liver retractor have been placed and the patient is appropriately positioned, the robot is docked. We routinely position the robotic cart at the patient's right side. The camera port is docked first using robotic arm three (R3). A 30° robotic scope is inserted into the abdomen in the 30° down position. The target anatomy, in this case the stomach, is selected and the robotic targeting process is completed to align the camera port with the robotic column. The remaining robotic arms (R1, R2, R4) are then docked. A 12–8 mm reducer is placed in the 12-mm trocar initially. A robotic vessel sealer (R4) and two Cadiere graspers (R1, R2) are then introduced into the abdomen under direct visualization. The assistant port can be used for retraction, suction, and insertion of sponges or needles as necessary.

The surgery begins with identifying a point 4 cm proximal to the pylorus along the greater curvature of the stomach. A Cadiere grasper (R2) is then used to elevate the greater curvature of the stomach at this point and provide medial retraction. An atraumatic grasper may be used to provide lateral counter traction of the gastrocolic ligament. The vessel sealer is then used to divide the gastrocolic ligament until the lesser sac is entered. Division of the gastrocolic ligament is then carried superiorly to the angle of His using the vessel sealer (see Fig. 3). As dissection is carried out superiorly, the gastrosplenic ligament is divided to mobilize the gastric fundus from the spleen and off the left crus of the diaphragm. To aid in mobilization of the fundus, the second Cadiere grasper (R1) can be used to grasp the greater curvature and roll the stomach by providing inferior and medial retraction. Full mobilization of the fundus is critical to avoid a large retained fundus as well as to correctly identify the gastroesophageal junction and identify any potential hiatal hernia. If a hiatal hernia is identified, it should be repaired at that time.

Fig. 3 Division of the gastrocolic ligament with the robotic vessel sealing device

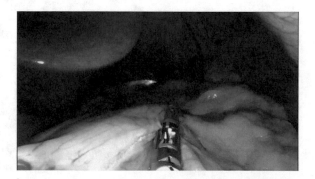

Once mobilization is complete, the anesthesiologist advances a 36-French ViSiGi™ bougie under direct visualization towards the pylorus. The bougie is positioned along the lesser curvature of the stomach and then placed to suction and secured. Stapling of the stomach is then begun using the robotic 60 mm SureForm™ stapler through the second robotic arm (R2). Although the stapler height varies depending on factors such as BMI, gender, and stomach thickness, typically, we start with a black load followed by two green loads and then blue loads for the remainder.

The first staple load with the robotic SureForm™ stapler is deployed across the gastric antrum approximately 5 cm proximal to the pylorus at a slight horizontal angle. During the second firing, care should be taken not to narrow the sleeve too much at the level of the incisura to prevent distal obstruction (see Fig. 4). During transection of the greater curvature of the stomach, particular attention is given to retracting the stomach laterally at the site of the transected vessels to prevent corkscrewing of the gastric sleeve. After the greater curvature is fully divided, the staple line is imbricated using a 2-0 barbed absorbable suture while the bougie remains in place.

After inspecting for hemostasis, the robot is undocked and moved away from the operative field. The Nathanson liver retractor is removed under direct visualization. The 12-mm robotic trocar site is then extended and dilated to allow for removal of the gastric specimen. The specimen is then sent for routine pathological evaluation. Although a specimen bag or wound protection device may be used, we do not routinely use such devices. The site of specimen removal is then closed using a #1 Vicryl suture with a laparoscopic trocar closure device before closing the skin at all trocar sites with 4-0 monocryl suture.

6   Clinical Outcomes

Complications following RSG are similar to those seen following LSG and are widely reported in the literature [20–22]. The overall 30-day mortality and morbidity following SG is reported to be 0% to 1.2% and 0% to 17.5%, respectively

Fig. 4 Stapling of stomach using robotic 60 mm SureForm™ stapling device

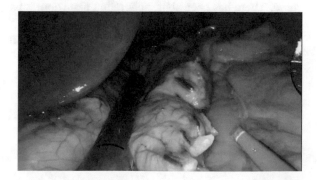

[23]. Complications specific to SG include bleeding, stenosis, portal thrombosis and leak. The most feared of these complications is the staple line leak because of its associated high morbidity and mortality and significantly increased health-care costs. The leak rate after sleeve gastrectomy has been reported between 0–6% [24–29].

Although there is a paucity of long-term data following RSG, there are a number of studies looking at 30-day outcomes. Many of these studies have demonstrated that robotic bariatric surgery has a similar safety profile when compared to laparoscopic bariatric surgery [21, 30, 31]. In a meta-analysis which included sixteen studies and 29,787 patients, Magouliotis et al. found that the RSG technique showed significantly higher mean operative time and increased length of hospital stay. Post-operative incidence of leakage, wound infection, and bleeding were comparable to LSG [20]. Some have suggested that RSG may have improved outcomes when compared with LSG [32]. In a propensity score-matched comparative analysis of the 2015–2016 MBSAQIP database, Sebastian et al. reported that postoperative bleeding and blood transfusion are significantly reduced in bariatric surgery when using a robotic platform [32].

However, other studies have suggested that RSG may be associated with increased complications when compared with LSG. In a review of the MBSAQIP database, Fazl-Alizadeh et al.'s report found no significant difference in 30-day mortality between RSG and LSG (0.02% vs. 0.01%, P=0.88). However, RSG was associated with higher serious morbidity (1.1% vs. 0.8%, P<0.01), higher leak rate (1.5% vs. 0.5%, P<0.01), and higher surgical site infection rate (0.7% vs. 0.4%, P=0.01) [33] (see Table 1).

In a more recent review of the 2016 MBSAQIP database, Lundberg et al. report no difference in serious adverse events or mortality when comparing laparoscopic and robotic sleeve gastrectomy. However, RSG was found to have a higher rate of organ space infection when compared to LSG (odds ratio 2.07). Otherwise, RSG did not significantly differ from LSG save for a longer median operative time (89 vs. 63 min, respectively, P<0.0001) [34] (see Table 2).

Although RSG is still an overall safe and effective procedure, consideration should be given to these findings of increased complications when selecting the approach to SG. The increased complications may be explained by the use of older technology in previously reported outcomes as well as an undefined learning curve. There has been some suggestion that robotic bariatric surgery outcomes are improving over time making it reasonable to expect that we may continue to see an improvement in the safety profile and benefits of the robotic platform in bariatric surgery [8]. Additional research with prospective randomized trials is needed to confirm these findings (Table 3).

Table 1 Risk-adjusted analysis of postoperative outcomes after robotic sleeve gastrectomy versus laparoscopic sleeve gastrectomy [12]

Complications	LSG (N =70,293)	RSG (N = 4781)	AOR	95% CI	P value
30-day mortality	17 (0.02%)	1 (0.01%)	0.85	0.11–6.46	0.88
Serious morbidity	550 (0.8%)	52 (1.1%)	1.40	1.05–1.86	<0.01
Postoperative leak	318 (0.5%)	74 (1.5%)	3.42	2.65–4.42	<0.01
Acute renal failure	40 (0.1%)	0 (0%)	–	–	–*
Renal insufficiency	54(0.1%)	4(0.1%)	1.12	0.40–3.11	0.82
Urinary tract infection	222 (0.3%)	10 (0.2%)	0.66	0.35–1.25	0.20
Unplanned intubation	70 (0.1%)	6 (0.1%)	1.26	0.54–2.90	0.58
Ventilator dependency	25 (0.0%)	5 (0.1%)	2.87	0.92–6.21	0.07
Pneumonia	90 (0.1%)	3 (0.1%)	0.48	0.15–1.54	0.22
Any respiratory complications	158 (0.2%)	13 (0.3%)	1.21	0.68–2.13	0.51
Pulmonary embolism	64 (0.1%)	8 (0.2%)	1.84	0.88–3.85	0.10
Deep vein thrombosis	118 (0.2%)	12 (0.3%)	1.50	0.82–2.72	0.18
Venous thromboembolism	172 (0.2%)	19 (0.4%)	1.63	1.01–2.62	0.04
Superficial SSI	172 (0.2%)	13 (0.3%)	1.09	0.62–1.92	0.75
Deep SSI	15 (0.02%)	0 (0%)	–	–	–*
Organ space SSI	111 (0.2%)	19 (0.4%)	2.51	1.54–4 10	<0.01
Dehiscence	14 (0.01%)	1 (0.02%)	1.03	0.13–7.89	0.97
Any SSI	310 (0.4%)	33 (0.7%)	1.55	1.08–2.23	0.01
Sepsis	60 (0.1%)	5 (0.1%)	1.23	0.49–3.08	0.64
Bleeding disorders requiring transfusion	376 (0.5%)	22 (0.5%)	0.86	0.56–1.32	0.50
Reoperation	582 (0.8%)	53 (1.1%)	1.34	1.01–1.78	0.04
Readmission	2,302 (3.3%)	198 (4.1%)	1.27	109–1.47	<0.01

Table 2 Outcomes of robotic versus laparoscopic sleeve gastrectomy based on MBSAQIP [E]. SLR = staple-line reinforcement; RSG = robot-assisted sleeve gastrectomy; LSG = laparoscopic sleeve gastrectomy; SAE = significant adverse event; OR = odds ratio; CI = confidence interval; OSI = organ space infection. * Based on separate Mann Whitney rank sums tests, X2, or Fisher's exact tests, with $P < 0.05$ denoting statistical significance and no adjustment for the multiple comparisons

Primary outcomes

	SAEn(%)	OSIn (%)	Bleedingn (%)	Mortality at 30 dn (%)
Conventiona laparoscopic (n = 100,341)	None: 281 (1.2)	None: 34 (0.2)	None: 140 (0.6)	None: 18 (0.08)
	SLR only: 729 (1.3)	SLR only: 74 (0.1)	SLR only: 224 (0.4)	SLR only: 37 (0.07)
	Oversew only: 107 (1.2)	Oversew only: 10 (0.1)	Oversew only: 50 (0.6)	Oversew only: 5 (0.06)
	Both: 136 (1.0%)	Both: 14 (0.1)	Both: 47 (0.4)	Both: 6 (0.05)
	Total: 1253 (1.3)	Total: 132 (0.1)	Total: 461 (0.5)	Total: 66 (0.07)
Robotic-assisted (n = 7385)	None: 21 (1.1)	None: 6 (0.3)	None: 6 (0.3)	None: 2 (0.1)
	SLR only: 35 (1.0)	SLR only: 7 (0.2)	SLR only: 15 (0.4)	SLR only: 3 (0.08)
	Oversew only: 7 (1.2)	Oversew only: 3 (0.5)	Oversew only: 3 (0.5)	Oversew only: 0
	Both: 17 (1.3)	Both: 4 (0.3)	Both: 2 (0.2)	Both: 0
	Total: 80 (1.1%)	Total: 20 (0.3%)	Total: 26 (0.4%)	Total: 5 (0.07%)
P value*	0.14	0.79	**0.003**	0.49
Total (N = 107,726)	None: 302 (0.3)	None: 40 (0.04)	None: 146 (0.2)	None: 20 (0.02)
	SLR only: 764 (0.7)	SLR only: 81 (0.08)	SLR only: 239 (0.2)	SLR only: 40 (0.04)
	Oversew only: 114 (0.1)	Oversew only: 13 (0.01)	Oversew only: 53 (0.05)	Oversew only: 5 (0.005)
	Both: 183 (0.2%)	Both: 18 (0.02%)	Both: 49 (0.05%)	Both: 6 (0.006%)

Table 3 Cost analysis of robotic sleeve gastrectomy (R-SG) compared with laparoscopic sleeve gastrectomy (L-SG). SG = sleeve gastrectomy; LOS = length of stay; NS = nonsignificant; OR = operating room. Based on separate Mann–Whitney rank sum tests due to the skewed distributions, with P < 0.05 denoting statistical significance, and no adjustment for multiple testing

	Robotic SG (n = 39)	Laparoscopic SG (n = 59)	P	Total (n = 98)
LOS Direct cost	$704.60	$687.48	NS	$694.29
OR time direct cost	$1340.65	**$1111.83**	**<0.0001**	$1202.89
Supplies direct cost	$3263.75	$3119.57	NS	$3176.95
Total costs	$3263.75	$4918.88	NS	$5074.13

7 Future Directions

Although robotic surgery offers superior technology and many potential advantages, there is no level 1 evidence to suggest that it is superior to laparoscopy for bariatric procedures. Additionally, concerns over cost and increase operative times remain [5, 6]. However, with development of new robotic platforms and technology and the introduction of competition into the robotic surgery market, it is reasonable to expect an improvement in both cost and efficiency, as well as a potential improvement in outcomes. To assess the outcomes and further determine the effectiveness of robotic bariatric surgery, it is essential to continually track outcomes. Most robotic outcome studies in bariatric surgery are based on the MBSAQIP database. Unfortunately, the MBSAQIP database does not collect robotic specific data. Creation of multi-institutional robotic specific databases or adding robotic specific data to national databases such as MBSAQIP will help further define the safety profile and advantages of robotic bariatric surgery.

8 Conclusion

Robotic sleeve gastrectomy is a safe and effective treatment for patients with morbid obesity. The operative steps are similar to that of a laparoscopic sleeve gastrectomy. The robotic approach to sleeve gastrectomy offers potential advantages such as 3-dimensional visualization, improved surgeon dexterity, and increased degrees of motion which may be particularly beneficial in super morbid obese patients. Outcomes are comparable to laparoscopic sleeve gastrectomy. Further studies are needed before meaningful conclusions can be made on whether robotic sleeve gastrectomy is advantageous or not.

References

1. Nguyen NT, Nguyen B, Gebhart A, Hohmann S. Changes in the makeup of bariatric surgery: a national increase in use of laparoscopic sleeve gastrectomy. J Am Coll Surg. 2013;216:252–7.
2. Gonzalez R, Nelson LG, Gallagher SF, Murr MM. Anastomotic leaks after laparoscopic gastric bypass. Obes Surg. 2004;14(10):1299–307.
3. Ali M, MEl Chaar M, Ghiassi S, Rogers AM. American Society for Metabolic and Bariatric Surgery updated position statement on sleeve gastrectomy as a bariatric procedure. Surg Obes Relat Dis. 2017;13(10):1652–1657.
4. Masoomi H, Kim H, Reavis KM, Mills S, Stamos MJ, Nguyen NT. Analysis of factors predictive of gastrointestinal tract leak in laparoscopic and open gastric bypass. Arch Surg. 2011;146(9):1048–51.
5. Fourman MM, Saber AA. Robotic bariatric surgery: a systemic review. Surg Obes Relat Dis. 2012;8(4):483–8.
6. Li K, Zou J, Tang J, Di J, Han X, Zhang P. Robotic versus laparoscopic bariatric surgery: a systematic review and meta-analysis. Obes Surg. 2016;26(12):3031–44.

7. Estimate of Bariatric Surgery Numbers, 2011–2018. Gainesville: The American Society of Metabolic and Bariatric Surgeons; c2018 [updated 2018 Jun; cited2019 Dec 1]. https://asmbs.org/resources/estimate-ofbariatric-surgery-numbers.

8. Lundberg PW, Wolfe S, Seaone J, Claros L, Stoltzfus J, El Chaar M. Robotic gastric bypass is getting better: first results from the Metabolic and Bariatric Surgery Accreditation and Quality Improvement Program. Surg Obes Relat Dis. 2018;14(9):1240–5.

9. P. Bhatia, V. Bindal, R. Singh, et al. Robot-assisted sleeve gastrectomy in morbidly obese versus super obese patients JSLS 2014; 18 (3)

10. Lin S, Jiang HG, Chen ZH, Zhou SY, Liu XS, Yu JR. Meta-analysis of robotic and laparoscopic surgery for treatment of rectal cancer. World J Gastroenterol. 2011;17(47):5214–20.

11. O'Neill M, Moran PS, Teljeur C, et al. Robot-assisted hysterectomy compared to open and laparoscopic approaches: systematic review and meta-analysis. Arch Gynecol Obstet. 2013;287(5):907–18.

12. Moser F, Horgan S. Robotically assisted bariatric surgery. Am J Surg. 2004;188(4A Suppl):38–44.

13. Jacobsen G, Berger R, Horgan S. The role of robotic surgery in morbid obesity. J Laparoendosc Adv Surg Tech A. 2003;13(4):279–83.

14. Bhatia P, Bindal V, Singh R, et al. Robot-assisted sleeve gastrectomy in morbidly obese versus super obese patients. JSLS. 2014;18(3)

15. El Chaar M, Gacke J, Ringold S, Stoltzfus J. Cost analysis of robotic sleeve gastrectomy (R-SG) compared with laparoscopic sleeve gastrectomy (L-SG) in a single academic center: debunking a myth! Surg Obes Relat Dis. 2019;15(5):675–9.

16. Suh I, Mukherjee M, Oleynikov D, Siu K-C. Training program for fundamental surgical skill in robotic laparoscopic surgery: Int. Robot: J. Med; 2011.

17. Tausch TJ, Kowalewski TM, White LW, McDonough PS, Brand TC, Lendvay TS. Content and construct validation of a robotic surgery curriculum using an electromagnetic instrument tracker. J Urol. 2012;188(3):919–23.

18. Arain NA, Dulan G, Hogg DC, Rege RV, Powers CE, Tesfay ST, Hynan LS, Scott DJ. Comprehensive proficiency-based inanimate training for robotic surgery: reliability, feasibility, and educational benefit. Surg Endosc. 2012;26(10):2740–5.

19. Dulan G, Rege RV, Hogg DC, Gilberg-Fisher KK, Tesfay ST, Scott DJ. Content and face validity of a comprehensive robotic skills training program for general surgery, urology, and gynecology. Am J Surg.

20. Magouliotis DE, Tasiopoulou VS, Sioka E, Zacharoulis D. Robotic versus Laparoscopic Sleeve Gastrectomy for Morbid Obesity: a Systematic Review and Meta-analysis. Obes Surg. 2017;27(1):245–53.

21. Acevedo E, Mazzei M, Zhao H, Lu X, Soans R, Edwards MA. Outcomes in conventional laparoscopic versus robotic-assisted primary bariatric surgery: a retrospective, case-controlled study of the MBSAQIP database. Surg Endosc. 2019.

22. Ayloo S, Buchs NC, Addeo P, Bianco FM, Giulianotti PC. Robot-assisted sleeve gastrectomy for super-morbidly obese patients. J Laparoendosc Adv Surg Tech. A2011;21(4):295–9.

23. Fischer L, Wekerle AL, Bruckner T, et al. BariSurg trial: sleeve gastrectomy versus Roux-en-Y gastric bypass in obese patients with BMI 35–60 kg/m2—a multi-centre randomized patient and observer blind non-inferiority trial. BMC Surg 2015;15:87. 1656 M. Ali et al./Surgery for Obesity and Related Diseases. 2017;13:1652–1657.

24. Ferrer-Marquez M, Belda-Lozano R, Ferrer-Ayza M. Technical controversies in laparoscopic sleeve gastrectomy. Obes Surg. 2012;22:182–7.

25. Burgos AM, Braghetto I, Csendes A, et al. Gastric leak after laparoscopic-sleeve gastrectomy for obesity. Obes Surg. 2009;19:1672–7.

26. Gagner M, Buchwald JN. Comparison of laparoscopic sleeve gastrectomy leak rates in four staple-line reinforcement options: a systematic review. Surg Obes Relat Dis. 2014;10(4):713–23.

27. Chang SH, Stoll CR, Song J, et al. The effectiveness and risks of bariatric surgery: an updated systematic review and meta-analysis, 2003–2012. JAMA Surg. 2014;149:275–87.
28. Banka G, Woodard G, Hernandez-Boussard T, et al. Laparoscopic vs open gastric bypass surgery: differences in patient demographics, safety, and outcomes. Arch Surg. 2012;147:550–6.
29. Aggarwal S, Kini SU, Herron DM. Laparoscopic sleeve gastrectomy for morbid obesity: a review. Surg Obes Relat Dis. 2007;3:189–94.
30. Clapp B, Liggett E, Jones R, Lodeiro C, Dodoo C, Tyroch A. Comparison of robotic revisional weight loss surgery and laparoscopic revisional weight loss surgery using the MBSAQIP database. Surg Obes Relat Dis. 2019;15(6):909–19.
31. Papasavas P, Seip RL, Stone A, Staff I, Mclaughlin T, Tishler D. Robot-assisted sleeve gastrectomy and Roux-en-y gastric bypass: results from the metabolic and bariatric surgery accreditation and quality improvement program data registry. Surg Obes Relat Dis. 2019;15(8):1281–90.
32. Sebastian R, Howell MH, Chang KH, et al. Robot-assisted versus laparoscopic Roux-en-Y gastric bypass and sleeve gastrectomy: a propensity score-matched comparative analysis using the 2015–2016 MBSAQIP database. Surg Endosc. 2019;33(5):1600–12.
33. Fazl Alizadeh R, Li S, Inaba CS, et al. Robotic versus laparoscopic sleeve gastrectomy: a MBSAQIP analysis. Surg Endosc. 2019;33(3):917–22.
34. Lundberg PW, Stoltzfus J, El Chaar M. 30-day outcomes of robot-assisted versus conventional laparoscopic sleeve gastrectomy: First analysis based on MBSAQIP. Surg Obes Relat Dis. 2019;15(1):1–7.

Laparoscopic Sleeve Gastrectomy in Situs Inversus Totalis

Mohammed A. Bawahab

1　Introduction

Situs inversus totalis (SIT) is a rare genetic autosomal recessive disorder, 1st time described in 1600 by Fabricius [1] with an incidence of 1 in 5000–20,000 live births [2] This mutation, anatomically described as 270° counterclockwise rotation of the intraabdominal organs, is also known as mirror image rotation [3, 4]. Most of SIT patients can live normally without associated organ abnormalities, though cardiac, lung, and/or intestinal anomalies can be present including atrial or ventricular septal defects, bronchiectasis, single lung absence, and duodenal stenosis or atresia, respectively [5].

SIT can also be a component of Kartagener syndrome (KS) which is made up of bronchiectasis, chronic sinusitis, and SIT. The main problems encountered in this syndrome is due to the defective movement of cilia, leading to recurrent chest infections, and infertility [6]. However, since the introduction of laparoscopy to the field of bariatric surgery, operating on such patients has become a more straight forward feat [7].

2　How to Perform the Procedure

Firstly, the patient should be admitted in the morning of surgery day having fasted for eight hours. After intubation and induction of general anesthesia, the patient will be positioned in semilithotomy (french) reverse Trendelenburg position. CO_2

M. A. Bawahab (✉)
Upper GI, Laparoscopic, and Bariatric Surgeon, Department of Surgery, College of Medicine, King Khalid University, Abha, Saudi Arabia
e-mail: mbawahab@kku.edu.sa

insufflation is then started using a veress needle at palmar's space. After adequate gas insufflation an 11 mm bladeless trocar will be inserted at the supraumblical region, which will contain a 10 mm 30° scope which will be used for examination of the peritoneal cavity. The monitor is positioned at the patients' right shoulder, while the surgeon stands between the patients' legs, with the nursing assistant on the patients' left side (mirror image of the typical positioning for a gastric sleeve). A 15 mm bladeless trocar is then inserted at the left upper quadrant, while a 12 mm bladeless trocar is inserted at the right upper quadrant, Iron med laparoscopic liver retractor is then used to lift up the hepatic lobe (Fig. 1). Dissection is then started by taking down the gastrocolic ligament using the left sided trocar, just proximal to the pylorus, all the way up to the base of the right diaphragmatic crus, with meticulous dissection of the gastosplenic ligament. 1st stapling is done using an Endo GIA black articulating, while reload with Tri-staple Technology 60 mm (extrathick) is done just proximal to the pylorus. A 36F calibrating tube is then inserted orally by the anesthesiologist under direct vision all the way up to the pylorus, followed by stapling of the rest of the stomach using a purple Endo GIA articulating reload with Tri-staple Technology 60 mm and ending about 2 cm lateral to the GE Junction. Staple line reinforcement is recommended using 10 mm Endo clips at the overlap and bleeding areas, afterwards, the calibrating tube is pulled out to the level of the GE Junction and 150 ml methylene blue leak test is then performed. The tube can then be removed completely. Interrupted 2.0 vicryl gastropexy stitches are then done between the sleeved stomach and the

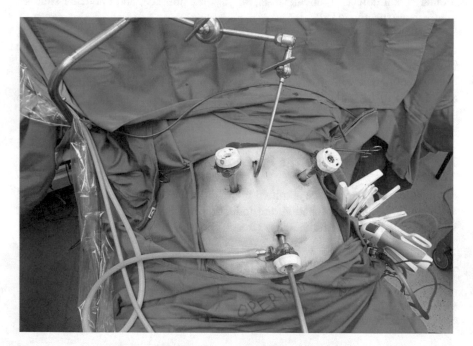

Fig. 1 Trocars and liver retractors placement

Table 1 A brief review of the studies of laparoscopic sleeve gastrectomy with situs inversus totalis

	Age/gender	Body mass index (BMI) before operation (kg/m²)	Preoperative diagnostic method	The need for additional trocars	Operation time (mean operation	Kartagner syndrome	Previous operation	Surgical procedure	Postoperative complicatons
Wittgrove et al. (1998) [7] first case	38/F	47.8 kg/m²	ECO/X-ray chest	No	300 min (159)	No	No	LRYGB	No
Ahmed et al. (2006) [5]	47/F	58.1 kg/m²	RCG/X-ray chest/CT scan	No	160 min (105)	No	No	LRYGB	No
Tsepelidis et al. (2015) [8]	51/F	43 kg/m²	NA	No	120 min (NA)	No	No	LRYGB	No
Slier et al. (2014) [9]	39/M	44 kg/m²	USG/X-ray chest/gastroscopy/ECG	No	76 min (50–93)	No	No	LRYGB	No
Stier et al. (2014) [9]	51/F	54.2 kg/m²	USG/X-ray chest/gastroscopy/ECG	No	61 min (16–87)	No	No	LSG	No
Catheline et al. (2006) [10	19/M	76 kg/m²	ECG/gastroscopy/X-ray chest/USG	Yes	NA	No	No	LSG	No
Deutseh et al. (2012) [11]	39/F	42 kg/m¹	Ahdominal CT	No	NA	No	Open gastric banding	LSG	Suture line
Genscr et al. (2015) [12]	52/F	49 kg/m²	ECG/X-ray chest/CT scan	No	52 min (45–60) (il was learned via e-mail)	Yes	No	Trans-umbilical SILSG	No
Samaan et al. (2008) [14]	29/M	56 kg/m	ECG	No	NA	No	No	LAGB	Band erosion
Malar et al. (2008) [15]	28/M	51 kg/m²	ECG/Barium graphy/X-ray ehest/USG	No	NA	No	No	LAGB	No
Taskin et al. (2008) [16]	20/F	44.9 kg/m²	ECG/X-niy chest/USG	Yes	90 min	No	BIB	LAGB + LC	No

(continued)

Table 1 (continued)

Pauli et al. (2008) [17]	47/F	60 kg/m²	X-ray chest/chest and abdominal CT scan	Yes	105 min	Yes	No	LAGB	No
Ersoy et al. (2005) [13]	33/F	53 kg/m²	ECG/gastroscopy/X-ray chest/USG	No	NA	No	No	LAGB	No
Current Study (20 15)	21/F	41.8 kg/m²	ECG/gastroscopy/X-ray chest/USG	No	78 min (28–60)	Noo	No	LSG	No

BIB bioenterie intragastric ballon, *BMI* body mass index, *CT* compound tomography, *DM* diabetes mellitus, *ECG* electrocardiography, *HT* hypertension, *LAGB* laparoscopic adjustable gastric banding, *LC* laparoscopic cholecystectomy, *LRYGB* laproscopic Roux-en-Y gastric bypass, *LSG* laparoscopic sleeve gastrectomy, *NA* not available, *OSAS* obstructive sleep apnea syndrome, *SILSG* single incision laparoscopic sleeve gastrectomy, *USG* abdominal ultrasonography

pre-pancreatic facia to keep the stomach aligned. A 5 mm Neleton free gravity drain is then inserted at the right upper quadrant with the tip near the GE Junction. The excised stomach is then removed from the 15 mm trocar port. Both 12 and 15 mm port sites would be closed using 1 vicryl Endo closure. The skin is then closed at all port sites with 3.0 monocryl in a subcuticular fashion with surgeon pore dressing done.

3   Discussion

Obesity is a worldwide health problem and has been on a continuous rise as has been stated by the world health organization (WHO) [8]. Challenges that may face surgeons in bariatric surgery are many, one of these challenges being Situs Inverses Totalis which is usually discovered preoperatively during patient work up for surgery or incidentally during the procedure. Preoperative diagnosis gives the patient a better chance for a more complete cardiopulmonary assessment, and better planning opportunity for the surgeon for patient positioning and proper operating theater setup, obtaining instruments needed which may reduce technical challenges during the procedure and the operative time [9]. Longer operative time will be faced if intraoperative diagnosis of SIT is made, which in turn required a later adaptation and surgeon position changes [10]. The surgeon may need to add additional trocars if needed, as seen by the literature review we conducted. Trocars were found to be added for the following reasons: concomitant laparoscopic cholecystectomy for incidental gall stones, severely morbid obesity with higher BMI, and patients with Kartagener syndrome who need to be on a low insufflation pressure [9, 11, 12]. SIT does not increase bariatric surgery complication specially if it is done by an experienced laparoscopic bariatric surgeon [13].

4   Conclusion

Laparoscopic sleeve gastrectomy and other bariatric surgeries can be done safely in SIT patients, however proper preoperative assessment and evaluation is needed. Preoperative diagnosis of SIT has a positive impact on patient management. Patients with Kartagener syndrome need to be evaluated by a pulmonologist and anesthetist preoperatively (Table 1).

References

1. Akbulut S, Caliskan A, Ekin A, Yagmur Y. Left-sided acute appendicitis with situs inversus totalis: review of 63 published cases and report of two cases. J Gastrointest Surg. 2010;14(9):1422–8.
2. Rungsakulkij N, Tangtawee P. Fluorescence cholangiography during laparoscopic cholecystectomy in a patient with situs inversus totalis: a case report and literature review. BMC Surg. 2017;17(1):43.

3. Douard R, Feldman A, Bargy F, Loric S, Delmas V. Anomalies of lateralization in man a case of total situs inversus. Surg Radiol Anat. 2001;22(5–6):293–7.
4. Nelson MJ, Pesola GR. Left lower quadrant pain of unusual cause. J Emerg Med. 2001;20(3):241–5.
5. Varano N. Situs inversus: review of the literature, report of four cases and analysis of the clinical implications. J Int Coll Surg. 1960;33:131–48.
6. Yazar FM, Emre A, Akbulut S, Urfalıoğlu A, Cengiz E, Sertkaya M, et al. Laparoscopic sleeve gastrectomy in situs inversus totalis: a case report and comprehensive literature review. Indian J Surg. 2016;78(2):130–5.
7. Spiegel H-U, Skawran S. From longitudinal gastric resection to sleeve gastrectomy—revival of a previously established surgical procedure. J Gastrointest Surg. 2011;15(1):219–28.
8. Worni M, Guller U, Maciejewski ML, Curtis LH, Gandhi M, Pietrobon R, et al. Racial differences among patients undergoing laparoscopic gastric bypass surgery: a population-based trend analysis from 2002 to 2008. Obes Surg. 2013;23(2):226–33.
9. Taskin M, Zengin K, Ozben V. Concomitant laparoscopic adjustable gastric banding and laparoscopic cholecystectomy in a super-obese patient with situs inversus totalis who previously underwent intragastric balloon placement. Obes Surg. 2009;19(12):1724–6.
10. Wittgrove A, Clark G. Laparoscopic gastric bypass for morbid obesity in a patient with situs inversus. J Laparoendosc Adv Surg Tech. 1998;8(1):53–5.
11. Catheline JM, Rosales C, Cohen R, Bihan H, Fournier JL, Roussel J, et al. Laparoscopic sleeve gastrectomy for a super-super-obese patient with situs inversus totalis. Obes Surg. 2006;16(8):1092–5.
12. Pauli EM, Wadiwala II, Rogers AM. Laparoscopic placement of an adjustable gastric band in a super-super obese patient with situs inversus. Surg Obes Relat Dis. 2008;4(6):768–9.
13. Genser L, Tayar C, Eddine IK. Trans-umbilical single incision laparoscopic sleeve gastrectomy in a patient with situs inversus totalis and kartagener syndrome: video report. Obes Surg. 2015;25(10):1985–6.

Banded Sleeves

Mohit Bhandari

1 Introduction

Bariatric surgery has emerged as the only feasible long-term solution for the treatment of obesity [1]. Long-term studies show that surgery causes a significant long-term loss of weight, recovery from diabetes, improvement in cardiovascular risk factors, and a mortality reduction [2–5].

There has been an explosion in the number of bariatric surgical procedures performed worldwide. 61 countries that contributed to the International Federation for Surgical Obesity (IFSO) global registry {2019} with a total of 833,687 surgical procedures covering a data of 2,94,530 gastric bypasses, 3,91,423 sleeves, 30,914 one anastomosis gastric bypass and 70,085 gastric banding procedures. 47% of these procedures were sleeve gastrectomies [6].

Surgical treatment of morbid obesity has witnessed a significant evolution since the advent of laparoscopy. Laparoscopic Sleeve Gastrectomy (LSG) was originally intended as a bridging procedure for super obese patients [7] awaiting definitive bariatric intervention, but has evolved into a stand-alone procedure encouraged by early postoperative results and owing to its technical simplicity in performing LSG compared to Roux-en- Y Gastric Bypass (RYGB), it has become the most performed surgery in the world overtaking RYGB [8]. Though early results seem encouraging, long term results show significant weight regain requiring revisional surgery [9].

Dilation is part of the natural history of these operations. To address this issue, Fobi introduced the placement of a ring/band around the pouch of the Gastric

M. Bhandari (✉)
Head of Department At the Mohak Bariatric and Robotic Surgery Center, SAIMS University, Indore, India
e-mail: drmohitbhandari@gmail.com

Bypass (GBP) to stabilize the size of the reservoir in the GBP operation [10, 11]. This resulted in better and sustained weight loss as compared to the non-banded GBP [12]. The same concept was applied to the LSG by placing a ring/band loosely around the proximal sleeve. This resulted in better and sustained weight loss compared to the non-banded sleeve [13–15]. Placing this ring/band enhances three mechanisms that result in weight loss maintenance:

1. the restriction of a small pouch is maintained.
2. the early satiety due to the full sense effect caused by food in the pouch dilating the gastroesophageal junction with stimulation of the vagus nerves is maintained and
3. the forced compliance of the patient having to eat slowly, chew the food thoroughly, and stop eating when full all contribute to the effectiveness of the BSG. This better outcome of weight loss and maintenance is at an acceptable cost of a low incidence of ring/band erosion, slippage, and solid food intolerance in a small group of patients [16].

2   Procedure

The Laparoscopic Banded Sleeve Gastrectomy (BSG) operation is performed with the patient placed in the supine reverse Trendelenberg position. With the surgeon to the right of the patient, pneuma-peritoneum is achieved using a Veress needle. A supraumbilical 12 mm port is placed for the optics. A second 10 mm port is placed under vision in line with the optical port in the left midclavicular line. Two 5 mm ports are placed in the right and left the subcostal region in the mid-clavicular line (Fig. 1) A Nathanson liver retractor is placed for retracting the liver.

Creation of the Sleeve Gastrectomy (SG) starts with mobilizing the omentum along the greater curvature of the stomach (Fig. 2), starting at a point 1–2 cm from the pylorus up to the gastroesophageal junction, exposing the left crus of the diaphragm. The sleeve is formed by transecting the stomach, starting from 3–4 cm from the pylorus using a green Ethicon Endo-stapler (Johnson and Johnson) (Fig. 3). The stapled resection of the stomach is continued with blue staplers alongside a 38 French bougie in the stomach leaving a sleeve estimated at 90–110 cc in size.

A peri-gastric window is then made in the lesser omentum 3–4 cm from the esophagogastric junction and careful dissection is carried out around the sleeve pouch. Through this window, a silastic ring of number 8 which is approx. 2.7 cm in diameter is passed and locked in place. The Ring must be loose around the pouch (Fig. 4). The ring is then sutured to the staple line on the greater curvature of the sleeve with non-absorbable sutures. Hemostasis is usually achieved using clips and in case of severe bleeding with staple line suturing. Typically no drains are placed.

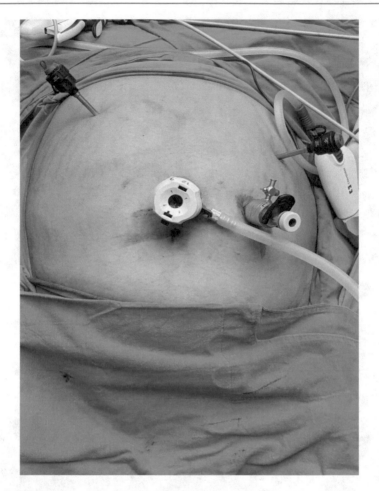

Fig. 1 Port position

3   Pre- Intra- and Post-Operative Management

Patients who seek treatment at our centre are usually advised of all the various options for the management of obesity. Presentations are complemented by printed handouts that explain the various treatment options. We follow the 1991 NIH criteria [17] with the modifications for Asian patients for qualifying patients for surgery. The exceptions to these criteria apply to patients who seek endoscopic bariatric operations, revision bariatric operations, or for whom the indication for surgery is Type 2 Diabetes.

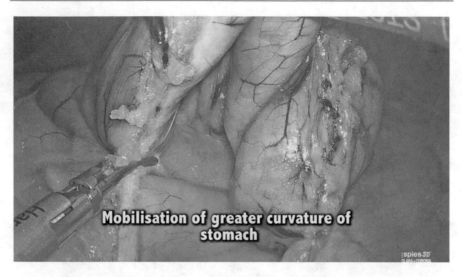

Fig. 2 Mobilisation

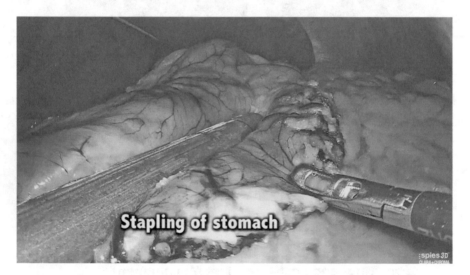

Fig. 3 Stapling of stomach

The type of procedure offered to a patient is guided by an algorithm. This algorithm is based on evidence-based medicine and experience from our own data. The Body Mass Index (BMI), age, gender, comorbid conditions, previous surgeries, social history, and the patient's understanding and wishes are all taken into consideration. Various consents for treatment are obtained as per hospital protocols. Consent is also taken for the use of patient's redacted data for research purposes. Preoperatively all patients are usually evaluated by multiple disciplinary teams

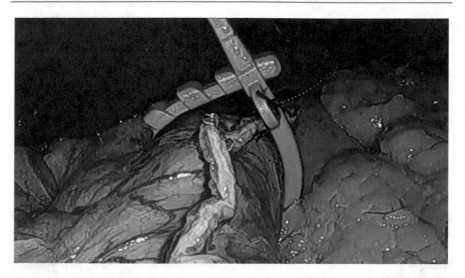

Fig. 4 Banded sleeve

that include a bariatric physician, bariatric surgeon, pulmonologist, cardiologist, anaesthesiologist, and as indicated by other consultants. Bariatric Physician sees the patient initially and obtains a detailed history and does an examination with emphasis on determining any risk factors and comorbid conditions usually associated with obesity such as diabetes, hypertension, sleep apnea, osteoarthritis, liver disorders, bleeding disorders, polycystic ovarian disease, Gastroesophageal reflux disease (GERD) and other social, physical, psychological and economic problems. Preoperative laboratory investigations include but are not limited to complete blood count, blood tests that include electrolytes, urea, glucose, and calcium levels. Liver function tests, including Bilirubin, protein, Albumin is routinely determined. Lipid Profile, thyroid profile, HbA-1c, C-peptide, serology-HIV, and Hepatitis B and C tests are done. Radiological investigations include chest x-rays, abdominal CT scan, and Ultrasound. Electrocardiography, echocardiography, pulmonary function tests and arterial blood gas are routinely done. All the investigations are reviewed by the surgeon and/or a member of the multi-disciplinary team to make sure the patient is a safe and good candidate for surgery.

Once the patient and the surgeon have decided on the operation to be done, the patient consents for surgery. Consent is also obtained from all patients to use their redacted information for analysis, presentation, and publications as needed. Patients are admitted the day before surgery and are kept on a clear liquid diet and then NPO for at least six hours before the operation. All patients get a dose of prophylactic antibiotics preoperatively. Compression devices are used during the operation. Ambulation is initiated within four hours of return of the patient from surgery. All patients get low molecular weight heparin prophylaxis for 24 hour or until the patient is ambulating frequently. In high risks patients, this prophylaxis is continued for six weeks. Patients are started on sips of water 4 hours after the surgery and advanced to a liquid diet the following day if vital parameters are normal. Patients are usually discharged on the third postoperative day with instructions on how to advance their diet. All patients are placed on proton pump inhibitors for six months. Vitamins and other mineral supplements are prescribed for life long use. Patients are seen at three months, six months, twelve months, and yearly thereafter. Nutritional counseling is done and evaluation of the quality of life and blood chemistries are monitored at six months, 12 months, and yearly thereafter.

4   Results

We have performed a total of 1121 BSG. We have six-year follow up comparative data of BSG v LSG for 68 and 152 patients respectively [14]. The groups were extremely well-matched at baseline for all relevant characteristics. Both groups experienced major, durable weight loss throughout 6 years, with significant changes from baseline. While in BSG nadir weight was achieved at 3 years, in LSG nadir it was at 1 year and patients have gradually started gaining weight from thereafter (Table 1). Maximum %EWL achieved was 90% at 3 years in BSG from there on plateaued and %EWL at the end of 6 years in 82.25% whereas in LSG maximum % EWL was at 1 year, plateaued for a year and from 2nd-year patients started regaining weight and at the end of 6 years, %EWL was 50.25%. There is a total of 32% difference in %EWL in BSG v LSG at 6 years (Table 2). Follow up was 70.5% and 64.4% IN BSG AND LSG respectively (Table 3). Failure rate which is defined as % EWL less than 50% at 3 years is 11.1% and 0% and at 6 years is 46.9% and 0% in LSG and BSG respectively (Table 4). Resolution of diabetes was 75.7 and 58%, Hypertension was 64% and 49.1%, OSA was 80% and 55% respectively in BSG and LSG.

Resolution of type 2 diabetes, defined as normal fasting blood glucose levels ($\leq$110 mg/dL), HbA1C levels below 6.5 mmol/L and no longer taking type 2 diabetes medications [18].

Remission of hypertension can be defined as systolic and diastolic blood pressure <140 mm Hg and 90 mm Hg, respectively, without any medications based on blood pressure monitoring unit [19].

There is no major difference in nutrient deficiencies in both groups. During our 5-year follow-up, no BSG patient underwent any additional operations, whereas 19 SG patients had elective revisional bariatric procedures (3 at 3 yr, 16 at 4 yr), for inadequate weight loss or weight regain. These failed SG operations were converted to 11 banded gastric bypasses, 6 one-anastomosis gastric bypasses, and 2 repeat SGs.

5   Band Complications

Of the total 1121 BSG performed at our center band complications were seen in 26(2.3%) patients.

Table 1 Weight loss outcome in BSG vs LSG at 6 years

Weight loss outcome						
	06 M	1 yr	2 yr	3 yr	4 yr	5 yr	yr
BSG	95.24 ± 12.71	4.84 ± 11.27	76.88 ± 10.28	75.15 ± 10.26	8.3 ± 10.14	79.5 ± 11.01	80.48 ± 10.85
LSG	89.49 ± 14.14	81.75 ± 12.70	82.12 ± 13.05	4.15 ± 13.89	8.58 ± 14.75	92.22 ± 16.17	95.23 ± 15.87

Table 2 % EBWL loss outcome in BSG vs LSG at 6 years

% EBWL loss outcome							
	06 M	1 yr	2 yr	3 yr	4 yr	5 yr	yr
BSG	5.47 ± 5.64	4.17 ± 7.21	88.09 ± 8.06	90.57 ± 8.11	5.33 ± 7.38	3.20 ± 8.57	2.25 ± 8.49
LSG	57.46 ± 5.152	3.68 ± 9.43	3.18 ± 15.64	8.48 ± 20.07	8.58 ± 16.36	52.98 ± 16.59	50.25 ± 18.92

Table 3 Follow up data (BSG vs LSG)

Follow up data # and % F/U							
	06 M	1 yr	yr	yr	yr	5 yr	yr
BSG (68)	68 (100%)	66 (97.0%)	3 (92.6%)	8 (85.2%)	54 (79.4%)	0 (73.5%)	46 (70.5%)
SG (152)	152 (100%)	48 (97.3%)	142 (93.4%)	34 (88.1)	111 (73.0%)	102 (67.1%)	98 (64.4%)

Table 4 Failure rate at 3 and 6 years (BSG vs LSG)

	Three years			Six years		
	Less than 50%	50–75%	Above75%	Less than 50%	50–75%	Above75%
BSG	(0) 0%	(2) 3.5%	(56) 96.5%	(0) 0%	(4) 8.3%	(44) 91.7%
SG	(15)11.1%	(66)47.4%	(53)39.5%	(46)46.9%	(46)46.9%	(9)9.1%

These are grouped as.

1. Band erosion—5 (19.23%)
2. Band slippage—4 (15.38)
3. Stricture—16 (61.5%)
4. Food intolerance—1 (3.8%).

Of the 5 people with band erosion all of them were removed endoscopically and in four patients with band slippage laparoscopic band removal was done. Of sixteen patients with stricture in six band removal was done and converted to gastric bypass, in eight patients laparoscopic band removal was done and in two patients laparoscopic band removal with endoscopic dilatation was done. One patient who had food intolerance issues had the band removed laparoscopically.

6   Weight Loss and Complications After Banded Sleeve in Other Studied and Comparative Analysis

We have compared this data in terms of excess weight loss and a total percentage of weight loss with other existent studies. At 6 years, the cohort of patients operated at our centre had percentage excess weight loss. The total percentage weight loss at 6 years for the banded group was 82.25 and 50.25% for the non-banded group.

Failure rate which is defined as % EWL less than 50% at 3 years is 11.1% and 0% and at 6 years is 46.9% and 0% in LSG and BSG respectively.

The banded sleeve group maintained much better weight loss which increased progressively from 3 until 5 years.

In the series on banded sleeve published by Luc Lemmens et al., %EWL at 5 years was 57.8 ± 25 and 86.7 ± 11.9 in the non-banded group and BLSG, respectively [13].

These results show that in the non-banded group, 35.2% of the patients have < 50%EWL at the 5 years follow-up, whereas none of the banded sleeves treated patients had < 50%EWL.

In a series published by Jodok Fink et al., he has reported better weight loss by Banded sleeve [20].

Total weight loss in their series was equal in the early follow-up but significantly better in BSG, 3 and 5 years after surgery (BSG versus SG at 3 yr $38.7\% \pm 7.8$, n = 33 versus 31.9 ± 10.7, n = 33, $P = 0.002$; BSG versus SG at 5 yr $37.6\% \pm 8.5$, n = 27 versus 29.5 ± 12.9, n = 23, $P = 0.008$).

We have reported band complications of 2.3%, whereas Lemmens et al. reported band-related complications of 4.1% which required band removal or readjusting.

7 Conclusions

The banded sleeve is a safe and feasible procedure. Considering the excellent weight loss maintenance results seen after the banded sleeve procedure, banding of the sleeve makes sense. We need long term data from multiple institutions on complications from the banded sleeve and its efficacy.

A randomised control trial between banded and non-banded sleeves with long term results will be the key to answers we sought regarding the efficacy and complications of banded sleeve.

References

1. Kissler HJ, Settmacher U. Bariatric surgery to treat obesity. Semin Nephrol. 2013;33(1):75–89. https://doi.org/10.1016/j.semnephrol.2012.12.004.
2. Maciejewski ML, Arterburn DE, Van Scoyoc L, et al. Bariatric Surgery and Long-term Durability of Weight Loss. JAMA Surg. 2016;151(11):1046–55. https://doi.org/10.1001/jamasurg.2016.2317.
3. Kashyap SR, Gatmaitan P, Brethauer S, Schauer P. Bariatric surgery for type 2 diabetes: weighing the impact for obese patients. Cleve Clin J Med. 2010;77(7):468–76. https://doi.org/10.3949/ccjm.77a.09135.
4. Benraouane F, Litwin SE. Reductions in cardiovascular risk after bariatric surgery. Curr Opin Cardiol. 2011;26(6):555–61. https://doi.org/10.1097/HCO.0b013e32834b7fc4.
5. Adams TD, Mehta TS, Davidson LE, Hunt SC. All-Cause and Cause-Specific Mortality Associated with Bariatric Surgery: A Review. Curr Atheroscler Rep. 2015;17(12):74. https://doi.org/10.1007/s11883-015-0551-4.
6. Ramos A, Kow L, Brown W, Welbourn R, Dixon J, Kinsman ER, Walton P. 5th IFSO Global Registry Report 2019.
7. Iannelli A, Dainese R, Piche T, Facchiano E, Gugenheim J. Laparoscopic sleeve gastrectomy for morbid obesity. World J Gastroenterol. 2008;14(6):821–7. https://doi.org/10.3748/wjg.14.821.

8. Ozsoy Z, Demir E. Which Bariatric Procedure Is the Most Popular in the World? A Bibliometric Comparison [published correction appears in Obes Surg. 2018 Mar 16]. Obes Surg. 2018;28(8):2339–2352. https://doi.org/10.1007/s11695-018-3163-6.
9. Clapp B, Wynn M, Martyn C, Foster C, O'Dell M, Tyroch A. Long term (7 or more years) outcomes of the sleeve gastrectomy: a meta-analysis. Surg Obes Relat Dis. 2018;14(6):741–7. https://doi.org/10.1016/j.soard.2018.02.027.
10. Fobi MA, Lee H. The surgical technique of the Fobi-Pouch operation for obesity (the transected silastic vertical gastric bypass). Obes Surg. 1998;8(3):283–8. https://doi.org/10.1381/096089298765554485.
11. Fobi M. Why the operation I prefer is silastic ring vertical gastric bypass. Obes Surg. 1991;1(4):423–6. https://doi.org/10.1381/096089291765560854.
12. Bhandari M, Bhandari S, Mishra A, Mathur W, Dixit A. Comparison between banded and nonbanded Roux-En-Y gastric bypass with 2-year follow-up: a preliminary retrospective analysis. Obes Surg. 2016;26(1):213–8. https://doi.org/10.1007/s11695-015-1929-7.
13. Lemmens L, Van Den Bossche J, Zaveri H, Surve A. Banded sleeve gastrectomy: better long-term results? a long-term cohort study until 5 years follow-up in obese and superobese patients. Obes Surg. 2018;28(9):2687–95. https://doi.org/10.1007/s11695-018-3248-2.
14. Bhandari M, Mathur W, Kosta S, Mishra AK, Cummings DE. Banded versus nonbanded laparoscopic sleeve gastrectomy: 5-year outcomes. Surg Obes Relat Dis. 2019;15(9):1431–8. https://doi.org/10.1016/j.soard.2019.04.023.
15. Tognoni V, Benavoli D, Bianciardi E, et al. Laparoscopic sleeve gastrectomy versus laparoscopic banded sleeve gastrectomy: first prospective pilot randomized study. Gastroenterol Res Pract. 2016;2016:6419603. https://doi.org/10.1155/2016/6419603.
16. Fobi M, Lee H, Igwe D, et al. Band erosion: incidence, etiology, management and outcome after banded vertical gastric bypass. Obes Surg. 2001;11(6):699–707. https://doi.org/10.1381/09608920160558632.
17. Gastrointestinal surgery for severe obesity. Consens Statement. 1991;9(1):1–20.
18. Schauer PR, Burguera B, Ikramuddin S, et al. Effect of laparoscopic Roux-en Y gastric bypass on type 2 diabetes mellitus. Ann Surg. 2003;238(4):467–85. https://doi.org/10.1097/01.sla.0000089851.41115.1b.
19. Schiavon CA, Bersch-Ferreira AC, Santucci EV, et al. Effects of Bariatric Surgery in Obese Patients With Hypertension: The GATEWAY Randomized Trial (Gastric Bypass to Treat Obese Patients With Steady Hypertension) [published correction appears in Circulation. 2019 Oct;140(14):e718]. *Circulation.* 2018;137(11):1132-1142. https://doi.org/10.1161/CIRCULATIONAHA.117.032130.
20. Fink JM, von Pigenot A, Seifert G, Laessle C, Fichtner-Feigl S, Marjanovic G. Banded versus nonbanded sleeve gastrectomy: 5-year results of a matched-pair analysis. Surg Obes Relat Dis. 2019;15(8):1233–8. https://doi.org/10.1016/j.soard.2019.05.023.

Buttressing the Sleeve

Safwan Taha

1   Introduction

Ever since staplers were introduced to the gastrointestinal tract surgery arsenal, a vigilant search was started for techniques and\or gadgets that increased their safety [1, 2]. Buttressing the staple line was one of those techniques that drew particular attention from bariatric surgeons who implemented it late in the last century and published data about it in the early 2000s, starting with laparoscopic Roux-en-Y gastric Bypass (RYGB) [3, 4] and, eventually, laparoscopic sleeve gastrectomy (LSG) [5–7] with special emphasis on its two most feared inherent complications; bleeding [8, 9] and leak [10–12].

Staple line leak post LSG is a potentially serious complication that has been reported in 1.5–3% of cases [13]. It can result in grave morbidities, and even mortality, if not promptly recognized and properly managed [14].

The main cause of staple line leak following LSG is the markedly increased intraluminal pressure in the sleeve tube beyond the ability of the staples to hold the integrity of the staple line (also known as burst pressure), resulting in disruption of the staple line and, consequently, leak. This phenomenon was clearly described in several publications that also tested it under controlled environments on animal models both with and without buttressing materials. Most of those studies reported a significantly higher burst pressure for tissues that were reinforced with buttressing material [15–17], (Fig. 1). It is believed that buttressing achieves this result through distributing the tension across a wider surface area of the gastric edge,

S. Taha (✉)
Consultant Metabolic and Bariatric Surgeon, Mediclinic Airport Road Hospital,
Abu Dhabi, UAE
e-mail: Safwan.Taha@Mediclinic.ae

© The Editor(s) (if applicable) and The Author(s), under exclusive license to Springer   261
Nature Switzerland AG 2021
S. Al-Sabah et al. (eds.), *Laparoscopic Sleeve Gastrectomy*,
https://doi.org/10.1007/978-3-030-57373-7_28

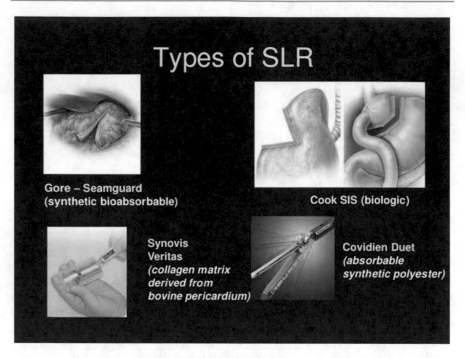

Fig. 1 Burst pressure increases significantly with buttressing

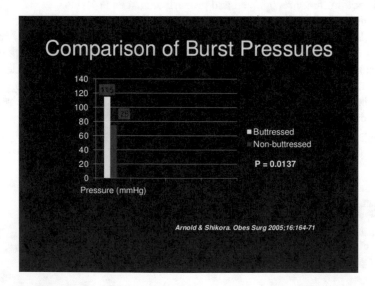

Fig. 2 The ideal "B" configuration of the staple

increasing the burst pressure of the staple line beyond that of the gastric body itself in the process [18].

2 Technical Aspects

Technical aspects of the procedure also play a decisive role to its outcome especially when it comes to post-operative leak. Of particular relevance of all those factors is choosing the appropriate staple height that corresponds to the thickness of the part of stomach to be stapled (Table 1), which is why all manufacturers provide their recommendations for the staple height that is most suitable for deployment on the specific parts of stomach in relation to its tissue thickness [17]. More attention should be paid to this point when the surgeon chooses to use a buttressing material, since the latter increases the thickness of the tissue to be buttressed, adding twice the thickness of the buttressing layer to the original tissue thickness, with a possible upgrade of the staple height, to make sure that the staples will go through all the four layers, 2 tissue and 2 buttressing, and deploy properly forming the ideal, complete "B" configuration [18–21] (Fig. 2). As examples, the bovine pericardial strip (Peri-Strips, Synovis Surgical Innovations) adds a total thickness of 0.8 mm, the absorbable synthetic Polyglycolide/Trimethylene

Table 1 Summary statistics for gastric tissue thickness

	Antrum thickness (mm)	Midbudy thickness (mm)	Fundus thickness (mm)
Female ($N = 15$)			
Mean + SU	3.09 ± 062	2.64 ± 0.60	1.72 ± 0.59
MeantSD (Elariny)	3.09 ± 0.553	2.34 ± 0349	1.61 ± 0279
Min	2.00	2.00	1.05
Max	407	4 00	2.83
Quartile 1–25th %	2.63	2.23	1.32
Quartile 2–50th %	3.10	2,50	1.50
Quartile 2–75th %	3.53	2.88	2.03
Male ($N = 11$)			
MeantSD	3.I2 ± 0.8I	2.57 ± 0.42	1.67 ± 0.32
MeantSD (Elanny)	3.17 ± 0.324	2.6 ± 0.391	1 81 ± 0453
Min	2.45	2.12	1.24
Max	5.39	3.46	2.28
Quartile 1–25th %	2.72	2.29	1.37
Quartile 2–50th %	2.92	2.45	1.65
Quartile 2–75th %	3.21	2.82	1.85

SD standard deviation

Fig. 3 Types of products
used for buttressing

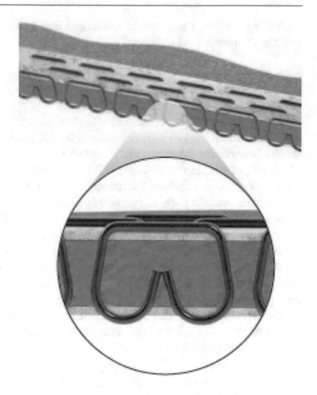

Carbonate buttress material (Seamguard Bioabsorbable, W. L. Gore & Associates) adds a total thickness of 0.5 mm while the absorbable Glycolide Diaxonone Trimethylene Carbonate product that comes integrated\pre-loaded onto the Stapler Cartridge (Covidien) adds a total thickness of 0.14 mm. Consideration of the additional thickness of the buttressing material used is of paramount relevance to the safety of the procedure since stapling through a "tissue plus buttress" complex that is too thick for the chosen stapler height will result in deformed staple formation and\or tissue injury, while deploying a stapler on a "tissue plus buttress" complex that is too thin for its height can result in instantaneous staple line leakage [15–17].

3   Buttressing for Bleeding

The other major complication of LSG is post-operative bleeding which can be either intra- or extraluminal. Intraluminal bleeding from the staple line is rather uncommon and usually presents with signs and symptoms of upper gastrointestinal bleeding including hematemesis and\or melena stools depending on the severity and duration of the bleeding [22]. Diagnosis and management of intraluminal bleeding follows the standard algorithm for upper gastrointestinal bleeding, including blood transfusion, if needed.

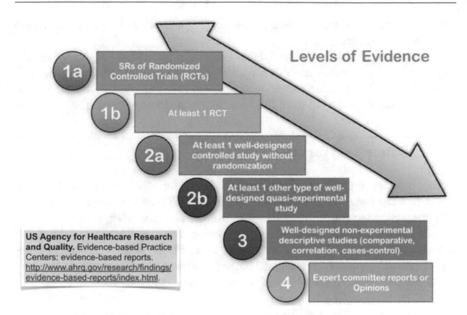

Fig. 4 Levels of evidence

Extraluminal bleeding can present as an "acute" episode with full blown clinical picture of hypovolemia and\or significant serial drop of hemoglobin or assume a subclinical course that presents mainly as relative tachycardia, mild pallor and dizziness, especially on standing up quickly.

Acute bleeding is reported with a frequency that ranges from 1.7% [23] to 2.8% [24] and usually requires return to the operating room (OR) with some sort of operative intervention, mostly laparoscopic. Subclinical bleeding, on the other hand, occurs in up to 7.7% of cases [24] and is managed quite effectively in a conservative manner.

Although some studies concluded that buttressing didn't produce a favorable effect on bleeding following LSG [25, 26], most investigators, by far, agree that buttressing of the staple line in LSG reduces bleeding compared to patients that receive no buttressing [8, 12, 27–29]. Some studies showed more favorable results for some types of buttressing materials against the others when it comes to bleeding [30, 31] but there were too many variables involved in those studies to support this finding. It is noteworthy that such a superiority was not reproduced in several other similar studies. When compared to over sewing, the other technique that reduces staple line bleeding in LSG, buttressing was found to produce similar, or better, hemostatic outcomes without the inherent complications of over sewing, namely longer operative time [12, 27] and stenosis of the sleeve tube lumen [32]. Over sewing was also found to be associated with a significantly higher rate of post-operative nausea and vomiting to the point that it increased the duration of the symptoms during the first hours after surgery and prevented early oral intake compared to buttressing [33].

Furthermore, buttressing of the staple line was reported not only to reduce the rate of staple line bleeding itself directly, but also significantly reduced the number of surgical clips required to achieve hemostasis [34, 35] and the overall rate of post-LSG complications [6] including bleeding-related re-operation [29].

4   Buttressing for Leaks

Unlike bleeding, the role of buttressing in reducing the incidence of leak from the staple line has been, for a long time, controversial. Several investigators reported that buttressing the staple line didn't improve the outcome when it came to leaks [26, 36, 37]. There has been, however, growing evidence lately that buttressing actually reduces the incidence of staple line leak in LSG, with an increasing number of researchers reporting a significant improvement in leak rates with buttressing of the staple line when compared to non-buttressing [6, 38–42].

5   Results from the MBSAQIP

One extremely controversial report that caused a lot of noise, when published in 2016, was the first report from the Metabolic and Bariatric Surgery Accreditation and Quality Improvement Program (MBSAQIP) [43]. The researchers went through the MBSAQIP data registry for 189,477 LSG cases that were performed from 2012 to 2014, assessed the effect of various surgical techniques used in them on the 30-day outcomes, and evaluated their impact on weight loss and comorbidities one year following the procedure. From that report, they were able to conclude that staple line reinforcement (SLR) was associated with an increased leak rate. So many variables, however, were involved in the design of this study, which questioned the credibility of this conclusion. More than 1600 surgeons, each with their own different techniques and preferences, performed the procedures at 720 centers, each with their own different protocols and set up. Furthermore, a wide range of different consumables were used by different surgeons\centers, making it very difficult to identify the factor(s) that could have contributed to the relatively higher rate of leak reported in this study following LSG with SLR (0.96%) compared to no SLR (0.65%). Strangely enough, the researchers reported that staple line leak was directly, and significantly, related to a bougie size; that is less than 38 F (0.96%) compared to more than 38 F (0.80%), but they still managed to contribute the higher incidence of leak to buttressing the staple line. It is worth mentioning that a later, well-structured study of the MBSAQIP database proved that this, rather surprising conclusion was actually unfounded. The researchers went through the MBSAQIP Participant Use File data for 198,339 primary LSG cases that were performed during the years 2015–2016, assessed all the variables that were related to leak rate and used multiple bivariate analyses to evaluate the

30-day outcomes. They concluded that buttressing was associated with reduced rates of bleeding and reoperations but not with a higher incidence of leak [29].

6   Previous Evidence

Cesana et al., in 2018, published the results of their analysis of the predictors of leak in 1738 consecutive LSG procedures and concluded that buttressing of the staple line significantly reduced the risk of bleeding ($P < 0.05$) [44]. Gagner and Kemmeter studied the leak rate following LSG with 5 different staple line reinforcement methods though a systemic review of all the papers that were published between 2012 and 2016 and concluded that buttressing was not only associated with a lower rate of leak compared with no reinforcement, but also that its effectiveness was significantly better when compared to that of over-sewing or sealants [45].

7   Conclusion

8   Types of buttressing materials that are coomercially available (Fig. 3)

The main buttressing materials that are currently used in bariatric surgery are (alphabetically):

- Neoveil, an absorbable polyglycolic acid felt; Gunze Medical. This is the material that is used in Medtronic's latest released "Pre-loaded" Reinforced cartridges with Tristapler technology.
- Peristrips Dry; permanent bovine pericardial strips; Baxter Healthcare (Formerly Synovis)
- Peristrips Dry with Veritas; remodelable collagen matrix strips; Baxter Healthcare (Formerly Synovis)
- Seamguard; a synthetic bioabsorbable glycolide trimethylene carbonate copolymer; WL Gore & Associates.
- Surgisis Biodesign; Remodelable small intestinal submucosa strips that are coated with fructose self-adhesive; Cook Medical.

However, it is important to note that very few direct comparisons of one material to another have been reported. In one, nonrandomized, study, bovine pericardial strips were compared with polyglycolide/trimethylene carbonate buttress material. This study found a significantly greater incidence of leaks in the latter group; but importantly, the authors used the same stapler (3.5 mm staple height) in both groups [46] and, because the polyglycolide/trimethylene carbonate product is significantly thinner than the bovine pericardial product, the increased leak rate may be attributable to their use of the same stapler with buttress materials of significantly different thicknesses.*

Other large series that compared essentially the same products reported contradicting outcomes with varying levels of evidence [31, 45]; Fig. 4.

References

1. Nguyen NT, Longoria M, Chalifoux S, Wilson SE. Bioabsorbable staple line reinforcement for laparoscopic gastrointestinal surgery. Surg Technol Int. 2005;14:107–11.
2. Downey DM, Ali S, Goldblatt MI, Saxe JM, Dolan JP. Gastrointestinal staple line reinforcement. Surg Technol Int. 2007;16:55–60.
3. Shikora SA, Kim JJ, Tarnoff ME. Reinforcing gastric staple-lines with bovine pericardial strips may decrease the likelihood of gastric leak after laparoscopic Roux-en-Y gastric bypass. Obes Surg. 2003;13(1):37–44.
4. Miller KA, Pump A. Use of bioabsorbable staple reinforcement material in gastric bypass: a prospective randomized clinical trial. Surg Obes Relat Dis. 2007;3(4):417–21.
5. Assalia A, Ueda K, Matteotti R, Cuenca-Abente F, Rogula T, Gagner M. Staple-line reinforcement with bovine pericardium in laparoscopic sleeve gastrectomy: experimental comparative study in pigs. Obes Surg. 2007;17(2):222–8.
6. Daskalakis M, Berdan Y, Theodoridou S, Weigand G, Weiner RA. Impact of surgeon experience and buttress material on postoperative complications after laparoscopic sleeve gastrectomy. Surg Endosc. 2011;25(1):88–97.
7. Cunningham-Hill M, Mazzei M, Zhao H, Lu X, Edwards MA. The Impact of Staple Line Reinforcement Utilization on Bleeding and Leak Rates Following Sleeve Gastrectomy for Severe Obesity: a Propensity and Case-Control Matched Analysis. Obes Surg. 2019;29(8):2449–63.
8. Zafar SN, Felton J, Miller K, Wise ES, Kligman M. Staple line treatment and bleeding after laparoscopic sleeve gastrectomy. JSLS. 2018;22(4).
9. Mocanu V, Dang J, Ladak F, Switzer N, Birch DW, Karmali S. Predictors and outcomes of bleed after sleeve gastrectomy: an analysis of the MBSAQIP data registry. Surg Obes Relat Dis. 2019;15(10):1675–81.
10. Parikh M, Issa R, McCrillis A, Saunders JK, Ude-Welcome A, Gagner M. Surgical strategies that may decrease leak after laparoscopic sleeve gastrectomy: a systematic review and meta-analysis of 9991 cases. Ann Surg. 2013;257(2):231–7.
11. Abou Rached A, Basile M, El Masri H. Gastric leaks post sleeve gastrectomy: review of its prevention and management. World J Gastroenterol. 2014;20(38):13904–10.
12. Wang Z, Dai X, Xie H, Feng J, Li Z, Lu Q. The efficacy of staple line reinforcement during laparoscopic sleeve gastrectomy: A meta-analysis of randomized controlled trials. Int J Surg. 2016;25:145–52.
13. Bashah M, Khidir N, El-Matbouly M. Management of leak after sleeve gastrectomy: outcomes of 73 cases, treatment algorithm and predictors of resolution. Obes Surg. 2020;30(2):515–20.
14. Leonard-Murali S, Nasser H, Ivanics T, Shakaroun D, Genaw J. Perioperative Outcomes of Roux-en-Y Gastric Bypass and Sleeve Gastrectomy in Patients with Diabetes Mellitus: an Analysis of the Metabolic and Bariatric Surgery Accreditation and Quality Improvement Program (MBSAQIP) Database. Obes Surg. 2020;30(1):111–8.
15. Downey DM, Harre JG, Dolan JP. Increased burst pressure in gastrointestinal staple-lines using reinforcement with a bioprosthetic material. Obes Surg. 2005;15:1379–83.
16. Arnold W, Shikora SA. A comparison of burst pressure between buttressed versus non-buttressed staple-lines in an animal model. Obes Surg. 2005;15:164–71.

17. Baker RS, Foote J, Kemmeter P, Brady R, Vroegop T, Serveld M. The science of stapling and leaks. Obes Surg. 2004;14:1290–8.
18. Shikora SA. The use of staple-line reinforcement during laparoscopic gastric bypass. Obes Surg. 2004;14:1313–20.
19. Assalia A, Ueda K, Matteotti R, et al. Staple-line reinforcement with bovine pericardium in laparoscopic sleeve gastrectomy: experimental comparative study in pigs. Obes Surg. 2007;17:222–8.
20. Consten EC, Gagner M, Pomp A, Inabnet WB. Decreased bleeding after laparoscopic sleeve gastrectomy with or without duodenal switch for morbid obesity using a stapled buttressed absorbable polymer membrane. Obes Surg. 2004;14:1360–6.
21. Basu NN, Leschinskey D, Heath DI. The use of Seamguard to buttress the suture repair of a staple line leak following laparoscopic gastric bypass for obesity. Obes Surg. 2008;18:896–7.
22. Kourosh S, Daniel WB, Arya S, Shahzeer K. Complications associated with laparoscopic sleeve gastrectomy for morbid obesity: a surgeon's guide. Can J Surg. 2013;56(5):347–52.
23. De Angelis F, Abdelgawad M, Rizzello M, Mattia C, Silecchia G. Perioperative hemorrhagic complications after laparoscopic sleeve gastrectomy: four-year experience of a bariatric center of excellence. Surg Endosc. 2017;31(9):3547–51.
24. Spivak H, Azran C, Spectre G, Lidermann G, Blumenfeld O. Sleeve Gastrectomy Postoperative Hemorrhage is Linked to Type-2 Diabetes and Not to Surgical Technique. Obes Surg. 2017;27(11):2927–32.
25. Albanopoulos K, Alevizos L, Flessas J, et al. Reinforcing the staple line during laparoscopic sleeve gastrectomy: prospective randomized clinical study comparing two different techniques Preliminary Results. Obes Surg. 2012;22:42–6.
26. Simon TE, Scott JA, Brockmeyer JR, Rice RC, Frizzi JD, Husain FA, Choi YU. Comparison of staple-line leakage and hemorrhage in patients undergoing laparoscopic sleeve gastrectomy with or without Seamguard. Am Surg. 2011;77(12):1665–8.
27. Shah SS, Todkar JS, Shah PS. Buttressing the staple line: a randomized comparison between staple-line reinforcement versus no reinforcement during sleeve gastrectomy. Obes Surg. 2014;24(12):2014–20.
28. Guerrier JB, Mehaffey JH, Schirmer BD, Hallowell PT. Reinforcement of the Staple Line during Gastric Sleeve: A Comparison of Buttressing or Oversewing, versus No Reinforcement- A Single-Institution Study. Am Surg. 2018;84(5):690–4.
29. Demeusy A, Sill A, Averbach A. Current role of staple line reinforcement in 30-day outcomes of primary laparoscopic sleeve gastrectomy: an analysis of MBSAQIP data, 2015–2016 PUF. Surg Obes Relat Dis. 2018;14(10):1454–61.
30. David Spector, Zvi Perry, Tracy Konobeck, Daniel L Mooradian, Scott Shikora. Comparison of hemostatic properties between collagen and synthetic buttress materials used in staple line reinforcement in a swine splenic hemorrhage model. Technological Leadership Institute (2011).
31. Shikora SA, Mahoney CB. Clinical Benefit of Gastric Staple Line Reinforcement (SLR) in Gastrointestinal Surgery: a Meta-analysis. Obes Surg. 2015;25:1133–41.
32. Guerrier JB1, Mehaffey JH, Schirmer BD, Hallowell PT. Reinforcement of the staple line during gastric sleeve: a comparison of buttressing or oversewing, versus no reinforcement—a single-institution study. Am Surg. 2018;84(5):690–4.
33. Ruiz-Tovar J, Zubiaga L, Muñoz JL, Llavero C. Incidence of postoperative nausea and vomiting after laparoscopic sleeve gastrectomy with staple line reinforcement with oversewing and staple line inversion vs buttressing material: A randomized clinical trial. Int J Surg. 2018;59:75–9.
34. Angrisani L, Lorenzo M, Borrelli V, et al. The use of bovine pericardial strips on linear stapler to reduce extraluminal bleeding during laparoscopic gastric bypass: prospective randomized clinical trial. Obes Surg. 2004;14:1198–202.

35. Nguyen NT, Longoria M, Welbourne S, et al. Glycolide copolymer staple-line reinforcement reduces staple site bleeding during laparoscopic gastric bypass: a prospective randomized trial. Arch Surg. 2005;140:773–8.
36. Chen B, Kiriakopoulos A, Tsakayannis D, Wachtel MS, Linos D, Frezza EE. Reinforcement does not necessarily reduce the rate of staple line leaks after sleeve gastrectomy. A review of the literature and clinical experiences. Obes Surg. 2009;19(2):166–72.
37. Timucin Aydin M, Aras O, Karip B, Memisoglu K. Staple line reinforcement methods in laparoscopic sleeve gastrectomy: comparison of burst pressures and leaks. JSLS. 2015;19(3).
38. Yo LS, Consten EC, Quarles van Ufford HM, Gooszen HG, Gagner M. Buttressing of the staple line in gastrointestinal anastomoses: overview of new technology designed to reduce perioperative complications Dig Surg. 2006;23(5–6):283–91.
39. Glaysher M, Khan OA, Mabvuure NT, Wan A, Reddy M, Vasilikostas G. Staple line reinforcement during laparoscopic sleeve gastrectomy: does it affect clinical outcomes? Int J Surg. 2013;11(4):286–9.
40. Al Hajj GN, Haddad J. Preventing staple-line leak in sleeve gastrectomy: reinforcement with bovine pericardium vs. oversewing. Obes Surg. 2013;23(11):1915–21.
41. Durmush EK1, Ermerak G, Durmush D. Short-term outcomes of sleeve gastrectomy for morbid obesity: does staple line reinforcement matter? Obes Surg. 2014;24(7):1109–16.
42. Iossa A, Abdelgawad M, Watkins BM, Silecchia G. Leaks after laparoscopic sleeve gastrectomy: overview of pathogenesis and risk factors. Langenbecks Arch Surg. 2016;401(6):757–66.
43. Berger ER, Clements RH, Morton JM, Huffman KM, Wolfe BM, Nguyen NT, Ko CY, Hutter MM. The Impact of Different Surgical Techniques on Outcomes in Laparoscopic Sleeve Gastrectomies: The First Report from the Metabolic and Bariatric Surgery Accreditation and Quality Improvement Program (MBSAQIP). Ann Surg. 2016;264(3):464–73.
44. Cesana G, Cioffi S, Giorgi R, Villa R, Uccelli M, Ciccarese F, Castello G, Scotto B, Olmi S. Proximal Leakage After Laparoscopic Sleeve Gastrectomy: an Analysis of Preoperative and Operative Predictors on 1738 Consecutive Procedures. Obes Surg. 2018;28(3):627–35.
45. Gagner M, Kemmeter B. Comparison of laparoscopic sleeve gastrectomy leak rates in five staple-line reinforcement options: a systematic review. Surg Endosc. 2020;34(1):396–407.
46. Shikora SA, Kim JJ, Tarnoff ME. Comparison of permanent and nonpermanent staple line buttressing materials for linear gastric staple lines during laparoscopic Roux-en-Y gastric bypass. Surg Obes Relat Dis. 2008;4(6):729–34.

Sleeve and Ventral Hernias

Meshari Almuhanna and Wei-Jei Lee

1   Introduction

Obesity is a major risk factor for many metabolic diseases, including diabetes, cardiovascular disease, sleep apnea, musculoskeletal disorders and some cancers. The number of obese people is increasing worldwide; according to WHO since the number of obese people nearly tripled [1]. Surgical treatment of Obesity (Bariatric Surgery) is concomitantly increasing worldwide [2]. Bariatric surgeries that are most commonly performed are laparoscopic sleeve gastrectomy (LSG) followed by Roux-en-Y gastric bypass (RYGB) [3].

There is a strong association between developing ventral hernia and obesity [4, 5]. Furthermore, obesity in itself also increases the risk and failure of ventral hernia repair. Being obese and having ventral hernia makes performing bariatric surgery a challenge. Can it be done in concomitant with LSG is the question. In this chapter we will focus on what is the best approach for an obese patient with ventral hernia who has chosen to undergo an LSG.

M. Almuhanna (✉)
Bariatric & Metabolic Surgery Unit, Department of General Surgery, Jaber Al-Ahmad Al-Sabah Hospital, Kuwait, Kuwait
e-mail: almuhanna@moh.gov.kw

M. Almuhanna · W.-J. Lee
Asia-Pacific Endoscopic Bariatric and Metabolic Surgical Center, Min-Sheng General Hospital, Taoyuan, Taiwan

S. Al-Sabah et al. (eds.), *Laparoscopic Sleeve Gastrectomy*,
https://doi.org/10.1007/978-3-030-57373-7_29

2   Prevalence, Incidence and Cost of Ventral Hernia

Ventral hernia (VH) is defined as an anterior abdominal wall fascia defect with protrusion of internal content [6]. Incidence of VH is increased between the 3rd and 6th decade of life and highest between 41–50 years of age. Incisional hernia and umbilical hernia are both the most common type of VH. Umbilical hernia is common in male (M:F – 1.5:1) where incisional hernia is more common in females (F:M 2.3:1) [4]. It has also been proven that there is a significant association between smoking, alcohol, obesity and VH.

Obesity is a major risk factor for developing VH but the incidence of VH varies by location due to different etiological factors [4]. Incisional hernia is a common long-term complication of abdominal surgery with an incidence of 3–13% of laparotomy incisions [5]. Priti Prasad et al. reported a series of 200 cases of VH of hospital admissions and found the most common type to be incisional hernia (41%) followed by umbilical (32%), paraumbilical (17%) and epigastric (10%) [4]. In another report, Jaykar, R.D. et al. also found that the most common VH is incisional hernia with an incidence of 41% of hospital admission [5]. Infra-umbilical incisional hernia (42%) was the most common site of incisional hernia followed by umbilical incisional hernia (32%). He found the mean age of VH to be 41 years of age, with male to female ratio 1:1.9. Other than obesity, constipation was the major predisposing risk factor of developing VH. They also noticed that small defects (<2 cm) presented early with complication [5]. Poulose BK et al. found the number of inpatient VH repairs (VHR) in the United States increased from 126,548 in 2001 to 154,278 in 2006. Furthermore, an estimate of 348,000 outpatient VHRs were done in 2006 [7]. This is burden on healthcare systems, although the majority of cases were performed as an emergency [8]. The cost of VHR for 2006 in US was $3.2 billion. Incidence of VHR is rising, and by reducing the recurrence rate alone, it would save $32 million dollar in the US alone for each 1% reduction in operation [7]. Raquel Maia et al. in their review article, confirmed that obesity alone is a risk factor for both primary and incisional hernia. Further, obese individuals are at a high risk of having co-morbidities which significantly increase the risk of perioperative complications and recurrence rates of VHR [9]. In addition, there is a positive correlation between the size of the hernia defect and obesity: the higher the body mass index (BMI), the bigger the defect size [9]. Similarly, the recurrence rate is also higher in obese people with a higher BMI [9, 10]. Furthermore, obesity itself is an independent risk factor of longer hospital stay, surgical site infection, recurrence and re-admission after VHR [11, 12].

3   Diagnosis and Classification of Ventral Hernia in Obese Patients

The clinical presentation of ventral hernias varies depending on the size and location of the hernia and weather it is symptomatic (pain, bulge, discomfort) or asymptomatic. A complete history and physical examination are very important for obese patients with ventral hernias. In non-obese patients, ventral hernia can be easily diagnosed but in obese patients it usually requires additional imaging studies to diagnose. Murphy KP et al. found in his study that physical examination of obese patients with suspected ventral hernia are difficult to diagnose and the best modality for diagnoses is to do abdominopelvic computed tomography (CT) [13]. It helps identifying the hernia site, size and the content of the hernia sac in both acute and elective circumstances (Figs. 1 and 2).

In classification of VH, they are classified into primary abdominal wall hernia and incisional hernia bases on the recommendation of the European Hernia Society (EHS) classification [14, 15].

4   Primary Abdominal Wall Hernia

The classification of primary abdominal wall hernia is based on localization and size of the hernia (Table 1).

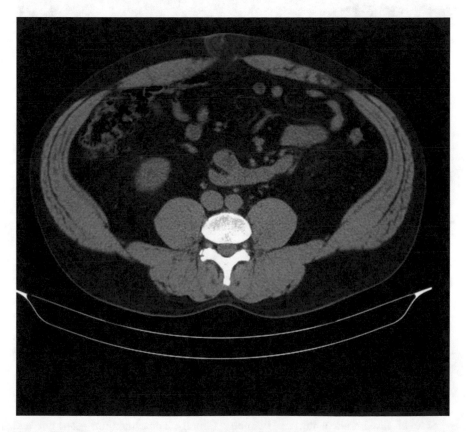

Fig. 1 CT scan of obese patient with ventral hernia showing omental content without sign of complication

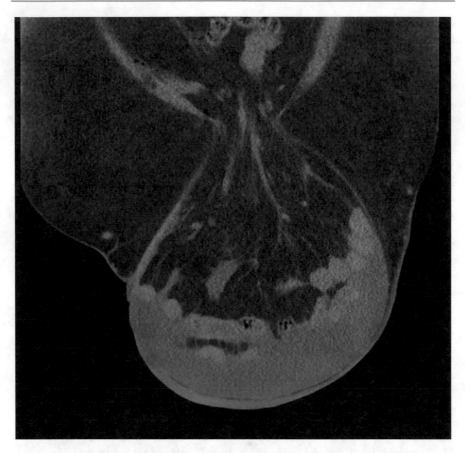

Fig. 2 CT scan of obese patient with panniculus abdomen and ventral hernia for more than 5 years, with sign of complication as the bowel incarcerated in hernia sac with reactional fluid

Table 1 European Hernia Society (EHS) classification of primary abdominal wall hernias

EHS Primary abdominal wall hernia classification		Diameter in cm	Small < 2 cm	Medium ≥ 2–4 cm	Large ≥ 4 cm
Midline	Epigastric				
	Umbilical				
Lateral	Spigelian				
	Lumbar				

- Localization of the hernia two midline (epigastric and umbilical) and two lateral hernias (Spighelian and lumbar)
- Size of the hernia using the diameter (small < 2 cm, medium ≥ 2–4 cm and large ≥ 4 cm).

5   Incisional Hernia

Classification of incisional abdominal wall hernias based on localization of the hernia: medial or midline zone and the lateral zone (Table 2).

Table 2 European Hernia Society (EHS) classification of incisional abdominal wall hernias

EHS Incisional Hernia Classification			
Midline	Subxiphoidal	M1	
	Epigastric	M2	
	Umbilical	M3	
	Infraumbilical	M4	
	Suprapublic	M5	
Lateral	Subcostal	L1	
	Flanks	L2	
	Iliac	L3	
	Lumbar	L4	
Recurrent incisional hernia?	Yes ○ No ○		
Length cm	Width cm		

Width	W1	W2	W3
cm	<4 cm	≥4 – 10 cm	≥10 cm
	○	○	○

5.1   Medial or Midline Zone

The borders of the medial or midline area are defined as:

(1) cranial: the xyphoid
(2) caudal: the pubic bone
(3) lateral: the lateral margin of the rectal sheath.

All incisions made between the lateral margin of the rectus sheath are midline hernias. Midlines hernias are further subdivided into subgroup (5 M zones) as it is believed that hernias close to bony structures have high risk of recurrence and pose specific therapeutic approach (Fig. 3).

M1: subxiphoidal (from the xyphoid till 3 cm caudally).
M2: epigastric (from 3 cm below the xyphoid till 3 cm above the umbilicus).
M3: umbilical (from 3 cm above till 3 cm below the umbilicus).
M4: infraumbilical (from 3 cm below the umbilicus till 3 cm above the pubis).
M5: suprapubic (from pubic bone till 3 cm cranially).

5.2   Lateral Hernias (Flank Hernias)

Any incisions lateral to the lateral margin of the rectus sheath are lateral hernias (Fig. 4).

Fig. 3 Classification of midline incisional hernias between the two lateral margins of the rectus muscle sheaths, which is divided into five zones

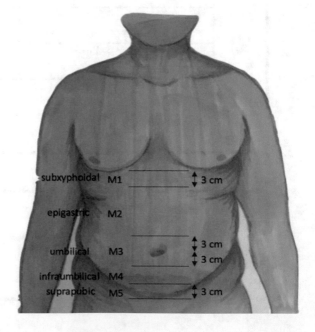

Fig. 4 Classification of lateral incisional hernias, four zones (L1–L4) lateral of the rectus muscle sheaths

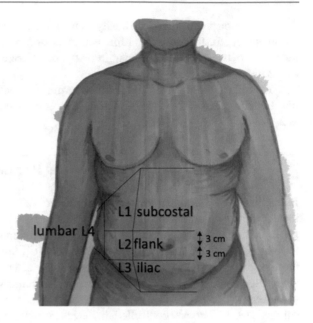

The borders of the lateral hernia are defined as:

(1) cranial: the costal margin
(2) caudal: the inguinal region.
(3) medially: the lateral margin of the rectal sheath
(4) laterally: the lumbar region.

So, the four lateral hernia zones on each side are:

L1: Subcostal (between the costal margin and a horizontal line 3 cm above the umbilicus)
L2: Flank (lateral to the rectal sheath in the area 3 cm above and below the umbilicus)
L3: Iliac (between a horizontal line 3 cm below the umbilicus and the inguinal region)
L4: Lumbar (latero-dorsal of the anterior axillary line).

6   Size of the Hernia

Grid format used to describe the size of incisional hernias measure the width and length. Width of the hernia is defined as the greatest horizontal distance in cm between the lateral margins of the hernia defect on both sides. In case of multiple incisional hernia, the width is measured between the two most lateral located hernias with the most lateral edges. The length of incisional hernias is measured by the greatest distance in cm vertically between the most cranial and most caudal margins (Fig. 5). In case of multiple hernia caused by a single incision, the length measured between the cranial margin of the most cranial defect and distal margin of the most distal defect (Fig. 6).

To avoid the confusion of incisional hernia size with the size of primary hernia (small, medium and large), code taxonomy was chosen as: W1 < 4 cm, W2 ≥ 4–10 cm, W3 ≥ 10 cm.

7   Indication and Risks of Ventral Hernia Repair

Indication for ventral hernia repair is for the relief of symptoms (pain, acute incarceration, enlargement and skin problem). In case of large ventral hernias, pre-operative optimization of the pulmonary function is very important in order to reduce the risk of pulmonary complications [16]. Smoking is known to increase the risk of surgical site infection and recurrence after hernia repair [12, 17]. It is recommended to stop smoking 4 weeks prior to surgery to decrease the incidence of pulmonary complications and reduce the incidence of leak in Gastrointestinal surgery [18, 19]. Poorly controlled diabetes is a risk factor for post-operative complications in ventral hernia repair [11]. Glycosylated hemoglobin (HbA1c) is used as a test for checking the patients' diabetic control.

The key for successful outcomes in ventral hernia repair is to reduce the risk factors of ventral hernia with weight reduction, control of diabetes and cessation of smoking with optimizing the nutritional parameters.

Fig. 5 Grid format of incisional hernia for single defect

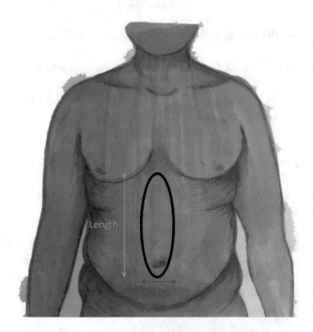

Fig. 6 Grid format of incisional hernia for multiple defects

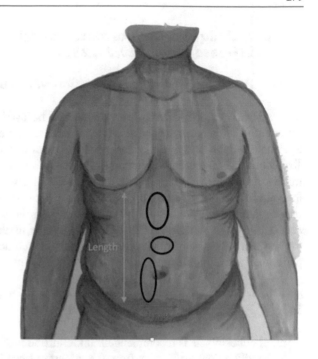

Laparoscopic or laparoscopic assisted ventral hernia repair is favorable over open hernia repair in obese patients. Advantages of laparoscopic ventral hernia repair (LVHR) include fewer surgical site infection, less pain postoperatively, 5 days faster return to work compared to open ventral hernia repair (OVHR), but no significant difference has been made in recurrence rate between LVHR and OVHR [20–22]. Prophylactic antibiotics as a single dose of first-generation Cephalosporin (cefazoline) is recommended to be given pre-operatively, in case of allergy to Cephalosporin, Clindamycin or Vancomycin can be given. There is no strong recommendation on bowel preparation or urinary catheterization unless surgery will take a long time [20]. Deep vein thrombosis prophylaxis is recommended for obese patients as it lowers incidence of pulmonary embolism [23, 24].

Although LVHR is recommended for VH repair in obese patients, there are some contraindications of LVHR, including defect size greater than 15 cm, high risk patients, loss of domain (hernia sac contains more 30% of abdominal content and solid organ), active enterocutaneous fistula, need to remove prosthetic mesh and small defect but large hernia sac [20, 21, 23]. Patients with small defects but large hernia sacs maintained for a long period (such as in Fig. 2) may have respiratory distress after repairing the ventral hernia and reducing the sac content into the abdomen.

8 Technique of Laparoscopic Ventral Hernia Repair in Obese Patient [20, 21, 23]

8.1 Position of Trocar and Creation of Pneumoperitoneum

Veress needle or open Hasson's technique can be used for creation of pneumoperitoneum. It is recommended that Veress needle or first port should be inserted at Palmer's point away as much as possible from expected adhesion. First trocar size should be 10 mm to accommodate the camera and mesh insertion, while other trocars should be inserted under vision. In dealing with midline incision trocars inserted on the left side of the patient, ideally 3 or more trocars in line with optimal distance from the defect 16–18 cm to expose the whole hernia sac and allow accessibility for adhesiolysis and proper fixation of the mesh. Site and size of trocars can be chosen based on the surgeons preference and expertise. In obese patients, it is preferable to use long bariatric length instruments.

9 Principles of Adhesiolysis

Limited adhesiolysis is recommended. It should be limited to freeing the adhesion near the abdominal wall, away from the adherent bowel. Adhesiolysis can be performed using sharp and blunt dissection, limiting the use of energy devices for hemostasis. Bowel should be inspected at the end of adhesiolysis. In case of iatrogenic bowel injury without significant enteric fluid leakage, it can be repaired followed by hernia repair and mesh fixation.

For safe adhsiolysis, many maneuvers can be used:

- Traction/counter traction technique
- Angled/flexible camera
- Moving scope among ports
- Outside pressure over the abdominal wall to reduce the hernia sac
- Careful sharp dissection under vision and close to abdominal wall
- Limit the use of energy devices
- Reposition patient table and ports if needed
- Maintain the camera clean
- Repeat inspection of bowel at the end of adhesiolysis.

10 Measurement of Hernia Defect

Size of hernia is a significant risk of recurrence. It is important to measure the size of the hernia defect accurately. Accurate measurement helps to choose the prober size for the mesh. Dynamic rather than static measurement for ventral hernia defect is recommended. To determine the size of the defect it should be measured vertically and transversely. The most accurate method of measurement of ventral hernia defects is intracorporeal rather than extracorporeal due to the thickness of the abdominal wall, which can cause an overestimation of the defect size. Intracorporeal method can be accomplished using two spinal needle placed through the abdominal wall. Using a sterile ruler, intracorporeal measurement is done using the largest diameter of the defect transversally and vertically. This method reduces the overestimation of the hernia defect which may result in large sized mesh that will be more difficult to handle, allowing the bowel to incarcerate and bulge into the defect.

11   Closure of Hernia Defect and Intraperitoneal Onlay Mesh (IPOM) Fixation

Suturing the defect in-order to reduce the hernia size to the smallest size possible thus may reduce the bulging and risk of seroma formation, which may decrease the risk of infection. The suture material should be nonabsorbable. It is recommended to reconstruct the linea alba or any defect combined to IPOM, this augmentation repair is termed IPOM-PLUS. Mesh size should be used to cover the defect with an overlap at the edge of the defect by at least 3–4 cm in all directions. Large mesh size (e.g. 30 cm × 30 cm) can be inserted through 10 or 12 mm ports by rolling up tightly. For very large size mesh (e.g. 35 cm × 30 cm), a 15 mm port should be used. It is important to avoid mesh-skin contact. Mesh fixation can be done by suturing or tacker device with no difference in recurrence rate.

12   Technique of Open Ventral Hernia Repair [10, 25, 26]

Although LVHR for obese patients with ventral hernia is better than open approach, some scenarios need to be approached using the open technique. These include emergency surgery for hernias with complications, loss of domain, very large defects that need component separation and the need for resection panniculus. It is advised that all ventral hernia should be repaired using mesh. There are four types of mesh placement in open technique, ranked by the best approach with least recurrence and surgical site infection rates as follow (Fig. 7):

- Retrorecuts also named sublay, retromuscular repair or Rives-Stoppa (preperitoneal mesh placement)
- Open intra-peritoneal onlay mesh (underlay)
- Onlay (place the mesh on anterior fascia)
- Inlay (place the mesh on hernia defect).

Fig. 7 Site of mesh
placement in Open and
Laparoscopic Technique of
ventral hernia repair

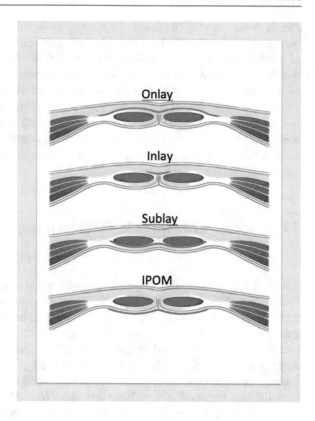

13   Concurrent LSG with LVHR

LSG and LVHR can be done during the same procedure in selected patients.
Most cases done in patients with a BMI less than 50 kg/m^2 and a defect size less
than 10 cm (Fig. 1). Raziel A et al. reported a series of 54 cases of concomitant bariatric and ventral/incisional hernia surgeries in morbidly obese patients
with a mean BMI of 44 kg/m^2 and a mean age of 50 years, with the majority of
cases being LSG (48 cases). They did not encounter mesh infection or major
complications directly related to LVHR within a 5 year follow up [27]. Moolla
et al. reported on a matched analysis from Metabolic and Bariatric Surgery
Accreditation and Quality Improvement Program (MBSAQIP) database in the
USA of 430,225 cases in which 1.1% (4690) of them had concurrent LVHR. He
was able to find that LVHR is safer with LSG (2718 cases) than with LRYGB
(1930 cases) in terms of readmission, reoperation and major complications with
30 days [28]. Marzouk et al. in their study of LVHR combined with LSG in 15
obese patients with a mean BMI 45.2 kg/m^2 and ventral hernia less than 10 cm,
found that LSG combined with LVHR is safe and feasible in carefully selected
patients [29]. In Praveen Raj P et al.'s retrospective study on 156 cases of bariatric surgery concomitant with LVHR, 120 of them had LSG with an average BMI

Table 3 Details of included studies of Concurrent LSG with LVHR

Author	Number of LSG + LVHR	Mean age (years)	Mean BMI kg/m²S	Size of defect (cm)	Recurrence rate (%)	Major complication (%)
Raziel A et al.	48	53	44.2	–	1.8	–
Muhammad Moolla et al. (MBSAQIP)	2718	49	46	–	–	3.2
Marzouk et al.	15	42.7	45	2.63	6.6	–
Praveen Raj P et al.	120	43.94 ± 11.41	43.64 ± 6.8	3.58 ± 3.36	<1	–
Eid GM et al.	20	–	<50	<8	10	–

of 43 kg/m² and included both primary and recurrent VH (average size of hernia 3.58 ± 3.36 cm). After a follow up of 12 months, they were able to demonstrate that LSG is safe in combination with hernia repair [30] (Table 3).

14 LSG with Sequential LVHR

Eid GM et al. gave a suggested algorithm on how to treat morbidly obese patients presenting with ventral hernia [31]. The study classified patients on favorable and unfavorable anatomical hernias. Favorable anatomical hernias are defined as hernias located in the center, with a size less than 8 cm, BMI less than 50 kg/m², body wall thickness less than 4 cm with gynecoid body habit and a reducible hernia. Unfavorable anatomical hernias on the other hand are defined as hernias that are lateral, size larger than 8 cm, BMI more than 50 kg/m², body wall thickness more than 4 cm with android body habit and unreducible hernia. They found that all symptomatic hernias should have hernia repair first prior to bariatric surgery. Asymptomatic patients with favorable anatomy can have concomitant LVHR and bariatric surgery, while patients with unfavorable anatomy should have bariatric surgery followed by LVHR [31]. In Fig. 2, the patient underwent concurrent LSG and open VHR. However, the patients died 2 months later due to respiratory failure. Finally, obese patients with asymptomatic VH and unfavorable anatomy should have LSG first, followed by VHR.

15 Conclusion

There is a strong association between obesity and ventral hernia. The most common type of ventral hernia is incisional hernia followed by umbilical hernia. Obesity does not only increase the risk of developing ventral hernia, but also increases the risk of perioperative complications and recurrence rates. For small umbilical or incisional hernias, concurrent LSG and VH repair can be done safely. However, a sequential LSG followed by VH repair is recommended for patients with an asymptomatic VH with unfavorable anatomy or significant medical problems, such as large size (10 cm), BMI > 50, small hernia defect with large sac, poorly controlled diabetes, heavy smokers, etc. Complexity of ventral hernia associated with obesity requires careful approach for such a treatment. Currently, there is no consensus on the best treatment options for obese patients with ventral hernias. Successful treatment should be individualized based on patient's symptoms and concerns.

References

1. https://www.who.int/news-room/fact-sheets/detail/obesity-and-overweight. Accessed 01 July 2020
2. Buchwald H, Oien DM. Metabolic/bariatric surgery world-wide 2011. Obes Surg. 2013;23(4):427–36.
3. Angrisani L1, Santonicola A, Iovino P, Formisano G, Buchwald H, Scopinaro N. Bariatric surgery worldwide 2013. Obes Surg. 2015;25(10):1822–32.
4. Priti PraSad Shah, Shama Shaikh, Sunil Panchabhai, Prevalence of anterior abdominal wall hernia and its associated risk factors. Int J Anat Radiol Surg. 2016;5(3): SO07–10.
5. Jaykar RD, Varudkar AS, Akamanchi AK. A clinical study of ventral hernia. Int Surg J. 2017;4(7):2326–9.
6. Townsend RC, Beauchamp BD, Mattox MEK. Clinical surgery of hernia. Sabiston textbook of surgery, vol II, 19th ed. Elsevier; 2016, p. 1128.
7. Poulose BK, Shelton J, Phillips S, et al. Epidemiology and cost of ventral hernia repair: making the case for hernia research. Hernia. 2012;16(2):179–83. https://doi.org/10.1007/s10029-011-0879-9.
8. Smith J, Parmely JD. Ventral Hernia. [Updated 2019 Jan 16]. In: StatPearls [Internet]. Treasure Island (FL): StatPearls Publishing; 2020 January. https://www.ncbi.nlm.nih.gov/books/NBK499927/.
9. https://www.sages.org/wiki/ventral-hernia-obesity/. Accessed 01 June 2020
10. Maia R, Salgaonkar H, Lomanto D, Shabbir A. Ventral hernia and obesity: is there a consensus? Ann Laparosc Endosc Surg. 2019;4:17.
11. Goodenough CJ, Ko TC, Kao LS, et al. Development and validation of a risk stratification score for ventral incisional hernia after abdominal surgery: hernia expectation rates in intra-abdominal surgery (the HERNIA Project). J Am Coll Surg. 2015;220(4):405–13. https://doi.org/10.1016/j.jamcollsurg.2014.12.027.
12. Danzig MR, Stey AM, Yin SS, Qiu S, Divino CM. Patient profiles and outcomes following repair of irreducible and reducible ventral wall hernias. Hernia. 2016;20(2):239–47. https://doi.org/10.1007/s10029-015-1381-6.
13. Murphy KP, O'Connor OJ, Maher MM. Adult abdominal hernias. AJR Am J Roentgenol. 2014;202(6):W506–11. https://doi.org/10.2214/AJR.13.12071.
14. Bittner R, Bain K, Bansal VK, et al. Update of guidelines for laparoscopic treatment of ventral and incisional abdominal wall hernias (International Endohernia Society (IEHS))—Part A. Surg Endosc. 2019;33:3069–139. https://doi.org/10.1007/s00464-019-06907-7.
15. Muysoms FE, Miserez M, Berrevoet F, et al. Classification of primary and incisional abdominal wall hernias. Hernia. 2009;13(4):407–14. https://doi.org/10.1007/s10029-009-0518-x.

16. Lindmark M, Strigård K, Löwenmark T, Dahlstrand U, Gunnarsson U. Risk Factors for Surgical Complications in Ventral Hernia Repair. World J Surg. 2018;42(11):3528–36. https://doi.org/10.1007/s00268-018-4642-6.
17. Kaoutzanis C, Leichtle SW, Mouawad NJ, et al. Risk factors for postoperative wound infections and prolonged hospitalization after ventral/incisional hernia repair. Hernia. 2015;19(1):113–23. https://doi.org/10.1007/s10029-013-1155-y.
18. Thomsen T, Tønnesen H, Møller AM. Effect of preoperative smoking cessation interventions on postoperative complications and smoking cessation. Br J Surg. 2009;96(5):451–61. https://doi.org/10.1002/bjs.6591.
19. Cooke DT, Lin GC, Lau CL, et al. Analysis of cervical esophagogastric anastomotic leaks after transhiatal esophagectomy: risk factors, presentation, and detection. Ann Thorac Surg. 2009;88(1):177–85. https://doi.org/10.1016/j.athoracsur.2009.03.035.
20. https://www.sages.org/publications/guidelines/guidelines-for-laparoscopic-ventral-hernia-repair/. Accessed 01 June 2020
21. Bittner R, Bain K, Bansal VK, et al. Update of Guidelines for laparoscopic treatment of ventral and incisional abdominal wall hernias (International Endohernia Society (IEHS))-Part A [published correction appears in Surg Endosc. 2019 Jul 12]. Surg Endosc. 2019;33(10):3069–39. https://doi.org/10.1007/s00464-019-06907-7.
22. Patel PV, Aziz M. Merchant. Bariatr Surg Pract Patient Care. 2014:61–65. http://doi.org/10.1089/bari.2014.0008.
23. Bittner R, Bingener-Casey J, Dietz U, et al. Guidelines for laparoscopic treatment of ventral and incisional abdominal wall hernias (International Endohernia Society (IEHS)—Part 1. Surg Endosc. 2014;28:2–29. https://doi.org/10.1007/s00464-013-3170-6.
24. Freeman AL, Pendleton RC, Rondina MT. Prevention of venous thromboembolism in obesity. Expert Rev Cardiovasc Ther. 2010;8(12):1711–21. https://doi.org/10.1586/erc.10.160.
25. https://www.sages.org/wiki/ventral-hernia-obesity/. Accessed 10 June 2020
26. Bougard H, et al. HIG (SA) Guidelines for the Management of Ventral Hernias. South African journal of surgery Suid-Afrikaanse tydskrif vir chirurgie. 2016;54:S1–29.
27. Raziel A, Sakran N, Szold A, Goitein D. Concomitant bariatric and ventral/incisional hernia surgery in morbidly obese patients. Surg Endosc. 2014;28(4):1209–12. https://doi.org/10.1007/s00464-013-3310-z.
28. Moolla M, Dang J, Modasi A, et al. Concurrent Laparoscopic Ventral Hernia Repair with Bariatric Surgery: a Propensity-Matched Analysis. J Gastrointest Surg. 2020;24(1):58–66. https://doi.org/10.1007/s11605-019-04291-0.
29. Marzouk AMSM, Ali HOE. Laparoscopic ventral hernia repair combined with sleeve gastrectomy in morbidly obese patients: early outcomes. Surg J (N Y). 2019;5(3):e87–91. Published 2019 Aug 28. https://doi.org/10.1055/s-0039-1694979.
30. Praveen Raj P, Bhattacharya S, Saravana Kumar S, Parthasarathi R, Cumar B, Palanivelu C. Morbid obesity with ventral hernia: is concomitant bariatric surgery with laparoscopic ventral hernia mesh repair the best approach? An experience of over 150 cases. Surg Obes Relat Dis. 2019;15(7):1098–103. https://doi.org/10.1016/j.soard.2019.04.027.
31. Eid GM, Wikiel KJ, Entabi F, Saleem M. Ventral hernias in morbidly obese patients: a suggested algorithm for operative repair. Obes Surg. 2013;23(5):703–9. https://doi.org/10.1007/s11695-013-0883-5.

Sphincter Augmentation and Management of Gastroesophageal Reflux with the LINX® Device and Sleeve Gastrectomy

Helmuth T. Billy, Terry L. Simpson, Masoud S. Chopan and Yuchen You

1   Introduction

Laparoscopic Sleeve Gastrectomy has become one of the most popular primary operations for the treatment of morbid obesity worldwide. Between 2013 and 2015 sleeve gastrectomy accounted for 40.7% of all primary bariatric procedures performed internationally [1]. In some parts of the world and in countries with the highest rates of morbid obesity, sleeve gastrectomy is the most common bariatric procedure performed, reaching 60% of recorded operations [2]. The popularity of sleeve gastrectomy as a primary operation for the treatment of morbid obesity is easily understood. The operation is straightforward and simple to perform when compared to duodenal switch or the well-established Roux Y gastric

H. T. Billy (✉)
Metabolic and Bariatric Surgery, St. John's Regional Medical Center, Oxnard, CA, USA
e-mail: Htbilly@gmail.com

H. T. Billy
Metabolic and Bariatric Surgery, Community Memorial Hospital, Ventura, CA, USA

H. T. Billy
Bariatric Surgery, Hamad General Hospital, Doha, Qatar

T. L. Simpson
Ventura Advanced Surgical Associates, Ventura, CA, USA
e-mail: Tsimpson@gmail.com

M. S. Chopan · Y. You
Department of Surgical Education, Community Memorial Hospital, Ventura, CA, USA
e-mail: Mchopan@cmhshealth.com

Y. You
e-mail: You1@cmhshealth.com

© The Editor(s) (if applicable) and The Author(s), under exclusive license to Springer Nature Switzerland AG 2021
S. Al-Sabah et al. (eds.), *Laparoscopic Sleeve Gastrectomy*,
https://doi.org/10.1007/978-3-030-57373-7_30

bypass. Sleeve gastrectomy can be routinely performed as an outpatient operation and does not involve anatomical rearrangement or surgical anastomoses. Sleeve gastrectomy has no risk of internal hernia. Malnutrition secondary to malabsorption does not occur. It also has a relatively short operative time of 20–30 min. For high-risk patients such as individuals suffering from end stage renal and liver disease, the super morbidly obese and the elderly, sleeve gastrectomy is an ideal and safe operation with which to achieve adequate weight loss [3].

Sleeve gastrectomy can be routinely performed in an outpatient setting, increasing the available facilities performing bariatric surgery. By augmenting the number of operations being performed as outpatient procedures and increasing the number of facilities capable of performing bariatric operations, sleeve gastrectomy has a direct and positive impact on the number of patients having potential access to care. With respect to weight loss outcomes, sleeve gastrectomy has been shown to achieve results comparable to Roux Y Gastric bypass [4, 5]. Individuals who fail to achieve their goals or who regain sufficient weight are easily revised to an alternative more aggressive operation as a second stage procedure. Sleeve gastrectomy therefore has multiple reasons to maintain its popularity as a desirable operation for the treatment of obesity and can be expected to be performed in high numbers for the foreseeable future.

Despite the success and widespread popularity of sleeve gastrectomy, symptomatic reflux is now a commonly recognized side effect of the operation. Esophageal reflux, esophagitis and possible Barrett's esophagus following sleeve gastrectomy has resulted in an ongoing controversy regarding the long-term complications after this operation. Magnetic sphincter augmentation is a simplified approach to address post-operative reflux following sleeve gastrectomy. The majority of symptomatic reflux patients have been typically converted to Roux-en-Y gastric bypass following sleeve gastrectomy. This approach destroys the benefits of sleeve gastrectomy, subjecting the patient to a lifetime risk of internal hernia, dumping syndrome, reactive hypoglycemia, malabsorption, malnutrition and intussusception. Magnetic sphincter augmentation preserves the anatomic benefits of sleeve gastrectomy while eliminating post-operative reflux and will be the focus of discussion in this chapter. The utilization of sphincter augmentation and the LINX® device is a straightforward, simple and low risk operation that eliminates esophageal reflux, preserving the multiple benefits offered by sleeve gastrectomy over gastric bypass procedures.

2   The Controversy of Gastroesophageal Reflux Following Sleeve Gastrectomy

Gastroesophageal reflux following sleeve gastrectomy is not unusual. As recently as 2014 the pathophysiology and anatomic changes exacerbating reflux was still poorly understood. Although the problem was well recognized, most patients reporting symptoms were treated rather successfully with simple PPI therapy. Asymptomatic GERD following sleeve gastrectomy for the most part was not treated. Studies exploring the association Between GERD and sleeve gastrectomy were small, single-center series and examined symptomatic reflux as only a secondary outcome measure. Resolution or control of reflux with PPI therapy typically eliminated reflux symptoms and did not result in secondary screening with esophageal endoscopy. Patients with asymptomatic reflux were not the subject of further investigation. These early small studies stimulated significant debate regarding the significance of GERD following sleeve gastrectomy and whether the problem was more widespread. The question as to whether reflux documented prior to sleeve gastrectomy should be considered a contraindication for patients considering sleeve gastrectomy has been an ongoing source of discussion.

The 2017 publication by Genco reporting their findings that erosive esophagitis and Barrett's esophagus following sleeve gastrectomy was significantly higher than what had been reported in the most current literature ignited an intense debate on the issue of the relationship of GERD and sleeve gastrectomy [6]. To further complicate the debate, severe reflux that is resistant to medical treatment has become the leading cause for reoperation following sleeve gastrectomy. The most common operation for this problem has become the conversion of sleeve gastrectomy to RYGB. This approach leads to a permanent destruction of the sleeve gastrectomy and the benefits of sleeve gastrectomy are forever lost [4, 5]. Genco's 2017 report redirected scrutiny toward the relationship between sleeve gastrectomy and GERD and in particular the possible contribution sleeve gastrectomy related reflux might have on any progression towards Barrett's esophagus. The renewed controversy generated by the Genco paper came shortly after The Fifth International Consensus Conference for Sleeve Gastrectomy concluded that there was still no consensus among expert surgeons regarding the absolute contraindication of GERD prior to sleeve gastrectomy [2].

GERD is still the primary risk factor for Barret's Esophagus. Despite the debate surrounding sleeve gastrectomy and postoperative GERD, the practice of routine pre- and postoperative endoscopic screening for esophagitis and BE is also very varied between practices. There is no standardization as to how to perform the sleeve gastrectomy and as a result surgical technique and outcomes vary tremendously. The tremendous differences between surgical technique and the ensuing results and outcome regarding postoperative GERD are also unknown. Although patients are consented for the risk of GERD following sleeve gastrectomy, there is no standard of care or consensus agreement as to the informed consent requirements regarding the risks of progressive esophagitis following sleeve gastrectomy or Barrett's esophagitis in particular. The relative lack of case reports demonstrating progression of Barrett's esophagus to adenocarcinoma following sleeve gastrectomy contribute to the poor understanding regarding long term complications following sleeve gastrectomy. Despite two decades of performing sleeve gastrectomy, variations in surgical technique and the effect these variations may play in the incidence of reflux and are still yet to be determined [7].

As the current popularity of sleeve gastrectomy continues to increase, the major drawback and controversy associated with this operation will continue to be the potential development or worsening of gastroesophageal reflux disease postoperatively. It is well established that the Achilles heel of sleeve gastrectomy is the ongoing confirmation in publications reporting that sleeve gastrectomy can worsen preexisting, or cause "de novo" GERD [6–8]. There is also a widespread variation and discrepancy in preoperative criteria with some centers not offering SG to those with GERD and some who do. If sleeve gastrectomy leads to worsening GERD in a subset of patients, there may be severe unintended consequences for patient outcomes and implications for long-term GERD-related complications in those individuals. This chapter explores the proper preoperative evaluation and management and technique when utilizing Magnetic sphincter augmentation with the LINX® device in eliminating reflux either preoperatively or postoperatively in appropriate patients considering and undergoing sleeve gastrectomy.

3   The Anatomic Susceptibility for Reflux After Sleeve Gastrectomy

The physiologic advantage magnetic sphincter augmentation provides when addressing post-operative reflux following sleep gastrectomy is based on the work by Korn and Stein and their 1997 model of lower esophageal sphincter function [8]. The lower esophageal sphincter is not constructed with an annular muscular ring typical in classical sphincter anatomy but rather between perpendicularly located muscular bands. In the human gastroesophageal junction two distinct anatomic structures exist creating a complimentary set of forces that create a functional sphincter. Along the lesser curve side is a looping set of muscular fibers, the clasp fibers, and opposite these fibers are a long set of oblique positioned sling fibers (Fig. 1). The intersection and arrangement of these fibers create the high pressure zone of the lower esophagus that can be measure manometrically. The location and integrity of these fibers is crucial to maintaining a functional lower esophageal sphincter. In order for the sphincter to remain closed both sets of muscular fibers must be in contact with each other and not disrupted.

Removal of the greater curvature such as occurs with sleeve gastrectomy, occurs in close proximity to the angle of His and the location of the greater curvature sling fibers. By removing and resecting the greater curvature in this manner, the contact and strength of the looped esophageal sphincter mechanism and sling fibers is disrupted (Fig. 2).

It has been reported that almost 45% of obese patients suffer from gastroesophageal reflux disease [9]. The association between gastroesophageal reflux disease and morbid obesity is not well understood however an increased incidence of hiatal hernia resulting in dilation of the gastric cardia can also interfere with the clasp and sling fibers discussed by Korn. In addition, esophageal dysfunction is reported and described in as high as 60% of patients with obesity [10].

Csendes, et al. reported that reflux symptoms are common in bariatric surgery patients with 79% presenting with heartburn and 66% with regurgitation following sleeve gastrectomy. Shauer, et al. reported that the incidence of GERD is as high as 50–100% in patients with severe esophagitis submitted for gastric bypass.

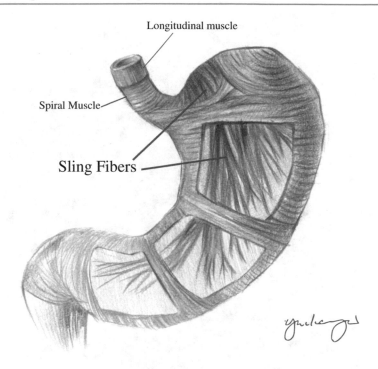

Fig. 1 Orientation of the Sling fibers of the gastroesophageal junction creates a unique anti-reflux valve mechanism that can be disrupted following sleeve gastrectomy

Laparoscopic sleeve gastrectomy is a well accepted surgical treatment for obesity and utilizes staplers to resect the greater curvature, effectively removing the entire fundus through the gastric cardia just lateral to the esophagus. By transecting through the angle of His near the esophago- gastric junction a critical modification of the anatomy occurs. The sling fibers are partially transected and certainly reduced in numbers. In converting to a straight tubular segment, long term reflux producing damage can occur simply by cutting through and partially damaging the sling fibers. The sling fibers as a result are misaligned and the sphincter loses its proper contact and strength. This has been demonstrated to create an imbalance of the lower esophageal sphincter mechanism between the sling fibers and clasp fibers. The efficiency and natural balance between the sling fibers and clasp fibers is disrupted and an incompetent lower esophageal sphincter is the clinical result in many cases.

Braghetto et al. in 2010 demonstrated the manometric changes of the lower esophageal sphincterafter sleeve gastrectomy in obese patients [11]. In his prospective study of 20 sleeve gastrectomy patients, all had a normal total and abdominal length before sleeve gastrectomy however following sleeve gastrectomy the abdominal length and total length of the high pressure zone at the esophagogastric junction (EGJ) were adversely affected. Six patients had normal

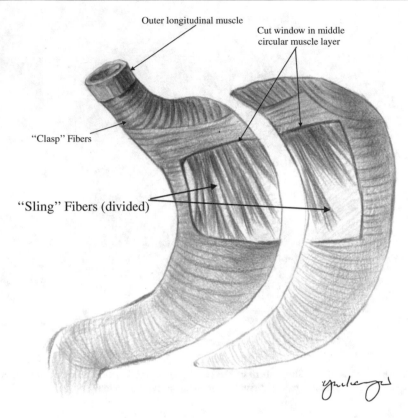

Outer longitudinal muscle

Cut window in middle
circular muscle layer

"Clasp" Fibers

"Sling" Fibers (divided)

Fig. 2 Orientation of the Sling fibers of the gastroesophageal junction creates a unique anti-reflux valve mechanism that can be disrupted following sleeve gastrectomy

total and abdominal LES length (total length > 3.5 and abdominal length > 1 cm). With regards to the other 14 patients, five patients had total length = 3.5 cm but an abdominal length < 1 cm and nine patients had a total < 3.5 cm and an abdominal length equal to 0.5 cm. Resting LES pressures in the cohort decreased significantly before, and six months after sleeve gastrectomy. More investigation into the mechanism of action causing these changes is needed since at least a partial resection of the sling fibers can occur when performing a transection near the angle of His during a sleeve gastrectomy. It is hypothesized that this partial resection results in an imbalance between the lateral and longitudinal forces necessary to sustain a competent lower esophageal sphincter.

The most important barriers that protect the esophagus from reflux is the Lower Esophageal Sphincter (LES) (Fig. 3). There is sufficient evidence to demonstrate that the LES is modified when a sleeve gastrectomy is performed. Division of the sling fibers and provoking a decrease in the LES resting pressure, as shown

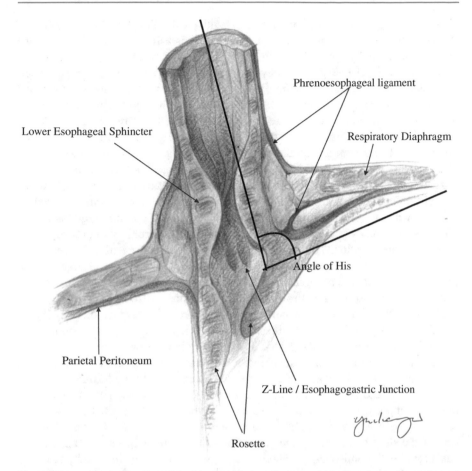

Fig. 3 The anatomic location of the Linx device in order to position it at the gastroesophageal junction overlying the lower esophageal sphincter. Dissection will require a 360° dissection and takedown of the phrenoesophageal ligament and mobilization of the lower esophageal sphincter into the abdomen

by Braghetto's group may very well be the critical change affecting reflux [12]. Manometric changes occurring in the LES after sleeve gastrectomy demonstrates the physiologic change. Braghetto's study revealed a mean LES resting pressure (LESRP) decreasing significantly after SG from 14.2 ± 5.8 to 10.5 ± 6.06 mmHg ($P = 0.01$). Fifteen percent of patients maintained normal lower esophageal resting pressure (23.1 ± 3.7 mmHg) while 85% were hypotensive producing a mean resting pressure of only 8.3 ± 2.6 mmHg. After sleeve gastrectomy, the length of the high-pressure zone of the LES was also critically affected. 45% of patients now had a shortened total LES length (shorter than 3.5 cm) and 70% of patients now had an abdominal length less than 1 cm [11]. The presence of increased GERD, clear endoscopic evidence of erosive esophagitis, and dilatation of the gastric cardia was also observed after sleeve gastrectomy increasing the likelihood that the changes affecting LES function contributed to the outcome [12].

Laparoscopic sleeve gastrectomy has been accepted as an option for surgical treatment for obesity. It should come as no surprise that a large percentage of patients undergoing sleeve gastrectomy will develop both symptomatic and asymptomatic reflux. Sleeve gastrectomy modifies the anatomy of the esophagogastric junction in a significant way. The decrease in gastric luminal volume, by converting it to a straight tubular segment and partially transecting some of the sling fibers, contributes to a dysfunctional esophageal sphincter mechanism. Magnetic Sphincter Augmentation, rather than revision to gastric bypass, restores the physiologic function of the LES and addresses the mechanism of reflux directly without subjecting the patient to additional risks commonly associated with gastric bypass operations. Revision from sleeve gastrectomy to gastric bypass eliminates the function, physiology and nutritional advantage of the sleeve gastrectomy in a nearly irreversible way. Conversion from a sleeve gastrectomy to gastric bypass because of an incompetent LES results in limited treatment options should complications arise. Problems that are unique to Roux Y Gastric bypass such as carbohydrate intolerance, dumping syndrome, marginal ulceration and reactive hypoglycemia have significantly reduced therapeutic options should they occur as a complication of the gastric bypass operation following conversion.

The human gastroesophageal sphincter maintains it critical function due to the arrangement and architecture of the muscular"clasp" and "sling" fibers surrounding the gastroesophageal junction and gastric cardia. Sleeve gastrectomy produces an important decrease in LES pressure, which can promote the appearance of reflux symptoms and esophagitis after the operation due to the partial resection of the sling fibers during the gastrectomy. Magnetic Sphincter Augmentation can preserve the anti-obesity benefits of sleeve gastrectomy in a safe, effective and reproducible way and at the same time eliminate pathologic reflux despite the alterations in LES function which occur following sleeve gastrectomy.

4   Magnetic Sphincter Augmentation and Resolution of GERD Following Sleeve Gastrectomy

The LINX® is the only Magnetic Sphincter Augmentation device commercially available and approved for use in the treatment of reflux disease. The LINX® procedure requires minimal surgical dissection and introduces a standardized procedure for patients with significant medically recalcitrant GERD. Clinical trials have shown that augmentation of the lower esophageal sphincter is effective in decreasing esophageal acid exposure resulting in reduced symptoms and eliminating or significantly reducing daily PPI dependence. Safety concerns typically arise with questions regarding device erosions and migrations have proven to be rare and can be resolved with device explantation. These uncommon events have not been associated with any device related mortality and in the event they occur do not eliminate conversion to gastric bypass as a final option for treatment.

The concept is simple as the mechanical device is designed to augment the physiologic barrier to reflux created by the clasp and sling fibers of the lower esophageal sphincter (LES). This is accomplished through the use of magnetic force. The LINX® is particularly suitable to augmenting the injured lower esophageal sphincter by adding a circular mechanism of action to the clasp and oblique sling fibers which currently make up the physiology of the sphincter (Fig. 4). In order to function as a relaxing and constricting augmentation of the natural LES, the LINX® is designed based on a series of biocompatible titanium beads with magnetic cores hermetically sealed inside. The beads are connected individually with independent titanium wires which allow the ring to be both flexible and expandable. In its resting, relaxed position, each bead is in contact with adjacent beads via the individual magnetic cores. The beads can move independent of the adjacent beads, creating an adjustable ring that does not compress the esophagus. The range of motion complements the natural oblique and lateral fibers of the LES by adding a third circumferential ring created by the LINX®. The LINX® is therefore able to accommodate a wide array of physiologic situations including swallowing, belching, and vomiting. For reflux to occur, the intragastric pressure must overcome the resistance to opening of both the patient's native LES pressure and the magnetic bonds of the device.

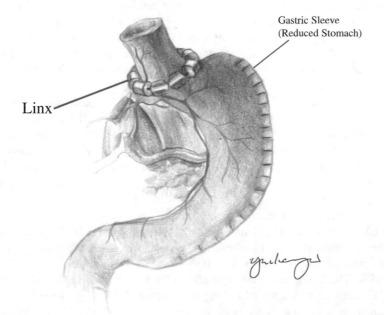

Fig. 4 Final location of the Linx device following sleeve gastrectomy for severe post operative gastroesophageal reflux disease

Once implanted the device becomes encapsulated in fibrous tissue but remains separated from and not incorporated into the esophagus itself. It remains a distinct and separate implant. The LINX® can be explanted by releasing the fibrous capsule overlying each bead.

Utilization of Magnetic Sphincter Augmentation as a treatment for severe reflux following sleeve gastrectomy was reported by Hawasli in 2016 [13]. In addition Desart and Ben David reported the first case series of seven patients having undergone anti reflux therapy using the LINX® system in 2015 [14]. These early reports had greatly improved gastroesophageal reflux symptoms 2–4 weeks following implantation of the device. Significant and successful improvement in the severity and frequency of their reflux, regurgitation, epigastric pain, fullness, dysphagia, and cough symptoms was uniformly reported postoperatively compared to their initial preoperative evaluation. There were no reported perioperative complications and Magnetic Sphincter Augmentation appeared to be a safe and effective option for the treatment of severe reflux following sleeve gastrectomy.

5   Operative Concerns and Patient Selection

Fear of device erosion is the primary concern voiced by surgeons preferring conversion to Roux Y gastric bypass over magnetic sphincter augmentation in patients with severe intractable reflux. Most surgeons today have had no experience with the Angelchik device however it is commonly discussed as a historical reference for concern regarding safety of gastroesophageal devices. More recently, adjustable gastric banding which was widely used as an a minimally invasive weight loss device, is cited as another example demonstrating adverse outcomes and device erosions when placing implantable devices at the gastric cardia near the gastroesophageal junction.

Device erosion in adjustable gastric banding is a commonly experienced complication of the device. Occurring primarily in the first 18 months following implantation, the complication was a significant issue, often leaving the lower esophagus and proximal stomach with a significant inflammatory reaction There was typically a perforation that required repair and as a result subsequent bariatric operations were more difficult and at times challenging. In contrast however, esophageal erosion following magnetic sphincter augmentation with the LINX® device has remained a relatively uncommon and rare occurrence. The safety profile of LINX® was studied in a multicenter review of the first 1000 implants which had been performed at multiple hospitals around the world. This study included the 82 hospitals involved in the first 1000 device implants. The readmission rate was 1.3%. There was a 3.4% reoperation rate and a 5.6% endoscopic dilation rate [15]. Erosion was reported in only one patient (0.1%). All reoperations were performed on a non-emergent basis for device removal and 36 patients underwent device removal. The most common symptoms requiring device removal was dysphagia and recurrence of reflux symptoms. Another recent study focusing on reoperations following LINX® reported a median follow-up of 48 months and a device removal rate of 6.7%. 11 of 164 patients who underwent a laparoscopic LINX® implant were explanted at a later date. Of the main presenting symptom requiring device removal was regurgitation or heartburn in 46%, dysphagia in 37%, and chest pain in 18%. Only two patients (1.2%) developed a full-thickness erosion of the esophageal wall with partial endoluminal penetration of the device [16]. Device explant occurred at 12–24 months after initial implant in 82% of the patients that required explant.

Bonevina, et al. reported 6 year follow up on 100 patients who had undergone implantation of a LINX® device for treatment of GERD. There were no reported device erosions or migrations in the study group [17]. Several additional series have reported various erosion rates as a low occurance. Alicuban, et al. published a 2018 review of the worldwide experience of device erosion following magnetic sphincter augmentation [18]. Their review of all devices placed worldwide from February 2007 to July 2017 included 9453 devices identified in the manufacturers database. In a total of 9453 device implants, only 29 reported cases of erosion were discovered. The risk of erosion was determined to be 0.3% at four years after implantation. Explantation was commonly done via a combined endoscopic followed by a delayed laparoscopic removal. At 58 days post removal there were no complications. Of the 29 patients, 24 patients had returned to baseline and four patients reported mild persistent dysphagia.

Erosion following magnetic sphincter augmentation is a relatively rare occurrence. The device is designed to be implanted after careful measurement using a calibration tool. Devices that are more commonly associated with erosion were small 12 bead devices which were found to have a 4.93% erosion rate. Our own series of utilization of the LINX® device for treatment of severe reflux following sleeve has limited use to devices with 15 or 17 beads with no erosion over the past three years. Alicuban identified that most patients with erosions presented between 1 and 4 years after device implantation. Only a very few patients presented with erosions within the first year following implantation. 26 months was the median time to erosion in the review. The most common presenting symptom was dysphagia in 26 patients (90%) followed by chest pain in 7 patients. Reflux, cough, vomiting and weight loss were other, less common symptoms. At 1 year after implantation The risk of erosion was 0.05% increasing to 0.3% at 4 years post implantation.

Risk factors for developing erosion have been discussed and identification of these risk factors may lead to a lower erosion rate in patients following sleeve gastrectomy. Device size mismatch appears to be the most common risk factor which is easily modified to decrease the risk following implantation. Smaller devices are more commonly associated with the development of erosions. The LINX® device was available in sizes ranging from 11 to 17 beads. Our most commonly implanted size for treatment of reflux following sleeve gastrectomy is evenly divided between 15 beads and 17 bead sizes. Alibuban identified in their review of over 9000 implanted devices that the centers with the highest utilization of smaller devices also reported the highest erosion rates of 4–20 times other centers. Larger sized devices appear to have similar efficacy in obtaining reflux control as smaller devices with a lower reported rate of erosion [18]. The 12 bead device was responsible for 62% of erosions and is no longer available commercially.

It is important to utilize proper technique when determining device size. To obtain the optimal size, we recommend the technique popularized by Lipham. There are two visual cues which improve proper device selection. A specific sizing device is positioned around the esophagus prior to device selection. The sizer is specifically designed to encircle the esophagus and locks gently with a magnetic link to itself. When the device rests comfortably around the esophagus and when no compression is noted the surgeon then ratchets the sizer down until it releases itself from its magnetic link. The size of the release is noted and two sizes above this release size number is the appropriate size for device choice. The two sizes are compared from these two visual evaluations and if there is a discrepancy the larger of the two sizes is selected.

Surgical technique may also play a significant role in the avoiding or development of erosion following LINX® implantation. Early operative technique supported a minimal esophageal dissection, however, current operative technique favors a full hiatal dissection. Better exposure of the distal esophagus and proximal stomach allows complete evaluation of the crura, improved and more accurate crural repair can be achieved, reduction of any hiatal hernia and avoidance of injury to the posterior esophageal wall.

Patient specific risk factors may also play a role including conditions contributing to tissue weakening and breakdown. Connective tissue disorders, steroid use, poorly controlled diabetes, and immunosuppression are all conditions that must be considered prior to any decision for sphincter augmentation.

6   Preoperative Evaluation

Patients with significant reflux following sleeve gastrectomy are candidates for magnetic sphincter augmentation and preservation of the benefits of sleeve gastrectomy. Evaluation for possible sphincter augmentation device placement is straightforward. Diagnostic testing is recommended for patients with GERD [19]. Essential preoperative testing prior to LINX® placement includes esophagogastroduodenoscopy (EGD), ambulatory pH monitoring, esophageal high-resolution manometry, and esophagram [19, 20]. Each testing modality has a specific role in the clinical evaluation and appropriateness of possible magnetic sphincter augmentation. No single test alone can substitute for the overall clinical appropriateness of device placement in any single patient [21].

Evaluation of individual anatomy, motility and evidence of GERD must be defined in each individual patient preoperatively. As outlined above each initial evaluation includes upper GI swallow (esophagram) in order to elicit radiographic evidence of reflux. In addition, this study is essential to evaluate the gastric sleeve for signs of proximal dilation, narrowing or obstruction of the angularis incisura, kinking, twisting or other evidence of a mechanical etiology possibly contributing to reflux. Comparison of this study to any previously obtained postoperative studies is useful to determine if significant changes are present from studies done early after surgery. Patients with evidence of mechanical obstruction are not good candidates for magnetic sphincter augmentation with the LINX® device.

Preoperative esophagoduodenoscopy is essential and performed in all patients. Esophagodudenoscopy, preferentially by the operating surgeon, is needed to evaluate the severity of any esophagitis. Biopsy to evaluate for helicobacter pylori is done at the time of EGD as well as biopsy of the gastroesophageal junction to evaluate for possible Barrett's changes. EGD can assess the Los Angeles classification for severity of reflux and visualize the extent to which any bile reflux is occurring. Preoperative treatment of severe esophagitis can be initiated. Once the assessment by EGD and upper GI swallow is complete, and if the patient appears appropriate for further evaluation, an esophageal manometry study is arranged. A BRAVO pH study can be ordered but in many patients this can be reserved for cases where the presence of GERD is only reported by history or is still unclear.

7   Esophageal High-resolution Manometry

In addition to upper endoscopy and esophageal pH testing, a preoperative evaluation should include high resolution manometry. Normal esophageal motility is essential in avoiding post-operative dysphagia following magnetic sphincter augmentation. Post-operative dysphagia is the most common cause for device explantation in patients undergoing MSA. Evaluation of the quality of esophageal function via manometry testing is the only modality available to determine if esophageal motility meets the minimum criteria for a good outcome following device placement [20, 22]. Esophageal transnasal high resolution manometry measures the pressure in the upper and lower esophageal sphincters, measures the effectiveness and coordination of peristalsis, and detects abnormal contractions. Differentiation between pure GERD and other esophageal motility disorders can be accomplished via high resolution manometry and can be used to evaluate and exclude esophageal motility disorders such as achalasia, esophageal spasm, and lower esophageal sphincter hypotension and hypertension [20].

8   Surgical Technique

Surgical technique utilizes the same positioning and trocar placement as with sleeve gastrectomy. The patient can be positioned either supine or in the French position. Generally, there are four trocars and a fifth incision for placement of a retractor to expose the hiatus. Meticulous lysis of adhesions is done to expose the esophagus, the hiatus of the diaphragm and the gastric body.

The critical steps in the exposure of the distal esophagus are as follows.

a. Complete exposure of the right crus, the left crus and division of the phrenoe-sophageal ligament.
b. Reduction of any hiatal hernia and distalization of the esophagus to decrease the chance of recurrence.
c. Identification of the posterior vagus nerve.
d. Removal of all tubes/bougies from the esophagus and release and retraction like penrose drains to avoid stretching the esophagus. The esophagus must be in the resting state.
e. Placement of the LINX® system sizer between the posterior vagus nerve and the esophagus.
f. Repeat the measurement using the LINX® system sizer multiple times to confirm size and accuracy and prevent placement of the wrong size device.
g. The LINX® device is then selected and introduced into the abdomen.
h. The LINX® is placed around the esophagus but anterior to the posterior vagus nerve (between the esophagus and nerve).
i. The LINX® system is magnetically locked into place.
j. Repair and re approximation of the posterior crural defect is completed.

Our technique is described in the following paragraphs with corresponding images to clarify the technique. The first step after dissection and exposure of the upper foregut and positioning of appropriate liver retraction is division of the gastrohepatic ligament and visualization of the right crus (Figs. 5 and 6). The right crus is carefully dissected to preserve the fascial integrity overlying the crus while gaining entry into the mediastinum (Figs. 7 and 8). The dissection is carried anteriorly to allow division of the peritoneum on the anterior surface of the gastroesophageal junction below the insertion of the phrenoesophageal ligament (Fig. 9). A wide exposure of the esophageal hiatus is performed to maximize exposure in order to insure against injury to the esophageal structure which can occur when trying to utilize a minimal dissection approach (Figs. 10 and 11).

The lateral surface of the left crus is freed from any scar or retained fundus which has occurred as a result of previous dissection at the angle of His. Complete exposure of the posterior confluence of the right and left crus is accomplished.

Fig. 5 Initial dissection and release of the liver from residual adhesions from previous sleeve gastrectomy

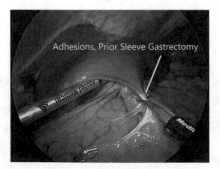

Fig. 6 Initial dissection is to define the right crus, releasing it from previous scar

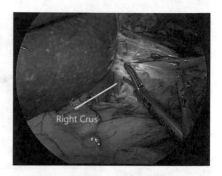

Fig. 7 Dissection of the right crus and takedown of the phrenoesophageal ligament and exposure of previous crural repair sutures in order to perform a complete 360° dissection of the gastroesophageal junction

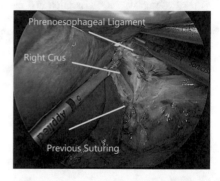

Fig. 8 Removal of all previous crural repair sutures to expose the posterior retro-esophageal space and the posterior vagus nerve

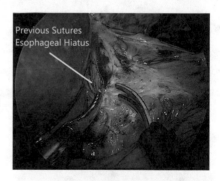

Fig. 9 Complete dissection of the angle of His and release of the esophagus ateriorly

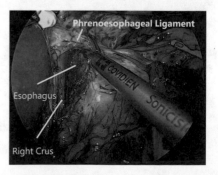

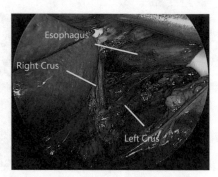

Fig. 10 Complete 360° dissection and retraction of the esophagus using a penrose drain will avoid injury to the esophagus and facilitate exposure of the posterior vagus nerve which must be dissected to create a path for the sphincter augmentation device between the esophagus and the vagus neve at the gastroesophageal junction

Fig. 11 Completed 360° dissection

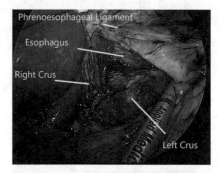

Fig. 12 Posterior vagus nerve exposed

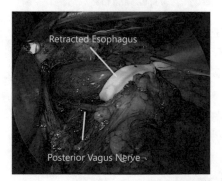

Preparation of the retroesophageal window is completed to facilitate placement of a penrose drain. The penrose drain is used for retraction of the gastric cardia in order to maximize exposure while dissecting the distal esophagus and crural structures. Once the dissection is complete the identification of the posterior vagus nerve can proceed (Fig. 12).

Fig. 13 Completing dissection of the posterior vagus nerve as close to the gastroesophageal junction as possible. The sphincter augmentation device will be positioned in the path between the posterior vagus nerve and the esophagus

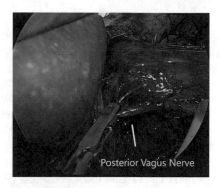

Posterior Vagus Nerve

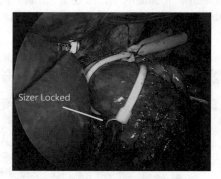

Sizer Locked

Fig. 14 Proper positioning of the sizing guide is essential. The sizing device is positioned as far distal as possible against the gastroesophageal junction. Selecting the proper size is done by allowing the magnetic lock to secure in place on the sizing guide and then gently ratcheting the sizing guide closed until the magnetic lock spontaneously releases itself

The gastrohepatic ligament was previously opened above and below the hepatic branch to facilitate the preparation of the retroesophageal window is extended as necessary. A penrose drain can be passed if necessary to improve exposure and dissection using the drain as a retractor (Fig. 13).

Gentle dissection from the right side is made toward the left crus just above the crural decussation to identify the posterior vagus nerve.

A tunnel is then created between the vagus and the posterior esophageal wall, and the Penrose drain is repositioned and passed in a left-to-right direction.

The circumference of the esophagus is measured to determine the proper size of the LINX® device to be implanted. The sizing tool is a laparoscopic instrument with a soft, circular curved tip actuated by the surgeon using the handset on the instrument (Fig. 14). The handset contains a number that changes as the instrument is ratcheted down onto the esophagus. The number corresponds to the size range of the LINX® device. The sizing tool is placed around the esophagus in the dissected space between the esophageal wall and the posterior vagus nerve bundle (Fig. 15). As it is tightened it will spontaneously release allowing the surgeon to see the corresponding number associated with the point of release. The surgeon adds "2" to the number indicated to determine the appropriate device size (Fig. 16).

Once the appropriate LINX® device has been selected, it is introduced through the posterior tunnel and positioned between the esophagus and the posterior vegus nerve (Fig. 17). The opposing ends are then brought to the anterior surface of the esophagus and connected together by engaging the two clasps (Figs. 18, 19, 20 and 21).

The decision to proceed with a posterior crural repair depends on the size of the hernia that is found intraoperatively (Fig. 22). Operative time is generally less than 1 hour. Patients are discharged the same day of surgery or on the first postoperative day and are counseled to gradually return to a normal diet and to discontinue use of acid suppression medication (Figs. 23, 24, 25 and 26).

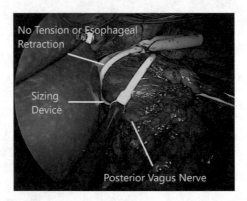

Fig. 15 It is essential to release any esophageal retraction and preform the sizing test under a zero tension, relaxed esophagus. Once the sizing guide releases itself from the magnetic lock the surgeon examines the guide to determine the proper size of the Linx device. In this example the sizing guide released at "15". The proper size Linx device would be to add "2" to the measured size which would indicate a size "17" device would be the proper device to choose

Fig. 16 Sizing device size

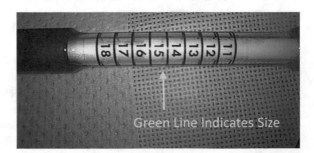

Fig. 17 Positioning of the
Linx device between the
posterior vagus nerve and
the esophagus at the gastro
esophageal junction

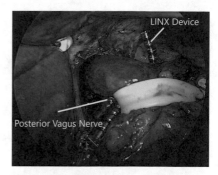

Fig. 18 Locking the Linx
device in place using two
locking sutures attached to
the device. I properly locked
device will resist opening and
will sit in a relaxed position
on the distal esophagus

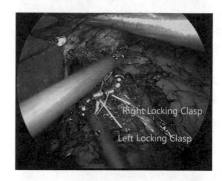

Fig. 19 Proper orientation of
the Linx device in place

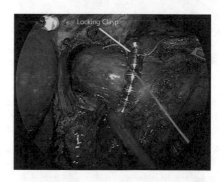

Fig. 20 The device is relaxed
and there is only gentle
compression on the lower
esophageal sphincter

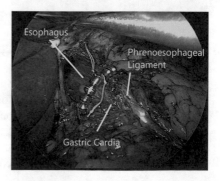

Fig. 21 The device should not appear tight when in the proper position and should rest at the gastroesophageal junction on the distal most position of the esophagus

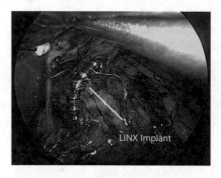

Fig. 22 Final completed positioning of the Linx device. The Linx passes between the posterior vagus nerve and the esophagus. The posterior crural defect has been closed and there is no tension on the esophagus at the site of the implant

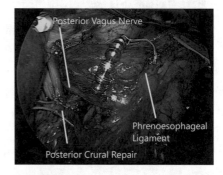

Fig. 23 Completed implantation of a Linx sphincter augmentation device at the lower esophageal junction following sleeve gastrectomy

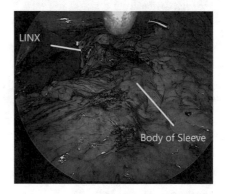

9   Discussion

The controversy of worsening reflux following post sleeve gastrectomy and GERD is now well established [23]. Development of new-onset GERD following LSG is observed in as many as 8.6–22% of patients [24, 25]. The increasing rate of reflux following sleeve gastrectomy is alarming and some authors have reported unacceptable and high rates of reflux related transition to Barrett's esophagus.

Fig. 24 The proper position and appearance of a Linx device following implantation after sleeve gastrectomy

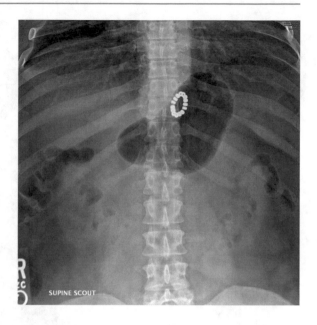

The LINX® gained FDA approval in 2012. Magnetic sphincter augmentation is now an important option to consider among patients who have undergone sleeve gastrectomy who subsequently develop severe and pathologic reflux disease. The division and injury of sling fibers comprising the major anti reflux mechanism at the gastroesophageal junction result in anatomic changes that are not favorable for performing a Nissen or Toupet fundoplication. As a result, fundoplication following sleeve gastrectomy is nearly impossible to perform due to the limited amount of fundus tissue remaining. Implantation of a LINX® device occurs at the gastroesophageal junction, through tissue and operative planes that are typically undisturbed during sleeve gastrectomy. This may be a more favorable less complicated approach to the problem of post sleeve gastrectomy reflux than the current recommendation of conversion to gastric bypass.

Conversion to a gastric bypass following sleeve gastrectomy produces a reduction in acid exposure-related symptoms with high success rates but comes with the increased morbidity associated with revision surgery [26, 27]. The routine conversion of patients to Roux-Y gastric bypass creates an unnecessary risk of internal hernia, marginal ulceration, reactive hypoglycemia and other complications which are entirely avoidable with the implantation of a sphincter augmentation device. Surgical options that attempt to address the mechanism of postoperative reflux have historically been limited to the repair of a hiatal hernia as fundoplication is typically impossible after sleeve gastrectomy. Magnetic Sphincter augmentation can also be used in patients following sleeve gastrectomy with no clinical evidence of hiatal hernia or who do not desire conversion to a bypass procedure [28, 29]. Magnetic sphincter augmentation is an underutilized procedure and may be the most exciting and straightforward treatment option for the patient developing

Fig. 25 Proper location and positioning of Linx device on post operative barium swallow. There is a gentle narrowing at the gastroesophageal junction and no evidence of reflux following placement

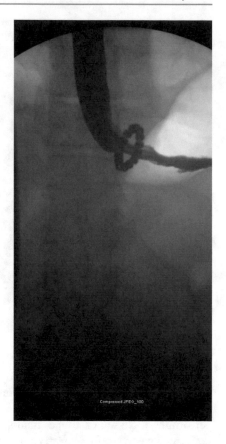

GERD after sleeve gastrectomy. MSA is the only procedure that restores LES function after sleeve gastrectomy. Roux Y gastric bypass does not create an anti reflux mechanism, rather it provides a drainage function that decreases reflux related incidents but does not nothing to improve or restore the antireflux function of the lower esophageal sphincter. Roux Y gastric bypass is well documented to have its own rate of postoperative GERD, does not restore LES function and is at best an unpredictable procedure for the treatment for reflux following sleeve gastrectomy.

There are now several series demonstrating improved outcomes following magnetic sphincter augmentation following sleeve gastrectomy. Device erosions and other complications following magnetic sphincter augmentation are rare and erosion rates of less than 0.5% are well established [30, 31]. Magnetic sphincter augmentation achieves at least 50% improvement in reflux related symptoms in patients undergoing implantation for routine reflux related symptoms and medical therapy can be discontinued in up to 90% of patients [24]. Magnetic sphincter augmentation after sleeve gastrectomy for GERD has the potential to be a less morbid solution with better short and long term outcomes for the difficult problem of reflux following sleeve gastrectomy. MSA is well tolerated and can be performed on an

Fig. 26 The contrast flows easily through the Linx device with no significant delay of contrast transiting through the device. There is no evidence of esophageal pooling or delay clearing the distal esophagus

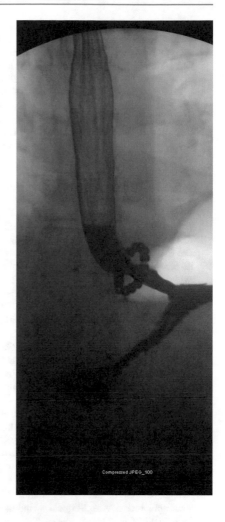

outpatient basis with immediate results. The risk of anastomotic leakage and post-operative staple line bleeding associated with conversion to Roux-Y gastric bypass is completely avoided. Magnetic sphincter augmentation is a safe and effective procedure with a low complication rate. MSA achieves complete restoration of LES function and is completely reversible should postoperative dysphagia result in difficult eating or discomfort [32, 33]. Conversion to Roux-Y gastric bypass can and should be preserved as a last resort option for the majority of successful sleeve gastrectomy patients who have developed post-operative reflux symptoms.

References

1. Higa KH, Welbourn J, Dixon R, et al. P. IFSO Global Registry Report. International Federation for the Surgery of Obesity and Metabolic Disorders. 2017.

2. Berger ER, Huffman KM, Fraker T, et al. Prevalence and risk factors for bariatric surgery readmissions: Findings from 130,007 admissions in the metabolic and bariatric surgery accreditation and quality improvement program. Ann Surg. 2018;267:122–31.
3. Gagner M, Hutchinson C, Rosenthal R. Fifth international consensus conference: current status of sleeve gastrectomy. Surg Obes Relat Dis. 2016;12:750–6.
4. Peterli R, Wölnerhanssen BK, Peters T, et al. Effect of laparoscopic sleeve gastrectomy vs laparoscopic Roux-en-Y gastric bypass on weight loss in patients with morbid obesity: the SM-BOSS randomized clinical trial. JAMA. 2018;319:255–65.
5. Salminen P, Helmio M, Ovaska J, et al. Effect of laparoscopic sleeve gastrectomy vs laparoscopic Roux-en-Y gastric bypass on weight loss at 5 years among patients with morbid obesity: the SLEEVEPASS randomized clinical trial. JAMA. 2018;319:241–54.
6. Genco A, Soricelli E, Casella G, et al. Gastroesophageal reflux disease and Barrett's esophagus after laparoscopic sleeve gastrectomy: a possible, underestimated long-term complication. Surg Obes Relat Dis. 2017;13:568–74.
7. Wright FG, Duro A, Medici JR, et al. Esophageal adenocarcinoma five years after laparoscopic sleeve gastrectomy. A case report. Int J Surg Case Rep. 2017;32:47–50.
8. Korn O, Stein H, Richter T, Liebermann-Meffert D. Gastroesophageal Sphincter, a Model. Dis Esophagus. 1997;10:105–9.
9. El-Serag H. The association between obesity and GERD: a review of the epidemiological evidence. Dig Dis Sci. 2008;53:2307–12.
10. Jaffin BW, Knoepflmacher P, Greenstein R. High prevalence of asymptomatic esophageal motility disorders among morbidly obese patients. Obes Surg. 1999;9:390–5.
11. Braghetto I, Lanzarini E, Korn O, et al. Manometric changes of the lower esophageal sphincter after sleeve gastrectomy in obese patients. Obes Surg. 2010;20(3):357–62.
12. Braghetto I, Csendes A, Korn O, et al. Gastroesophageal reflux disease after sleeve gastrectomy. Surg Laparosc Endosc Percutan Tech. 2010;20(3):148–53.
13. Hawasli A, Tarakji M, Tarboush M. Laparoscopic management of severe reflux after sleeve gastrectomy using the LINX®system: Technique and one year follow up case report. Int J Surg Case Rep. 2017;30:148–51.
14. Desart K, Rossidis G, Michel M. T Lux, Ben-David K, gastroesophageal reflux management with the LINX® system for gastroesophageal reflux disease following laparoscopic sleeve gastrectomy. J Gastrointest Surg. 2015;19(10):1782–6.
15. Lipham JC, Taiganides PA, Louie BE, Ganz RA, DeMeester TR. Safety analysis of first 1000 patients treated with magnetic sphincter augmentation for gastroesophageal reflux disease. Dis Esophagus. 2015;28:305–11.
16. Asti E, Siboni S, Lazzari V, Bonitta G, Sironi A, Bonavina L. Removal of the magnetic sphincter device. Surgical technique and results of a single-center cohort study. Ann Surg. 2017;265(5):941–5.
17. Bonavina L, Saino G, Bona D, Sironi A, Lazzari V. One hundred consecutive patients treated with magnetic sphincter augmentation for gastroesophageal reflux disease: 6 years of clinical experience from a single center. J Am Coll Surg. 2013;217(4):577–85.
18. Alicuben ET, Bell RCW, Jobe BA, Buckley FP 3rd, Daniel Smith C, Graybeal CJ, Lipham JC. Worldwide experience with erosion of the magnetic sphincter augmentation device. J Gastrointest Surg. 2018;22(8):1442–7.
19. Katz PO, Gerson LB, Vela MF. Guidelines for the diagnosis and management of gastroesophageal reflux disease. Am J Gastroenterol. 2013;108:308–28.
20. Kahrilas PJ, Shaheen NJ, Vaezi MF, Hiltz SW, Black E, Modlin IM, Johnson SP, Allen J, Brill JV; American Gastroenterological Association. American Gastroenterological Association Medical Position Statement on the management of gastroesophageal reflux disease. Gastroenterology. 2008;135:1383–91.
21. ASGE Standards of Practice Committee; Muthusamy VR, Lightdale JR, Acosta RD, Chandrasekhara V, Chathadi KV, Eloubeidi MA, Fanelli RD, Fonkalsrud L, Faulx AL, Khashab MA, Shaukat A, Wang A, Cash B, DeWitt JM. The role of endoscopy in the management of GERD. Gastrointest Endosc. 2015;81:1305–10.

22. Badillo R, Francis D. Diagnosis and treatment of gastroesophageal reflux disease. World J Gastrointest Pharmacol Ther. 2014;5:105–12.
23. Melissas J, Braghetto I, Molina JC, et al. Gastroesophageal reflux disease and sleeve gastrectomy. Obes Surg. 2015;25(12):2430–5.
24. Saino G, Bonavina L, Lipham JC, et al. Magnetic sphincter augmentation for gastroesophageal reflux at 5 years: final results of a pilot study show long-term acid reduction and symptom improvement. J Laparoendosc Adv Surg Tech A. 2015;25(10):787–92.
25. Howard DD, Caban AM, Cendan JC, Ben-David K. Gastroesophageal reflux after sleeve gastrectomy in morbidly obese patients. Surg Obes Relat Dis. 2011;7(6):709–13.
26. Altieri MS, Pryor AD. Gastroesophageal reflux disease after bariatric procedures. Surg Clin North Am. 2015;95(3):579–91.
27. Zhang L, Tan WH, Chang R, et al. Perioperative risk and complications of revisional bariatric surgery compared to primary Roux-en-Y gastric bypass. Surg Endosc. 2015;29(6):1316–20.
28. Soricelli E, Iossa A, Casella G, et al. Sleeve gastrectomy and crural repair in obese patients with gastroesophageal reflux disease and/or hiatal hernia. Surg Obes Relat Dis. 2013;9(3):356–61.
29. Chen RH, Lautz D, Gilbert RJ, et al. Antireflux operation for gastroesophageal reflux after Roux-en-y gastric bypass for obesity. Ann Thorac Surg. 2005;80(5):1938–40.
30. Ganz RA, Peters JH, Horgan S. Esophageal sphincter device for gastroesophageal reflux disease. N Engl J Med. 2013;368(21):2039–40.
31. Bauer M, Meining A, Kranzfelder M, Jell A, Schirren R, Wilhelm D, et al. Endoluminal perforation of a magnetic antireflux device. Surg Endosc. 2015;29(12):3806–10.
32. Parmar AD, Tessler RA, Chang HY, Svahn JD. Two-stage explantation of a magnetic lower esophageal sphincter augmentation device due to esophageal erosion. J Gastrointest Surg Laparoendosc Adv Surg Tech A. 2017;27(8):829–33.
33. Yeung BPM, Fullarton G. Endoscopic removal of an eroded magnetic sphincter augmentation device. Endoscopy. 2017;49(7):718.

Omentopexy in Laparoscopic Sleeve Gastrectomy

Mohanned-Al-Haddad

1   Background

Sleeve gastrectomy (SG) was first performed by Hess in 1988 as part of a as a component of the malabsorptive procedure, the biliopancreatic diversion with duodenal switch [1]. The promising results of SG in terms of weight loss and resolution of comorbidities as a first stage, combined with a low rate of complications, has encouraged the global emergence and monumentally rapid spread of SG as a standalone procedure. In 2009, the American Society for Metabolic and Bariatric Surgery (ASMBS) issued a position statement recommending laparoscopic sleeve gastrectomy (LSG) as a standalone bariatric procedure [2]. Currently, LSG and Roux-en-Y gastric bypass are the most commonly performed bariatric procedures in United States and Asia/Pacific regions [3]. However, despite having a comparatively lower morbidity rate among bariatric procedures, LSG has several postoperative complications, both acute and chronic. Moreover, the alteration of gastric anatomy, a loss of ligamentous fixation, and the progressive rotation of the stable line associated with this procedure are widely believed to be the reasons for the formation of a twisted or spiral stomach in a condition similar to organoaxial gastric volvulus [4]. The resulting functional narrowing, despite a fairly normal luminal diameter, has been linked with a wide range of postoperative gastrointestinal symptoms, such as nausea, vomiting, and gastroesophageal reflux disease (GERD). In response, the use of omentopexy during LSG is believed by many bariatric surgeons to play a major role in solving this problem [4], and this approach is used routinely in an attempt to regain the normal anatomic fixation of the new

Mohanned-Al-Haddad (✉)
Jaber Al-Ahmed Al-Sabah Hospital, Kuwait, Kuwait
e-mail: dr.moq8@hotmail.co.uk

greater curvature of the sleeved stomach to the gastrocolic and gastrosplenic ligaments.

2   Clinical Benefits of the Omentum

Various surgical specialties uses the omentum in their practices. Due to its intrinsic features, the omentum not only inhances the healing process in the setting of inflammation, it also has the ability to halt bleeding through direct pressure and acceleration of the formation of fibrin clots [5]. Considering these remarkable properties, surgeons are using the omentum to close perforations in the gastrointestinal tract and to reinforce gastrointestinal anastomosis. Also, it has been shown that the omentum has a role in heart repair following myocardial infarction because of its capability for angiogenesis and smooth muscle production [6]. In addition, a recent study concluded that laparoscopic placement of a peritoneal dialysis catheter using omentopexy minimise catheter obstruction and migration [7].

3   Omentopexy in Sleeve Gastrectomy

3.1   Definition

The neutral orientation of the stomach is maintained by four anchoring ligaments: gastrophrenic, gastrosplenic, gastrocolic, and gastrohepatic. Use of the omentum by omentopexyin LSG entails the suturing the free end of the greater omentum—the gastrocolic and gastrosplenic ligaments—to the gastric suture line on the new greater curvature of the sleeved stomach to resume its normal anatomic position in an effort to improve postoperative food tolerance, slow gastric emptying (GE), and reduce symptoms of GERD.

3.2   Operative Technique

The patient is positioned in the 30-degree reverse Trendelenburg position with legs abducted. A 5-port technique is used, including a 5-mm port inserted in the epigastrium for liver retraction, a 10-mm port inserted supraumbilicaly slightly to the left for the camera, a 12-mm right hypochondrial midclavicular port and a 15-mm left hypochondrial midclavicular port, and a 5-mm left anterior axillary line port for the assistant surgeon.

Once all the steps for LSG are completed, the integrity of the stable line is confirmed by the methylene blue test and hemostasis of the staple line is secured. Then the divided free edge of the omentum—the gastrocolic and gastrosplenic ligaments—is identified and sutured it to the stable line of the sleeved stomach in a continuous fashion. Using polydioxanone sutures (PDS) 2–0, the suturing starts

2 cm distal to gastroesophageal junction to the antrum, until approximately 2 cm proximal to the pylorus, leaving 1 cm distance between each suture line to avoid ischaemia.

4 Effect on Food Intolerance and Gastroesophageal Reflux Disease

Although the relationship between LSG and GERD is still a matter of discussion, several studies have correlated LSG with worsening GERD. In a study by De Groote et al. In which they performed a systemic review to compare various bariatric procedures and their effect on GERD, LSG was found to aggravate postoperative GERD [8]. Loss of efficacy of the antireflux barrier, twisting of the gastric remnant, decreased gastric compliance, and decreased lower esophageal sphincter pressure have all been suggested as possible factors associated with the development of postoperative GERD [9–13].

Various surgical techniques have been suggested to reduce the postoperative food intolerance and symptoms of GERD, most of which are proposed to minimise gastric malposition resulting from loss of ligmentous fixation. A study by Daes et al. demonstrated that the correct alignment of the gastric sleeve is maintained by equidistant stapling of the anterior and the posterior walls to prevent coiling [14]. However, asymmetrical staples leading to the formation of twisted sleeve is always a possibility, and therefore omentopexy of the gastric remnant is believed to counteract such a twist.

In 2015, the first randomised study ofomentopexyin LSG compared 2 patients groups (omentopexy vs. no-omentopexy) in terms of decreased postoperative food intolerance and gastrointestinal symptoms, and no significant difference was found between groups [15]. In contrast, growing evidence suggests that the impact of omentopexy on the reduction of postoperative gastrointestinal symptoms has been observed in many recent studies. A retrospective study by Arslan E et al. concluded that omentopexy can in fact reduce the incidence of gastric volvulus by reducing the gastric mobility and restoring the stomach back to its natural anatomic position [15]. Currently, the association of omentopexy in the reduction of food intolerance and GERD symptoms is still controversial, and increasing evidence supports the key role of this surgical technique on reducing the incidence of postoperative GERD.

5 Effect on Gastric Emptying

Unsurprisingly, small gastric volume is believed to be associated with rapid GE because of rapid gastric distension. Acceleration of GE for food and liquid following SG has been shown on scintigraphy [16, 17]., Fixation of the omentum to the new greater curvature of the stomach to restore the natural anatomic position has been observed to slow GE [15]. However, data are insufficient to support this claim. Therefore, in the opinion of these authors, further studies with strong evidence are still needed to substantiate the association of omentopexy with reduced GE.

6   Conclusion

Surgical technique is one of the main factors in the postoperative outcome of gastrointestinal symptoms. Reattaching the omentum to the new greater curvature of the sleeved stomach in an effort to restore the natural anatomic position is becoming increasingly popular among bariatric surgeons to address this issue. Although, the impact of omentopexy on food tolerance, GE, and GERD was observed in various studies, further randomised studies are needed to draw a definitive conclusion. Therefore, we recommend the use of omentopexy for select patients undergoing LSG who are at higher risk of developing gastric coiling or gastric twist as observed interoperatively.

References

1. Hess DS, Hess DW. Obes Surg. 1998;8:267–82.
2. Clinical Issues Committee of the American Society for Metabolic and Bariatric Surgery. Surg Obes Relat Dis. 2010; 6:1–5.
3. Peterli R, Borbély Y, Kern B, Gass M, Peters T, Thurnheer M,et al. Early results of the Swiss Multicentre Bypass orSleeve Study (SM-BOSS): a prospective randomized trialcomparing laparoscopic sleeve gastrectomy and Roux-en-Ygastric bypass. Ann Surg. 2013; 258:690–4; discussion 695.
4. Elbalshy MA, Fayed AM, Abdelshahid MA, Alkhateep YM. Role of staple line fixation during laparoscopic sleeve gastrectomy. Int Surg J. 2018 Jan; 5:156–61.
5. Campbell BG. Harnessing the healing properties of the omentum. ACVSc college science week: Washington State University; 2009.
6. Marino M, Snyder B. Two sides of the omentum. Lens: Vanderbilt Medical Center. 2007: A New Way of Looking at Science.
7. Cao W, Tu C, Jia T, Liu C, Zhang L, Zhao B, et al. Prophylactic laparoscopic omentopexy: a new technique for peritoneal dialysis catheter placement. Ren Fail. 2019;41:113–7.
8. De Groot NL, Burgerhart JS, Van De Meeberg PC, de Vries DR, Smout AJ, Siersema PD. Systematic review: the effects of conservative and surgical treatment for obesity on gastrooesophageal reflux disease. Aliment Pharmacol Ther. 2009; 30:1091–102.
9. Rosenthal RJ, Diaz AA, Arvidsson D, et al. International Sleeve gastrectomy expert panel consensus statement: best practice guidelines based on experience of > 12,000 cases. Surg Obes Relat Dis. 2012; 8:8–19.
10. Kleidi E, Theodorou D, Albanopoulos K, Menenakos E, Karvelis MA, Papailiou J, et al. The effect of laparoscopic sleeve gastrectomy on the antireflux mechanism: can it be minimized? Surg Endosc. 2013;27:4625–30.
11. Braghetto I, Lanzarini E, Korn O, Valladares H, Molina JC, Henriquez A. Manometric changes of the lower esophageal sphincter after sleeve gastrectomy in obese patients. Obes Surg. 2010;20:357–62.
12. Mandeville Y, Van Looveren R, Vancoillie PJ, Verbeke X, Vandendriessche K, Vuylsteke P, et al. Moderating the enthusiasm of sleeve gastrectomy: up to fifty percent of reflux

symptoms after ten years in a consecutive series of one hundred laparoscopic sleeve gastrectomies. Obes Surg. 2017;27:1797–803.

13. Filho AMM, Silva LB, Godoy ES, Falcão AM, de Quadros LG, Zotarelli Filho IJ, et al. Omentopexy in sleeve gastrectomy reduces early gastroesophageal reflux symptoms. Surg Laparosc Endosc Percutan.

14. Daes J, Jimenez ME, Said N, Daza JC, Dennis R. Laparoscopic sleeve gastrectomy: symptoms of gastroesophageal reflux can be reduced by changes in surgical technique. Obes Surg. 2012;22:1874–9.

15. Afaneh C, Costa R, Pomp A, Dakin G. A prospective randomized controlled trial assessing the efficacy of omentopexy during laparoscopic sleeve gastrectomy in reducing postoperative gastrointestinal symptoms. Surg Endosc. 2015;29:41–7.

16. Arslan E, Banli O, Sipahi M, et al. Effects and results of omentopexy during laparoscopic Sleeve Gastrectomy. Surg Laparosc Endosc Percutan Tech. 2018; 28(3):174–77.

17. Kandeel AA, Sarhan MD, Hegazy T, Mahmoud MM, Ali MH. Comparative assessment of gastric emptying in obese patients before and after laparoscopic sleeve gastrectomy using radionuclide scintigraphy. Nucl Med Commun. 2015;36:854–62.

18. Melissas J, Daskalakis M, Koukouraki S, Askoxylakis I, Metaxari M, Dimitriadis E, et al. Sleeve gastrectomy-a "food limiting" operation. Obes Surg. 2008;18:1251–6.

Sleeve Gastrectomy and Gallstones Disease

Hanan M. Alghamdi

1   Introduction

Obesity is an established risk factor for gallstone formation, furthermore, rapid weight loss increases the likelihood of developing gallbladder stone. Both risks contribute to biliary disease complications in bariatric surgery. Laparoscopic Sleeve Gastrectomy (SG) is the most common bariatric surgery performed worldwide, hence the increased gravity of any complication that may occur post operatively, moreover, the possible cumulative risk of biliary complications related to rapid weight loss [1]. However, there is relative scarcity of published data on SG and gallstones, with most of the research on this topic coming from the earlier bariatric procedures, namely gastric bypass and adjustable gastric band.

2   Obesity and the Risk of Gallstone

Obesity is a worldwide health problem which causes serious diseases including the risk of developing gallstone (Cholelithiasis risk) [2, 4]. The risk is more established in the female population than male patients, especially with higher body mass index (BMI) [5]. It has been proven that women with a BMI of 30 kg/m2 or more have at least double the risk as those of normal BMI for gallstone formation [6–12].

In a large cohort study that included nearly 90,000 women followed for a period of 8 years, it was able find that a significant increase in the incidence of

H. M. Alghamdi (✉)
HBP & Bariatric Surgeon, Imam Abdulrhman Bin Faisal University, Dammam, Saudi Arabia
e-mail: hmalghamdi@iau.edu.sa

gallstone disease was established with increasing BMI, particularly in women with a BMI of 30 kg/m2 or more, with an exponential increase in the incidence of gall-stones from a rate of 3.7 to 7.4 times with higher BMI in women as compared to women with normal BMI [12].

3   Rapid Weight Loss and the Risk of Gallstone

Strong evidence of an increased risk for gallstones among the obese came from clinical studies of individuals subjected to very low-calorie diets and having rapid weight loss with an estimated risk of 10–25% [13–17]. The rationale behind this is rapid mobilization of cholesterol from adipose tissue stores and excess cho-lesterol excretion from the liver leading to bile supersaturation with cholesterol. Furthermore, fasting has been associated with reduced gallbladder contractility, a sequala of dietary fat restriction, leading to gallbladder stasis and favoring gall-stone formation. In contrast, increasing the dietary fat by a small amount induces better gallbladder emptying and may reduce the risk of gallstone formation in patients undergoing rapid weight loss [18]. Fluctuation of BMI due to repeated dieting may also play an added role in gallstone formation [19, 20].

During follow-up, the Nurses' Health Study cohort found an increased risk of gallstone formation, with a 44% increase in women who lost 4 to 10 kg and a 94% increase in women who lost more than 10 kg, compared to those whose weight loss was less than 4 kg [12].

In the first U.S. National Health and Nutrition Examination Survey, a history of dieting (however unknown degree of weight loss) among women was associated with a raised incidence of hospitalization with gallstones during a 10 year follow-up (67%; P = 0.001) [21].

An association of gallstone disease and obesity in men has been more difficult to establish, probably due to the fact that gallstone disease is generally more rare in men. In an ultrasonographic study from Copenhagen County, Denmark, men with a history of more than one weight loss treatment (with weight loss of more than 5 kg) had a statistically significant increased prevalence of gallstone disease (11.0% compared with 5.2% in normal diet) [9].

4   Pathophysiology and Type of Gallstones Formation in Obesity

Cholesterol gallstones comprise 80% of all gallbladder stones in Western countries [22]. More specifically, obesity related gallstones are predominantly of the cho-lesterol type and are formed when there is a disproportion in substance compos-ing bile, partly due to the increase in the activity of 3-hydroxy-3-mthylglutaryl coenzyme A reductase (HMGCoA), leading to increased secretion of biliary cho-lesterol [23]. Generally, there are three physical conditions described that contrib-ute to the formation of cholesterol gallstones, however, they do not necessarily all exist at the same time [Table 1] [24, 25]. Cholesterol crystal formation (visible by microscopy) followed by sludge formation (visible by gallbladder ultrasonography) are thought to be necessary precursors for cholesterol gallstone formation. Gallbladder hypomotility is measured by increased fasting volume, decreased ejection fraction, and increased contracted volume [27–29].

Several prenucleation and antinucleating proteins (mechanism 2), perhaps derivatives of gallbladder mucin, have been implicated as kinetic factors. Interestingly, Gustafsson et al. found that, by obtaining gallbladder bile during bariatric surgery and percutaneous aspiration postoperatively after weight loss, crystallization promoting compound like "Mucin" are of great importance in the development of cholesterol Crystals. Patients are therefore transiently at risk for gallbladder stones during the active weight reduction phase, which usually consists of the first 6–12 months, after which the risk diminishes after 2 years [30].

5 Incidence of Cholecystectomy in Sleeve Gastrectomy

Routine bariatric surgery is generally associated with a low frequency of postoperative cholecystectomy, however, it is highest early after surgery and is mainly determined by the amount of excess weight loss within the first 3 months. As a sequalae, several studies discouraged routine prophylactic cholecystectomy at the time of bariatric surgery in asymptomatic patients [31].

In the largest retrospective series to date, with a 5 year follow-up period, Altieri et al. found that cholecystectomy was required postoperatively, most prominently following LSG in 167 (10.1%) of 1650 patients, with lower numbers seen following RYGB (Roux-en-Y Gastric Bypass) making up 1931 (9.7%) patients out of 19,996, as well as LAGB (laparoscopic adjustable Gastric Band) compromising 989 (6.5%) patients from 15,301. Based on a multivariable Cox proportional hazard mode, risk factors for subsequent cholecystectomy included younger age, female sex, race, and some co-morbidities and complications ($P < 0.05$). Further, they concluded that patients should be counseled preoperatively about this risk and contemplate the use of Ursodiol biliary prophylaxis [32].

Table 1 Mechanism of cholesterol gallbladder formation in obesity and weight loss

Physical mechanism	Affect
The first physical mechanism: cholesterol supersaturation of bile	Leading to preconditioning of cholesterol crystallization
The second physical mechanism: the presence of a kinetic defect	Causing acceleration of cholesterol crystal nucleation and increase in supersaturated bile
The third physical mechanism: hypomotility of gallbladder	Bile increased cholesterol supersaturation, stasis in the gallbladder, and cholesterol crystallization leading to gallstone formation

6   Biliary Complications Post LSG

Most research on biliary complications have come from large studies on RYGB. In a study of 3765 patients who underwent bariatric surgery, around 138 (3.6%) patients developed postoperative biliary complications. The mean time from surgery to biliary complication was seen to be 1.8 ± 1.4 years. The main biliary complications were chronic cholecystitis (70.2%) and to a lesser extent, acute cholecystitis (18.1%), acute pancreatitis (9.4%), choledocholithiasis (5.7%), and jaundice (2.8%). The interventions were laparoscopic (n = 134, 97.0%) and open (n = 1, 0.7%) cholecystectomy [33]. Similar studies with longer prospective follow up (3 years) post open RYGB included 40 morbidly obese patients free of gallbladder disease preoperatively. Eleven of these patients (28.9%) developed cholelithiasis, four (10.5%) experienced biliary pain, and 2 suffered from acute biliary pancreatitis (5.3%). The treatment for these patients involved laparoscopic cholecystectomy. There were no deaths encountered post-op, which makes it a reasonable conclusion to perform a cholecystectomy during RYGB in the presence of cholelithiasis, or following this procedure if gallstones develop [34].

The most recent systematic review and meta-analysis of 42 studies with a cumulative sample size of 729,642 patients was able to show an incidence rate of biliary complications to be 5.54 cases/1000 patient year: SD = ± 6.87 (Table 2). Sleeve gastrectomy had the highest complications rate equal to 5.66 cases/1000 patient year; SD = ± 9.06 compared to all other procedures. This was probably because none of the SG studies included ursodiol use. The most common biliary complications encountered were biliary colic or biliary dyskinesia with 3.04 cases/1000 patient year: (SD = ± 2.67). Acute cholecystitis made up 1.44 cases/1000 patient year (SD = ± 2.13), acute pancreatitis was 0.11 cases/1000 patient year (SD = ± 0.2), and common bile duct stones showed an incidence of 0.34 cases/1000 patient year (SD = ± 0.53). The complication rate tended to be exponential to the severity of weight loss [Table 2] [35].

7   Cholecystectomy: When to Operate?

Presently there is no consensus on the best timing to perform a cholecystectomy for asymptomatic gallstones in individuals undergoing bariatric surgery, with widespread variation in practice. This can be explained by a lack of high-quality studies and the lack of randomized control trials, especially covering LSG. This controversy is null when the patient presents with symptomatic gallstone given that the standard practice would be to perform a cholecystectomy before or commitment to their bariatric procedure [36].

There are three possible approaches to deal with the risk of biliary complications and asymptomatic gallstones:

Table 2 Incidence of biliary complication post bariatric surgery

Bariatric Technique, UDCA & Biliary complications	Mean total patient year	(±SD)	Mean number of cases/1000 patient year	(±SD)
RYGB	62,116.02	226,168.85	5.27	6.12
LSG	4771.36	5907.47	5.66	9.06
LAGB	2819.17	766.23	1.02	1.08
BPD/DS	6059.50	1908.48	5.53	2.11
UDCA	3176.17	2584.51	4.1	3.37
NO UDCA URSODIOL	10,912.36	17,963.78	5.67	9.82
Global biliary complications	135,581	598,964.17	5.54	6.87
Biliary colic or dyskinesia	61,952.22	232,429.74	3.04	2.67
Acute cholecystitis	167,371.45	740,115.82	1.44	2.13
Acute pancreatitis	11,938.94	19,571.46	0.11	0.2

1. Prophylactic (Routine) Cholecystectomy
2. Selective (Elective) Cholecystectomy
3. Conventional (expectant) Cholecystectomy

8   Prophylactic (Routine) Cholecystectomy

Refers to performing laparoscopic cholecystectomy in all patients at the time of initial surgery, regardless of the presence or absence of gallstones. In earlier concerns, there has been an increased incidence of biliary complications after bariatric surgery compared to the general population. Another important concern is that the diagnosis of microlithiasis is difficult, while the incidence might be higher than expected.

The risk for postoperative complications was lower when the procedure was performed concomitantly with bariatric surgery compared to those performed post- (RD = −0.09; 95% CI − 0.13, − 0.05) or pre-bariatric surgery (RD = −0.05; 95% CI − 0.08, − 0.01). Furthermore, the risk for reoperation was lower for patients that underwent concomitant cholecystectomy (RD = −0.02; 95% CI − 0.05, − 0.00). The reason for cholecystectomy having a higher risk postoperatively is thought to be because 36.2% of the cholecystectomy indications following bariatric procedures were acute cholecystitis or involved choledochotomy for common bile duct exploration [35]

Worni et al. retrospectively analyzed 70,287 adults that underwent RYGB which reported only 9.1% of the patients had undergone concomitant cholecystectomy. However, the proportion of patients undergoing concomitant cholecystectomy decreased significantly from 26.3% in 2001 to 3.7% in 2008. Due to increased postoperative complications, interventions, mortality, and longer hospital stay they did not recommend concomitant cholecystectomy [37–39].

This approach was challenged by the fact that patients submitted to bariatric surgery have a low incidence rate of biliary complications, and concomitant cholecystectomy increases the risk for postoperative complications, cost and operative time. Subsequent reports and a major meta-analysis covered 13 studies analyzing the rate and morbidity of subsequent cholecystectomy in 6,048 patients who underwent RYGB without concomitant cholecystectomy. The rate of subsequent cholecystectomy was 6.8% (95% CI, 5.0–8.7%). The rate of subsequent cholecystectomy due to biliary colic or gallbladder dyskinesia was 5.3%; due to cholecystitis, 1.0%; choledocholithiasis, 0.2%; and biliary pancreatitis, 0.2%. The mortality rate after subsequent cholecystectomy was 0% (95% CI, 0–0.1%). The surgery-related complication rate after subsequent cholecystectomy was 1.8% (95% CI, 0.7–3.4%) while the risk of suffering from a cholecystectomy-related complication was 0.1% (95% CI, 0.03–0.3%) in patients undergoing RYGB without concomitant cholecystectomy. An important recommendation was to avoid prophylactic concomitant cholecystectomy during RYGB in patients without cholelithiasis, with the procedure exclusively reserved for patients with symptomatic biliary disease [36].

9 Elective (Selective) Cholecystectomy:

The approach involves performing concomitant laparoscopic cholecystectomy only in patients with gallstones pre/intraoperatively, even if asymptomatic. Many of the reasons that make it an appealing approach is that there is an assumed higher incidence of symptomatic disease as compared to patients without gallstones.

Hamed et al. performed cholecystectomy in 16.9% of patients during RYGB and compared the outcomes to those who did not have concomitant surgery. The result showed significantly longer operative time, longer hospital stays, and higher major morbidity in those with concomitant cholecystectomy.

There was, however, no specific morbidities causally related to cholecystectomy [40].

10 Conventional (Expectant) Cholecystectomy Approach

This involves expectant management with or without prophylactic administration of UDCA until the symptoms develop. Thus, cholecystectomy is performed only when symptoms arise. The advantage of this approach is that surgery is performed after a significant weight loss is achieved allowing surgical risk and technical difficulties to subside after the weight loss procedure.

Several studies showed a low incidence rate (only 9.84%) of patients after RYGB without prophylactic UDCA requiring subsequent cholecystectomy and they concluded that the natural history of patients with asymptomatic gallstones undergoing bypass is very much like the natural history of asymptomatic gallstones in the general population [41].

11 Ursodeoxycholic Acid (UDCA) Prophylaxis

The role of UDCA in prevention of gallstones is well established in the literature. It works by acting at the cholesterol and mucin levels in the bile (decreasing bile saturation) and improving gallbladder emptying.

In a randomized clinical trial, although a small sample was included, 51 obese women and 17 obese men all received a 16-week, 520-kcal-per-day weight-loss program. Gallstones formation was reported in 0 of 18 of the ursodeoxycholic acid-treated group, 2 of 14 of the aspirin-treated group and significantly in 5 out of 19 of the placebo-treated group [14].

12 UDCA Efficacy in Post Bariatric Surgery

12.1 Dose, Frequency

The ideal dose of UDCA to markedly and significantly reduce gallstone formation from 32 to 2% proved to be 600 per day, provided prophylactically twice daily in divided doses for 6 months after RGBP-induced rapid weight loss. This intervention further decreases the morbidity of this potentially life-saving operation. However, UDCA can reduce gallstone formation with no further risk reduction when using higher doses of 1200 mg daily (6%) [42].

There was weak evidence that the duration of UDCA prophylaxis is proportional to the BMI preoperatively, with no strong evidence available and the best recommendation to support 6 month prophylaxis period in all patients.

Consensus from an earlier systemic review of eight studies incorporating 1355 patients demonstrated lower incidence of gallstone formation in patients taking UDCA in relation to different bariatric procedures, doses of administered UDCA, and time from bariatric surgery. Adverse events were similar in both groups. Fewer patients required cholecystectomy in the UDCA group and no deaths were reported [43].

The only randomized clinical trial that has been published to date among SG patients investigated gallstone prevention with UDCA in 37 patients randomized to the UDCA treatment arm and 38 patients to no treatment. The results at 6 months demonstrated that the UDCA group had a statistically significant lower incidence of gallstones ($p = 0.032$) while at 1 year no significant difference in gallstones between the two groups was detected. The overall gallstone formation rate was 29.8% [44].

13 Disadvantages of UDCA

Other than the higher cost inferred on patients, some side effects can be seen with UDCA usage, e.g. diarrhea, skin rash and aggravation of liver diseases that the patient needs to be informed about and could be a limiting factor in its use [43].

14 Summary

Obesity and rapid weight loss after LSG contribute to the risk of gallstone formation and the likelihood of developing biliary disease complications.

There is relative scarcity of published data on LSG and biliary disease and a limitation of this review is that most of the included studies were a retrospective cohort that mostly came from RYGB studies. These studies characteristics may explain the high heterogeneity noted in some analysis.

Clearly the data showed low incidence of biliary complications after bariatric surgery. Prophylactic cholecystectomy currently has no indications, even in the presence of asymptomatic gallstones due to the fact that it may increase the risk of postoperative complications and the mean operative time. However, if cholecystectomy is not performed before or at the time of the LSG, patients should be carefully followed with special attention for biliary complications. Commonly, indication for cholecystectomy post-bariatric surgery is due to acute biliary complications, which despite being unusual, infer a higher risk for postoperative complications and reoperations. If a patient presents with biliary symptoms at the time of bariatric surgery, surgeons should considerer cholecystectomy before or concomitantly.

Given the current popularity of the sleeve. Future controlled trials are required for evidence of higher power. In addition, a standardized usage of ursodiol for each type of bariatric technique should also be assessed in further studies. The use of UDCA in a dose of 300 mg taken twice daily for 6 months significantly reduces or prevents gallstone formation and is highly recommended in asymptomatic gallstones.

15 Conclusion

Sleeve gastrectomy is an increasingly performed procedure worldwide and is viewed by many experts as a valid option for weight reduction and resolution of metabolic comorbidity. Post-operative biliary disease is a serious risk, however prophylactic cholecystectomy is not indicated while UDCA prophylaxis is indicated especially in asymptomatic gallstones. Longer term, and comparative data are still needed.

References

1. Angrisani L, Santonicola A, Lovino P et al. IFSO worldwide survey 2016: primary, endoluminal, and revisional procedures. OBES SURG. 2018; 28:3783–94.
2. Scragg RK, McMichael AJ, Baghurst PA. Diet, alcohol, and relative weight in gall stone disease: a case-control study. Br Med J (Clin Res Ed). 1984; 288(6424):1113–19.
3. Erlinger S. Gallstones in obesity and weight loss. Eur J Gastroenterol Hepatol. 2000; 12(12):1347–52.
4. Maclure KM, Hayes KC, Colditz GA, et al. Weight, diet, and the risk of symptomatic gallstones in middle-aged women. N Engl J Med. 1989;321(9):563–9.
5. World Health Organization. Obesity: preventing and managing the global epidemic. Part I. The problem of overweight and obesity. WHO Technical Report Series No. 894. WHO: Geneva. 2000:5–15.
6. Barbara L, Sama C, Morselli Labate AM, Taroni F, Rusticali AG, Festi D, et al. A population study on the prevalence of gallstone disease: the Sirmione study. Hepatology. 1987;7:913–7.
7. Layde PM, Vessey MP, Yeates D. Risk factors for gall-bladder disease: a cohort study of young women attending family planning clinics. J Epidemiol Community Health. 1982;36(274–8):7.
8. The epidemiology of gallstone disease in Rome, Italy. Part II. Factors associated with disease. The Rome Group for Epidemiology and Prevention of Cholelithiasis (GREPCO). Hepatology. 1988; 8:907–13.
9. Jorgensen T. Gallstones in a Danish population. Relation to weight, physical activity, smoking, coffee consumption, and diabetes mellitus. Gut. 1989; 30:528–34.
10. Maurer KR, Everhart JE, Knowler WC, Shawker TH, Roth HP. Risk factors for gallstone disease in the Hispanic populations of the United States. Am J Epidemiol. 1990;131:836–44.
11. Sichieri R, Everhart JE, Roth HP. Low incidence of hospitalization with gallbladder disease among blacks in the United States. Am J Epidemiol. 1990;131:826–35.
12. Stampfer MJ, Maclure KM, Colditz GA, Manson JE, Willett WC. Risk of symptomatic gallstones in women with severe obesity. Am J Clin Nutr. 1992;55:652–8.
13. Yang H, Petersen GM, Roth MP, Schoenfield LJ, Marks JW. Risk factors for gallstone formation during rapid loss of weight. Dig Dis Sci. 1992; 37:912–8.]
14. Broomfield PH, Chopra R, Sheinbaum RC, Bonorris GG, Silverman A, Schoenfield LJ, et al. Effects of ursodeoxycholic acid and aspirin on the formation of lithogenic bile and gallstones during loss of weight. N Engl J Med. 1988;319:1567–72.
15. Liddle RA, Goldstein RB, Saxton J. Gallstone formation during weight-reduction dieting. Arch Intern Med. 1989;149:1750–3.
16. Festi D, Orsini M, Bassi SL, Cerel C, Sangermano A, Parenti M, et al. Risk of gallstone formation during rapid weight loss: protective role of gallbladder motility (Abstract). Gastroenterology. 1992;102:A311.
17. Hoy K, Blank B, Grasset E, Schamacher D, Ritch D, Heymsfield S. Cholelithiasis in obese patients before and after short term weight loss (Abstract). Int J Obesity. 1991;15(Suppl 3):20.
18. Gebhard RL, Prigge WF, Ansel HJ, Schlasner L, Ketover SR, Sande D, et al. The role of gallbladder emptying in gallstone formation during diet-induced rapid weight loss. Hepatology. 1996; 24:544–8. Weight.
19. Erlinger S. Gallstones in obesity and weight loss. Eur J Gastroenterol Hepatol. 2000;12(12):1347–52.
20. Everhart JE. Contributions of obesity and weight loss to gallstone disease. Ann Intern Med. 1993;119(10):1029–35.
21. Sichieri R, Everhart JE, Roth HP. A prospective study of hospitalization with gallstone disease among women: role of dietary factors, fasting period, and dieting. Am J Public Health. 1991;81:880–4.

22. Bennion LJ, Grundy SM. Risk factors for the development of cholelithiasis in man. N Engl J Med. 1978;299(21):1161–7.
23. Trotman BW, Petrella EJ, Soloway RD, Sanchez HM, Morris TA, 3rd, Miller WT. Evaluation of radiographic lucency or opaqueness of gallstones as a means of identifying cholesterol or pigment stones. Correlation of lucency or opaqueness with calcium and mineral. Gastroenterology. 1975; 68:1563–6.]
24. Busch N, Matern S. Current concepts in cholesterol gallstone pathogenesis. Eur J Clin Invest. 1991; 21:453–60.
25. Hay DW, Carey MC. Pathophysiology and pathogenesis of cholesterol gallstone formation. Semin Liver Dis. 1990; 10:159–70.
26. Paumgartner G. Sauerbruch T. Gallstones: pathogenesis. Lancet. 1991;338:1117–21.
27. Bennion LJ, Grundy SM. Effects of obesity and caloric intake on biliary lipid metabolism in man. J Clin Invest. 1975;56:996–1011.
28. Angelin B, Einarsson K, Ewerth S, Leijd B. Biliary lipid composition in obesity. Scand J Gastroenterol. 1981;16:1015–9.
29. Reuben A, Qureshi Y, Murphy GM, Dowling RH. Effect of obesity and weight reduction on biliary cholesterol saturation and the response to chenodeoxycholic acid. Eur J Clin Invest. 1986;16:133–42.
30. Gustafsson U1, Benthin L, Granström L et al. Changes in gallbladder bile composition and crystal detection time in morbidly obese subjects after bariatric surgery. Hepatology. 2005; 41(6):1322–8.
31. Tsirline VB, Keilani ZM, El Djouzi S, Phillips RC, Kuwada TS, Gersin K, Simms C, Stefanidis D. How frequently and when do patients undergo cholecystectomy after bariatric surgery? Surg Obes Relat Dis. 2014 Mar−Apr; 10(2):313–21.
32. Altieri MS, Yang J, Nie L, Docimo S, Talamini M, Pryor AD et al. Incidence of cholecystectomy after bariatric surgery. Surg Obes Relat Dis. 2018; 14(7):992–6.
33. Chang J, Corcelles R, Boules M, Jamal MH, Schauer PR, Kroh MD. Predictive factors of biliary complications after bariatric surgery. Surgery for Obesity and Related Diseases. 2016;12(9):1706–10.
34. Nagem RG, Lázaro-da-Silva A, de Oliveira RM, Morato VG. Gallstone-related complications after Roux-en-Y gastric bypass: a prospective study. Hepatobiliary Pancreat Dis Int. 2012 Dec 15; 11(6):630−5.
35. Tustumi F, Bernardo WM, Santo MA. Ivan cecconello. cholecystectomy in patients submitted to bariatric procedure: a systematic review and meta-analysis. OBES SURG. 2018; 28: 3312–20.
36. Warschkow R, Tarantino I, Ukegjini K, et al. Concomitant cholecystectomy during laparoscopic Roux-en-Y gastric bypass in obese patients is not justified: a meta-analysis. Obes Surg. 2013;23(3):397–407.
37. Worni M, Guller U, Shah A, et al. Cholecystectomy concomitant with laparoscopic gastric bypass: a trend analysis of the nationwide inpatient sample from 2001 to 2008. OBES SURG. 2012;22:220–9.
38. Villegas, L., Schneider, B., Provost, D. Craig Chang, Daniel Scott, Thomas Sims, BS et al. Is routine cholecystectomy required during laparoscopic gastric bypass? OBES SURG. 2004; 14:206–11.
39. Fobi M, Lee H, Igwe D, et al. Prophylactic cholecystectomy with gastric bypass operation: incidence of gallbladder disease. OBES SURG. 2002;12:350–3.
40. Hamad GG, Ikramuddin S, Gourash WF, et al. Elective cholecystectomy during laparoscopic Roux-En-Y gastric bypass: is it worth the wait? OBES SURG. 2003;13:76–81.
41. Bernabé M Quesada, Gustavo Kohan, Hernán E Roff, Carlos M Canullán, Luis T Chiappetta Porras. Management of gallstones and gallbladder disease in patients undergoing gastric bypass. World J Gastroenterol. 2010; 16(17):2075–9.
42. Sugerman HJ, Brewer WH, Shiffman ML, Brolin RE, Fobi MA, Linner JH, et al. A multicenter, placebo-controlled, randomized, double-blind, prospective trial of prophylactic

ursodiol for the prevention of gallstone formation following gastric-bypass-induced rapid weight loss. Am J Surg. 1995 Jan; 169(1):91–6; discussion 96–7.

43. Magouliotis DE, Tasiopoulou VS, Svokos AA, Svokos KA, Chatedaki C, Sioka E, Zacharoulis D. Ursodeoxycholic acid in the prevention of gallstone formation after bariatric surgery: an updated systematic review and meta-analysis. OBES SURG. 2017;27:3021–30.

44. Adams LB, Chang C, Pope J, Kim Y, Liu P, Yates A. Randomized, prospective comparison of ursodeoxycholic acid for the prevention of gallstones after sleeve gastrectomy. Obes Surg. 2016;26(5):990–4.

LSG Under Block Anesthesia (PVB)

Mohamad Hayssam Elfawal, Saleh Kanawati
and Diya Aldeen Mohammed

1 Introduction

Laparoscopic sleeve gastrectomy (LSG) remains the gold standard technique to achieve and maintain long term weight loss among the overweight population. The current trend is to perform LSG under general anesthesia (GA) because of several factors, including good muscle relaxation which allows better manipulation of laparoscopic tools, but this cannot be attained safely among severely co-morbid obese patients where GA carries a high risk of complications or is considered a contraindication, and therefore, paravertebral blockade (PVB) could offer a safe alternative.

2 Review on General Anesthesia

2.1 General Overview

Almost all surgeries of the modern era share a common procedure that is anesthesia. The Oxford dictionary defines anesthesia as "Insensitivity to pain, especially as artificially induced by the administration of gases or the injection of drugs before surgical operations." The act of abolishing surgical pain was always sought

M. H. Elfawal (✉)
Clinical Assistant Professor of Surgery, CEO New You Center, Director Fellowship Program Bariatric and Metabolic Surgery at Beirut Arab University, Beirut, Lebanon
e-mail: hayssamfawal@gmail.com

S. Kanawati
Department of Anesthesia, Chairman Department of Anesthesia, Makassed General Hospital, Beirut, Lebanon

D. A. Mohammed
Bariatric Surgeon, New You Center, Beirut, Lebanon

© The Editor(s) (if applicable) and The Author(s), under exclusive license to Springer Nature Switzerland AG 2021
S. Al-Sabah et al. (eds.), *Laparoscopic Sleeve Gastrectomy*,
https://doi.org/10.1007/978-3-030-57373-7_33

out throughout history, but it was in the nineteenth century that discoveries about certain anesthetic agents made anesthesia possible and reproducible [1]. To date, advancements in the field of anesthesia grow and evolve to try and perfect this procedure for a better and safer patient experience.

The objectives of anesthesia are to provide analgesia and amnesia during an operative event. To achieve these objectives, the anesthesiologist can perform different types of anesthesia depending on the situation presented, and these are [2]:

1. General anesthesia
2. Neuraxial anesthesia (Spinal, Epidural)
3. Nerve Block
4. Regional (local) anesthesia

2.2   General Anesthesia in the Obese/bariatric Population

Obesity is well known for the overall risks it imparts on an individual, ranging from an increased risk of metabolic syndrome to an increased risk in cardiovascular events and overall mortality [3]. In the normal population, complications can occur with the use of general anesthesia either perioperatively or postoperatively, as stated earlier. However, obese patients, in whom comorbid diseases are frequently encountered, are even more drastically impacted by general anesthesia in this regard [4]. According to previously published data, the incidence of postoperative complications, ranging from the harmless vomiting to the fatal myocardial ischemia, are all somewhat higher in the obese surgical patient [5].

The increased risk of perioperative complications stems from the concept that morbidly obese patients possess unique pathophysiologic changes that makes this population particularly more vulnerable to life threatening issues [5].

Obese patients are characterized by an increased extracellular volume owing to an enlarged cardiopulmonary vascular system, as well as increased metabolic demands. This change ultimately leads to an increase in lung resistance and consequently a decrease in lung compliance, causing decreased ventilation and hypoxemia [5]. In addition to the hypervolemia, mechanical barriers such as excess fatty tissue especially around the neck and trunk also negatively affect respiratory function leading to hypoxia [6]. Furthermore, reduced compliance of the diaphragm, an important muscle for respiration, occurs during laparoscopic abdominal surgery under general anesthesia, partly from the gases used to expand the abdomen, and partly from the drugs used during anesthesia that cause a loss of muscular tone [6]. This reduced diaphragmatic compliance, as well as a documented cephalad diaphragmatic displacement in obese patients undergoing bariatric surgery, raises the risk of basal atelectasis and ultimately the prevalence of chest infections [7]. That is why obese patients are prone to develop respiratory complications and special care is taken in general anesthetic protocols involving these patients for this reason [8].

Moving on from the respiratory standpoint, obesity by itself is a risk factor for coronary artery disease, and hence these patients pose an increased risk of angina pectoris, heart failure, and even sudden death. Fatty infiltration of the cardiac conduction system may as well increase the risk of cardiac arrhythmias [7].

As a conclusion, this patient population represents a particular challenge for the anesthesiologist. The presence of a vast difference in published data regarding the matter results in difficulty establishing a well inscribed and universal general anesthesia regimen or even predict its outcome. That is why general anesthesia for the morbidly obese patient is still regarded as holding a higher risk for major complications than the general population [8].

3   Review on Paravertebral Block (PVB)

Paravertebral nerve blockade (PVB) is an old technique that is being rejuvenated and revisited for not only perioperative and post-operative pain relief but as a sole anesthetic technique in many thoraco-abdominal surgeries.

Hugo Sellheim of Leipzig in 1905 was the pioneer concerning the concept of paravertebral block, which was later refined by Lawen (1911) and Kappis (1919) [9].

This technique was formally introduced by Eason and Wyatt (1979) with their paper "paravertebral block-a reappraisal" [10]. However, it was really over the last 20 years that paravertebral block generated interest initially for the patients undergoing breast surgery, inguinal hernia repair and most recently bariatric procedures [11].

4   Anatomy

The paravertebral space in general is not well defined in anatomy books and references, it was first described however by Macintosh and Bryce Smith in their book about local anesthesia in 1962 [12].

This space extends from T1 to the lumbar vertebral column, it is a wedge shaped area posteriorly bounded by the superior costo-transverse ligament, antero-laterally by the parietal pleura and medially by the posterolateral aspect of the vertebra and intervertebral foramen (Fig. 1) [11].

The space communicates medially with the epidural space via the intervertebral foramen and it is continuous with the intercostal space as well [10].

There are anatomical variations of the nerve in the lateral part of the space. In some of Eason and Wyatt's dissections the nerve was shown to divide into multiple parts which may or may not re-join, and in one case it was seen to deviate downwards to become an intercostal nerve running along the top of the rib below [10].

In that space the spinal nerve root exits the intervertebral foramen to give the dorsal and ventral rami, the sympathetic chain lies anteriorly to the intercostal

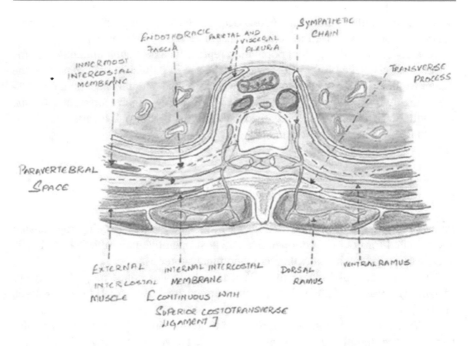

Fig. 1 Anatomy of the paravertebral space. [11] *Source* Batra RK, Krishnan K, Agarwal A. Paravertebral block. J AnaesthesiolClinPharmacol. 2011;27(1):5–11.(11)

nerve communicating with it via the rami communicants. This explains why blockade of that space causes, sensory and sympathetic block [13].

Also it was noted by Lönnqvist in 1992 that the paravertebral space is sealed off caudally at the thoraco-lumbar junction by the psoas muscle, by instilling dye via a catheter inserted in the paravertebral space at the 12th thoracic vertebrae level. This explains why the spread of the block to a level lower than T12 is unlikely [14].

Furthermore the endothoracic fascia which lies between the parietal pleura and the innermost intercostal muscle divides the paravertebral space into two fascial compartments, the extra pleural compartment anteriorly and the subendothoracic paravertebral compartment posteriorly (Fig. 2) [15].

4.1 Indication

Perioperative anesthesia or analgesia is the most frequent indication.

In anesthesia however indications are generally for breast surgery, [16–18] inguinal hernia repair [19, 20] among other general surgeries, lithotripsy [21] and video assisted thoracic surgeries [22].

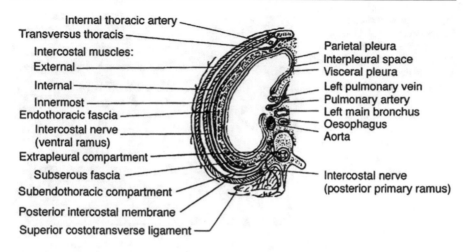

Internal thoracic artery
Transversus thoracis
Intercostal muscles:
External
Internal
Innermost
Endothoracic fascia
Intercostal nerve
(ventral ramus)
Extrapleural compartment
Subserous fascia
Subendothoracic compartment
Posterior intercostal membrane
Superior costotransverse ligament

Parietal pleura
Interpleural space
Visceral pleura
Left pulmonary vein
Pulmonary artery
Left main bronchus
Oesophagus
Aorta

Intercostal nerve
(posterior primary ramus)

Fig. 2 Fascial compartments of the paravertebral space. [15] *Source* Karmakar, M. K., Kwok, W. H., & Kew, J. (2000). Thoracic paravertebral block: Radiological evidence of contralateral spread anterior to the vertebral bodies. British Journal of Anaesthesia, 84(2), 26.(15)

Single injection paravertebral blocks can be used for surgeries with mild to moderate pain [23] such as hernioplasties and minimally invasive cardiac surgeries [24].

For minor abdominal surgeries such as prostatectomies [25], laparoscopic cholecystectomies and hysterectomies bilateral single paravertebral blocks are needed. Alternatively, a continuous bilateral block is used for major surgeries whether abdominal (pancreatectomy, colectomies…), cardiac or pelvic (cystectomy, hysterectomy, nephrectomies…) by placement of a PV catheter [26] (Table 1).

Table 1 Indications of paravertebral blocks and the level at which they should be performed

	Continuous PVBs	Single PVBs
Breast	T1-T2 (axillary dissection)	T2-T6
Esophagectomy\bariatric surgery	Bilateral T2-T3	-
Thoracotomy including video assisted thoracic surgery (VATS)	T4-T5	-
Liver resection	Bilateral T6-T7	-
Umbilical hernia	Bilateral T8	Bilateral T7-T9
Abdominal surgery	Bilateral T8-T9	-
Pelvic surgery	Bilateral T11-T12	T10-L1

Source Chelly, J. E. (2012). Paravertebral blocks. Anesthesiology Clin, 30, 75–90.(2-).

Fig. 3 Lindgren needles.
[27] Source: James, C. D.,
& Bowers, J. R. (1968).
Aid to lumbar paravertebral
sympathetic block.
Anaesthesia, 23(4), 644–645

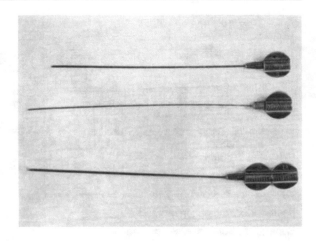

4.2 Techniques

Over time several techniques have been described concerning paravertebral block, including: blind, nerve stimulator guided and Ultrasound guided technique.

Irrespective of the technique, first the patient needs to be properly positioned ideally in a sitting position with his back in flexion; however it also can be performed with the patient in the lateral decubitus position especially in trauma patients [10].

Light sedation is given prior to the block with a combination of midazolam and fentanyl; however it could be performed with no preceding sedation [10].

The choice of needle is key, in 1968 Bryce and Bowers [27] found that Lindgren needles (Fig. 3) which were initially used for carotid and femoral angiograms, are ideal due to their straight shaft, large bore and rigidity which allows for an accurate placement.

However, Eason and Wyatt used a Tuohy needle, which is the needle that is standardized for the use in paravertebral blockade (Fig. 4) [10].

4.2.1 Blind Technique

The patient should be sitting up or placed on his lateral side. After scrubbing and cleaning the site, a skin weal is raised with local anesthetic solution 3 cm lateral from the anatomical midline. The Tuohy needle is advanced through the wheal at a 90 degree angle until striking the transverse process of the vertebra inferior to the spinal process palpated at a depth of 2.5–3.5 cm. When bone is felt the needle is redirected in a cephalad direction and advanced until passing above the transverse process (1–1-5 cm) and do so until the superior costotransverse ligament is passed (Fig. 5). This will manifest in loss of resistance when the needle enters areolar tissue of the paravertebral space, the needle is then aspirated to make sure that neither the Dural space nor the pleura nor a blood vessel has been punctured. Local anesthesia is then administered or a catheter inserted if a prolonged block is needed [10].

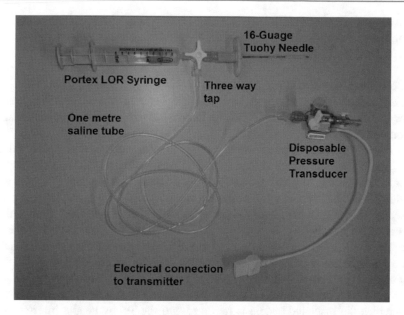

Fig. 4 The disposable epidural pressure measurement system. [28] *Source* N. Vaughan, V. N. Dubey, M. Y. K. Wee, and R. Isaacs. Devices for accurate placement of epidural Tuohy needle for Anaesthesia administration. Mech. Sci., 5, 1–6, 2014

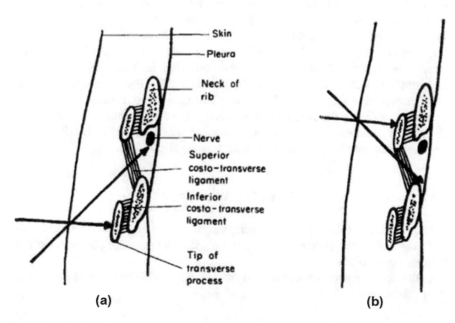

Fig. 5 Longitudinal section to show direction of needle: (a) above, (b) below. [10] *Source* Eason, M., & Wyatt, R. (1979). Paravertebral thoracic block-a reappraisal. Anaesthesia, 34(7), 638–642)

However, unpredictability of spread, failure rate and complications has prompted the modification of this technique to ensure more accuracy in defining the paravertebral space.

4.2.2 Neurostimulation Technique

This technique in paravertebral blockade has been in use since 1998, since it allows more accurate localization of the intercostal nerve and thus lowers complication rate [29].

A nerve stimulator with an initial current of 5 mA and 9 V is connected to a 21G insulated needle which is then advanced perpendicularly to the skin. First the contraction of the Paraspinal muscles is detected, which subsequently ceases when the needle reaches the costo-transverse ligament. After piercing the latter, a proper muscular response is noted, being that of the intercostal muscles. The needle is then adjusted into a position to allow muscular response while reducing the current. The intensity is directly related to the distance between the tip of the needle and the intercostal muscle. The position of the needle is considered optimal when the current is between 0.4–0.8 mA [29].

The distance between the skin and the paravertebral space is then measured, after which the insulated needle is removed and the Tuohy needle inserted at the same depth measured [15].

4.2.3 Ultrasound Guided Technique

The utilization of ultrasound as a guide has enhanced the accuracy of needle and subsequent catheter placement into the paravertebral space. A linear array transducer is placed 2.5 cm laterally to the spinous process in an oblique axis and the goal is to obtain a sonographic image consisting of the pleura (anteriorly), the cototransverse ligament (posteriorly) and the bony prominences (Fig. 6) [30]. Thus the ultrasound technique permits the visualization of the needle, the spread of the anesthetic solution and direct vision of the placement of the catheter.

After visualizing the landmarks, the needle is inserted into the paravertebral space, then the anesthetic solution is deposited which translates by the parietal pleura bulging anteriorly on the ultrasound image (Fig. 7) [31].

4.3   Mechanism and Spread of Anesthetic

Ipsilateral Block of the somatic and sympathetic nerves is achieved by local anesthetic injection in the paravertebral space including the posterior ramus in multiple adjacent dermatomes.

In that area the nerves are devoid of fascial sheath which facilitates penetration of anesthetic agents [32].

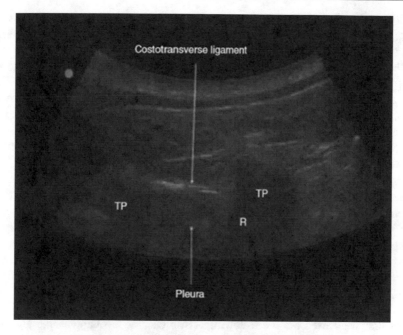

Fig. 6 Sonogram of the paravertebral space. [30] *Source* Luyet, C., Eichenberger, U., Greif, R., Vogt, A., Farkas, Z. S., & Moriggl, B. (2009). Ultrasound-guided paravertebral puncture and placement of catheters in human cadavers: An imaging study. British Journal of Anaesthesia, 102(4), 534–539

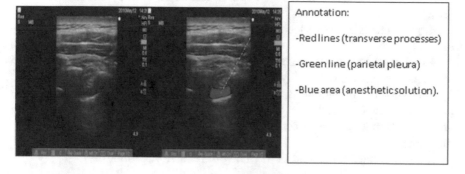

Fig. 7 Local anesthetic injection in the paravertebral space. [31] *Source* Bondár, A., Szűcs, S., &Iohom, G. (2010). Thoracic paravertebral blockade. Medical Ultrasonography, 12(3), 223–227

Concerning longitudinal spread it is thought that a single paravertebral space blocked can result in anesthesia of a mean of 5 dermatomes somatic wise, and a mean of 8 dermatomes sympathetic wise [33].

This ipsilateral spread of the anesthetic agent is through the heads of the ribs along the vertebral bodies [34].

It also has been demonstrated that injections ventral to the endothoracic fascia facilitates longitudinal spread versus unpredictable spread in case of dorsal infiltration [35].

Concerning the contralateral spread of the block, it was proven that one of the ways this is possible is by the drug penetrating the epidural space through the intervertebral foramen [36].

Between the pleura and the endothoracic fascia there's the subserous fascia which acts as a channel of communication between the paravertebral spaces on both sides, anterior to the vertebral body, which provides another possibility for the spread of the block to the contralateral side [16].

4.4 Anesthetic Drugs

Drugs that were used are the following: (Bupivacaine,levobupivacaine and ropivacaine) alone or with either epinephrine, Fentanyl,Clonidine or corticosteroids, and lidocaine with or without epinephrine.

The dose depends on the surgery and the number of dermatomes that are required to block, but as a general consensus 15 ml in adults is enough to cover 3 dermatomes, and 0.5 mg/kg in children will cover 4 dermatomes [13].

So it is proven that at least 3 to 4 spaces can be covered by one blocked level [10].

Bupivacaine is an amide local anesthetic that can produce long lasting anesthesia [37].

As adjuncts to bupivacaine, fentanyl and clonidine can be added which reduce the local anesthetic dose initially administered.

Average onset of anesthesia is around 30 min, and enhancement postoperative pain relief is noticed. However, their use can be limited by their side effects which are nausea/vomiting when it comes to fentanyl and hypotension concerning clonidine [38].

Lasts in average for around 14 to 15 h with relative variations [39].

4.5 Complications

In 2001 Naja and Lonnqvist prospectively studied the failure and complications rates of paravertebral blockade in 620 adults. Failure rate was 6.1% in adults, while the complications were the following [40] (Table 2).

They reported also that pneumothorax and vascular puncture risk were higher when it comes to bilateral block.

Table 2 Complication rate of paravertebral block

Complication	Rate (%)
Inadvertent vascular puncture	6.8
Hypotension	4
Intrathecal\epidural spread	1
Pleural puncture	0.8
Pneumothorax	0.5

Source Naja MZ, Lonnqvist PA. Somatic paravertebral nerve blockade: incidence of failed block and complications. Anaesthesia. 2001;56:1184–8 (102)

In 2005, a case of contralateral Harlequin and ipsilateral Horner syndrome was documented post paravertebral block for a breast operation and it was thought to be due to the spread of analgesics to the stellate ganglion [41].

Also a case of pulmonary hemorrhage was seen in a patient that underwent a paravertebral block, however, this patient suffered from a previous thoracic surgery which resulted in paravertebral space fibrosis, making loss of resistance less evident [42].

This technique lacks systemic toxicity by the anesthetic drug due to the moderately slow absorption time (Tmax = 15-30 min) [43]; however there's one documented case where the patient suffered a seizure following systematic spread [44].

4.6   Paravertebral Blockade (PVB) vs General Anesthesia (GA) a Review of Data

4.6.1 Abdominal Surgeries

Multiple authors compared GA to PVB in different abdominal surgeries. In all reviewed articles, superiority of the PVB technique was noticed, whether through the decrease in post op vomiting, pain or any post op adverse events. Some of those most important articles discussing that are listed in Table 3 [35, 46–51].

4.6.2 First Paravertebral Block in Sleeve Gastrectomy

Kanawati et al. conducted a case series in 2015 where they performed a paravertebral block on 5 patients undergoing sleeve gastrectomy. A bilateral block was performed, with 4–5 ml of local anesthetic infiltrated at the thoracic level from T6 through T11, guided by a nerve stimulator. The nerve stimulator was used as well to secure a cervical block to relieve shoulder pain in these patients brought on by abdominal insufflation for laparoscopy. Patients were hemodynamically stable, conscious and cooperative throughout the operation. In that case series paravertebral block proved to be a satisfactory alternative to general anesthesia [45].

In our study (unpublished data), a total of 210 participants were included of which 48 constituted the PVB group and 162 patients composed the GA group. Both groups were similar in baseline demographic factors, with patients in PVB

Table 3 Characteristics and outcomes reported from studies that used PVB in abdominal and urological surgeries

Author	Surgery	General anesthesia control (n)	Intervention (n)	Outcome
Akcaboy et al. (46)	Open inguinal herniorrhaphy	30	Unilateral TPVB (30)	Faster readiness for discharge And longer mean duration of analgesia in PVB group No difference in patient nor surgeon satisfaction between groups
Hadzic et al. [19]	Open inguinal herniorrhaphy	24	Unilateral TPVB (24)	More nausea in GA group, however only one patient vomited No difference in post op pain
Agarwal et al. [47]	laparoscopic cholecystectomy	25	Bilateral TPVB + GA	Lower 24 h morphine intake and less post op nausea and vomiting in TPVB group
Naja et al. [35]	laparoscopic cholecystectomy	30	Bilateral TPVB + GA	Fewer patients requiring analgesics supplementation in TPVB group, however no difference concerning post op nausea and vomiting
Moussa [48]	Donorhepatectomy	12	Bilateral TPVB + GA (12)	Lower morphine consumption and less post op nausea and vomiting with TPVB
Abou Zeid et al. [49]	Ventral hernia repair	30	Bilateral TPVB (30)	Lesser analgesic intake, shorter hospital stay and less post op nausea in TPVB group
Elm Ak et al. [50]	Percutaneous nephrolithotomy	28	Unliteral TPVB + GA (27)	Higher patient satisfaction and lower 24 h morphine intake with the TPVB technique 3 failed TPVB(excluded)
Borle et al. [51]	Percutaneous nephrolithotomy	24	Unilateral TVPB + GA (24)	Lower post op fentanyl consumption in the TPVB group One patient with hydropneumothorax in each group

Legend: TPVB: thoracic paravertebral block; GA: General anesthesia.

suffering from higher number and advanced stage of comorbidities than the GA group. Mean operative time was similar in between the two groups. Intra-operative complications were scarce among both study groups. GA group requested a second dose of analgesia earlier than PVB group, When comparing pain management post-op, In the Post Anesthesia Care Unit, the patients in the PVB group did not ask for pain killers, as compared to GA group where at least 20% of the patients asked for an additional analgesia dose, There was a significant statistical difference in the number of doses received by the two groups when compared for analgesia requirements in the postoperative period. This reflects the important effect of the paravertebral blockade in post-operative analgesia on top of its role as an anesthetic technique. After at least 1 year postoperatively, the mean percentage of excess weight were similar.

References

1. Robinson DH, Toledo AH. Historical development of modern Anesthesia. J Invest Surg. 2012;25(3):141-s9.
2. Potyk DK, Raudaskoski P. Overview of anesthesia for primary care physicians. WJM.1998;168(6).
3. Segula D. Complications of obesity in adults: a short review of the literature. Malawi Med J. 2014 Mar; 26(1).
4. American society of anesthesiologists (ASA) [internet]. 905 16th Street, N.W. Suite 400 Washington, DC. 20006. Updated in October 15, 2014, cited in July 19, 2019. Available form: https://www.asahq.org/standards-and-guidelines/asa-physical-status-classification-system.
5. Tassoudis V, Ieropoulos H, Karanikolas M, Vretzakis G, Bouzia A, Mantoudi E. et al. Bronchospasm in obese patients undergoing elective laparoscopic surgery under general anesthesia. Springer Plus. 2016; 5(1).
6. Piskin O, Altinsoy B, Cimencan M, Aydin B, Okyay D, Kucukosman G. The effect of bariatric anaesthesia on postoperative pulmonary functions. J Pak Med Assoc. 2017;67(4):561–7.
7. Goulding ST, Hovell BC. Anaesthetic experience of vertical banded gastroplasty. Br J Anaesth. 1995;75(3):301–6.
8. Lindauer B, Steurer MP, Müller MK, Dullenkopf A. Anesthetic management of patients undergoing bariatric surgery: two year experience in a single institution in Switzerland. BMC Anesthesiology. 2014; 14(1).
9. Richardson J. Fin-de-siecle renaissance of Paravertebral analgesia. Pain Rev. 1997.
10. Eason M, Wyatt R. Paravertebral thoracic block-a reappraisal. Anaesthesia. 1979;34(7):638–42.
11. Batra RK, Krishnan K, Agarwal A. Paravertebral block. J Anaesthesiol Clin Pharmacol. 2011;27(1):5–11.
12. Macintosh RR, Bryce-Smith R. Local analgesia-abdominal surgery, 2nd edn. 1962; p. 26. Livingstone, Edinburgh.
13. Richardson J, Lönnqvist PA. Thoracic paravertebral block. Br J Anaesth. 1998;81(2):230–8.
14. Lönnqvist PA, Hildingsson U. The caudal boundary of the thoracic paravertebral space. Anaesthesia. 1992;47(12):1051–2.
15. Karmakar MK, Kwok WH, Kew J. Thoracic paravertebral block: radiological evidence of contralateral spread anterior to the vertebral bodies. Br J Anaesth. 2000;84(2):263–5.
16. Weltz CR, Greengrass R, Klein S. A randomized prospective trial comparing paravertebral block and general anesthesia for operative treatment of breast cancer. 2001 Jan.

17. Buggy DJ, Kerin MJ. Paravertebral analgesia with Levobupivacaine increases postoperative flap tissue oxygen tension after immediate Latissimus Dorsi breast reconstruction compared with intravenous opioid analgesia. Anesthesiology. 2004;100(2):375–80.
18. Buckenmaier CC, Steele SM, Nielsen KC, Martin AH, Klein SM. Bilateral continuous paravertebral catheters for reduction mammoplasty. Acta Anaesthesiol Scand. 2002;46(8):1042–5.
19. Hadzic A, Kerimoglu B, Loreio D. Paravertebral blocks provide superior same-day recovery over general anesthesia for patients undergoing inguinal hernia repair. Survey of Anesthesiology. 2006;50(6):274.
20. Klein SM, Pietrobon R, Nielsen KC, Steele SM, Warner DS, Moylan JA, et al. Paravertebral somatic nerve block compared with peripheral nerve blocks for outpatient inguinal herniorrhaphy. Reg Anesth Pain Med. 2002;27(5):476–80.
21. Jamieson BD, Mariano ER. Thoracic and lumbar paravertebral blocks for outpatient lithotripsy. J Clin Anesth. 2007;19(2):149–51.
22. Soni AK, Conacher ID, Waller DA, Hilton CJ. Video-assisted thoracoscopic placement of paravertebral catheters: a technique for postoperative analgesia for bilateral thoracoscopic surgery. J Cardiothorac Vasc Anesth. 1995;9(6):778.
23. Ganapathy S, Nielsen KC, Steele SM. Outcomes after paravertebral blocks. Int Anesthesiol Clin. 2005;43(3):185–93.
24. Tsai T, Rodriguez-Diaz C, Deschner B, Thomas K, Wasnick JD. Thoracic paravertebral block for implantable cardioverter-defibrillator and laser lead extraction. J Clin Anesth. 2008;20(5):379–82.
25. Ben-David B, Swanson J, Nelson JB, Chelly JE. Multimodal analgesia for radical prostatectomy provides better analgesia and shortens hospital stay. J Clin Anesth. 2007;19(4):264–8.
26. Chelly JE. Paravertebral Blocks Anesthesiology Clin. 2012;30:75–90.
27. James CD, Bowers JR. Aid to lumbar paravertebral sympathetic block. Anaesthesia. 1968;23(4):644–5.
28. Vaughan N, Dubey VN, Wee MYK, Isaacs R. Devices for accurate placement of epidural Tuohy needle for Anaesthesia administration. Mechanical Sciences. 2014 Feb; 5(1):1–6.
29. Naja Z, Maaliki H, Al-Tannir M, El-Rajab M, Ziade F, Zeidan A. Repetitive paravertebral nerve block using a catheter technique for pain relief in post-herpetic neuralgia. Br J Anaesth. 2006;96(3):381–3.
30. Luyet C, Eichenberger U, Greif R, Vogt A, Farkas ZS, Moriggl B. Ultrasound-guided paravertebral puncture and placement of catheters in human cadavers: an imaging study. Br J Anaesth. 2009;102(4):534–9.
31. Bondár A, Szűcs S, Iohom G. Thoracic paravertebral blockade. Medical Ultrasonography. 2010;12(3):223–7.
32. Richardson J, Sabanathan S, Jones J, Shah RD, Cheema S, Mearns AJ. A prospective randomized comparison of preoperative and continuous balanced epidural or paravertebral bupivacaine on post-thoracotomy pain, pulmonary function and stress responses. Br J Anaesth. 1999;83:387–92.
33. Cheema SPS, Ilsley D, Richardson J, Sabanathan S. A thermographic study of paravertebral analgesia. Anaesthesia. 1995;50:118–21.
34. Moore DC. Intercostal nerve block: spread of India ink injected to the ribs costal groove. Br J Anaesth. 1981;53:325.
35. Naja MZ, Ziade MF, Rajab ME, Tayara KE, Lönnqvist PA. Varying anatomical injection points within the thoracic paravertebral space: Effect on spread of solution and nerve blockade. Anaesthesia. 2004;59(5):459–63.
36. Kappis M. Sensibilitat und lokale anasthesie im chirurgischen gebeit der bauchkokle mit besonderer berucksichtigung der splanchnicusanasthesie. Beitr Klin Chir. 1919;115:161–75.
37. Kopacz DJ, Allen HW, Thompson GE. A comparison of epidural levobupivacaine 0.75% with racemic bupivacaine for lower abdominal surgery. Anesth Analg. 2000; 90:642–8.

38. Burlacu CL, Frizelle HP, Moriarty DC, Buggy DJ. Fentanyl and clonidine as adjunctive analgesics with levobupivacaine in paravertebral analgesia for breast surgery. Anaesthesia. 2006;61(10):932–7.
39. Finnetry O, Carney J, Mcdonnel JG. Trunk blocks for abdominal sugery. Anaesthesia. 2010;65:76–83.
40. Naja MZ, Lonnqvist PA. Somatic paravertebral nerve blockade: incidence of failed block and complications. Anaesthesia. 2001;56:1184–8.
41. Burlacu CL, Buggy DJ. Coexisting harlequin and Horner syndromes after high thoracic paravertebral anesthesia. Br J Anaesth. 2005;95:822–4.
42. Thomas PW, Sanders DJ, Berrisford RG. Pulmonary haemorrhage after percutaneous paravertebral block. Br J Anaesth. 1999;83:668–9.
43. Lonnqvist PA. Plasma concentrations of lignocaine after thoracic paravertebral blockade in infants and children. Anaesthesia. 1993; 48:958–60.
44. Snowden CP, Bower S, Conacher ID. Plasma bupivacaine levels in paravertebral blockade in adults. Anaesthesia. 1994; 49:546.
45. Kanawati S, Fawal H, Maaliki H, Naja ZM. Laparoscopic sleeve gastrectomy in five awake obese patients using paravertebral and superficial cervical plexus blockade. Anaesthesia. 2015;70:993–5.
46. Akcaboy EY, Akcaboy ZN, Gogus N. Comparison of paravertebral block versus fast-track general anesthesia via laryngeal mask airway in outpatient inguinal herniorrhaphy. J Anesth. 2010;24:687–93.
47. Agarwal A, Batra RK, Chhabra A, et al. The evaluation of efficacy and safety of paravertebral block for perioperative analgesia in patients undergoing laparoscopic cholecystectomy. Saudi J Anaesth. 2012;6(344–9):31.
48. Moussa A. Opioid saving strategy: bilateral single-site thoracic paravertebral block in right lobe donor hepatectomy. Middle East J Anesthesiol. 2008;19:789–801.
49. Abou Zeid HA, Al-Ghamdi AMA, Abdel-Hadi MS-A, Zakaria HM, Al-Quorain AAA, Shawkey MN. Bilateral paravertebral block in advanced schistosomal liver disease: a prospective study. Saudi J Gastroenterol. 2004; 10:67–77.
50. Ak K, Gursoy S, Duger C, et al. Thoracic paravertebral block for postoperative pain management in percutaneous nephrolithotomy patients: a randomized controlled clinical trial. Med Princ Pr. 2013;22:229–33.
51. Borle AP, Chhabra A, Subramaniam R, et al. Analgesic efficacy of paravertebral bupivacaine during percutaneous nephrolithotomy: an observer blinded, randomized controlled trial. J Endourol. 2014;28:1085–90.

Elderly High Risk Patients Undergoing Laparoscopic Sleeve Gastrectomy

Kashif Saeed, Emanuele Lo Menzo, Samuel Szomstein and Raul J. Rosenthal

1   Scope of the Problem

1.1   Increasing of the Elderly Population

The definition of "elderly" has varied over time and according to the regional life expectancy. In most developed countries, age more than 65 years is considered elderly, although in developing nations this age is 60 years [1]. Life expectancy has increased substantially in all parts of the world and over the last century it has more than doubled [2]. According to the WHO, life expectancy at birth globally increased from 66.5 years in 2000 to 72 years in 2016 [3] and in the US has almost increased by 10 years from 69.9 years in 1959 to 78.87 years in 2019 [4].

Life expectancy is expected to continue to increase due to continued advancement in health and improvement in living conditions around the world. With increase in life expectancy, the proportion of elderly population will inevitably increase. According to recent statistics, there were 703 million people of age 65 years and older worldwide in 2019, and this number is projected to double by 2050 [5]. In the United States, the population of 65 years and older is projected to nearly double from 52 million in 2018 to 95 million by 2060 [6].

K. Saeed · E. Lo Menzo · S. Szomstein · R. J. Rosenthal (✉)
Department of General Surgery and Director, Bariatric and Metabolic Institute,
Cleveland Clinic Florida, 2950 Cleveland Clinic Blvd, Weston, FL 33331, US
e-mail: rosentr@ccf.org

© The Editor(s) (if applicable) and The Author(s), under exclusive license to Springer
Nature Switzerland AG 2021
S. Al-Sabah et al. (eds.), *Laparoscopic Sleeve Gastrectomy*,
https://doi.org/10.1007/978-3-030-57373-7_34

1.2 Prevalence of Obesity and Related Comorbidities in the Elderly

Obesity is a global pandemic that is affecting people of all ages. With the increase in the elderly population, it is no wonder that the number of obese older individuals will increase as well. In fact, elderly subjects are more prone to develop obesity due to decreased resting energy expenditure [7, 8] and physical decline. In the US about 35% of adults aged 65 and over were obese in 2007–2010, representing over 8 million adults aged 65–74, and almost 5 million adults aged 75 and over, and this number is predicted to double by 2050 [9].

Elderly subjects are more likely to develop obesity-associated comorbidities, as with increase in age there is decline in physiologic reserves [10] and obesity further accentuates this risk. In fact, the incidence of both diabetes and HTN surges in older individuals as the BMI increases. Increased age and obesity are considered strongest factors for uncontrolled arterial hypertension and its incidence will rise the growth of the elderly obese population [11]. Similar trends are observed between elevated BMI and the risk of developing diabetes [12], coronary artery disease [13], and stroke [14]. Obesity has also been determined to be a major contributor to increase in incidence of osteoarthritis [15], erectile dysfunction, urinary incontinence [16] and decline in renal function in older individuals [17]. In addition to the physical decline, elderly obese compared to non-obese are at increased risk of cognitive decline. One study found that for every 1.0 increase in BMI at age 70 years, Alzheimers disease risk increased by 36% [18].

1.3 Risks of Surgery in the Elderly

There are no contraindications per se for major surgery in elderly patients, and in fact, the number of surgical procedures is 55% higher in persons over the age of 65 than in persons below the age of 65 [19]. Increasing age causes a decline in physiologic function of almost every organ system of the body, making it more susceptible to the stress of surgery [20]. This has been well demonstrated in the literature, with reported rates of 28% morbidity and 2.3% mortality after surgery in elderly and in patients above 80 years, postoperative morbidity of 51% and mortality of 7% [21, 22]. Despite this evidence, however, bariatric surgery continues to have low risk of complication and mortality, less than colonic surgery, cholecystectomy, and appendectomy [23].

1.3.1 Bariatric Surgery in Elderly

Two decades ago, bariatric surgery was not recommended in patients aged 60 years or older. The recommendations were based on the available evidence of increased mortality and morbidity, and less favorable outcomes in terms of weight loss in older patients undergoing bariatric surgery. In 1977, Printen and Mason reported an 8% mortality rate in patients older than 50 years, compared with a 2.8% mortality rate in patients younger than 50 years and recommended against surgery above 50 years [24]. In 1985 the NIH Consensus Conference on Obesity [25], and in 1987, a study by Grace, regarded age greater than 50 years as a potential contraindication to bariatric surgery [26]. Livingston et al. in 2002 recommended against bariatric surgery for those aged 55 years or older due to threefold-higher mortality rate relative to younger patients [27]. Flum et al. in 2005 reported a mortality rate of 11.1% at 1 year for patients aged > 65 and recommended against it in elderly [28].

With the advent of laparoscopy and the improvement in pre, peri and postoperative care, surgical morbidity and mortality in elderly from bariatric surgery improved and bariatric surgery was increasingly accepted as a treatment of obesity in the elderly.

From 1999 to 2005 2.7% of all bariatric surgeries were performed in elderly subjects. This number increased to 10% from 2009 to 2013 [29]. Sosa et al. in 2004 reported that patients > 60 years of age undergoing laparoscopic bariatric surgery have higher but acceptable levels of morbidity and mortality and significant improvement in co-morbidities, and recommended it in elderly [30]. Papasavas et al. in 2004 showed that laparoscopic bariatric surgery is a safe and well tolerated surgical option for the treatment of morbid obesity in patients > 55 years [31].

2   Sleeve Gastrectomy: Procedure of Choice

The popularity of bariatric surgery in the elderly population increased exponentially with the advent of laparoscopic sleeve gastrectomy (LSG) as a stand-alone procedure in 2004. LSG with its technical simplicity, shorter operative time, and acceptable rate of co-morbidities improvement and weight loss is currently the surgery of choice for elderly obese patients worldwide. This has been recognized in the 2016 International Consensus Conference on Sleeve Gastrectomy [32]. Early studies by Van Rute et al. [33] and Leivonen et al. [34] that compared LSG in elderly with younger patients reported similar complications rate and acceptable reduction in weight and improvement in co-morbidities. The additional increase in popularity of LSG among elderly patients was also attributed to recognition of LSG by Medicare in the US in 2012 [35].

LSG can be performed safely in the elderly with an acceptable low rate of complications. These complications can be reduced further by careful patient selection [36]. The reduction of complications is also related to the performance of such procedures by an experienced surgeon within a Center of Excellence with appropriate resources, and with the availability of a multidisciplinary team.

Patient characteristics considered high risk for bariatric surgery are highly vari-able. In a group of 381 patients undergoing LSG Husain et al. found that male sex, preoperative $BMI \geq 60$ kg/m^2, smoker within the last year, deep vein thrombosis, therapeutic anticoagulation, and abnormal serum albumin < 3.5 g/dL are risk fac-tors associated with severe complications [37]. Also attempts were made to stratify the patient population risk by using standardized scoring systems. The obesity sur-gery mortality risk score (OS-MRS), proposed by De Maria et al. was used and validated in patients undergoing gastric bypass surgery [38]. More recent studies doubted the ability of such scores to accurately predict risk of postoperative com-plications in LSG [39, 40].

A bariatric specific score risk calculator was recently developed by the Metabolic and Bariatric Surgery Accreditation and Quality Improvement Program (MBSAQIP). This calculator uses 20 patient predictors, such as age, American Society of Anesthesiologists Physical Status classification, and preoperative body mass index (BMI) to predict the likelihood that patients will experience any of nine different outcomes within the first 30 days after an operation [41].

Optimization of co-morbidities before LSG can further reduce complications. It is highly important that all elderly individuals should have a comprehensive geriatric preoperative assessment before undergoing bariatric surgery in order to identify any potential risks and address accordingly. Batsis et al. detailed the ways to assess elderly individuals undergoing bariatric surgery and listed the character-istics of ideal candidates for bariatric surgery, which is beyond the scope of this chapter [42].

2.1   Intraoperative Difference in Elderly

No significant intraoperative differences have been described between elderly patients undergoing LSG and younger individuals. In fact, both young and older individuals undergoing bariatric surgery have similar length of operative procedure time [43]. Due to increase in tissue friability, decrease in physiologic reserves, and increased chances of adhesion formation in the elderly, operative time can be expected to be longer, but no differences were observed. Bartosiak et al. reported a mean operative time of 82.1 min for the elderly and 77 minutes for younger patients undergoing LSG [43].

The only exception pertains to the presence of a hiatal hernia, which could be more common in the elderly. In one study, 46.7% of older patients required hiatal hernia repair versus 8.3% in younger counterparts [44, 45]. Also, the intra-operative complications are comparable between the two populations [43]. There is, however, in some studies a potential but non-statistically significant trend of increased intraoperative complications in septuagenarians [45].

3   Postoperative Care in the Elderly

Based on the different physiologic needs and higher prevalence of comorbidities, the postoperative care of the elderly bariatric patient may differ. Among the different levels of care, likely more ICU admissions can be expected. ICU admission in general has been linked to both preoperative and perioperative factors. Older age, male gender, higher BMI, OSA and open surgery are at increased risk of requiring ICU admission. Less important is the type of procedure, as no difference was observed between LSG and gastric bypass in terms of need for ICU admission postoperatively [46, 47]. In a study by Khidir et al., the number of comorbidities, a diagnosis of OSA, and ASA score were found to predict the need for post-LSG ICU admission [48].

On the other end, ERAS protocol after bariatric surgery is associated with decreased length of stay, and cost reduction without increase in perioperative morbidity or readmission rates [49, 50]. Though ERAS has not been studied exclusively in elderly obese undergoing SG, its implementation in other laparoscopic gastrointestinal surgeries has been proven beneficial in older patients [51]. Given the simplicity of LSG, ERAS can be safely implemented in elderly patients undergoing LSG. Length of stay after LSG in elderly does not appear to be different as compared to the younger population. In fact, depending on institution protocols, it varies from 1 to 4 days [52, 53, 54, 55].

4   Postoperative Mortality and Morbidity

LSG in carefully selected patients in elderly is a very safe procedure. With increase in age, it is expected that complications and mortality rate will also increase [56]. However, multiple studies have demonstrated the safety of LSG in the elderly and a comparable rate of complications and mortality to the younger population.

Early 30-day mortality after LSG has remained very low and approaches zero [43]. Goldberg et al. reported a slightly higher rate of mortality in elderly, but the absolute increase is very small, much less than 1% [57, 58, 59].

Early complications remain a serious concern when operating on elderly patients. Increasing age is associated with increase in morbidity following LSG [60, 61]. Though increase is present, it is within the acceptable range and comparable to younger patients undergoing LSG. Early 30-day morbidity has been reported to be around 8 to 12% [45, 59, 55, 43, 62]. The increase is seen mainly in medical complications as opposed to surgical complications [61]. Susmallian et al. reported a total number of complications of 8.86% but among those, 3.10% were in relation to aggravation of previous medical diseases [63]. Also in a study by Charles et al., surgical complications in patients undergoing LSG less than 65 years and greater than 65 years of age were 1.4% and 1.3%, respectively, while medical complications increased from 3.10 to 6.60% as patients age moved above 65 years [61]. Among medical complications, cardiac, pulmonary, and renal are significantly more in elderly [59]. A recent study from Poland showed an early morbidity rate of 8.9% for elderly and 6.7% for younger patients, and the most common was bleeding in both groups [64].

Similar to early complications, late complications also occur at an acceptable rate in the elderly. GERD is one of the most common mid and long term complications of LSG. Due to an increased incidence of hiatal hernias in the elderly, it is expected to have more incidence of GERD in the elderly, but studies have shown comparable rates to younger patients [55]. Due to a decreased tendency in tissue healing abilities [65], higher BMI [66], loss of muscle mass [67] and high prevalence of comorbidities that increase intra-abdominal pressure, there is in general a higher prevalence of incisional hernias in the elderly [68]. But as with other laparoscopic procedures, LSG does not have an increased incidence of ventral hernia compared to younger individuals. Similarly the rate of dysphagia and stricture were not different between the elderly and the younger population [53].

Nevo et al. compared early versus late morbidity between elderly and younger patients undergoing LSG and showed similar rates of complications. Early morbidity rate was 10.6% among the elderly and 10.7% in younger patients with similar rate of leaks, re-bleeding and re-operation. Late complications (i.e. GERD, stricture, ventral hernia) were also similar [53].

Increased incidence of osteoporotic fractures has been reported after bariatric surgery. In general, this risk is less after LSG than after gastric bypass. Although this particular complication has not been directly studied in the elderly cohort, extrapolating from the results on a younger population, the risk of osteoporotic fractures should be lower in patients undergoing LSG compared to gastric bypass [69].

Elderly subjects are expected to be at higher risk of malnutrition [70], especially of micronutrients after bariatric surgery. However, close monitoring and proper supplementation can prevent and treat the above-mentioned deficiencies. In a recent study, there was no difference in micronutrient deficiencies between groups [71].

5 Postoperative Outcomes

5.1 Excess Body Weight Loss

The percentage of excess body weight loss (%EBWL) tends to be less after LSG in elderly as compared to younger patients [72]. %EBWL ranges from 50 to 70% at 12-month follow-up, which is statistically less than that in younger patients [43, 64, 63].

Although the weight loss tends to be inferior in the elderly, the amount of weight loss achieved and the consequent comorbidity resolution is still quite significant [73]. Several mechanisms have been offered to explain the more modest weight loss in the elderly. First of all, the increasing age is associated with decrease in body muscle mass and increase in fat mass, referred to as sarcopenic obesity [67]. Loss of muscle mass along with certain other factors [7, 8] results in decrease in resting metabolic rate. In addition, due to physical decline, active energy expenditure decreases rapidly with age and contributes significantly to overall decrease in energy expenditure [7]. Also, the ability of the body to mobilize fat decreases in the elderly and thus leads to accumulation of fat [74]. Hormonal alterations in females after menopause have been associated with an increase in abdominal adiposity and thus less %EBWL, as evidenced by greater %EBWL in premenopausal women compared to menopausal women after bariatric surgery [75]. All these factors are postulated to contribute to less %EBWL in the elderly but further studies need to be done to determine other factors and mechanisms that lead to less %EBWL in the elderly after bariatric surgery compared to younger counterparts.

5.2   Comorbidities Improvement

The positive metabolic effects of LSG have been well described in the elderly population. This improvement is more significant for elderly as they have more burden of co-morbidities and have much significant impact on quality of life compared to younger patients. Even in some elderly, individual reduction in the amount of medication used postoperatively is significantly higher compared to young patients [76]. Despite significant reduction in the severity of comorbidities, the total resolution of comorbidities have been reported to be less in elderly. This can be attributed to more permanent organ damage in elderly due gradual decline in physiological reserve with aging [77]. and presence of comorbidities for a longer time.

Arterial hypertension improvement has been reported in the range of 50 to 80% [78, 45, 55]. Interestingly, some studies reported a more significant improvement than in younger patients, based on the more significant reduction of HTN medications in the elderly [79]. In a recent study, HTN improvement for elderly was 73.1% for older and 69.2% for younger patients [64]. In another recent study 72.5% of older individuals showed improvement in HTN [58]. Froylich et al. reported a decrease in anti-hypertensive medication on average from 1.6 to 1.0 [52, 80].

Similarly to HTN, the use of diabetic medications decreases substantially in the elderly after LSG. Although compared to younger patients, the complete resolution of DM is less, the relative improvement of the disease is more substantial as the elderly have a more severe burden of disease itself. The improvement has been reported in the range of 30 to 80% [64, 55, 45]. In a study by Danan et al. 65% of older individuals reported improvement of diabetes [58], and 50% improvement by Bianco et al. [80].

As for other comorbidities, the elderly population presents an improvement in obstructive sleep apnea (OSA) to a less significant degree as compared to younger patients. Burchett et al. reported that 27% of elderly patients showed improvement or resolution compared to 37% of the younger group after LSG [55]. Navarrete et al. showed significantly higher improvement or resolution of OSA (60.8% of elderly) but still statistically lower than in younger patients (76%) [62]. Hyperlipidemia also follows the same pattern of improvement of HTN and DM after bariatric surgery [55, 53]. Danan et al. showed 47.1 improvement in hyperlipidemia in older individuals [58].

Elderly at baseline have more severe arthritis compared to younger patients. Complete resolution is less compared to younger patients, but the amount of improvement is greater in the elderly. In one recent study, improvement was seen in 27% of older and 34% of younger patients [55].

5.3 Quality of Life Improvement

Compared to in the younger population, obesity has more quality limiting effects on the elderly due to age-related frailty and burden of comorbidities. In a study by Lainas et al., using the SF-36 Questionnaire, significant improvement was seen in physical health and mental health scores [81]. As LSG is a safer bariatric procedure in elderly, it can lead to significant improvement in quality of life [82, 83].

With significant improvement in co-morbidities, it is expected that bariatric surgery will improve life expectancy in the elderly compared to non-surgical weight loss measures. However, more studies are needed before drawing definitive conclusions on the life expectancy of elderly patients after bariatric surgery.

6 LSG in Septuagenarians and Elderly Super Obese

Septuagenarians have higher baseline comorbidities; consequently, there is a potential for higher complication rate in such patients undergoing LSG as compared to those less than 70. This difference, however, is still within acceptable range, and the benefits of bariatric surgery are still present. As previously mentioned, the longer operative time reported was due to the higher incidence of hiatal hernia requiring concomitant repair. Also, the planned post-procedure ICU admission incidence increased in septuagenarians.

In a study by our institution, bariatric surgery in those age > 70 years was associated with a slightly higher but acceptable rate of complications [84, 85]. Pechman et al has reported that LSG in age > 70 years was associated with increased length of stay, slight increase in morbidity, unplanned or prolonged intubation, progressive renal insufficiency, and increased transfusion requirement [86]. Smith et al. showed that although the overall complications are more as compared to patients less than 69 years of age, the rate of severe complications is still less than 5% [87].

Weight loss and remission of comorbidities is modest but comparable to those less < 70 years of age [45]. A study from our institution evaluating LSG in a population of age > 75 reported a %EBWL of 56%, 50.9%, and 43.9% at 1– 2–, and 3–5 year follow-up, respectively. These weight loss results are slightly less than those in patients less than 70 years, but still significant [36, 85].

In conjunction with older age, a higher BMI is associated with higher complication rates [88]. Minhem et al. showed that complication rates were higher in older super obese patients (10%) compared to younger super obese patients (7%) [89]. In spite of these higher expected complications rates, the weight loss results are still significant. Daigle et al. reported EBWL of 48.3% after 37 months [90].

7   LSG Compared to Gastric Bypass in Elderly

Before the widespread use of LSG, laparoscopic Roux-en-Y gastric bypass (LRYGB) and laparoscopic adjustable gastric band (LAGB) were the most common procedures performed in the elderly. Similar to younger counterparts, the overall complications of the LRYGB in elderly present higher morbidity compared to LSG [61]. With the LAGB having fallen out of favor and the increased morbidity of the LRYGB, LSG has become the procedure of choice in the elderly.

In general, there is higher weight loss after LRYGB [91] and higher resolution of comorbidities compared to LSG, but at the cost of higher mortality and morbidity [92, 93, 94, 95].

A study by Janik et al. of 3371 matched patients showed that LRYGB compared to LSG in the elderly presents a higher leak rate (0.33 vs. 0.12%), 30 day readmission (6.08 vs. 3.74%), 30 day re-operation (2.49 vs. 0.89%), longer hospital stay (2.3 vs. 1.9%), increased operative time (122 vs. 84%) and increased rate of SSI (0.8 vs. 0.24) [96]. Similarly, Xu et al. reported that risk of both early and late complications are increased in the elderly. In this study, the elderly undergoing LRYGB are 1.75 and 1.63 times more prone to early and late complications as compared to the elderly undergoing LSG [97].

As previously reported, the %EBWL was less with LSG, but comparable to LRYGB. In a study by Moon et al., the elderly undergoing SG had a 60.8% EBWL after 24 months while those undergoing LRYGB had %EBWL of 67% after 24 months [95]. Regarding comorbidities improvement, RYGB has higher remission of type 2 diabetes mellitus (DM) and improvement in hyperlipidemia compared to LSG [98, 99]. Nevertheless, the ratio risk benefit with the SG remains superior to the LRYGB.

8   Conclusions

In conclusion, LSG in the elderly population seems safe and effective. Patient selection is paramount to reduce the morbidity of a population already at higher risk. Larger and longer studies are necessary to assess the benefits of bariatric surgery in terms of life expectancy.

References

1. WHO|Proposed working definition of an older person in Africa for the MDS Project. 2016 Oct 20 [cited 2020 May 3]. Available from: https://www.who.int/healthinfo/survey/ageingdefnolder/en/.
2. Roser M, Ortiz-Ospina E, Ritchie H. Life expectancy. Our World in Data [Internet]. 2013; Available from: https://ourworldindata.org/life-expectancy.
3. GHO|By category|Life expectancy and Healthy life expectancy—Data by WHO region. [cited 2020 May 3]; Available from: https://apps.who.int/gho/data/view.main.SDG2016LEXREGv?lang=en.
4. Woolf SH, Schoomaker H. Life expectancy and mortality rates in the United States, 1959–2017. JAMA [Internet]. 2019 Nov 26;322(20):1996–2016. Available from: http://dx.doi.org/https://doi.org/10.1001/jama.2019.16932.
5. World Population Ageing 2019: Highlights. Available from: https://www.un.org/en/development/desa/population/publications/pdf/ageing/WorldPopulationAgeing2019-Highlights.pdf.
6. Estimates P. Demographic turning points for the United States: Population projections for 2020 to 2060. Available from: https://www.census.gov/content/dam/Census/library/publications/2020/demo/p25-1144.pdf.
7. Alfonzo-González G, Doucet E, Bouchard C, Tremblay A. Greater than predicted decrease in resting energy expenditure with age: cross-sectional and longitudinal evidence. Eur J Clin Nutr [Internet]. 2006 Jan;60(1):18–24. Available from: http://dx.doi.org/https://doi.org/10.1038/sj.ejcn.1602262.
8. Johannsen DL, Ravussin E. Obesity in the elderly: is faulty metabolism to blame? Aging health [Internet]. 2010 Apr 1;6(2):159–67. Available from: http://dx.doi.org/https://doi.org/10.2217/ahe.10.12.
9. Fakhouri THI, Ogden CL, Carroll MD, Kit BK, Flegal KM. Prevalence of obesity among older adults in the United States, 2007–2010. NCHS Data Brief [Internet]. 2012 Sep;(106):1–8. Available from: https://www.ncbi.nlm.nih.gov/pubmed/23102091.
10. Alvis BD, Hughes CG. Physiology considerations in geriatric patients. Anesthesiol Clin [Internet]. 2015 Sep;33(3):447–56. Available from: http://dx.doi.org/https://doi.org/10.1016/j.anclin.2015.05.003.
11. Calhoun DA, Jones D, Textor S, Goff DC, Murphy TP, Toto RD, et al. Resistant hypertension: diagnosis, evaluation, and treatment: a scientific statement from the American Heart Association Professional Education Committee of the Council for High Blood Pressure Research. Circulation [Internet]. 2008 Jun 24;117(25):e510–26. Available from: http://dx.doi.org/https://doi.org/10.1161/CIRCULATIONAHA.108.189141.
12. Barnes AS. The epidemic of obesity and diabetes: trends and treatments. Tex Heart Inst J [Internet]. 2011;38(2):142–4. Available from: https://www.ncbi.nlm.nih.gov/pubmed/21494521.
13. Rexrode KM, Buring JE, Manson JE. Abdominal and total adiposity and risk of coronary heart disease in men. Int J Obes Relat Metab Disord [Internet]. 2001 Jul;25(7):1047–56. Available from: http://dx.doi.org/https://doi.org/10.1038/sj.ijo.0801615.

14. Abbott RD, Behrens GR, Sharp DS, Rodriguez BL, Burchfiel CM, Ross GW, et al. Body mass index and thromboembolic stroke in nonsmoking men in older middle age. The Honolulu Heart Program. Stroke [Internet]. 1994 Dec;25(12):2370–6. Available from: http://dx.doi.org/https://doi.org/10.1161/01.str.25.12.2370.

15. Cicuttini FM, Spector TD. Osteoarthritis in the aged. Epidemiological issues and optimal management. Drugs Aging [Internet]. 1995 May;6(5):409–20. Available from: http://dx.doi.org/https://doi.org/10.2165/00002512-199506050-00007.

16. Riedner CE, Rhoden EL, Ribeiro EP, Fuchs SC. Central obesity is an independent predictor of erectile dysfunction in older men. J Urol [Internet]. 2006 Oct;176(4 Pt 1):1519–23. Available from: http://dx.doi.org/https://doi.org/10.1016/j.juro.2006.06.049.

17. Hsu C-Y, Iribarren C, McCulloch CE, Darbinian J, Go AS. Risk factors for end-stage renal disease: 25-year follow-up. Arch Intern Med [Internet]. 2009 Feb 23;169(4):342–50. Available from: http://dx.doi.org/https://doi.org/10.1001/archinternmed.2008.605.

18. Gustafson D, Rothenberg E, Blennow K, Steen B, Skoog I. An 18-year follow-up of overweight and risk of Alzheimer disease. Arch Intern Med [Internet]. 2003 Jul 14;163(13):1524–8. Available from: http://dx.doi.org/https://doi.org/10.1001/archinte.163.13.1524.

19. Thomas DR, Ritchie CS. Preoperative assessment of older adults. J Am Geriatr Soc [Internet]. 1995 Jul;43(7):811–21. Available from: http://dx.doi.org/https://doi.org/10.1111/j.1532-5415.1995.tb07058.x.

20. Karakoc D. Surgery of the Elderly Patient. Int Surg [Internet]. 2016 Mar;101(3–4):161–6. Available from: https://www.internationalsurgery.org/doi/https://doi.org/10.9738/INTSURG-D-15-00261.1.

21. Turrentine FE, Wang H, Simpson VB, Jones RS. Surgical risk factors, morbidity, and mortality in elderly patients. J Am Coll Surg [Internet]. 2006 Dec;203(6):865–77. Available from: http://dx.doi.org/https://doi.org/10.1016/j.jamcollsurg.2006.08.026.

22. Susmallian S, Barnea R, Weiss Y, Raziel A. Outcome of bariatric surgery in older patients. Surg Obes Relat Dis [Internet]. 2018 Nov;14(11):1705–13. Available from: http://dx.doi.org/https://doi.org/10.1016/j.soard.2018.08.007.

23. Aminian A, Brethauer SA, Kirwan JP, Kashyap SR, Burguera B, Schauer PR. How safe is metabolic/diabetes surgery? Diabetes Obes Metab [Internet]. 2015 Feb;17(2):198–201. Available from: http://dx.doi.org/https://doi.org/10.1111/dom.12405.

24. Printen KJ, Mason EE. Gastric bypass for morbid obesity in patients more than fifty years of age. Surg Gynecol Obstet [Internet]. 1977 Feb;144(2):192–4. Available from: https://www.ncbi.nlm.nih.gov/pubmed/835056.

25. Health implications of obesity. National Institutes of Health Consensus Development Conference Statement. Ann Intern Med [Internet]. 1985 Dec;103(6 (Pt 2)):1073–7. Available from: https://www.ncbi.nlm.nih.gov/pubmed/4062128.

26. Grace DM. Patient selection for obesity surgery. Gastroenterology Clinics of North America [Internet]. 1987 Aug 31;16(3):399–413. Available from: https://europepmc.org/article/med/3325422.

27. Livingston EH, Huerta S, Arthur D, Lee S, De Shields S, Heber D. Male gender is a predictor of morbidity and age a predictor of mortality for patients undergoing gastric bypass surgery. Ann Surg [Internet]. 2002 Nov;236(5):576–82. Available from: http://dx.doi.org/https://doi.org/10.1097/00000658-200211000-00007.

28. Flum DR, Salem L, Elrod JAB, Dellinger EP, Cheadle A, Chan L. Early mortality among Medicare beneficiaries undergoing bariatric surgical procedures. JAMA [Internet]. 2005 Oct 19;294(15):1903–8. Available from: http://dx.doi.org/https://doi.org/10.1001/jama.294.15.1903.

29. Gebhart A, Young MT, Nguyen NT. Bariatric surgery in the elderly: 2009–2013. Surg Obes Relat Dis [Internet]. 2015 Mar;11(2):393–8. Available from: http://dx.doi.org/https://doi.org/10.1016/j.soard.2014.04.014.

30. Sosa JL, Pombo H, Pallavicini H, Ruiz-Rodriguez M. Laparoscopic gastric bypass beyond age 60. Obes Surg [Internet]. 2004 Nov;14(10):1398–401. Available from: http://dx.doi.org/https://doi.org/10.1381/0960892042583833.

31. Papasavas PK, Gagné DJ, Kelly J, Caushaj PF. Laparoscopic Roux-En-Y gastric bypass is a safe and effective operation for the treatment of morbid obesity in patients older than 55 years. Obes Surg [Internet]. 2004 Sep;14(8):1056–61. Available from: http://dx.doi.org/https://doi.org/10.1381/0960892041975541.

32. Gagner M, Hutchinson C, Rosenthal R. Fifth International Consensus Conference: current status of sleeve gastrectomy. Surg Obes Relat Dis [Internet]. 2016 May;12(4):750–6. Available from: http://dx.doi.org/https://doi.org/10.1016/j.soard.2016.01.022.

33. van Rutte PWJ, Smulders JF, de Zoete JP, Nienhuijs SW. Sleeve gastrectomy in older obese patients. Surg Endosc [Internet]. 2013 Jun;27(6):2014–9. Available from: http://dx.doi.org/https://doi.org/10.1007/s00464-012-2703-8.

34. Leivonen MK, Juuti A, Jaser N, Mustonen H. Laparoscopic sleeve gastrectomy in patients over 59 years: early recovery and 12-month follow-up. Obes Surg [Internet]. 2011 Aug;21(8):1180–7. Available from: http://dx.doi.org/https://doi.org/10.1007/s11695-011-0454-6.

35. National Coverage Determination (NCD) for Bariatric Surgery for Treatment of Morbid Obesity (100.1) [Internet]. [cited 2020 Jun 6]. Available from: https://www.cms.gov/medicare-coverage-database/details/ncd-details.aspx?NCDId=57&ncdver=4&bc=AgAAgAAAAAAAA%3D%3D&.

36. Nor Hanipah Z, Punchai S, Karas LA, Szomstein S, Rosenthal RJ, Brethauer SA, et al. The outcome of bariatric surgery in patients aged 75 years and older. Obes Surg [Internet]. 2018 Jun;28(6):1498–503. Available from: http://dx.doi.org/https://doi.org/10.1007/s11695-017-3020-z.

37. Husain F, Jeong IH, Spight D, Wolfe B, Mattar SG. Risk factors for early postoperative complications after bariatric surgery. Ann Surg Treat Res [Internet]. 2018 Aug;95(2):100–10. Available from: http://dx.doi.org/https://doi.org/10.4174/astr.2018.95.2.100.

38. DeMaria EJ, Portenier D, Wolfe L. Obesity surgery mortality risk score: proposal for a clinically useful score to predict mortality risk in patients undergoing gastric bypass. Surg Obes Relat Dis [Internet]. 2007 Mar;3(2):134–40. Available from: http://dx.doi.org/https://doi.org/10.1016/j.soard.2007.01.005.

39. Coblijn UK, Lagarde SM, de Raaff CAL, de Castro SM, van Tets WF, Jaap Bonjer H, et al. Evaluation of the obesity surgery mortality risk score for the prediction of postoperative complications after primary and revisional laparoscopic Roux-en-Y gastric bypass. Surg Obes Relat Dis [Internet]. 2016 Sep;12(8):1504–12. Available from: http://dx.doi.org/https://doi.org/10.1016/j.soard.2016.04.003.

40. García-García ML, Martín-Lorenzo JG, Lirón-Ruiz R, Torralba-Martínez JA, García-López JA, Aguayo-Albasini JL. Failure of the Obesity Surgery Mortality Risk Score (OS-MRS) to Predict Postoperative Complications After Bariatric Surgery. A Single-Center Series and Systematic Review. Obes Surg [Internet]. 2017 Jun;27(6):1423–9. Available from: http://dx.doi.org/https://doi.org/10.1007/s11695-016-2506-4.

41. Bariatric Surgical Risk/Benefit Calculator [Internet]. American College of Surgeons. [cited 2020 May 14]. Available from: https://www.facs.org/quality-programs/mbsaqip/calculator.

42. Batsis JA, Dolkart KM. Evaluation of older Adults with obesity for bariatric surgery: Geriatricians' perspective. Journal of Clinical Gerontology and Geriatrics [Internet]. 2015 Jun 1;6(2):45–53. Available from: https://www.sciencedirect.com/science/article/pii/S2210833515000027.

43. Bartosiak K, Różańska-Walędziak A, Walędziak M, Kowalewski P, Paśnik K, Janik MR. The Safety and Benefits of Laparoscopic Sleeve Gastrectomy in Elderly Patients: a Case-Control Study. Obes Surg [Internet]. 2019 Jul;29(7):2233–7. Available from: http://dx.doi.org/https://doi.org/10.1007/s11695-019-03830-7.

44. Oor JE, Koetje JH, Roks DJ, Nieuwenhuijs VB, Hazebroek EJ. Laparoscopic Hiatal Hernia Repair in the Elderly Patient. World J Surg [Internet]. 2016 Jun;40(6):1404–11. Available from: http://dx.doi.org/https://doi.org/10.1007/s00268-016-3428-y.

45. Al-Kurd A, Grinbaum R, Mordechay-Heyn T, Asli S, Abubeih A 'a, Mizrahi I, et al. Outcomes of Sleeve Gastrectomy in Septuagenarians. Obes Surg [Internet]. 2018 Dec;28(12):3895–901. Available from: http://dx.doi.org/https://doi.org/10.1007/s11695-018-3418-2.

46. Morgan DJR, Ho KM, Armstrong J, Baker S. Incidence and risk factors for intensive care unit admission after bariatric surgery: a multicentre population-based cohort study. Br J Anaesth [Internet]. 2015 Dec;115(6):873–82. Available from: http://dx.doi.org/https://doi.org/10.1093/bja/aev364.

47. Nofal WH, Amer AM, Mansour WA. Proposal of a score to detect the need for postoperative intensive care unit admission after bariatric surgery. Egyptian Journal of Anaesthesia [Internet]. 2017 Oct 1;33(4):351–5. Available from: https://www.sciencedirect.com/science/article/pii/S1110184917302350.

48. Khidir N, El-Matbouly M, Al Kuwari M, Gagner M, Bashah M. Incidence, Indications, and Predictive Factors for ICU Admission in Elderly, High-Risk Patients Undergoing Laparoscopic Sleeve Gastrectomy. Obes Surg [Internet]. 2018 Sep;28(9):2603–8. Available from: http://dx.doi.org/https://doi.org/10.1007/s11695-018-3221-0.

49. Małczak P, Pisarska M, Piotr M, Wysocki M, Budzyński A, Pędziwiatr M. Enhanced Recovery after Bariatric Surgery: Systematic Review and Meta-Analysis. Obes Surg [Internet]. 2017 Jan;27(1):226–35. Available from: http://dx.doi.org/https://doi.org/10.1007/s11695-016-2438-z.

50. Lam J, Suzuki T, Bernstein D, Zhao B, Maeda C, Pham T, et al. An ERAS protocol for bariatric surgery: is it safe to discharge on post-operative day 1? Surg Endosc [Internet]. 2019 Feb;33(2):580–6. Available from: http://dx.doi.org/https://doi.org/10.1007/s00464-018-6368-9.

51. Crucitti A, Mazzari A, Tomaiuolo PM, Dionisi P, Diamanti P, Di Flumeri G, et al. Enhanced Recovery after Surgery (ERAS) is safe, feasible and effective in elderly patients undergoing laparoscopic colorectal surgery: results of a prospective single center study. Minerva Chir [Internet]. 2020 Feb 20; Available from: http://dx.doi.org/https://doi.org/10.23736/S0026-4733.20.08275-9.

52. Froylich D, Sadeh O, Mizrahi H, Kafri N, Pascal G, Daigle CR, et al. Midterm outcomes of sleeve gastrectomy in the elderly. Surg Obes Relat Dis [Internet]. 2018 Oct;14(10):1495–500. Available from: http://dx.doi.org/https://doi.org/10.1016/j.soard.2018.07.020.

53. Nevo N, Eldar SM, Lessing Y, Sabo E, Nachmany I, Hazzan D. Sleeve Gastrectomy in the Elderly. Obes Facts [Internet]. 2019 Oct 14;12(5):502–8. Available from: http://dx.doi.org/https://doi.org/10.1159/000502697.

54. Vinan-Vega M, Diaz Vico T, Elli EF. Bariatric Surgery in the Elderly Patient: Safety and Short-time Outcome. A Case Match Analysis. Obes Surg [Internet]. 2019 Mar;29(3):1007–11. Available from: http://dx.doi.org/https://doi.org/10.1007/s11695-018-03633-2.

55. Burchett MA, McKenna DT, Selzer DJ, Choi JH, Mattar SG. Laparoscopic sleeve gastrectomy is safe and effective in elderly patients: a comparative analysis. Obes Surg [Internet]. 2015 Feb;25(2):222–8. Available from: http://dx.doi.org/https://doi.org/10.1007/s11695-014-1421-9.

56. Arnold MR, Schlosser KA, Otero J, Prasad T, Lincourt AE, Gersin KS, et al. Laparoscopic Weight Loss Surgery in the Elderly: An ACS NSQIP Study on the Effect of Age on Outcomes. Am Surg [Internet]. 2019 Mar 1;85(3):273–9. Available from: https://www.ncbi.nlm.nih.gov/pubmed/30947773.

57. Goldberg I, Yang J, Nie L, Bates AT, Docimo S Jr, Pryor AD, et al. Safety of bariatric surgery in patients older than 65 years. Surg Obes Relat Dis [Internet]. 2019 Aug;15(8):1380–7. Available from: http://dx.doi.org/https://doi.org/10.1016/j.soard.2019.05.016.

58. Danan M, Nedelcu A, Noel P, Zulian V, Carandina S, Nedelcu M. Operative morbidity of laparoscopic sleeve gastrectomy in subjects older than age 65. Surg Obes Relat Dis [Internet]. 2019 Jan;15(1):8–11. Available from: http://dx.doi.org/https://doi.org/10.1016/j.soard.2018.10.009.

59. Hajer AA, Wolff S, Benedix F, Hukauf M, Manger T, Stroh C, et al. Trends in Early Morbidity and Mortality after Sleeve Gastrectomy in Patients over 60 Years : Retrospective Review and Data Analysis of the German Bariatric Surgery Registry. Obes Surg [Internet]. 2018 Jul;28(7):1831–7. Available from: http://dx.doi.org/https://doi.org/10.1007/s11695-018-3110-6.

60. Haskins IN, Ju T, Whitlock AE, Rivas L, Amdur RL, Lin PP, et al. Older Age Confers a Higher Risk of 30-Day Morbidity and Mortality Following Laparoscopic Bariatric Surgery: an Analysis of the Metabolic and Bariatric Surgery Quality Improvement Program. Obes Surg [Internet]. 2018 Sep;28(9):2745–52. Available from: http://dx.doi.org/https://doi.org/10.1007/s11695-018-3233-9.

61. Qin C, Luo B, Aggarwal A, De Oliveira G, Kim JYS. Advanced age as an independent predictor of perioperative risk after laparoscopic sleeve gastrectomy (LSG). Obes Surg [Internet]. 2015 Mar;25(3):406–12. Available from: http://dx.doi.org/https://doi.org/10.1007/s11695-014-1462-0.

62. Navarrete A, Corcelles R, Del Gobbo GD, Perez S, Vidal J, Lacy A. Sleeve gastrectomy in the elderly: A case-control study with long-term follow-up of 3 years. Surg Obes Relat Dis [Internet]. 2017 Apr;13(4):575–80. Available from: http://dx.doi.org/https://doi.org/10.1016/j.soard.2016.11.030.

63. Susmallian S, Raziel A, Barnea R, Paran H. Bariatric surgery in older adults: Should there be an age limit? Medicine [Internet]. 2019 Jan;98(3):e13824. Available from: https://dx.doi.org/10.1097/MD.0000000000013824.

64. Dowgiałło-Wnukiewicz N, Janik MR, Lech P, Major P, Pędziwiatr M, Kowalewski PK, et al. Outcomes of sleeve gastrectomy in patients older than 60 years: a multicenter matched case-control study. Wideochir Inne Tech Maloinwazyjne [Internet]. 2020 Mar;15(1):123–8. Available from: http://dx.doi.org/https://doi.org/10.5114/wiitm.2019.81450.

65. Gerstein AD, Phillips TJ, Rogers GS, Gilchrest BA. Wound healing and aging. Dermatol Clin [Internet]. 1993 Oct;11(4):749–57. Available from: https://www.ncbi.nlm.nih.gov/pubmed/8222358.

66. Sauerland S, Korenkov M, Kleinen T, Arndt M, Paul A. Obesity is a risk factor for recurrence after incisional hernia repair. Hernia [Internet]. 2004 Feb;8(1):42–6. Available from: http://dx.doi.org/https://doi.org/10.1007/s10029-003-0161-x.

67. Zamboni M, Rubele S, Rossi AP. Sarcopenia and obesity. Curr Opin Clin Nutr Metab Care [Internet]. 2019 Jan;22(1):13–9. Available from: http://dx.doi.org/https://doi.org/10.1097/MCO.0000000000000519.

68. Caglià P, Tracia A, Borzì L, Amodeo L, Tracia L, Veroux M, et al. Incisional hernia in the elderly: risk factors and clinical considerations. Int J Surg [Internet]. 2014 Aug 23;12 Suppl 2:S164–9. Available from: http://dx.doi.org/https://doi.org/10.1016/j.ijsu.2014.08.357.

69. Paccou J, Martignène N, Lespessailles E, Babykina E, Pattou F, Cortet B, et al. Gastric Bypass But Not Sleeve Gastrectomy Increases Risk of Major Osteoporotic Fracture: French Population-Based Cohort Study. J Bone Miner Res [Internet]. 2020 Mar 18; Available from: http://dx.doi.org/https://doi.org/10.1002/jbmr.4012.

70. Hoffman R. Micronutrient deficiencies in the elderly - could ready meals be part of the solution? J Nutr Sci [Internet]. 2017 Jan 12;6:e2. Available from: http://dx.doi.org/https://doi.org/10.1017/jns.2016.42.

71. Faucher P, Aron-Wisnewsky J, Ciangura C, Genser L, Torcivia A, Bouillot J-L, et al. Changes in Body Composition, Comorbidities, and Nutritional Status Associated with Lower Weight Loss After Bariatric Surgery in Older Subjects. Obes Surg [Internet]. 2019 Nov;29(11):3589–95. Available from: http://dx.doi.org/https://doi.org/10.1007/s11695-019-04037-6.

72. Soto FC, Gari V, de la Garza JR, Szomstein S, Rosenthal RJ. Sleeve gastrectomy in the elderly: a safe and effective procedure with minimal morbidity and mortality. Obes Surg [Internet]. 2013 Sep;23(9):1445–9. Available from: http://dx.doi.org/https://doi.org/10.1007/s11695-013-0992-1.

73. Ochner CN, Teixeira J, Geary N, Asarian L. Greater short-term weight loss in women 20–45 versus 55–65 years of age following bariatric surgery. Obes Surg [Internet]. 2013 Oct;23(10):1650–4. Available from: http://dx.doi.org/https://doi.org/10.1007/s11695-013-0984-1.

74. Lipid metabolism in the elderly [Internet]. [cited 2020 May 1]. Available from: https://www.nature.com/articles/1601033.pdf?origin=ppub.

75. Toth MJ, Tchernof A, Sites CK, Poehlman ET. Effect of menopausal status on body composition and abdominal fat distribution. Int J Obes Relat Metab Disord [Internet]. 2000 Feb;24(2):226–31. Available from: http://dx.doi.org/https://doi.org/10.1038/sj.ijo.0801118.

76. Kaplan U, Penner S, Farrokhyar F, Andruszkiewicz N, Breau R, Gmora S, et al. Bariatric Surgery in the Elderly Is Associated with Similar Surgical Risks and Significant Long-Term Health Benefits. Obes Surg [Internet]. 2018 Aug;28(8):2165–70. Available from: http://dx.doi.org/https://doi.org/10.1007/s11695-018-3160-9.

77. Clegg A, Young J, Iliffe S, Rikkert MO, Rockwood K. Frailty in elderly people. Lancet [Internet]. 2013 Mar 2;381(9868):752–62. Available from: http://dx.doi.org/https://doi.org/10.1016/S0140-6736(12)62167-9.

78. Giordano S, Victorzon M. Bariatric surgery in elderly patients: a systematic review. Clin Interv Aging [Internet]. 2015 Oct 13;10:1627–35. Available from: http://dx.doi.org/https://doi.org/10.2147/CIA.S70313.

79. Luppi CR-O, Balagué C, Targarona EM, Mocanu S, Bollo J, Martínez C, et al. Laparoscopic sleeve gastrectomy in patients over 60 years: impact of age on weight loss and co-morbidity improvement. Surg Obes Relat Dis [Internet]. 2015 Mar;11(2):296–301. Available from: http://dx.doi.org/https://doi.org/10.1016/j.soard.2014.05.021.

80. Bianco P, Rizzuto A, Velotti N, Bocchetti A, Manzolillo D, Maietta P, et al. Results following laparoscopic sleeve gastrectomy in elderly obese patients: a single center experience with follow-up at three years. Minerva Chir [Internet]. 2020 Apr;75(2):77–82. Available from: http://dx.doi.org/https://doi.org/10.23736/S0026-4733.18.07757-X.

81. Lainas P, Dammaro C, Gaillard M, Donatelli G, Tranchart H, Dagher I. Safety and short-term outcomes of laparoscopic sleeve gastrectomy for patients over 65 years old with severe obesity. Surg Obes Relat Dis [Internet]. 2018 Jul;14(7):952–9. Available from: http://dx.doi.org/https://doi.org/10.1016/j.soard.2018.03.002.

82. Major P, Matłok M, Pędziwiatr M, Migaczewski M, Budzyński P, Stanek M, et al. Quality of Life After Bariatric Surgery. Obes Surg [Internet]. 2015 Sep;25(9):1703–10. Available from: http://dx.doi.org/https://doi.org/10.1007/s11695-015-1601-2.

83. Janik MR, Rogula T, Bielecka I, Kwiatkowski A, Paśnik K. Quality of Life and Bariatric Surgery: Cross-Sectional Study and Analysis of Factors Influencing Outcome. Obes Surg [Internet]. 2016 Dec;26(12):2849–55. Available from: http://dx.doi.org/https://doi.org/10.1007/s11695-016-2220-2.

84. Ramirez A, Roy M, Hidalgo JE, Szomstein S, Rosenthal RJ. Outcomes of bariatric surgery in patients >70 years old. Surg Obes Relat Dis [Internet]. 2012 Jul;8(4):458–62. Available from: http://dx.doi.org/https://doi.org/10.1016/j.soard.2012.04.001.

85. Parmar C, Mahawar KK, Carr WRJ, Schroeder N, Balupuri S, Small PK. Bariatric Surgery in Septuagenarians: a Comparison with <60 Year Olds. Obes Surg [Internet]. 2017 Dec;27(12):3165–9. Available from: http://dx.doi.org/https://doi.org/10.1007/s11695-017-2739-x.
86. Pechman DM, Muñoz Flores F, Kinkhabwala CM, Salas R, Berk RH, Weithorn D, et al. Bariatric surgery in the elderly: outcomes analysis of patients over 70 using the ACS-NSQIP database. Surg Obes Relat Dis [Internet]. 2019 Nov;15(11):1923–32. Available from: http://dx.doi.org/https://doi.org/10.1016/j.soard.2019.08.011.
87. Smith ME, Bacal D, Bonham AJ, Varban OA, Carlin AM, Ghaferi AA, et al. Perioperative and 1-year outcomes of bariatric surgery in septuagenarians: implications for patient selection. Surg Obes Relat Dis [Internet]. 2019 Oct;15(10):1805–11. Available from: http://dx.doi.org/https://doi.org/10.1016/j.soard.2019.08.002.
88. Elbahrawy A, Bougie A, Loiselle S-E, Demyttenaere S, Court O, Andalib A. Medium to long-term outcomes of bariatric surgery in older adults with super obesity. Surg Obes Relat Dis [Internet]. 2018 Apr;14(4):470–6. Available from: http://dx.doi.org/https://doi.org/10.1016/j.soard.2017.11.008.
89. Minhem MA, Safadi BY, Habib RH, Raad EPB, Alami RS. Increased adverse outcomes after laparoscopic sleeve gastrectomy in older super-obese patients: analysis of American College of Surgeons National Surgical Quality Improvement Program Database. Surg Obes Relat Dis [Internet]. 2018 Oct;14(10):1463–70. Available from: http://dx.doi.org/https://doi.org/10.1016/j.soard.2018.06.023.
90. Daigle CR, Andalib A, Corcelles R, Cetin D, Schauer PR, Brethauer SA. Bariatric and metabolic outcomes in the super-obese elderly. Surg Obes Relat Dis [Internet]. 2016 Jan;12(1):132–7. Available from: http://dx.doi.org/https://doi.org/10.1016/j.soard.2015.04.006.
91. Praveenraj P, Gomes RM, Kumar S, Perumal S, Senthilnathan P, Parthasarathi R, et al. Comparison of weight loss outcomes 1 year after sleeve gastrectomy and Roux-en-Y gastric bypass in patients aged above 50 years. J Minim Access Surg [Internet]. 2016 Jul;12(3):220–5. Available from: http://dx.doi.org/https://doi.org/10.4103/0972-9941.183481.
92. Poelemeijer YQM, Liem RSL, Våge V, Mala T, Sundbom M, Ottosson J, et al. Gastric bypass versus sleeve gastrectomy: Patient selection and short-term outcome of 47,101 primary operations from the Swedish, Norwegian, and Dutch national quality registries. Ann Surg [Internet]. 2019 Mar 20; Available from: http://dx.doi.org/10.1097/SLA.0000000000003279.
93. Wang Y, Yi X, Li Q, Zhang J, Wang Z. The Effectiveness and safety of sleeve gastrectomy in the obese elderly patients: A systematic review and meta-analysis. Obes Surg [Internet]. 2016 Dec;26(12):3023–30. Available from: http://dx.doi.org/https://doi.org/10.1007/s11695-016-2396-5.
94. Giordano S, Victorzon M. Laparoscopic roux-en-y gastric bypass in elderly patients (60 Years or Older): A Meta-Analysis of Comparative Studies. Scand J Surg [Internet]. 2018 Mar;107(1):6–13. Available from: http://dx.doi.org/https://doi.org/10.1177/1457496917731183.
95. Moon RC, Kreimer F, Teixeira AF, Campos JM, Ferraz A, Jawad MA. Morbidity rates and weight loss after roux-en-y gastric bypass, sleeve gastrectomy, and adjustable gastric banding in patients older than 60 years old: which procedure to choose? Obes Surg [Internet]. 2016 Apr;26(4):730–6. Available from: http://dx.doi.org/https://doi.org/10.1007/s11695-015-1824-2.
96. Janik MR, Mustafa RR, Rogula TG, Alhaj Saleh A, Abbas M, Khaitan L. Safety of laparoscopic sleeve gastrectomy and Roux-en-Y gastric bypass in elderly patients - analysis of the MBSAQIP. Surg Obes Relat Dis [Internet]. 2018 Sep;14(9):1276–82. Available from: http://dx.doi.org/https://doi.org/10.1016/j.soard.2018.04.008.

97. Xu C, Yan T, Liu H, Mao R, Peng Y, Liu Y. Comparative safety and effectiveness of roux-en-y gastric bypass and sleeve gastrectomy in obese elder patients: a systematic review and meta-analysis. Obes Surg [Internet]. 2020 Apr 10; Available from: https://dx.doi.org/10.1007/s11695-020-04577-2.

98. Gray KD, Moore MD, Bellorin O, Abelson JS, Dakin G, Zarnegar R, et al. Increased metabolic benefit for obese, elderly patients undergoing roux-en-y gastric bypass vs sleeve gastrectomy. Obes Surg [Internet]. 2018 Mar;28(3):636–42. Available from: http://dx.doi.org/https://doi.org/10.1007/s11695-017-2904-2.

99. Huang C-K, Garg A, Kuao H-C, Chang P-C, Hsin M-C. Bariatric surgery in old age: a comparative study of laparoscopic roux-en-y gastric bypass and sleeve gastrectomy in an Asia centre of excellence. J Biomed Res [Internet]. 2015 Apr;29(2):118–24. Available from: http://dx.doi.org/https://doi.org/10.7555/JBR.29.20140108.

Postoperative Diet Progression for Laparoscopic Sleeve Gastrectomy

Dana AlTarrah

1   Introduction

Nutritional management and regular postoperative follow-up are vital for patients undergoing bariatric surgery and has been found to impact weight loss and long-term weight maintenance. Registered dietitians (RDs) and clinical nutritionists play an important role in establishing a bariatric dietary protocol to maximize weight loss, meet postoperative nutritional requirements, manage food intolerances and prevent nutritional complications [1–3].

To date, evidence-based diet progression guidelines following bariatric surgery are lacking, and although some guidelines have been published, there is no standardization for the postoperative nutritional management of bariatric patients [2–4]. Moreover, there is limited evidence on diet progression recommendations specifically for laparoscopic sleeve gastrectomy (LSG) patients, thus postoperative dietary guidelines tailored for Roux-en-Y Gastric Bypass (RYGB) are likewise recommended for LSG patients.

Dietary progression stages are highly patient-dependent and are predominantly personalized to meet patient's individual tolerance and nutritional requirements [4–6]. Hence, postoperative nutrition management protocols adopted by RDs and surgeons are found to differ in relation to the duration a patient remains at each diet stage and the type of fluids/foods offered [7].

Patients undergoing weight loss surgery including LSG must be prepared for lifelong dietary, behavioral and lifestyle changes. Routine follow-up appointments with RDs are crucial to ensure long-term postoperative success and reduce the risk

D. AlTarrah (✉)
Faculty of Public Health, Kuwait University, Kuwait City, Kuwait
e-mail: danah.altarrah@ku.edu.kw

S. Al-Sabah et al. (eds.), *Laparoscopic Sleeve Gastrectomy*,
https://doi.org/10.1007/978-3-030-57373-7_35

of potential postoperative complications [8, 9]. In agreement with postoperative Center of Excellence recommendations, follow-up appointments should be scheduled 1 to 2 weeks following surgery, and continue regularly every month until 3 months, followed by a 6 month, 9 month and yearly follow up, thereafter [4, 10].

2   Diet Progression: Stages

Dietary progression stages following LSG are based on nutritional needs and a gradual transition in food texture and consistency over a period of 1 to 2 months, until regular textures and solids are reintroduced and well tolerated [2, 4]. Postoperatively, patients are advised to slowly and gradually begin introducing clear liquids (non-calorie, decaffeinated, sugar-free, non-carbonated) for the first 1 to 2 days, and later advance to a full liquid diet (1 to 2 weeks) which includes fluids rich in protein, carbohydrates and dietary nutrients. Approximately 14 days following surgery, patients are advanced to pureed and soft solids for 3 to 4 weeks, and lastly firmer regular foods are introduced as tolerated by the patient. Suggested guidelines for the quantity and frequency of foods and/or fluids at each stage are displayed in Table 1. However, as mentioned earlier the progression of patients from one stage to the next, and the pace and duration spent at each diet stage are highly patient-dependent, even among patients undergoing the same weight loss procedure. In particular, due to the long surgical staple line and high prevalence of nausea reported following LSG, a slow and gradual diet progression plan is highly recommended for LSG patients [4–6]. Table 2 provides an in-depth description of diet stages for LSG patients.

Food intolerances are commonly experienced by bariatric patients during the early postoperative period. Although, food tolerances are found to vary widely between LSG patients, intolerances are found to peak at 6 months, and progressively improve. Therefore, it is necessary that patients are advised to chew food efficiently, and to provide patients with guidelines regarding foods that are frequently reported to increase intolerances, such as rice, milk, certain vegetables and red meats [11, 12]. Frequent postoperative nutritional follow-up and support is highly recommended to advise and educate patients about difficult foods and substitutions for such foods. For instance, rice may be replaced with potatoes, milk with yoghurt, and tougher red meats with white tender meat (poultry and fish), to ensure that patients consume a varied and nutritionally balanced diet from all food groups as the patients gradually introduce solids [7].

During the early postoperative diet stages, many patients may particularly develop an intolerance to protein-rich foods due to inadequate mastication, and a decrease in hydrochloric acid and proteolytic enzymes (e.g. pepsinogen). As a result, protein deficiency is a commonly reported macronutrient complication associated with LSG [4, 13]. Although protein recommendations for LSG patients remain unclear, patients are advised to include 60–80 g of protein in their diet [14]. However, in the case that patients are unable to incorporate protein-rich foods, protein supplementation (whey, whey isolate, or soy protein powder;

Table 1 Diet stages postoperatively and suggested foods/fluids and quantities

Diet stage	Postoperative day	Duration	Fluids/Foods	Amount and Frequency
Clear liquid	1 to 2 days	1 to 2 days	Water Coconut water Clear broth Herbal tea	30 – 50 ml every 20 – 30 min
Full liquid	2 to 16 days	10 to 14 days	Water Coconut water Blended and strained soup Skimmed milk and dairy alternatives Fruit juice diluted in water	80 – 100 ml every 60 – 90 min
Pureed	16 to 30 days	10 to 14 days	Water Skimmed milk blended with fruit Bread or biscuits soaked in milk Mashed food (rice, chicken, meat) Porridge Mashed and cooked fruit Blended grains	100 – 150 ml every 2 h
Soft	30 to 60 days	Less than 14 days	Water Cooked vegetables Boiled eggs and cooked meat Soft bread Milk and skimmed dairy Soft fruit	150 ml every 2 h

Adapted from Mechanick, J. I. et al., 2013, Aills, L. et al., 2008

25–30 g protein per serving) is regularly integrated within each dietary progression stage, taking into account patients' individual intake and nutritional needs. Appropriate chewing and meal portioning training sessions may be provided by RDs and the multidisciplinary nutrition education team to ensure protein intake is adequate, and patients meet their recommended daily fluid intake [3, 4].

Following the early diet progression stages, patients are advised to follow a nutritional pyramid developed by Moizé et al.,[14] to establish lifelong healthy dietary habits. The pyramid is comprised of five levels. The base focuses on the importance physical activity, vitamin and mineral supplementation, and adequate hydration. Patients are largely recommended to incorporate foods within the second and third level, which includes: protein-rich foods (meats, fish, dairy and eggs) to meet their recommended protein intake (60–80 g per day), in addition to fruits, vegetables and vegetable oils. Within the upper levels, patients are advised to limit their consumption of carbohydrate rich foods, such as cereals and legumes, and avoid foods high in saturated and trans fats, cholesterol, sugar, salt and alcohol [14, 15].

Table 2 Suggested guideline for diet progression stages following Laparoscopic Sleeve Gastrectomy

Diet stage[a]	Start	Fluids/Food	Guideline
Stage 1:	Postop days 1 and 2	**Clear liquids:** noncarbonated; no calories, no sugar, no caffeine	Postop day 1 patients may undergo a gastrograffin swallow test for leaks; once tested, patients are advised to begin taking small sips of water
Stage 2: *Begin supplementation:* Chewable multivitamin with minerals (2 per day) Chewable or liquid calcium citrate with vitamin D Sublingual, liquid, or nasal 350–500 µg vitamin B$_{12}$ Vitamin D$_3$, 3,000 IU total per day	Postop day 3 (discharge diet)	**Clear liquids** • Encourage patients to have salty fluids at home and solid liquids: Sugar-free ice pops/gelatin **Plus, full liquids:** sugar per serving in full liquids liquids	Patients should consume a minimum of 48–60 oz of total fluids per day; 24–32 oz or more clear liquids; plus 24–32 oz of any combination of full liquids; examples of full liquids listed below: • 1% or skim milk • Smooth tomato soup, no chunks, mixed with 1% or skim milk • Whey, whey isolate, or soy protein powder (limit 25–30 g protein per serving) mixed with 25–30 g protein per serving) mixed with • Lactaid milk, soymilk, or almond milk • Light yogurt or Greek yogurt • Less than 25 g of sugar per serving listed on label; no chunks of fruit • Plain yogurt
Stage 3: Week 1	Postop days 10–14	Increase clear liquids (total liquids 48–64 oz or more per day) and replace full liquids with soft, moist, diced, ground, or pureed protein sources as tolerated **Stage 3 protein sources:** Eggs, ground meats, ground or pureed poultry, soft, moist fish, added gravy, bouillon, light mayo to moisten, cooked beans, hearty bean soups, cottage cheese, low-fat cheese, yogurt	Protein food choices are encouraged for 3–6 small meals per day; patients may only be able to tolerate a couple of tablespoons at each meal/snack Encourage patients to chew food prior to swallowing ~20 chews per bite Encourage patients not to drink with meals and to wait ~30 min after each meal before resuming fluids Patients can supplement small amounts of soft protein intake with one full liquid as listed in stage 2 Patients are advised to use small utensils and to help control portions

(continued)

Table 2 (continued)

Diet stage[a]	Start	Fluids/Food	Guideline
Stage 3: Week 2	4 weeks postop	Advance diet as tolerated; if protein foods are well tolerated, add well-cooked soft vegetables and soft or peeled fruit	Adequate hydration is essential and a priority for all patients during the rapid weight loss phase • Patient should be encouraged to add fruits/vegetables in a texture that is tolerated; added fruits and vegetables and adequate hydration will help prevent constipation • Full liquids may be used for meal or snack replacement
Stage 3: Week 3 May switch to pill form of supplementation if liquid or chewable not tolerated; encourage liquid or chewable forms of supplements for at least 3 months	5 weeks postop	Continue to consume protein with some fruit or vegetable at each meal; some patients tolerate salads 1 month postop	Avoid rice, bread, and pasta until patient is comfortably consuming adequate protein (60 g)per day and fruits/vegetables Consider diet a to meet nutritional needs during rapid weight loss and healing phase Diet should ensure: Some protein sources 3–5 times a day with fruits and vegetables Postop supplementation; as hunger increases and patients are meeting the Dietary Reference Intake for protein and consuming fruits and vegetables, and whole grains can be introduced
Stage 4 Vitamin and mineral supplementation daily	As hunger increases and more food is tolerated	Healthy balanced solid food diet	Healthy, balanced diet consisting of adequate protein (plant or animal sources), fruits, vegetables, and whole grains; calorie needs based on individual needs Advise patients to eat from small plates and using small utensils to help control portions Patient should meet calorie needs based on height, weight and age

Adapted from Mechanick, J. I. et al., 2013, Aills, L. et al., 2008

[a]There is no standardization of diet stages. Patients' progression is highly dependent on their nutritional needs and food tolerances postoperatively

Moreover, to ensure that patients are well prepared for lifelong dietary and life-style changes, RD's and a nutrition education team work closely with patients to ensure that they are taught how to prepare meals to suit their tolerance at each dietary progression stage, and eat mindfully, chew food adequately, and ensure that patients recognize their sense of satiety. Keeping hydrated is likewise impor-tant and a nutrition priority to prevent dehydration and constipation. As such, patients are advised to sip small quantities of water throughout the day, avoid drinking fluids with meals, and ideally wait 30 min between meals [13].

3 Conclusion

Nutritional management during the postoperative period is imperative to ensure bariatric patients adhere to dietary progression guidelines, maintain their nutri-tional status and maximize weight loss [4, 14]. However, taking into considera-tion that no evidence-based nutrition guidelines for LSG have been developed, it is evident that more research is needed to better understand the nutritional needs of LSG patients in order to tailor an appropriate postoperative diet [10].

References

1. Endevelt R, Ben-Assuli O, Klain E, Zelber-Sagi S. The role of dietician follow-up in the suc-cess of bariatric surgery. Surg Obes Relat Dis. 2013;9(6):963–8.
2. Mechanick JI, Youdim A, Jones DB, Garvey WT, Hurley DL, McMahon MM, et al. Clinical practice guidelines for the perioperative nutritional, metabolic, and nonsurgical support of the bariatric surgery patient—2013 update: cosponsored by American Association of Clinical Endocrinologists, the Obesity Society, and American Society for Metabolic & Bariatric Surgery. Obesity. 2013; 21(S1):S1−S27.
3. Mechanick JI, Apovian C, Brethauer S, Garvey WT, Joffe AM, Kim J, et al. Clinical prac-tice guidelines for the perioperative nutrition, metabolic, and nonsurgical support of patients undergoing bariatric procedures–2019 update: cosponsored by American Association of Clinical Endocrinologists/American College of Endocrinology, The Obesity Society, American Society for Metabolic & Bariatric Surgery, Obesity Medicine Association, and American Society of Anesthesiologists. Surg Obes Rel Dis. 2019.
4. Aills L, Blankenship J, Buffington C, Furtado M, Parrott J. ASMBS allied health nutritional guidelines for the surgical weight loss patient. Surg Obes Relat Dis. 2008; 4(5):S73–S108.
5. Himpens J, Dapri G, Cadière GB. A prospective randomized study between laparoscopic gastric banding and laparoscopic isolated sleeve gastrectomy: results after 1 and 3 years. Obes Surg. 2006;16(11):1450–6.
6. Melissas J, Daskalakis M, Koukouraki S, Askoxylakis I, Metaxari M, Dimitriadis E, et al. Sleeve gastrectomy—a "food limiting" operation. Obes Surg 2008; 18(10):1251−56.
7. Bosnic G. Nutritional requirements after bariatric surgery. Crit Care Nurs Clin North Am. 2014; 26(2):255–262.
8. Costa LD, Valezi AC, Matsuo T, Dichi I, Dichi JB. Nutritional and metabolic evalua-tion of patients after one year of gastric bypass surgery. Revista do Colegio Brasileiro de Cirurgioes 2010; 37(2):96–101.

9. Sherf Dagan S, Goldenshluger A, Globus I, Schweiger C, Kessler Y, Kowen Sandbank G, et al. Sinai T. Nutritional recommendations for adult bariatric surgery patients: clinical practice. Advances in Nutrition 2017;8(2):382–394.

10. Snyder-Marlow G, Taylor D, Lenhard MJ. Nutrition care for patients undergoing laparoscopic sleeve gastrectomy for weight loss. J Am Dietetic Assoc 2010;110(4):600–607.

11. de Mello França DL, do Nascimento EA, Gravena AAF. Aspectos Gastrointestinais, Perda de Peso e uso de Suplementos Vitamínicos em Pacientes Pós-Operatório de Cirurgia Bariátrica. Saúde e Pesquisa 2011;4(1).

12. Moizé V, Andreu A, Flores L, Torres F, Ibarzabal A, Delgado S, et al. Long-term dietary intake and nutritional deficiencies following sleeve gastrectomy or Roux-En-Y gastric bypass in a mediterranean population. J Acad Nutr Dietetics 2013;113(3):400–410.

13. Kushner RF, Still CD. Nutrition and bariatric surgery. CRC Press: 2014.

14. Moizé VL, Pi-Sunyer X, Mochari H, Vidal J. Nutritional pyramid for post-gastric bypass patients. Obes Surg 2010;20(8), 1133–1141.

15. Preedy VR, Rajendram R, Martin CR (Eds.). Metabolism and pathophysiology of bariatric surgery: nutrition, procedures, outcomes and adverse effects. Academic Press: 2016.

Potential Benefits of the LSG

How Laparoscopic Sleeve Gastrectomy May Cause Weight Loss

Michel Gagner

Comprendre, ce n'est pas tout comprendre, c'est aussi reconnaître qu'il y a de l'incompréhensible. Edgar Morin, in La méthode, Éthique (2004).

Increased restriction, diminished acid output, and intensified gastric emptying.

At first, sleeve gastrectomy which evolved as a two stage procedure from laparoscopic duodenal switch, then to a stand-alone procedure for non super-obese patients, was recognized to be mostly, purely restrictive, in the early 2000's [1, 2]. In fact Marceau et al., when conversing about the open duodenal switch operation, was insinuating a parietal cell gastrectomy with modest restriction [3]. It also involved at that time a decrease in acid output from the stomach, as shown by the dramatic reduction in ulcer rate, witnessed after classical BPD from when a greater curvature gastrectomy was executed with, as Hess mentioned, one or two fingers breath from a regular bougie [4].

Sleeve size has been shown to have an effect on weight loss over time, a smaller bougie causes more weight loss in the long-term, however a smaller tube seem to cause significantly more GERD and morbi-mortality, so the right balance much be chosen [5–12]. Decreased gastric volume, initially, in the first months causes a decrease of caloric intake, 500 too 700 kcal per day are not unusual. Comparable analogies have been achieved by looking at volume of gastric resection and correlate with weight loss [13–15]. Similarly, larger gastric resection, correlates with diminish levels of serum ghrelin and higher GLP-1 [14]. This is best exemplified with re-sleeve gastrectomy, in which re-resection of the left stretched parts of the sleeve, causes more weight loss, on average 10 points of BMI [16, 17]. The antrum size is another variable that has been studied recently. It appears that

M. Gagner (✉)
Department of Surgery, Sacré-Coeur Hospital, Montréal, QC, Canada
e-mail: Gagner.Michel@cliniqueMichelGagner.com

© The Editor(s) (if applicable) and The Author(s), under exclusive license to Springer Nature Switzerland AG 2021
S. Al-Sabah et al. (eds.), *Laparoscopic Sleeve Gastrectomy*,
https://doi.org/10.1007/978-3-030-57373-7_36

smaller antrum may cause more weight loss later, and resolution of type-2 diabetes, and faster gastric emptying [18, 19].

1   Ghrelin Effect

Ghrelin is an orexigenic (i.e. appetite-stimulating) hormone chiefly secreted from gastric cells [20]. Flowing ghrelin increases rapidly prior to meals in humans and was assumed to be decisive for eating. Cummings et al. from the University of Washington have observed that patients post-RYGB appeared to have cessation of diurnal or pre-meal variation in circulating ghrelin [21]. Clinical observations reveals that patients often, in the initial postoperative period, feels lessened hunger sensation, sometimes seems to disregard to eat or have to force themselves to ingest proteins and calories.

Furthermore, sleeve gastrectomy eliminates a majority of ghrelin-producing gastric matter from the fundus and body, and it has been postulated that the absence of ghrelin, may be fundamental to weight loss witnessed following this intervention [22]. This proposition is reinforced by the observation that circulating ghrelin levels are decreased immediately postoperatively and maintained at 1 to 5 years in sleeve gastrectomy patients [23, 24]. Some authors have made a clear correlation between the amount of Ghrelin-Secreting Cells in the gastric fundus and Excess Weight Loss after Sleeve Gastrectomy [25]. Resection is very important, as two recent observations seem to confirm this hypothesis, firstly when ghrelin levels and hunger sensation are measured after Laparoscopic Sleeve Gastrectomy and compared with Laparoscopic Greater Curvature Plication in obese patients, ghrelin is dramatically less and correlates with healthier weight loss, as when a simple tube is created without resected gastric tissue. This may explains why plication fails more repeatedly [26]. Secondly, analogous findings are detected following metabolic hormones measurements after Endoscopic Sleeve Gastroplasty (ESG), an endoscopic greater curvature plication [27].

It has also been observed that ghrelin reduction is more profound and durable after sleeve gastrectomy than after Roux-en-Y gastric bypass, making it an important mechanism of weight loss after sleeves, it also seems to potentiate GLP-1 effect [28, 29]. Interestingly, some levels of ghrelin production remains after near total gastrectomy, and it seems to come from the pancreas, de novo pancreatic production of ghrelin is stimulated [30]. Ghrelin reductions following bariatric surgery were associated with decreased resting state activity in the hippocampus [31].

But, this is still controversial as some papers seem to indicate that Ghrelin is not necessarily related with weight loss in bariatric surgery, certainly after Roux-en-Y gastric bypass, and in animal models at least, the data's are not completely connected. For example, short-term results suggest that sleeved stomach without resection is as effective as sleeve gastrectomy in improving glucose control in type 2 diabetes mellitus Sprague–Dawley Rat model [32].

1.1 Other Gastrointestinal Hormone Secretion

A recent structured systematic review and meta-analysis was performed to evaluate changes in ghrelin, glucagon-like peptide-1 (GLP-1), peptide YY (PYY), and gastric inhibitory peptide (GIP) gut hormone levels in patients after sleeve gastrectomy, especially using randomized controlled trials and prospective observational studies evaluating pre and post-procedure hormones fasting ghrelin, postprandial GLP-1, postprandial PYY, and fasting GIP levels were comprised. A total of 28 studies (n = 653; 29.56% male) were counted in, with a mean age was 42 years, and an average follow-up of 12 months. Pre-sleeve BMI) was 46 kg/m2, with a post sleeve gastrectomy BMI of 34 representing an excess weight loss of 57% (P<0.001). Fasting ghrelin levels decreased, whereas postprandial GLP-1 and PYY increased after sleeve gastrectomy. Fasting GIP levels remained unchanged [36].

Some studies imply that these postoperative changes are driven by the increased rate of nutrient delivery in the gut after sleeve gastrectomy. Gastric emptying and intestinal nutrient delivery are augmented following sleeve gastrectomy patients, and as stated before is associated with increased secretion of the more distal intestinal hormones GLP-1 and peptide YY (PYY) [37-41]. Postprandial GLP-1 secretion is greatly heightened in rats and humans after some bariatric techniques, including sleeve gastrectomy, and has been widely hypothesized to promote reduced consumption, weight loss, and the restitutions in glucose homeostasis after sleeve. Wilson-Perez and colleagues found that sleeve gastrectomy-operated GLP-1 receptor-deficient rodents responded comparably to wild-type controls in terms of body weight and body fat loss, improved glucose tolerance, food intake reduction, and altered food choice. This study explain that GLP-1 receptor activity is not necessary for the metabolic improvements induced by sleeve gastrectmy [42]. Further, post-bariatric surgery hypoglycaemia (PBH) is more frequently observed in sleeve gastrectomy patients than previously recognized. In rats it was shown to have increased glycemic variability and hypoglycaemia after sleeve gastrectomy. Postprandial hypoglycaemia was specifically detected after liquid versus solid meals. Further, the blockade of GLP-1R signalling raises the glucose nadir but does not affect glycemic variability [43].

1.2 Other Molecular Changes

Growth hormone (GH) (12.32 vs. 50.97 pg/mL, p<0.001) and insulin-like growth factor IGFBP-2 levels (51.86 vs. 68.81 pg/mL, p<0.001) were significantly elevated after sleeve gastrectomy. BMI (52.2 vs. 40.1, p=0.001), insulin (19.4 vs. 8.8 mIU/L, p<0.001) and HOMA-IR index (6.5 to 2.5, p<0.001) were reduced after surgery. Lipid profile analysis revealed that total cholesterol (4.26 vs. 5.12 mmol/L, p<0.001) and high-density lipoprotein (HDL) (0.90 to 1.55 mmol/L, p<0.001) were increased, while triglycerides were decreased, after surgery (1.62 vs. 1.05 mmol/L p<0.001). GH, IGF-1, and IGFBP-2 were not correlated with insulin or lipid parameters [44].

Cytokine behaviour after sleeve gastrectomy as been studied, and as showed two prototype patterns: a concordant type, where cytokines behave the same way for all patients (notably IL-0 and TNFα), and a variable type, where different patterns of expression are seen for different patients (notably IL-8, IL-6 and IL-1RA). Analysis of the cytokines at the individual patient-level showed a strong four-way correlation between IL-1RA, GCSF, MIP-1β and MCP-1. As it holds for most patients and not just on average, this suggests that they form a network, which may play a central role in the response to gastro-intestinal injuries in humans [45].

1.3   Bile Acid Metabolism

Bile acids and their receptors like farnesoid X receptor (FXR) and G-protein coupled bile acid receptor (TGR5)) are significant mediators of metabolism. Bile acids have metabolic effects, and in mice deficient in the bile acid receptor FXR, effects of sleeve gastrectomy on body weight are annulled [46]. Hence, sleeve is associated with increased plasma bile acid concentrations in patients [47, 48]. TGR5 has also been in the associated with rodents studies of sleeve gastrectomy, such like Cummings et al. revealed that TGR5, the G-protein coupled bile acid receptor, is required for improved glucose regulation phenotype of sleeve in the mouse [49]. Sleeve gastrectmy in TGR5 knockout mice is related with changed bile acid pool configuration, which may have additional metabolic significances. Captivatingly, the TGR5 knockout animals following sleeve reacted similar to wild type animals with respect to glucose-stimulated insulin secretion. Therefore, this experiment deduces that some beneficial effects of sleeve related to glucose homeostasis are mediated through TGR5 [49]. Another study investigated the acute and short-term effects of bypass and sleeve on bile acid compositions and fibroblast growth factor 19 (FGF19) in obese individuals with T2DM and to evaluate any correlations between changes in these measures with glucose metabolic improvements. At 3 days post-operation, FGF19 levels increased significantly in both surgery groups. Fasting and postprandial increases from pre-operative values in secondary, conjugated, glycine-conjugated and secondary-conjugated bile acids correlated with decreases in the postprandial states of glucose (defined by area under the curve (AUC) over 120 min (AUC0-120 min)). Increases in postprandial primary-conjugated bile acids were found to be associated with decreases in HOMA-IR). However, increases in fasting and postprandial taurine-conjugated bile acids correlated with decreases in both basal insulin secretion rate and C-peptide level. After 3 months, fasting and postprandial increases in secondary, secondary-conjugated and non-12α-OH bile acids were found to correlate with increases in Stumvoll Insulin Sensitivity Index. Increases in both fasting and postprandial 12α-OH BAs were correlated with the decreases in glucose AUC (P = 0.04). Both bypass and sleeve gastrectomy attain increases in many bile acids species as early as 3 days post-procedure, which are sustained at 3 months post-operation. Rises in secondary bile acids and conjugated forms are correlated with early upgrades in glucose metabolism at 3 days post-operation. These along with 12α-OH BA correlated with improved glucose metabolism at 3 months post-operation, evoking they may contribute to the observed T2DM remission after sleeve gastrectomy [50].

1.4   Microbiome

Laparoscopic sleeve gastrectomy (LSG) causes a change in gut microbiota and is linked to the efficacy of the operation. In fact severely obese subjects subjected to sleeve gastrectomy had the composition and abundance of the microbiota and bile acids in faeces assessed by 16S ribosomal RNA sequencing, quantitative PCR and liquid chromatography-mass spectrometry. The increase in α-diversity and abundance of specific taxa, such as Rikenellaceae and Christensenellaceae, was strongly associated with reduced faecal bile acid levels. These changes had a significant association with excess weight loss and metabolic improvements. Sleeve gastrectomy is related with a reduction in faecal bile acids and superior richness of specific bacterial taxa and α-diversity that may promote the metabolic changes observed [51].

1.5   Central Nervous System Changes

Authors have compared whole brain activation in response to high-energy dense versus low-energy dense visual and auditory food cues before and approximately 4 months after Roux-en-Y Gastric Bypass and Sleeve Gastrectomy. In this study, they included two control groups: a low-calorie diet weight loss group and a non-treatment group. Relative to the control groups, the surgery groups showed increased dorsolateral prefrontal cortex and decreased parahippocampal/fusiform gyrus activation in response to high enery dense visual cues, suggesting greater cognitive dietary inhibition and decreased rewarding effects and attention related to high energy dense foods. Dorsolateral prefrontal cortex activation was significantly more increased in bypass than in sleeve. They found that postprandial rises in GLP-1 correlated with postsurgical decreases in bypass brain activity in the inferior temporal gyrus and the right middle occipital gyrus in addition to increases in the right medial prefrontal gyrus/paracingulate for high energy stimuli, suggesting involvement of these attention and inhibitory regions in satiety signalling post surgery [52].

1.6 Conclusion

Sleeve gastrectomy causes multiple hormonal, physiological alterations that decreases appetite, causes a reduction and change in foods, and brings cerebral differences that leads to weight loss [53].

References

1. Ren CJ, Patterson E, Gagner M. Early results of laparoscopic biliopancreatic diversion with duodenal switch: a case series of 40 consecutive patients. Obes Surg. 2000 Dec; 10(6):514–23.
2. Chu C, Gagner M, Quinn T, Voellinger DC, Feng JJ, Inabnet WB, Herron D, Pomp A: Two-stage laparoscopic BPD/DS. An alternative approach to super-super morbid obesity. Surgical Endoscopy 2002; S187.
3. Lagace M, Marceau P, Marceau S, Hould FS, Potvin M, Bourque RA, Biron S. Biliopancreatic diversion with a new type of gastrectomy: some previous conclusions revisited. Obes Surg. 1995;5:411–8.
4. Hess DS, Hess DW. Biliopancreatic diversion with a duodenal switch. Obes Surg. 1998;8:267–82.
5. Parikh M, Gagner M, Heacock L, Strain G, Dakin G, Pomp A. Laparoscopic sleeve gastrectomy: does bougie size affect mean %EWL? Short-term outcomes. Surgery for obesity and related diseases. 2008;4:528–33.
6. Atkins ER, Preen DB, Jarman C, Cohen LD. Improved Obesity Reduction and Co-morbidity Resolution in Patients Treated with 40-French Bougie Versus 50-French Bougie Four Years after Laparoscopic Sleeve Gastrectomy. Analysis of 294 Patients. Obes Surg. 2011; 22:97–104.
7. Spivak H, Rubin M, Sadot E, Pollak E, Feygin A, Goitein D. Laparoscopic sleeve Gastrectomy using 42-French Versus 32-French Bougie: The First-Year Outcome. Obes Surg. 2014;24:1090–3.
8. Cal P, Deluca L, Jakob T, Fernández E. Laparoscopic sleeve gastrectomy with 27 versus 39 Fr bougie calibration: a randomized controlled trial. Surg Endosc. 2015;30:1812–5.
9. Albaugh VL, Schauer PR, Aminian A: Chapter 6. How the sleeve gastrectomy works (Metabolically). In Gagner M, et al. Editors. The perfect sleeve Gastrectomy. Springer 2020, pp 63–78.
10. Wang Y, Yi XY, Gong LL, Li QF, Zhang J, Wang ZH. The effectiveness and safety of laparoscopic sleeve gastrectomy with different sizes of bougie calibration: a systematic review and meta-analysis. Int J Surg. 2018;49:32–8. https://doi.org/10.1016/j.ijsu.2017.12.005.
11. Sanchez Santos R, Corcelles R, Vilallonga Puy R, et al. Prognostic factors of weight loss after sleeve gastrectomy: Multi centre study in Spain and Portugal. Factores predictivos de pérdida ponderal tras la gastrectomía vertical. Estudio multicéntrico hispano-portugués. Cir Esp. 2017; 95(3):135–142. doi:https://doi.org/10.1016/j.ciresp.2017.02.002.
12. Palermo M, Gagner M. Why we think laparoscopic sleeve gastrectomy is a good operation: step-by-step technique. J Laparoendosc Adv Surg Tech A. 2020;30(6):615–8. https://doi.org/10.1089/lap.2020.0154.
13. Robert M, Pasquer A, Pelascini E, Valette P-J, Gouillat C, Disse E. Impact of sleeve gastrectomy volumes on weight loss results: a prospective study. Surg Obes Relat Dis. 2016;12:1286–91.
14. Sista F, Abruzzese V, Clementi M, Carandina S, Amicucci G. Effect of resected gastric volume on ghrelin and GLP-1 plasma levels: a prospective study. J Gastrointest Surg. 2016;20:1931–41.

15. D'Ugo S, Bellato V, Bianciardi E, Gentileschi P. Impact of resected gastric volume on post-operative weight loss after laparoscopic sleeve gastrectomy. Gastroenterol Res Pract. 2019; 2019:3742075. Published 2019 Dec 1. doi:https://doi.org/10.1155/2019/3742075.
16. Noel P, Nedelcu A, Eddbali I, Gagner M, Danan M, Nedelcu M. Five-year results after resleeve gastrectomy [published online ahead of print, 2020 Apr 24]. Surg Obes Relat Dis. 2020; S1550–7289(20)30205–7. doi:https://doi.org/10.1016/j.soard.2020.04.021.
17. Aiolfi A, Micheletto G, Marin J, Bonitta G, Lesti G, Bona D. Re-Sleeve for failed laparoscopic sleeve Gastrectomy: systematic review and meta-analysis. Surg Obes Relat Dis. DOI: https://doi.org/10.1016/j.soard.2020.06.007.
18. Omarov T, Samadov E, Coskun AK, Unlu A. Comparison of weight loss in sleeve gastrectomy patients with and without antrectomy: a prospective randomized study. Obes Surg. 2020;30(2):446–50.
19. Ömeroğlu S, Bozkurt E, Kaya C, et al. How does the extent of antral resection affect the residual gastric volume and excessive weight loss? Ann Ital Chir. 2019;90:208–12.
20. Kojima M, Hosoda H, Date Y, Nakazato M, Matsuo H, Kangawa K. Ghrelin is a growth-hormone-releasing acylated peptide from stomach. Nature. 1999;402:656–60.
21. Cummings DE, Weigle DS, Frayo RS, Breen PA, Ma MK, Dellinger EP, et al. Plasma ghrelin levels after diet-induced weight loss or gastric bypass surgery. N Engl J Med. 2002;346:1623–30.
22. Choi E, Roland JT, Barlow BJ, O'Neal R, Rich AE, Nam KT, et al. Cell lineage distribution atlas of the human stomach reveals heterogeneous gland populations in the gastric antrum. Gut. 2014;63:1711–20.
23. Karamanakos SN, Vagenas K, Kalfarentzos F, Alexandrides TK. Weight loss, appetite suppression, and changes in fasting and postprandial ghrelin and peptide-YY levels after Roux-en-Y gastric bypass and sleeve gastrectomy. Ann Surg. 2008;247:401–7.
24. Bohdjalian A, Langer FB, Shakeri-Leidenmühler S, et al. Sleeve gastrectomy as sole and definitive bariatric procedure: 5-year results for weight loss and ghrelin. Obes Surg. 2010;20(5):535–40.
25. Itlaybah A, Elbanna H, Emile S, et al. Correlation between the number of ghrelin-secreting cells in the gastric fundus and excess weight loss after sleeve gastrectomy. Obes Surg. 2019;29(1):76–83.
26. Dobrescu A, Copaescu C, Zmeu B, et al. Ghrelin levels and hunger sensation after laparoscopic sleeve gastrectomy compared with laparoscopic greater curvature plication in obese patients. Clin Lab. 2020; 66(5):https://doi.org/10.7754/Clin.Lab.2019.191012.
27. Lopez-Nava G, Negi A, Bautista-Castaño I, Rubio MA, Asokkumar R. Gut metabolic hormones changes after Endoscopic Sleeve Gastroplasty (ESG) Vs. Laparoscopic Sleeve Gastrectomy (LSG). Obes Surg. 2020; 30(7):2642–51.
28. Salman MA, El-Ghobary M, Soliman A, et al. Long-Term Changes in leptin, chemerin, and ghrelin levels following Roux-en-Y gastric bypass and laparoscopic sleeve gastrectomy. Obes Surg. 2020;30(3):1052–60.
29. Page LC, Gastaldelli A, Gray SM, D'Alessio DA, Tong J. Interaction of GLP-1 and ghrelin on glucose tolerance in healthy humans. Diabetes. 2018;67:1976–85.
30. Camacho-Ramírez A, Mayo-Ossorio MÁ, Pacheco-García JM, et al. Pancreas is a preeminent source of ghrelin after sleeve gastrectomy in Wistar rats [published online ahead of print, 2020 Jan 17]. Histol Histopathol. 2020; 18200.
31. Zhang Y, Ji G, Li G, et al. Ghrelin reductions following bariatric surgery were associated with decreased resting state activity in the hippocampus. Int J Obes (Lond). 2019;43(4):842–51.
32. Zhang W, Widjaja J, Yao L, Shao Y, Zhu X, Li C. Short-term results suggest that sleeved stomach without resection is as effective as sleeve Gastrectomy in improving glucose control in Type 2 Diabetes Mellitus Sprague-Dawley Rat Model. Biomed Res Int. 2020; 2020:9024923. Published 2020 May 1.

33. Chambers AP, Kirchner H, Wilson-Perez HE, Willency JA, Hale JE, Gaylinn BD, et al. The effects of vertical sleeve gastrectomy in rodents are ghrelin independent. Gastroenterology. 2013;144:50–5.
34. McFarlane MR, Brown MS, Goldstein JL, Zhao T-J. Induced ablation of ghrelin cells in adult mice does not decrease food intake, body weight, or response to high-fat diet. Cell Metab. 2014;20:54–60.
35. Kulkarni BV, LaSance K, Sorrell JE, Lemen L, Woods SC, Seeley RJ, et al. The role of proximal versus distal stomach resection in the weight loss seen after vertical sleeve gastrectomy. AJP: Regulatory, Integrative and Comparative Physiology. 2016; 311:R979–87.
36. McCarty TR, Jirapinyo P, Thompson CC. Effect of Sleeve Gastrectomy on Ghrelin, GLP-1, PYY, and GIP Gut Hormones: A Systematic Review and Meta-analysis. Ann Surg. 2020;272(1):72–80.
37. Peterli R, Steinert RE, Woelnerhanssen B, Peters T, Christoffel-Courtin C, Gass M, et al. Metabolic and hormonal changes after laparoscopic Roux-en-Y gastric bypass and sleeve gastrectomy: a randomized, prospective trial. Obes Surg. 2012;22:740–8.
38. Mallipedhi A, Prior SL, Barry JD, Caplin S, Baxter JN, Stephens JW. Temporal changes in glucose homeostasis and incretin hormone response at 1 and 6 months after laparoscopic sleeve gastrectomy. Surg Obes Relat Dis. 2014;10:860–9.
39. Papamargaritis D, le Roux CW, Sioka E, Koukoulis G, Tzovaras G, Zacharoulis D. Changes in gut hormone profile and glucose homeostasis after laparoscopic sleeve gastrectomy. Surg Obes Relat Dis. 2013;9:192–201.
40. Sista F, Abruzzese V, Clementi M, Carandina S, Cecilia M, Amicucci G. The effect of sleeve gastrectomy on GLP-1 secretion and gastric emptying: a prospective study. Surg Obes Relat Dis. 2017;13:7–14.
41. Alamuddin N, Vetter ML, Ahima RS, Hesson L, Ritter S, Minnick A, et al. Changes in fasting and prandial gut and adiposity hormones following vertical sleeve gastrectomy or Roux-en-Y-Gastric bypass: an 18-month prospective study. Obes Surg. 2016;27:1563–72.
42. Wilson-Perez HE, Chambers AP, Ryan KK, Li B, Sandoval DA, Stoffers D, et al. Vertical sleeve gastrectomy is effective in two genetic mouse models of glucagon-like Peptide 1 receptor deficiency. Diabetes. 2013;62:2380–5.
43. Evers SS, Kim KS, Bozadjieva N, et al. Continuous glucose monitoring reveals glycemic variability and hypoglycemia after vertical sleeve gastrectomy in rats. Mol Metab. 2020;32:148–59.
44. Al-Regaiey K, Alshubrami S, Al-Beeshi I, et al. Effects of gastric sleeve surgery on the serum levels of GH, IGF-1 and IGF-binding protein 2 in healthy obese patients. BMC Gastroenterol. 2020;20(1):199.
45. Trahtemberg U, Darawshe F, Elazary R, et al. Longitudinal patterns of cytokine expression at the individual level in humans after laparoscopic sleeve gastrectomy. J Cell Mol Med. 2020;24(12):6622–33.
46. Ryan KK, Tremaroli V, Clemmensen C, Kovatcheva-Datchary P, Myronovych A, Karns R, et al. FXR is a molecular target for the effects of vertical sleeve gastrectomy. Nature. 2014;509:183–8.
47. Jahansouz C, Xu H, Hertzel AV, Serrot FJ, Kvalheim N, Cole A, et al. Bile acids increase independently from hypocaloric restriction after bariatric surgery. Ann Surg. 2016;264:1022–8.
48. Steinert RE, Peterli R, Keller S, Meyer-Gerspach AC, Drewe J, Peters T, et al. Bile acids and gut peptide secretion after bariatric surgery: a 1-year prospective randomized pilot trial. Obesity (Silver Spring). 2013;21:E660–8.
49. McGavigan AK, Garibay D, Henseler ZM, Chen J, Bettaieb A, Haj FG, et al. TGR5 contributes to glucoregulatory improvements after vertical sleeve gastrectomy in mice. Gut. 2017;66:226–34.
50. Chen Y, Lu J, Nemati R, Plank LD, Murphy R. Acute changes of bile acids and FGF19 after sleeve gastrectomy and Roux-en-Y gastric bypass. Obes Surg. 2019;29(11):3605–21.

51. Ikeda T, Aida M, Yoshida Y, et al. Alteration in faecal bile acids, gut microbial composition and diversity after laparoscopic sleeve gastrectomy [published online ahead of print, 2020 May 20]. Br J Surg. 2020; https://doi.org/10.1002/bjs.11654.
52. Baboumian S, Pantazatos SP, Kothari S, McGinty J, Holst J, Geliebter A. Functional Magnetic Resonance Imaging (fMRI) of neural responses to visual and auditory food stimuli pre and post Roux-en-Y Gastric Bypass (RYGB) and Sleeve Gastrectomy (SG). Neuroscience. 2019;409:290–8.
53. Arble DM, Evers SS, Bozadjieva N, et al. Metabolic comparison of one-anastomosis gastric bypass, single-anastomosis duodenal-switch, Roux-en-Y gastric bypass, and vertical sleeve gastrectomy in rat. Surg Obes Relat Dis. 2018;14(12):1857–67.

Expected Weight Loss After the Sleeve

Rickesha L. Wilson and Ali Aminian

1 Introduction

There is strong and growing clinical evidence that metabolic and bariatric surgery have a significant impact on the overall metabolic health of recipients. As surgeons and other healthcare providers continue to strive to educate the public on the myriad of benefits, weight loss remains the primary motivation for those considering metabolic and bariatric surgery. Thus, it is important for the healthcare provider, and especially the metabolic and bariatric surgeon, to offer realistic expectations for weight loss for the patient seeking surgery. The sleeve gastrectomy is now the most commonly performed procedure, potentially due to its technical simplicity compared to other diversionary operations [1]. This chapter will describe the expected weight loss after sleeve gastrectomy at various time points following surgery as well as cover special circumstances for specific groups of patients.

2 Preoperative Weight Loss

Weight loss begins in the preoperative period. Studies suggest that baseline body mass index (BMI) as well as preoperative weight loss can be indicative of post-operative weight loss [2]. Steinbeisser et al. published results of a small surgical cohort of patients who underwent laparoscopic sleeve gastrectomy (SG) by a single surgeon in a community health practice. This study reported a significant difference in percent excess body weight lost (% EWL) and change in BMI between

R. L. Wilson (✉) · A. Aminian
Department of General Surgery, Bariatric and Metabolic Institute, Cleveland Clinic, Cleveland, OH, USA
e-mail: WILSONR13@ccf.org

patients who lost less than 5% EWL preoperatively and those who lost $\geq$ 5% EWL at 1-year follow-up: 50% versus 57% for %EWL and $-11.2 \, \text{kg/m}^2$ versus $-13.2 \, \text{kg/m}^2$ for change in BMI, postoperatively. On average, patients in this study had a 68% EWL and had a decrease in BMI of $16 \, \text{kg/m}^2$ at 1 year follow-up [2]. Watanabe et al. reported results of their retrospective evaluation of 247 patients who were compared based on preoperative weight loss. Total weight loss (%TWL) at 1 year for all patients was 31.9% overall and 29.3%, postoperatively. There was an inverse relationship between preoperative and postoperative %TWL. Those with preoperative %TWL of 0–3% versus greater than 10% TWL, had postoperative %TWL of 33% versus 27%, respectively [3]. Tan et al. also show that a very low calorie liquid diet does not impact total weight loss or excess BMI loss beyond 6 months after surgery and evidence is lacking for mandating a preoperative low calorie diet [4]. Therefore, the studies on the impacts of preoperative weight loss on total weight loss after surgery have been inconclusive.

3   Short-Term and Mid-Term Outcomes

As summarized in a position statement by the leading organization in weight loss surgery, the American Society of Metabolic and Bariatric Surgery (ASMBS), short-term results after SG reveal %EWL ranging from 53% to 88% and estimated BMI loss (%EBMIL) of 58% to 81% [5]. A systematic review and meta-analysis was performed by Osland et al. to evaluate short-term weight loss results of 9 unique randomized controlled trials (RCTs) comparing Roux-en-Y gastric bypass (RYGB) and SG procedures. Postoperative follow-up ranged from 3 months to 5 years and 437 out of 865 patients underwent SG, with %EWL ranging from 69% to 83% at 12 months [6]. Three studies included in this systematic review reported %TWL outcomes. Keidar et al. reported an average TWL of 24 kg at 3 months and 34 kg at 12 months after SG [7]. Peterli et al. reported a 36 to 37 kg TWL within the first 12 months [8], and Yang et al. report a TWL of 25 kg at 3 years after SG [9].

The Swiss Multicenter Bypass or Sleeve Study (SM-BOSS) randomized 217 patients to receive either SG or RYGB with the primary goal of measuring weight loss expressed as %EBMIL. For SG (n = 107), the EBMIL at years 1, 2, 3, and 4 was 72%, 72%, 69%, and 64%, respectively [10]. The STAMPEDE trial authors reported their outcomes of weight loss by change in BMI and for the SG cohort, the baseline, and years 1, 2, 3, and 4 BMI values changed from 36 to 27, 28, 28, and 28, respectively [11].

A large retrospective study of 1,395 patients by Ellatif and colleagues noted from 6 months to 1, 2, 3, and 4 years postoperatively that %EWL was 42, 52, 61, 73, and 67% (Fig. 1) [12]. Short and mid-term weight loss results are acceptable for patients undergoing SG and can be offered to patients depending on their specific weight loss goals and metabolic risk profile.

Weight loss result.

Variable	Postop. BMI (Kg/m^2)	% EWL
6 months	41 ± 9	42%
1 year	39 ± 7.2	53%
2 years	36 ± 6.6	61%
3 years	33 ± 5.6	73%
4 years	29 ± 4.7	67%
5 years	30 ± 5.9	61%
6 years	31 ± 6	59%
7 years	31 ± 7.2	57%

Percentage of excess weight loss (%EWL).

Fig. 1 Short-term to Long-term weight loss results in a study of 1395 patients after sleeve gastrectomy. Adapted from International Journal of Surgery, 2014–05-01, Volume 12, Issue 5, Pages 504–508

4   Long-Term Outcomes

Long-term results for weight loss after SG have been studied, however, the follow-up rates for study participants has been consistently low in the literature. The ASMBS offers results on the durability of weight loss after SG and highlight long-term outcomes from combined published data. At 5 years after SG, the weighted average %EWL is 58% (40 to 86%) and %EBMIL is 68% (46 to 78%) in a combined 953 patients. Excess weight loss at 6 to 9 years is 58% (n = 865), at 10 years is 53% (n = 32), and at ≥ 10 years is 28% (n = 70) [5].

A systematic review and meta-analysis was performed by Sharples et al. evaluating RCTs comparing the long-term (≥ 5 years) results of SG versus RYGB. Meta-analysis included 4 studies and 320 patients that reported a %EWL of 57.3% after SG compared to 65.7% for 309 RYGB patients [13]. The STAMPEDE trial comparing RYGB and SG and intensive medical therapy alone was not included in the previously mentioned meta-analysis due to different weight loss reporting measures. In the RCT by Schauer et al., after SG there was a reduction in BMI from 36 to 29 kg/m^2, a −18.5% change in body weight (kg), and a -12.2% change in waist circumference. These weight loss parameters were significant from baseline and superior compared to participants who only received medical therapy, however, slightly inferior to those participants in the RYGB cohort [11]. The SM-BOSS trial, after 5 years of follow-up, reported a %EBMIL of 61% for the SG cohort compared to 68% for the RYGB cohort, which was not significant after multiple comparisons adjustment [10].

The systematic review performed by O'Brien et al. highlights metabolic and bariatric procedures that published %EWL as well as other outcomes beyond 10 years [14]. This study was able to include only two studies reporting long-term weight loss outcomes after the SG procedure with a mean %EWL of 58% [15, 16].

Evaluating these studies, specifically, Arman et al. were able to maintain follow-up data on 65 of the 110 patients who originally underwent SG and 47 of those that kept their sleeve reconstruction. They report a 62.5% EBMIL for those who did not have revisional surgery and 81.7% for those 16 who underwent revisional surgery [15]. Felsenreich et al. were able to follow 32 of 53 patients who underwent SG without revision at 10 years and noted a %EWL of 53% and a %TWL of 26% [16].

Evidence certainly demonstrates that the SG procedure has superior weight loss outcomes compared to medical therapy or lifestyle intervention alone and weight loss results decrease over time but are maintained up to 5 years [5]. Long-term data from retrospective and prospective studies have captured %EWL ranging from 48% to 69% (Fig. 2) [17].

5 Weight Regain and Other Factors Affecting Weight Loss

Similar to other weight loss interventions, SG is subject to long-term weight regain in some patients secondary to compensatory behavioral and physiologic adaptations. Weight regain is difficult to define in the literature as studies do not consistently use one definition to define this phenomenon and often combine the term with others such as "insufficient weight loss" and SG "failure". A common definition of weight regain has been an increase in weight of 10kg from weight nadir. Insufficient weight loss is often defined as never having achieved %EWL of $\geq 50\%$. A systematic review by Lauti et al. found 9 heterogenous studies to report weight regain ranging from 6% at 2 years to 76% at 6 years [18]. This systematic review and other reviews also describe factors that have been found to contribute to weight regain for SG patients followed at least 2 years: namely initial sleeve size, sleeve dilatation over time, increased ghrelin levels, inadequate follow-up support, and maladaptive lifestyle behaviors [19].

Arman et al. demonstrated that 21% of the 110 patients undergoing SG required revision due to weight regain. At long-term follow-up of 11+years, the EBMIL was 82% for those undergoing revision versus 62% for those who kept the original sleeve construction [15].

Panella and colleagues correlated weight loss outcomes with gastric reservoir volumes after SG in 50 patients. Gastric volume was measured at 1 month, 1 year, and 5 years after surgery and measured to be 114 ml, 216 ml, and 367 ml, respectively. The %EWL at 1 and 5 years was 74.5% and 55.5%, the %EBMIL was 86% and 64%, and %TWL was 35.7 and 27.4% [20]. Long-term weight loss has not been shown to correlate with gastric volume after SG. A different study has shown that smaller bougie size of $\leq 6Fr$ and closer distance of the staple line to the pylorus (2 to 4 cm) was correlated with superior weight loss outcomes at 4 to 7 years after SG [12].

Eid et al evaluated long-term outcomes after SG in super obese patients (BMI $\geq$ 60 kg/m^2) who did not undergo a planned second stage operation after SG. Excess weight loss at 72, 84, and 96 months after LSG was 52%, 43%, and 46%, respectively, with an overall %EWL of 48%. The mean BMI decreased from 66 kg/m^2 to

Author	Number	Type study	% Follow-up	% EWL	Months of follow-up	Preoperative BMI (kg/m²)	BMI late after surgery
Himpens [16]	53	R	78	53	72	39.9	31.1
D'Hondt [17]	83	R	28	56	72	39.3	?
Eid [8]	74	P	93	48	72	66	43
Sarela [18]	20	P	65	69	96	45.8	32
Ellatif [19]	1395	R	37	57	84	46.0	31
Hirth [9]	16	R	88	59	84	43.5	?
Arman [13]	110	R	59	62	132	38.8	29.7
Felsenreich [10]	53	R	100	53	120	48.9	35.5
Gadiot [20]	272	P	72	54	96	44.8	34.8
Casella [11]	180	R	81	67	72	45.9	30.2

R Retrospective, P prospective, EWL excess weight loss, BMI body mass index

Fig. 2 Long-term results of weight loss after sleeve gastrectomy according to publications with follow-up equal or longer than 72 months. Adapted from Csendes, A., Burgos, A.M., Martinez, G. et al. Loss and Regain of Weight After Laparoscopic Sleeve Gastrectomy According to Preoperative BMI. *OBES SURG* 28, 3424–3430 (2018)

46 kg/m² [21]. Csendes et al. showed significant rates of weight regain for patients with BMI $\geq$ 40 kg/m². Specifically, in patients with an initial BMI $\geq$ 40 kg/m² , 15% of patients (n $=$ 20) had a BMI over 30 at 1 year and that increased to 85% of patients beyond 5 years. For those patients with a BMI $\geq$ 50 kg/m², 100% of patients (n $=$ 4) had a BMI > 30 kg/m² at 1 year and $\geq$ 6 years [17]. Patient education is important in patients with high BMIs ($\geq$40 kg/m²) who are considering SG for weight loss as they should be counseled that weight loss outcomes may not meet expectations and other metabolic procedures may be a better option.

Women seeking to become pregnant following SG can be counseled that long-term weight loss has not been shown to be negatively impacted by pregnancy, but studies are conflicting [22]. Bakr et al. evaluated 100 patients after SG with up to 5 years follow-up, and 25 patients who became pregnant within 3 years had a 54% EWL compared to the 52 patients who did not become pregnant and had a 64% EWL [23]. Weight loss results may be acceptable after pregnancy but, in some cases, may be inferior to those not becoming pregnant. Lastly, while SG is deemed safe in the pediatric and elderly populations, more studies are to be done to determine the long-term weight loss outcomes and if they differ from the adult population [24, 25].

6 Summary

In summary, sleeve gastrectomy is now the most commonly performed metabolic and bariatric procedure worldwide. Heterogeneity of studies in terms of BMI at the time of surgery, technical details including bougie size and resection of gastric antrum, along with various retention rates and follow-up times can significantly affect the reported weight loss estimates in the literature. Evidence shows that the expected weight loss in the long-term is 50% to 60% of excess weight, with an average long-term BMI reduction of 10 kg/m². Patients should be counseled on the potential of weight regain that is multifactorial—related to patient characteristics, operative technique, compensatory behavioral and physiologic adaptations, and more [26].

References

1. Angrisani L, Santonicola A, Iovino P, Vitiello A, Higa K, Himpens J, Buchwald H, Scopinaro N. IFSO worldwide survey 2016: Primary, endoluminal, and revisional procedures. Obes Surg. 2018;28:3783–94.
2. Steinbeisser M, McCracken J, Kharbutli B. Laparoscopic sleeve gastrectomy: Preoperative weight loss and other factors as predictors of postoperative success. Obes Surg. 2017;27:1508–13.
3. Watanabe A, Seki Y, Haruta H, Kikkawa E, Kasama K. Preoperative weight loss and operative outcome after laparoscopic sleeve gastrectomy. Obes Surg. 2017;27:2515–21.
4. Ying S, Tan T, Loi PL, et al. Preoperative weight loss via Very Low Caloric Diet (VLCD) and its effect on outcomes after bariatric surgery. Surg: Obes; 2020.
5. Azagury D, Papasavas P, Hamdallah I, Gagner M, Kim J. ASMBS position statement on medium- and long-term durability of weight loss and diabetic outcomes after conventional stapled bariatric procedures. Surg Obes Relat Dis. 2018;14:1425–41.
6. Osland E, Nutr B, Mphil D, Yunus RM, Khan S, Memon B. Weight loss outcomes in Laparoscopic Vertical Sleeve Gastrectomy (LVSG) versus Laparoscopic Roux-en-Y Gastric Bypass (LRYGB) procedures. Surg Laparosc Endosc Percutan Tech. 2017;27:8–18.
7. Keidar A, Hershkop KJ, Marko L, Schweiger C, Hecht L, Bartov N, Kedar A, Weiss R. Roux-en-Y gastric bypass vs sleeve gastrectomy for obese patients with type 2 diabetes: A randomised trial. Diabetologia. 2013;56:1914–8.
8. Peterli R, Borbély Y, Kern B, Gass M, Peters T, Thurnheer M, Schultes B, Laederach K, Bueter M, Schiesser M. Early results of the swiss multicentre bypass or sleeve study (SM-BOSS): A prospective randomized trial comparing laparoscopic sleeve gastrectomy and Roux-en-Y gastric bypass. Ann Surg. 2013;258:690–5.
9. Yang J, Wang C, Cao G, Yang W, Yu S, Zhai H, Pan Y. Long-term effects of laparoscopic sleeve gastrectomy versus roux-en-Y gastric bypass for the treatment of Chinese type 2 diabetes mellitus patients with body mass index 28–35 kg/m2. BMC Surg. 2015;15:1–7.
10. Peterli R, Wolnerhanssen BK, Peters T, et al. Effect of laparoscopic sleeve gastrectomy vs laparoscopic roux-en-y gastric bypass onweight loss in patients with morbid obesity the sm-boss randomized clinical trial. JAMA - J Am Med Assoc. 2018;319:255–65.
11. Schauer PR, Bhatt DL, Kirwan JP, et al. Bariatric Surgery versus —5-Year Outcomes. N Engl J Med. 2017;376:641–51.
12. Abd Ellatif ME, Abdallah E, Askar W, et al. Long term predictors of success after laparoscopic sleeve gastrectomy. Int J Surg. 2014;12:504–8.
13. Sharples AJ, Mahawar K. Systematic review and meta-analysis of randomised controlled trials comparing long-term outcomes of Roux-En-Y gastric bypass and sleeve gastrectomy. Obes Surg. 2020;30:664–72.
14. O'Brien PE, Hindle A, Brennan L, Skinner S, Burton P, Smith A, Crosthwaite G, Brown W. Long-term outcomes after bariatric surgery: a systematic review and meta-analysis of weight loss at 10 or more years for all bariatric procedures and a single-centre review of 20-year outcomes after adjustable gastric banding. Obes Surg. 2019;29:3–14.
15. Arman GA, Himpens J, Dhaenens J, Ballet T, Vilallonga R, Leman G. Long-term (11+years) outcomes in weight, patient satisfaction, comorbidities, and gastroesophageal reflux treatment after laparoscopic sleeve gastrectomy. Surg Obes Relat Dis. 2016;12:1778–86.

16. Felsenreich DM, Langer FB, Kefurt R, Panhofer P, Schermann M, Beckerhinn P, Sperker C, Prager G. Weight loss, weight regain, and conversions to Roux-en-Y gastric bypass: 10-year results of laparoscopic sleeve gastrectomy. Surg Obes Relat Dis. 2016;12:1655–62.
17. Csendes A, Burgos AM, Martinez G, Figueroa M, Castillo J, Díaz JC. Loss and regain of weight after laparoscopic sleeve gastrectomy according to preoperative BMI. Obes Surg. 2018;28:3424–30.
18. Lauti M, Kularatna M, Hill AG, MacCormick AD. Weight regain following sleeve gastrectomy—a systematic review. Obes Surg. 2016;26:1326–34.
19. Yu Y, Lou KM, Kalarchian MA, Ji M, Burke LE. Predictors of weight regain after sleeve gastrectomy: an integrative review. Surg Obes Relat Dis. 2019;15:995–1005.
20. Pañella C, Busto M, González A, Serra C, Goday A, Grande L, Pera M, Ramón JM. Correlation of gastric volume and weight loss 5 years following sleeve gastrectomy. Obes Surg. 2020. https://doi.org/10.1007/s11695-020-04445-z.
21. Eid GM, Brethauer S, Mattar SG, Titchner RL, Gourash W, Schauer PR. Laparoscopic sleeve gastrectomy for super obese patients: Forty-eight percent excess weight loss after 6 to 8 years with 93% follow-up. Ann Surg. 2012;256:262–5.
22. Rottenstreich A, Shufanieh J, Kleinstern G, Goldenshluger A, Elchalal U, Elazary R. The long-term effect of pregnancy on weight loss after sleeve gastrectomy. Surg Obes Relat Dis. 2018;14:1594–9.
23. Bakr AA, Fahmy MH, Elward AS, Balamoun HA, Ibrahim MY, Eldahdoh RM. Analysis of Medium-Term Weight Regain 5 Years After Laparoscopic Sleeve Gastrectomy. Obes Surg. 2019;29:3508–13.
24. Jackson WL, Lewis SR, Bagby JP, Hilton LR, Milad M, Bledsoe SE. Laparoscopic sleeve gastrectomy versus laparoscopic Roux-en-Y gastric bypass in the pediatric population: a MBSAQIP analysis. Surg Obes Relat Dis. 2020;16:254–60.
25. Janik MR, Mustafa RR, Rogula TG, Alhaj Saleh A, Abbas M, Khaitan L. Safety of laparoscopic sleeve gastrectomy and Roux-en-Y gastric bypass in elderly patients—analysis of the MBSAQIP. Surg Obes Relat Dis. 2018;14:1276–82.
26. Aminian A, Brethauer SA, Andalib A, Punchai S, Mackey J, Rodriguez J, Rogula T, Kroh M, Schauer PR. Can sleeve gastrectomy "cure" diabetes? long-term metabolic effects of sleeve gastrectomy in patients with type 2 diabetes. Ann Surg. 2016;264:674–81.

Other Potential Benefits of the Sleeve: Effects on Body Fat Setpoint

Alexis C. Sudlow, Dimitri J. Pournaras and Carel W. le Roux

1 Introduction

One of the challenges facing clinicians in treating obesity has been the oversimplification and characterisation of the disease in itself, as well as the mechanisms contributing to its development. Although obesity is typically viewed as a single disease state, it is more likely that an increase in adipose tissue is the result of a heterogeneous set of complex interactions and disorders which affect appetite, eating behaviours and critically, metabolism. Recognising the multifactorial causes of obesity have shed light on the challenge of adequately treating this complex disease with lifestyle interventions. These changes may be effective in producing weight loss however, weight loss through modifications in dietary or exercise habits have yet to demonstrate the ability to treat the set of diseases of obesity or to produce a sustained change in the signs of these diseases specifically, long term weight loss maintenance. Lifestyle interventions for those with significant obesity have consistently found that only 15% of patients are able to maintain a 10% weight loss over one year and in the majority of patients, most of the weight is regained within 3–5 years [1, 2]. Rather than seeing these figures as a sign of the futility of treating obesity, it should serve as a reminder to clinicians and patients that obesity is indeed a challenging disease to treat and weight regain should not be viewed as a personal failing rather as an indication that we

A. C. Sudlow (✉) · D. J. Pournaras
Department of Upper GI Surgery, Southmead Hospital, Bristol, UK
e-mail: asudlow@gmail.com

C. W. le Roux
Department of Experimental Pathology, University College Dublin, Dublin, Ireland
e-mail: carel.leroux@ucd.ie

© The Editor(s) (if applicable) and The Author(s), under exclusive license to Springer Nature Switzerland AG 2021
S. Al-Sabah et al. (eds.), *Laparoscopic Sleeve Gastrectomy*,
https://doi.org/10.1007/978-3-030-57373-7_38

must employ interventions that shift the body fat set point in order to see sustained results.

Bariatric surgery is an effective treatment for obesity which can be in part attributed to the fact that it treats several of the pathological processes driving obesity, including inducing profound metabolic changes which alter the homeostatic regulation of our body fat set point. This concept of the set point is thought to be one of the main contributory factors associated with the critical long-term weight loss maintenance which is responsible for the improvements in cardiovascular risk factors and associated improvement in all-cause mortality [3, 4].

With our growing understanding of the multisystemic effects of obesity comes an appreciation that weight is not the sole measure of the efficacy of a treatment for obesity however it remains a useful and quantifiable measure of the effect of an intervention. Considering weight loss alone however is an unhelpful metric. Weight loss in isolation is largely meaningless unless accompanied by a sustained period of weight loss maintenance which is largely responsible for the physiological changes contributing to control of comorbidity and ultimately, improved mortality. Outcomes from both lifestyle and surgical interventions would suggest that in evaluating the utility of a treatment, we should perhaps shift our perception to view weight loss and weight loss maintenance as two distinct entities, governed by discrete but interrelated homeostatic mechanisms.

2   Set Point Theory

The proposed mechanisms underlying weight regulation have long been dominated by an overly simplistic view that it is governed predominantly by a calculation of energy balance between caloric intake and energy expenditure. The biological plausibility of this explanation has seen it become near dogma not only within the wider population but the medical community as well, in spite of mounting evidence to support the fact that mechanisms regulating weight are likely a complex series of interactions between environmental and biological factors, many of which remain incompletely understood. Bariatric surgery has proven to be an effective treatment for obesity in its own right but it has also produced conditions whereby we can further expand our understanding of the homeostatic mechanisms regulating weight. Although procedures were initially classified according to the presumed mechanisms based on anatomical intentions of the operations such as malabsorptive or volume restrictive, mechanistic studies have demonstrated that there are a series of changes both centrally and within the gut responsible for not only weight loss but changes in metabolism and energy balance. While these findings have enlightened our general view of the complex regulatory mechanisms controlling hunger, satiety and weight regulation, they have also highlighted that it is very likely our current understanding and appreciation of the disease is only very rudimentary and there are many more unanswered questions. Unlike weight loss mediated by lifestyle or dietary intervention, patients losing weight following sleeve gastrectomy are able to maintain this weight loss even after they return to caloric intake similar to their preoperative levels. These findings would suggest that sleeve gastrectomy produces a sustained changes in central neurohormonal, metabolic and behavioural processes regulating weight.

One proposed element in the regulation of body weight is thought to be a centrally determined 'set point' which ensures that through various homeostatic mechanisms there are adjustments in food intake, energy expenditure or a combination of the two in order to maintain a certain inherent body fat mass. From a basic evolutionary perspective which is supported by the observed trend towards an increasing prevalence of obesity, this set point appears to be more attuned to the need of preventing starvation rather than obesity as starvation would pose a more imminent threat to life. There are a number of different purported mechanisms by which our bodies 'defend' this set amount of fat mass including regulatory feedback from specific body components such as fat mass and/or neurohormonal signalling. One such theory regarding a set point controlled by fat mass comes from one of the earliest investigations of the regulation of body weight, the Minnesota Starvation Experiment [5]. The researchers found following a period of starvation in participants without obesity, the degree of hyperphagia or overeating once the starvation period ended was proportional to the depletion of fat and muscle mass, suggesting that food intake and appetite may be in part driven by a homeostatic mechanism to maintain or in this case, restore lost fat and or muscle mass. This very early work indicated the possible presence of regulatory mechanisms based on a set point, as hyperphagia persisted only until the patients returned to the pre-intervention levels of fat and muscle mass. This basic concept appears to be supported by later research suggesting it was not necessarily signals from fat per se as the determining factor rather, neurohormones responding to variation in fat mass which were major contributors to our homeostatic control of body weight. The adipocyte derived hormone, leptin appears to play a potentially critical role in this regulatory pathway, serving as signal to the hypothalamus regarding nutritional status, energy balance and body weight. Although leptin mediates its activity via both orexigenic and anorectic neurons in the hypothalamus, leptin activity appears to be more closely related to preservation of body weight rather than prevention of obesity. In weight loss where it appears to have its greatest effect, as leptin levels fall with decreasing body weight and overall fat mass, there is a rise in NPY levels [6]. NPY is produced in the arcuate nucleus and is one of the most potent orexigenic hormones, mediating increased appetite and food intake. Similarly, changes in leptin receptor sensitivity, receptor mutations or resistance could also potentiate these effects with preserved leptin levels. It has been proposed that conditions which alter the leptin concentrations at which the hypothalamus perceives as a state of energy imbalance may change the intrinsic 'set point' however it is unclear how this is mediated [7].

3   Weight Regulation and Weight Loss Maintenance

The emergence of bariatric surgery as a treatment for obesity has deepened our understanding of the metabolic and homeostatic mechanisms involved in obesity and specifically how weight is regulated. The ability to produce significant weight loss which is sustained in the long term, unlike that seen with any lifestyle intervention has led to further development of the "set point" theory to describe how weight is maintained in both healthy weight patients and in those with obesity. The set point theory evolved from the idea that individuals possess an intrinsic mechanism for weight regulation by which their body appears to have a baseline weight around which there is little variation once they have reached adulthood. Without sustained and major changes in diet or lifestyle/activity levels, most individuals will maintain their weight around this set point which appears to have at least in part a genetic basis. This concept may serve to explain why without intervention such as bariatric surgery, the majority of patients may be able to lose weight with lifestyle measures initially but will struggle to maintain this in the long term.

4   Weight Loss and Weight Loss Maintenance Following Sleeve Gastrectomy

Given the relative late adoption of sleeve gastrectomy in comparison to other procedures, there is not as much long term data regarding weight loss compared to RYGB although evidence from studies with short to mid-term follow up would support that it produces roughly equivalent weight loss and similar levels of improvement or resolution of many obesity related comorbidities [8–10]. Although there is some variation in the individual pattern of weight loss, following sleeve gastrectomy the majority of patients will follow a similar trajectory with a period of rapid weight loss over the first year to 18 months followed by a period of weight loss plateau and eventual gradual regain. Longer term studies with follow up > 5 years would suggest %EWL in the range of 50–60% [11, 12]. Although it is recognised that following SG, some patients will regain some of the initial weight lost however, the critical element to recognise is that most weight loss is durable and is maintained around what appears to be a new "settling point". Looking at the natural pattern of weight gain over the course of an individual's life, there is a general and gradual trend towards increasing weight. Patients following SG follow this same pattern however now starting from a new, lower baseline weight and following a parallel trajectory.

Bariatric surgery was initially viewed as a treatment governed by the fundamental principles of volume restriction and malabsorption to produce weight loss. Our early understanding at the time of its effects with regards to the metabolic changes it evoked as well as the mechanisms by which it acted were incomplete. Although the procedures since then have also changed as evidenced by the widespread adoption of sleeve gastrectomy, perhaps the most critical shift in the field of bariatric surgery has been our greater appreciation of the complexity of obesity as a disease as well as the mechanisms of weight regulation and how this is affected by surgery. Mechanistic and behavioural studies have demonstrated that number of interrelated mechanisms including alterations in appetite and satiety, neurohormonal signalling as well as bile acid metabolism are key mediators of the effects of SG with regards to weight loss and improvements in metabolic dysfunction [13–15].

5 Behavioural Change Following SG Contributing to a Shift in the Set Point and Long Term Weight Loss

Although there are well recognised behavioural changes following SG which may play an important role in weight loss maintenance, the concept that it is solely the result of a decreased volume in food intake has been consistently demonstrated to be incorrect. In both human and rodent models, it is recognised that there is decreased food intake during the early postoperative period however weight loss persists after this transient change disappears [16, 17]. There are however recognised changes in eating behaviours which are more likely to be contributory factors in maintaining weight loss. In one study looking at rats undergoing bariatric surgery, there was a clear change in food preferences following SG and RYGB with a decrease in the intake of dietary fat as well as a preference for less calorie dense foods. Interestingly, only the rats undergoing SG subsequently displayed an avoidance after intragastric oil administration whereas the RYGB rats did not, suggesting that the development of food avoidance in the SG model may contribute to altered food choices [18]. These findings were supported by a further study which demonstrated a reduced preference for high fat containing foods as well as an alteration in nutrient sensing which lowered the satiety threshold, resulting in smaller meal size following SG [19]. In human studies, these changes in food preferences are more controversial. One study observed patients following SG and showed a 68% reduction in caloric intake not only a result of decreased volume but due to a preference for less calorie dense foods up to two years postoperatively [20]. These findings have been supported by further studies demonstrating changes in food preferences with patients post SG reporting sensing an increased intensity of sweet and fatty flavours which was accompanied by decreased enjoyment and desire for these same food groups [21]. Other studies showed no changes in food selection when more direct measures of behaviour were employed [22].

6 Neurohormonal Regulation of the Body Set Point

Given the observed changes in food preferences, appetite and eating behaviour, there has been an increasing focus on gut derived neurohormonal signalling which may underlie or potentiate these changes and how they contribute to weight loss maintenance. In the period following SG, there may be an adjustment of the pre-existing set point at which the body perceives there to be an energy deficit. Lowering this threshold would alter the point at which the normal homeostatic mechanisms normally preventing excessive weight loss would become active. The role of leptin has been extensively investigated with suggestions that there is the possibility of increased leptin receptor sensitivity or receptor upregulation which would counteract the normal hypothalamic response to falling leptin levels due to fat loss however, this has not been borne out by data from rat models [16]. Looking specifically at RYGB, there are studies which have served to support the role of leptin, demonstrating that leptin deficient mice lost less weight following bypass surgery. This finding would suggest that intact leptin signalling pathways are required to demonstrate the beneficial response to bariatric surgery however, its exact role in SG has yet to be elucidated [23]. Other potential neurohormonal mediators which have been proposed to have an important role in postoperative weight loss maintenance include PYY and GLP-1 which are both secreted by the L cells primarily found in the distal ileum. PYY is a key hypothalamic regulator of satiety mediated though its effects of delayed gastric emptying and reduced gastric acid secretion and is thought to potentially counteract the orexigenic effects of falling leptin levels in the postoperative period. Like PYY, GLP-1 has important and similar regulatory effects with regards to appetite but as an incretin hormone is also thought to potentiate many of the metabolic improvements in glycaemic control following SG. Both PYY and GLP-1 levels rise post sleeve gastrectomy which appears to be related to increased appetite suppression and improved weight loss [15, 24–26]. Resection of the gastric fundus in SG differentiates it from other commonly performed procedures such as RYGB or LAGB which is an important consideration when it comes to the neurohormonal changes it imparts as this is the primary location for the production of ghrelin which plays an important role in regulating hunger. A meta-analysis of 25 studies including two randomised controlled trials demonstrated decreased levels of ghrelin following SG however the implications for postoperative weight loss, weight loss maintenance and the metabolic implications are less clear [14, 15, 27]. Outcomes with RYGB are similar with regards to all of the aforementioned parameters despite the fact that it has been associated with maintained or increased ghrelin levels. Furthermore, studies in ghrelin deficient mice have demonstrated comparable outcomes following SG to wild type mice with regards to weight loss, food intake and dietary preferences, suggesting the effects of SG are ghrelin independent [28]. While these studies have not definitively demonstrated a causal role in weight loss following bariatric surgery, it is likely that neurohormonal changes related to ghrelin are part of a complex interaction of numerous factors in postoperative weight regulation.

7   Bile Acids and Long-Term Fat Mass Set Point Regulation

Changes in bile acid metabolism have also been identified as potential targets for inducing long term weight loss following SG. Studies have demonstrated an increase in serum bile acids following SG in rats which are thought to play an important role in metabolic regulation via their interaction with the nuclear receptor, farnesoid X receptor (FXR) [29]. FXR is a bile acid receptor and a key regulator in bile acid synthesis which also plays an important role in lipid and glucose metabolism [30]. This may be a key mediator, linking the alterations in bile acids following surgery to changes in glucose metabolism and plays a critical role in the postoperative remission of T2DM. The presence of this link was demonstrated when mice with a genetic disruption of FXR and diet induced obesity had attenuated weight loss and glycaemic control after a sleeve gastrectomy, suggesting the potential role of this pathway in mediating the effects of surgery [31]. Increased levels of bile acids may also contribute to an overall negative energy balance in the postoperative period via their effect on the bile acid receptor, TGR5 which results in increased oxygen consumption and energy expenditure. In rodent models following sleeve gastrectomy, increases in bile acids result in upregulation of TGR5 activity, mediating an increase in brown adipose tissue (BAT) thermogenesis [32]. BAT is involved in postprandial increases in thermogenesis and is thought to play a protective role against obesity. Overall energy expenditure has not been demonstrated to rise following SG however this increase in BAT thermogenesis may be sufficient to counteract the drop in total energy expenditure that is commonly observed following weight loss, thereby contributing to the maintenance of a new, lower weight set point. Experimental studies looking at non-invasive methods of measuring thermogenesis have supported this observation in human studies with patients following SG demonstrating increased BAT thermogenesis when measured with infrared thermography whereas there was no change evident following RYGB [33]. Although only preliminary, this data would support the possible role of SG in inducing changes in BAT activation and postoperative alterations in energy expenditure.

8   Conclusions

Sleeve gastrectomy has proven to be an effective method of inducing clinically significant weight loss, improving obesity related complications and cardiometabolic risk factors for mortality. Of critical importance in the success of SG as a procedure has been its ability to produce these changes which are sustained in the long-term however the mechanisms by which this occurs are incompletely understood. Long-term follow up data would suggest that these changes are in part the result of a re-setting of the intrinsic 'set point'. Studies using both rodent and human data indicate that this new, lower set point may cause the changes in eating behaviours, hunger and satiety. This may be mediated by complex interactions of neurohormonal and bile acid signalling both within the gut and centrally. An understanding of the regulatory pathways involved in the 'set point' may help identify means of improving surgical outcomes. This may also explain why patients immediately after surgery have profound reductions in hunger and increases in satiety, because they find themselves 25–30% above their new set point. As they reach their new set point their hunger and satiety may return to normal to allow them to maintain themselves at this new set point. This is therefore not a failure of the operation of its mechanisms but rather explains clinical observations. Clinicians can thus use the explanation of the body fat set point changes after sleeve gastrectomy to inform patients to help them achieve optimal long term health benefits.

References

1. Kraschnewski JL, et al. Long-term weight loss maintenance in the United States. Int J Obes (Lond). 2010;34(11):1644–54.
2. Weiss EC et al. Weight regain in U.S. adults who experienced substantial weight loss, 1999–2002. Am J Prev Med. 2007; 33(1):34–40.
3. Sjöström L, et al. Effects of bariatric surgery on mortality in Swedish obese subjects. N Engl J Med. 2007;357(8):741–52.
4. Peterli R, et al. Effect of laparoscopic sleeve gastrectomy vs laparoscopic Roux-en-Y gastric bypass on weight loss in patients with morbid obesity: the SM-BOSS randomized clinical trial. JAMA. 2018;319(3):255–65.
5. Keys A, et al, The biology of human starvation. 1950, The University of Minnesota Press.
6. Sahu A. Leptin signaling in the hypothalamus: emphasis on energy homeostasis and leptin resistance. Front Neuroendocrinol. 2003;24(4):225–53.
7. Flier JS. Clinical review 94: What's in a name? In search of leptin's physiologic role. J Clin Endocrinol Metab. 1998;83(5):1407–13.
8. Salminen P, et al. Effect of Laparoscopic Sleeve Gastrectomy Vs Laparoscopic Roux-en-Y gastric bypass on weight loss at 5 years among patients with morbid obesity: the sleevepass randomized clinical trial. JAMA. 2018;319(3):241–54.
9. Himpens J, Dobbeleir J, Peeters G. Long-term results of laparoscopic sleeve gastrectomy for obesity. Ann Surg. 2010;252(2):319–24.
10. Schauer PR, et al. Bariatric surgery versus intensive medical therapy for diabetes - 5-year outcomes. N Engl J Med. 2017;376(7):641–51.
11. Brethauer SA et al. Can diabetes be surgically cured? Long-term metabolic effects of bariatric surgery in obese patients with type 2 diabetes mellitus. Ann Surg. 2013; 258(4):628–36; discussion 636–7.
12. Braghetto I, et al. Is laparoscopic sleeve gastrectomy an acceptable primary bariatric procedure in obese patients? Early and 5-year postoperative results. Surg Laparosc Endosc Percutan Tech. 2012;22(6):479–86.
13. Pournaras DJ, le Roux CW. Are bile acids the new gut hormones? Lessons from weight loss surgery models. Endocrinology. 2013;154(7):2255–6.
14. Kalinowski P, et al. Ghrelin, leptin, and glycemic control after sleeve gastrectomy versus Roux-en-Y gastric bypass-results of a randomized clinical trial. Surg Obes Relat Dis. 2017;13(2):181–8.
15. Karamanakos SN, et al. Weight loss, appetite suppression, and changes in fasting and postprandial ghrelin and peptide-YY levels after Roux-en-Y gastric bypass and sleeve gastrectomy: a prospective, double blind study. Ann Surg. 2008;247(3):401–7.

16. Stefater MA et al. Sleeve gastrectomy induces loss of weight and fat mass in obese rats, but does not affect leptin sensitivity. Gastroenterology. 2010; 138(7):2426–36, 2436.e1–3.

17. Laurenius A, et al. Changes in eating behaviour and meal pattern following Roux-en-Y gastric bypass. Int J Obes (Lond). 2012;36(3):348–55.

18. Wilson-Pérez HE, et al. The effect of vertical sleeve gastrectomy on food choice in rats. Int J Obes (Lond). 2013;37(2):288–95.

19. Chambers AP, et al. Effect of vertical sleeve gastrectomy on food selection and satiation in rats. Am J Physiol Endocrinol Metab. 2012;303(8):E1076–84.

20. Coluzzi I, et al. Food intake and changes in eating behavior after laparoscopic sleeve gastrectomy. Obes Surg. 2016;26(9):2059–67.

21. Van Vuuren MAJ, et al. Taste, enjoyment, and desire of flavors change after sleeve gastrectomy-short term results. Obes Surg. 2017;27(6):1466–73.

22. Søndergaard Nielsen M, et al. Bariatric surgery does not affect food preferences, but individual changes in food preferences may predict weight loss. Obesity (Silver Spring). 2018;26(12):1879–87.

23. Hao Z, et al. Does gastric bypass surgery change body weight set point? Int J Obes Suppl. 2016;6(Suppl 1):S37-43.

24. Batterham RL, et al. Gut hormone PYY(3–36) physiologically inhibits food intake. Nature. 2002;418(6898):650–4.

25. Nannipieri M, et al. Roux-en-Y gastric bypass and sleeve gastrectomy: mechanisms of diabetes remission and role of gut hormones. J Clin Endocrinol Metab. 2013;98(11):4391–9.

26. Peterli R, et al. Metabolic and hormonal changes after laparoscopic Roux-en-Y gastric bypass and sleeve gastrectomy: a randomized, prospective trial. Obes Surg. 2012;22(5):740–8.

27. McCarty TR, Jirapinyo P, Thompson CC. Effect of sleeve gastrectomy on Ghrelin, GLP-1, PYY, and GIP Gut hormones: A systematic review and meta-analysis. Ann Surg; (2019).

28. Chambers AP, et al. The effects of vertical sleeve gastrectomy in rodents are ghrelin independent. Gastroenterology. 2013;144(1):50-52.e5.

29. Myronovych A, et al. Vertical sleeve gastrectomy reduces hepatic steatosis while increasing serum bile acids in a weight-loss-independent manner. Obesity (Silver Spring). 2014;22(2):390–400.

30. Claudel T, Staels B, Kuipers F. The Farnesoid X receptor: a molecular link between bile acid and lipid and glucose metabolism. Arterioscler Thromb Vasc Biol. 2005;25(10):2020–30.

31. Ryan KK, et al. FXR is a molecular target for the effects of vertical sleeve gastrectomy. Nature. 2014;509(7499):183–8.

32. Baraboi ED, et al. Metabolic changes induced by the biliopancreatic diversion in diet-induced obesity in male rats: the contributions of sleeve gastrectomy and duodenal switch. Endocrinology. 2015;156(4):1316–29.

33. Piquer-Garcia I, et al. Use of infrared thermography to estimate brown fat activation after a cooling protocol in patients with severe obesity that underwent bariatric surgery. Obes Surg. 2020;30(6):2375–81.

Quality of Life and Bariatric Surgery

Rawan El-Abd and Salman Al-Sabah

Quality of life includes mental, physical, and social well-being. Besides increased morbidity and mortality, obesity is also associated with reduced quality of life as reported by studies assessing Health-Related Quality of Life (HRQL) in patients with obesity, which report BMI to be associated with fatigue, chronic pain, and physical limitations, ultimately resulting in poor patient health perception and reduced quality of life (QOL) [1–7] that is more prominent in the female population [8].

The success of a bariatric intervention does not only relate to weight loss, but is also determined by its effect on QOL, behaviors of eating disorders, food tolerance, and resolution of co-morbidities. It is expected that after bariatric surgery quality of life improves due to weight loss, better function, and resolution of co-morbidities, however, the occurrence of side effects may hinder that. Such side effects include recurrent vomiting, regurgitation, or poor postoperative nutrient absorption [9, 10].

In fact, the great majority of studies in the literature conclude that HRQL improves drastically within months after bariatric surgery with maintained effect up to 10 years post-operatively in some patients [11–16]. If assessed before and after undergoing a bariatric procedure, patients score better post-operatively and can even score better than the "normal" general population, making bariatric surgery an intervention of great impact on QOL [11, 12]. The changes in HRQL after bariatric surgery are not absolute but rather they largely reflect periods of weight loss, weight regain, and weight stability. HRQOL greatly improves with a weight loss of 30% after bariatric surgery [17] and starts deteriorating as a patient regains weight [16]. Peak improvement is seen in the short-term (6–12 months) but tends to slowly decrease with time (1 to 6 years post operatively), which is greatly

R. El-Abd (✉) · S. Al-Sabah
Faculty of Medicine, Health Sciences Centre, Kuwait University, Jabriya, Kuwait
e-mail: rawanela@gmail.com

© The Editor(s) (if applicable) and The Author(s), under exclusive license to Springer Nature Switzerland AG 2021
S. Al-Sabah et al. (eds.), *Laparoscopic Sleeve Gastrectomy*,
https://doi.org/10.1007/978-3-030-57373-7_39

influenced by the total weight loss and side-effects of specific procedures [14, 18]. In extended follow-up studies, it was reported that the periods between 6 and 10 years postoperatively show stability in both body weight and HRQL scores [16] and that a maintained total weight loss of only 10% is sufficient for a positive long term outcome on HRQL. In fact, if assessed after 10 years, patients who underwent bariatric surgery show better outcomes on health perception, social interaction psychosocial functioning and depression than those who did not undergo an intervention [16].

Food tolerance, gastrointestinal health, and quality of life are different between surgeries. Sleeve Gastrectomy (SG) and Roux-en-Y Gastric Bypass (RYGB) show better effect on HRQL as compared to Gastric Banding (GB) with a significant relation to weight loss after each surgery [19, 20]. SG also results in better food tolerance, eating behavior, and gastrointestinal quality of life than RYGB and GB, which contribute to its favorable outcome on HRQL [9, 21]. Gastrointestinal quality of life is strongly correlated with food tolerance after surgery [19].

To assess the QOL of patients, different tools are available, the most studied are:

1   Medical Outcomes Survey Short Form 36S (SF-36)

This is a questionnaire of 36 items around 8 areas: physical functioning, social functioning, physical problems, emotional problems, mental health, energy, pain, and general perception of health. Results are reported into 2 categories: physical health and mental health. It is scored from 0 to 100 for each area [22–24].

2   Bariatric Analysis and Reporting Outcome System (BAROS) Score [25]

This score is done after a bariatric intervention and assess its effectiveness through examining 3 domains: weight loss, changes in co-morbidities, and quality of life. Each domain can have up to 3 points, with points deducted for complications or reoperations. It finally divides patients into 5 groups and determines the success or failure of the intervention. This score can be used to compare outcomes of different operations or surgeons and serve as a uniform assessment of outcomes.

3   The Bariatric Quality of Life Index (BQL)

This tool combines medical data of a patient with a questionnaire of 13 questions and 65 points. It measures a patient's QOL before and after a bariatric intervention. It was reported to be superior to other questionnaires (e.g., BAROS) [26, 27]. A study conducted to validate this questionnaire reported BQL to show a strong correlation with results of SF but less correlation with BAROS, EWL, and other questionnaires [26]. The verified version of BQL was also validated by a study on 466 patients [27].

4   The Food Tolerance Score (FT Q)/Quality of Alimentation Questionnaire

This questionnaire of 27 points was developed to assess food tolerance after bariatric surgery through assessing 4 components including: tolerance of different food types, timing and content of meals, frequency of vomiting/regurgitation, and patient satisfaction with alimentation. It is easy to use and useful when comparing food tolerance before and after surgery and between different procedures [18].

Quality of Life After Sleeve Gastrectomy

Several studies of different follow-up intervals have assessed the effect of sleeve gastrectomy on QOL and compared it to other procedures.

1. Short-Term Effect (1–3 years)

Kirkir et al. conducted a study on 562 patients undergoing SG with a mean follow up time of 7 months and showed the mean scores for QOL to be significantly increased after SG ($p<0.05$ to<0.001), with 19.6% of the study sample to be classified as excellent, 25.6% as very good, 34.9% as good, 15.3% as fair, and 4.6% as failure results on the updated BAROS scoring system. They concluded that SG is a very effective bariatric intervention for weight control and improvement in comorbidities and QOL in short- and mid-term [28]. Peterli et al. also conducted a prospective study to measure QOL of patients undergoing SG and RYGB using the BQL and other scores and showed QOL to improve significantly when comparing pre- and post-operative results at 1 and 2 years but results were poorer at 3 years. They reported a tendency of SG patients' QOL to improve shortly after the surgery but continue to deteriorate overtime; however, they concluded that both surgery types are equally effective in terms of weight loss, quality of life, and complication rate [29]. In addition, Fezzi et al. used the SF36 questionnaire for 78 consecutive patients undergoing SG. The patients completed the questionnaire pre-operatively and one year post-operatively. All areas of the questionnaire regarding patients' QOL showed significant improvement, and they concluded that SG is an effective procedure with measurable improvement in HRQOL as well as weight reduction [30]. Even more, Nadalini et al. [20] examined 110 patients using the SF36 questionnaire to assess the effects of 3 different surgeries; GB, RYGB, and SG. Patients completed the questionnaire pre-operatively and at mean of 3 years' post-operatively. All categories of the questionnaire showed significant improvement, except general and mental health, and satisfaction was greater in patients with higher EWL and in those who underwent RYGB or SG as compared to GB, with a significant relation to weight loss after each surgery. The authors also examined the possibility of different domains of the questionnaire being able to predict weight loss and found physical functioning domain to be a significant predictor of the weight lost after surgery independent of age, sex and type of surgery (p = 0.01).

2. Medium-Term Effect (4–5 years)

AlKhalifa et al. compared SG to GB in 48 patients and showed the former surgery to result in better food tolerance (P < 0.001) and better eating behaviors (P = 0.001) when compared with gastric banding after 1–4 years of follow-up. They also reported that SG patients showed significant improvement in all parameters of HRQOL except for mental health status [21]. Also, Flølo et al. [31] studied the effect of SG using SF36 on 168 patients and reported their outcomes at 5 years post-operatively, which showed patients to score better on mental and physical components of the questionnaire than the non-surgical cohort but not the general population. Strain et al., in addition, conducted a study on 77 patients undergoing SG by using the SF36 at 1, 3, and 5 years post-operatively and found QOL to initially improve but then deteriorate in most domains overtime which was associated with weight regain [32].

3. Long-Term Effect (6–10 years)

D'Hondt et al. [33] used the BAROS and SF36 questionnaires to investigate the effect of SG on quality of life of 83 patients up to 6 years post-operatively. They concluded that SG results in good to excellent improvement in HRQOL. The authors divided patients into 2 groups according to %EWL (<50 or >50) and found QOL to improve dramatically with significant differences in 2 domains: physical functioning and general health. According to the BAROS score, authors reported that 75 (90.4%) of their study participants scored a "good" to "excellent" score. They also reported that different groups of patients may experience different changes in their QOL depending on factors like the development of reflux or weight regain. They concluded that SG procedure results in good to excellent improvement in HRQL. Furthermore, Felsenrich et. al conducted a study to assess QOL of patients 10 years after SG through BQL and SF 36 questionnaires and found that symptomatic reflux, but not %EWL, impairs patients' long-term QOL after SG. BQL showed significant differences between patients with and without any symptoms of reflux but failed to detect a statistically significant difference between those with >50% or <50% %EWL. The results with SF36 also showed reflux to be a determinant of lower QOL but this score also found %EWL >50 to correlate with better QOL scores in 3 categories; these were less body pain (p = 0.02), better emotional role (p = 0.04), and better mental health (p = 0.04) [34].

Conclusion

In conclusion, sleeve gastrectomy as a bariatric surgery is associated with significant improvement in HRQL that is most prominent in the first months after surgery and can be maintained in the long term and up to 10 years, which is largely dependent on maintained weight loss and absence of gastroesophageal reflux disease.

References

1. Hsu LK, Mulliken B, McDonagh B, Krupa Das S, Rand W, Fairburn CG, et al. Binge eating disorder in extreme obesity. Int J Obes Relat Metab Disord. 2002;26(10):1398–403.
2. Fabricatore AN, Wadden TA, Sarwer DB, Faith MS. Health-related quality of life and symptoms of depression in extremely obese persons seeking bariatric surgery. Obes Surg. 2005;15(3):304–9.
3. Fine JT, Colditz GA, Coakley EH, Moseley G, Manson JE, Willett WC, et al. A prospective study of weight change and health-related quality of life in women. JAMA. 1999;282(22):2136–42.
4. Fontaine KR, Cheskin LJ, Barofsky I. Health-related quality of life in obese persons seeking treatment. J Fam Pract. 1996;43(3):265–70.
5. Larsson U, Karlsson J, Sullivan M. Impact of overweight and obesity on health-related quality of life–a Swedish population study. Int J Obes Relat Metab Disord. 2002;26(3):417–24.
6. Sullivan M, Karlsson J, Sjöström L, Backman L, Bengtsson C, Bouchard C, et al. Swedish obese subjects (SOS)--an intervention study of obesity. Baseline evaluation of health and psychosocial functioning in the first 1743 subjects examined. Int J Obes Relat Metab Disord. 1993; 17(9):503–12.
7. Mitchell JE, Selzer F, Kalarchian MA, Devlin MJ, Strain GW, Elder KA, et al. Psychopathology before surgery in the longitudinal assessment of bariatric surgery-3 (LABS-3) psychosocial study. Surg Obes Relat Dis. 2012;8(5):533–41.
8. Kubik JF, Gill RS, Laffin M, Karmali S. The impact of bariatric surgery on psychological health. J Obes. 2013;2013:837989.
9. Freeman RA, Overs SE, Zarshenas N, Walton KL, Jorgensen JO. Food tolerance and diet quality following adjustable gastric banding, sleeve gastrectomy and Roux-en-Y gastric bypass. Obes Res Clin Pract. 2014;8(2):e115-200.
10. Tack J, Deloose E. Complications of bariatric surgery: dumping syndrome, reflux and vitamin deficiencies. Best Pract Res Clin Gastroenterol. 2014;28(4):741–9.
11. Schok M, Geenen R, van Antwerpen T, de Wit P, Brand N, van Ramshorst B. Quality of life after laparoscopic adjustable gastric banding for severe obesity: postoperative and retrospective preoperative evaluations. Obes Surg. 2000;10(6):502–8.
12. Choban PS, Onyejekwe J, Burge JC, Flancbaum L. A health status assessment of the impact of weight loss following Roux-en-Y gastric bypass for clinically severe obesity. J Am Coll Surg. 1999;188(5):491–7.
13. Dymek MP, le Grange D, Neven K, Alverdy J. Quality of life and psychosocial adjustment in patients after Roux-en-Y gastric bypass: a brief report. Obes Surg. 2001;11(1):32–9.
14. Karlsson J, Sjöström L, Sullivan M. Swedish obese subjects (SOS)--an intervention study of obesity. Two-year follow-up of health-related quality of life (HRQL) and eating behavior after gastric surgery for severe obesity. Int J Obes Relat Metab Disord. 1998; 22(2):113–26.
15. Roger Andersen J, Aasprang A, Bergsholm P, Sletteskog N, Våge V, Karin NG. Health-related quality of life and paid work participation after duodenal switch. Obes Surg. 2010;20(3):340–5.
16. Karlsson J, Taft C, Rydén A, Sjöström L, Sullivan M. Ten-year trends in health-related quality of life after surgical and conventional treatment for severe obesity: the SOS intervention study. Int J Obes (Lond). 2007;31(8):1248–61.
17. Sarwer DB, Wadden TA, Moore RH, Eisenberg MH, Raper SE, Williams NN. Changes in quality of life and body image after gastric bypass surgery. Surg Obes Relat Dis. 2010;6(6):608–14.
18. Suter M, Calmes JM, Paroz A, Giusti V. A new questionnaire for quick assessment of food tolerance after bariatric surgery. Obes Surg. 2007;17(1):2–8.
19. Overs SE, Freeman RA, Zarshenas N, Walton KL, Jorgensen JO. Food tolerance and gastrointestinal quality of life following three bariatric procedures: adjustable gastric banding, Roux-en-Y gastric bypass, and sleeve gastrectomy. Obes Surg. 2012;22(4):536–43.

20. Nadalini L, Zenti MG, Masotto L, Indelicato L, Fainelli G, Bonora F, et al. Improved quality of life after bariatric surgery in morbidly obese patients. Interdisciplinary group of bariatric surgery of Verona (G.I.C.O.V.). G Chir. 2014; 35(7–8):161–4.
21. Al Khalifa K, Al AA. Quality of life, food tolerance, and eating disorder behavior after laparoscopic gastric banding and sleeve gastrectomy - results from a middle eastern center of excellence. BMC Obes. 2018;5:44.
22. Jenkinson C, Coulter A, Wright L. Short form 36 (SF36) health survey questionnaire: normative data for adults of working age. BMJ. 1993;306(6890):1437–40.
23. Ware JE, Jr., Sherbourne CD. The MOS 36-item short-form health survey (SF-36). I. Conceptual framework and item selection. Med Care. 1992; 30(6):473–83.
24. Brazier JE, Harper R, Jones NM, O'Cathain A, Thomas KJ, Usherwood T, et al. Validating the SF-36 health survey questionnaire: new outcome measure for primary care. BMJ. 1992;305(6846):160–4.
25. Oria HE, Moorehead MK. Updated Bariatric Analysis and Reporting Outcome System (BAROS). Surg Obes Relat Dis. 2009;5(1):60–6.
26. Weiner S, Sauerland S, Fein M, Blanco R, Pomhoff I, Weiner RA. The Bariatric Quality of Life index: a measure of well-being in obesity surgery patients. Obes Surg. 2005;15(4):538–45.
27. Weiner S, Sauerland S, Weiner R, Cyzewski M, Brandt J, Neugebauer E. Validation of the adapted Bariatric Quality of Life Index (BQL) in a prospective study in 446 bariatric patients as one-factor model. Obes Facts. 2009; 2 Suppl 1(Suppl 1):63–6.
28. Kirkil C, Aygen E, Korkmaz MF, Bozan MB. Quality of life after laparoscopic sleeve gastrectomy using baros system. Arq Bras Cir Dig. 2018;31(3):e1385.
29. Peterli R, Wölnerhanssen BK, Vetter D, Nett P, Gass M, Borbély Y, et al. Laparoscopic sleeve gastrectomy versus Roux-Y-gastric bypass for morbid obesity-3-year outcomes of the prospective randomized Swiss Multicenter Bypass Or Sleeve Study (SM-BOSS). Ann Surg. 2017;265(3):466–73.
30. Fezzi M, Kolotkin RL, Nedelcu M, Jaussent A, Schaub R, Chauvet MA, et al. Improvement in quality of life after laparoscopic sleeve gastrectomy. Obes Surg. 2011;21(8):1161–7.
31. Flølo TN, Andersen JR, Kolotkin RL, Aasprang A, Natvig GK, Hufthammer KO, et al. Five-year outcomes after vertical sleeve gastrectomy for severe obesity: a prospective cohort study. Obes Surg. 2017;27(8):1944–51.
32. Strain GW, Saif T, Gagner M, Rossidis M, Dakin G, Pomp A. Cross-sectional review of effects of laparoscopic sleeve gastrectomy at 1, 3, and 5 years. Surg Obes Relat Dis. 2011;7(6):714–9.
33. D'Hondt M, Vanneste S, Pottel H, Devriendt D, Van Rooy F, Vansteenkiste F. Laparoscopic sleeve gastrectomy as a single-stage procedure for the treatment of morbid obesity and the resulting quality of life, resolution of comorbidities, food tolerance, and 6-year weight loss. Surg Endosc. 2011;25(8):2498–504.
34. Felsenreich DM, Prager G, Kefurt R, Eilenberg M, Jedamzik J, Beckerhinn P, et al. Quality of Life 10 Years after sleeve gastrectomy: a multicenter study. Obes Facts. 2019;12(2):157–66.

LSG: Risks and Considerations

Risks Associated with Sleeve Gastrectomy

Aparna Govil Bhasker and Kamal Mahawar

Approximately 46% of all bariatric operations performed worldwide consist of Sleeve Gastrectomy (SG). Thus, making it the most commonly performed bariatric operation worldwide [1]. Technical ease, simplicity, no alteration of gastrointestinal continuity, and relative safety are some of the reasons behind its immense popularity. SG also has a lower learning curve as compared to gastric bypass procedures which are technically more challenging. In a review, the outcomes of sleeve gastrectomy were compared with other bariatric operations and the complication rate in the SG group was much lower than the gastric bypass group [2]. However, though less frequent, the complications after SG, especially leaks, can be devastating and very difficult to treat. It is, therefore, important that surgeons undergo appropriate training and mentoring before they start performing this procedure. Careful attention to a number of preoperative, intra-operative, and postoperative considerations is the only way to deliver safety. Newer surgeons should recognise that bariatric surgery poses a number of unique challenges that go beyond the general, technical expertise of the surgeon. Even surgeons well versed with other complex gastrointestinal procedures need to be involved with at least 50–100 bariatric procedures before independent practice. Best outcomes are delivered by surgeons who are appropriately trained and mentored and have a reasonable volume that allow for the maintenance of skills. Surgeons should consider teaming up with other surgeons if the volumes are low in their practice.

A. G. Bhasker (✉)
Bariatric and Laparoscopic Surgeon, Gleneagles Global Hospital, Parel, Mumbai, India
e-mail: draparnagovil@gmail.com

K. Mahawar
Consultant General & Bariatric Surgeon, Sunderland Royal Hospital, Sunderland, UK
e-mail: kmahawar@gmail.com

411
S. Al-Sabah et al. (eds.), *Laparoscopic Sleeve Gastrectomy*,
https://doi.org/10.1007/978-3-030-57373-7_40

The early complication rate after sleeve gastrectomy varies from 5.4 to 7.3%. The overall rate of severe complications after sleeve gastrectomy is approximately 1.2 to 2.2% and the 30 days readmission rate is reported as 2.8% [3–6]. Complications after sleeve gastrectomy can be classified as:

- Intra-operative complications—Anaesthesia related complications, Injury to internal organs, Haemorrhage
- Early complications (≤30 day)—Haemorrhage, Staple line leaks, Deep Vein Thrombosis and Pulmonary Embolism, Porto-mesenteric venous thrombosis, Trocar site herniation
- Late complications (>30 day)—Abscesses, Late leaks, Strictures, Twists and kinks, Gastro-esophageal reflux disease, Cholelithiasis, Iron and vitamin B 12 deficiency, Secondary hyperparathyroidism, Neuropathy.

Like any other surgery, complications after sleeve gastrectomy may be graded as per the Clavien Dindo classification and surgeons are encouraged to use them whilst reporting (Table 1).

It is crucial to not only pay attention to technical details but also diagnose and manage complications promptly to further improve the safety of this procedure. Currently, there is enormous variation amongst bariatric surgeons concerning various aspects of this procedure [8]. Future studies and consensus building exercises

Table 1 Clavien Dindo classification of surgical complications [7]

Grade	Definition
Grade I	Any deviation from the normal postoperative course without the need for pharmacological treatment or surgical, endoscopic, and radiological interventions Allowed therapeutic regimens are: drugs as antiemetics, antipyretics, analgetics, diuretics, electrolytes, and physiotherapy. This grade also includes wound infections opened at the bedside
Grade II	Requiring pharmacological treatment with drugs other than such allowed for grade I complications Blood transfusions and total parenteral nutrition are also included
Grade III Grade IIIa Grade IIIb	Requiring surgical, endoscopy or radiological intervention Intervention not under general anesthesia Intervention under general anesthesia
Grade IV Grade IVa Graade IVb	Life-threatening complication (including CNS complications)* requiring IC/ICU management Single organ dysfunction (including dialysis) Multiorgan dysfunction
Grade V	Death of a patient
Suffix "d"	If the patient suffers from a complication at the time of discharge, the suffix "d" (for "disability") is added to the respective grade of complication. This label indicates the need for a follow up to fully evaluate the complication

*Brain hemorrhage, ischemic stroke, subarrachnoidal bleeding, but excluding transient ischemic attacks. CNS, central nervous system; IC, intermediate care; ICU, intensive care unit

will need to identify the best options from amongst a range of practices being used worldwide.

Patients suffering from obesity pose a greater challenge when it comes to diagnosing severe early surgical complications. They may not present in the manner other general surgery patients do. Hence the onus is on the bariatric professionals to be extra-vigilant and pick up the subtle signs that may be the only indication of an impending catastrophe.

In general, unexplained tachycardia, tachypnoea, fever, pain, nausea, vomiting and not feeling well should prompt further evaluation. In particular, a heart rate of over 100 should alert the surgeon and a heart rate of > 120 should prompt further investigation or even a diagnostic laparoscopy as appropriate. A full blood count, CRP, urine routine, pro-calcitonin, X-ray studies of chest and abdomen, CT scan and other tests as appropriate may be performed as indicated clinically. In general, bariatric surgeons advise early laparoscopy in cases of persistent doubt and uncertainty.

Best outcomes are achieved when the complications are detected and treated early. Early action also helps to reduce the morbidity and mortality. Ensuing chapters in this section discuss the management of some of the commonest and most dreaded complications of this procedure in detail.

References

1. Welbourn R, Hollyman M, Kinsman R et al. Bariatric surgery worldwide: baseline demographic description and One-Year Outcomes from the Fourth IFSO global registry report 2018. Obes Surg. 2019 Mar; 29(3):782–95.
2. Trastulli S, Desiderio J, Guarino S, Cirocchi R, Scalercio V, Noya G, et al. Laparoscopic sleeve gastrectomy compared with other bariatric surgical procedures: a systematic review of randomized trials. Surg Obes Relat Dis. 2013;9:816–29.
3. Finks JF, Kole KL, Yenumula PR, English WJ, Krause KR, Carlin AM, Genaw JA, Banerjee M, Birkmeyer JD, Birkmeyer NJ Michigan Bariatric Surgery Collaborative, from the Center for Healthcare Outcomes and Policy. Predicting risk for serious complications with bariatric surgery: results from the Michigan Bariatric Surgery Collaborative. Ann Surg. 2011; 254:633–40.
4. Pradarelli JC, Varban OA, Ghaferi AA, Weiner M, Carlin AM, Dimick JB. Hospital variation in perioperative complications for laparoscopic sleeve gastrectomy in Michigan. Surgery. 2016;159:1113–20.
5. Birkmeyer NJ, Dimick JB, Share D, Hawasli A, English WJ, Genaw J, Finks JF, Carlin AM, Birkmeyer JD Michigan Bariatric Surgery Collaborative. Hospital complication rates with bariatric surgery in Michigan. JAMA. 2010; 304:435–42.
6. Berger ER, Huffman KM, Fraker T, Petrick AT, Brethauer SA, Hall BL, Ko CY, Morton JM. Prevalence and risk factors for bariatric surgery readmissions: findings from 130,007 admissions in the metabolic and bariatric surgery accreditation and quality improvement program. Ann Surgery. 2018;267:122–31.
7. Dindo D, Demartines N, Clavien PA. Classification of surgical complications: a new proposal with evaluation in a cohort of 6336 patients and results of a survey. Ann Surg. 2004;240(2):205–13.
8. Adil MT, Aminian A, Bhasker AG et al. Perioperative practices concerning sleeve gastrectomy—a survey of 863 surgeons with a cumulative experience of 520,230 Procedures. Obes Surg. 2020 Feb; 30(2):483–92.

Outcomes and Complications After Sleeve Gastrectomy

Shujhat Khan and Hutan Ashrafian ⓘ

1   Introduction

The SG does not involve intestinal bypass and is simply a restrictive procedure. The evolution from an open duodenal switch procedure to the laparoscopic sleeve gastrectomy that is now routinely performed was initially reserved for high risk, super-morbidly obese patients as a staged procedure. It was then subsequently adapted as a single-staged operation in those with a lower BMI. However, the beneficial effects of SG go beyond that of simply reducing obesity, and has positive effects on diabetes, dyslipidaemia, and hypertension.

2   Impact on Obesity

Studies have shown that SG can produce outcomes that are equivalent to or better than Roux-en-Y gastric bypass in alleviating obesity-related comorbidities [2]. Patients report an improvement in hypertension, type 2 diabetes, increased HDL levels, and reduction in uraemia levels, that were present even after 10 years [3]. Whilst these changes vary amongst the population, it appears that it typically occurs within 17 months [4–6]. However, after approximately 2–3 years, patients start to regain weight following the bariatric operation, although the amount of overall mass that patients lose varies within the literature, with some studies

S. Khan
Milton Keynes University Hospital, London, UK
e-mail: shujhat.khan15@imperial.ac.uk

H. Ashrafian (✉)
Institute of Global Health Innovation at Imperial College London, London, UK
e-mail: h.ashrafian@imperial.ac.uk

© The Editor(s) (if applicable) and The Author(s), under exclusive license to Springer   415
Nature Switzerland AG 2021
S. Al-Sabah et al. (eds.), *Laparoscopic Sleeve Gastrectomy*,
https://doi.org/10.1007/978-3-030-57373-7_41

Table 1 Meta-analysis demonstrating changes in weight (pooled mean (95% confidence interval)).

Time after surgery	Change in BMI	Change in EWL
6 months	−11.49 (−8.81 to −14.18)	−50.40 (−26.29 to −74.50)
12 months	−13.05 (−9.68 to −16.42)	−61.12 (−20.26 to −101.98)
24 months	–	−71.00 (−57.00 to −85.00)
36 months	−13.00 (−11.00 to −15.00)	−75.90 (−67.62 to −84.18)

Adapted from Pedroso et al. [1]. BMI = body mass index; EWL = excess weight loss

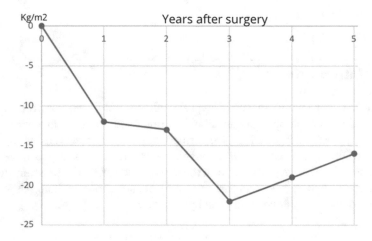

Fig. 1 Meta-analysis results assessing weight loss following bariatric operations. (GB = gastric bypass; AGB = adjustable gastric banding; SG = laparoscopic sleeve gastrectomy). Adapted from Chang et al. [16]

suggesting there is an estimated weight loss of 46% whilst others suggest estimated weight loss as high as 86% (Table 1, Fig. 1) [7–16].

3 Impact on Diabetes

Bariatric surgery is highly effective at improving outcomes in diabetic patients and has demonstrated superior results to medication alone [17]. Additionally, surgery can significantly improve microvascular and macrovascular effects which are often responsible for the complications of diabetes [18–20]. Approximately 56–59% of patients experience type 2 diabetes mellitus remission after a year following a SG operation, and the beneficial effects of the operation on diabetes continue long after a year, with 84–86% of patients noting remission after a 5-year period. However, it does appear that many patients will also relapse. The HBA1c level reduces significantly in the several months following a SG but starts to steadily increase again (Fig. 2) [21]. There is however conflicting evidence

Fig. 2 Change in HBA1c after sleeve gastrectomy over time. Adapted from McTigue et al. [21]

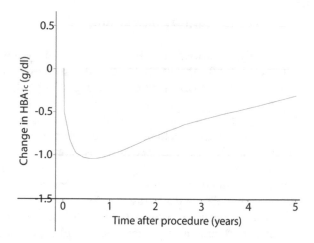

when comparing the effects of Roux-en-Y gastric bypass with SG. Whilst some studies report no significant difference between the two [22–24], others suggest Roux-en-Y will lead to a greater improvement in diabetes remission, and a more sustained improvement [21].

There are multiple different mechanisms contributing to the beneficial effect. Firstly, patients experience a hypocaloric state immediately following a bariatric operation aided by a restriction in caloric intake. Additionally, there is significant weight lost through the procedure, together, these play a fundamental role in influencing diabetes remission. This is exemplified when patients achieve comparable glycaemic changes whilst observing caloric restriction after a SG when compared with those who have similar caloric restriction without being operated upon [25].

4 Impact on Hypertension

There is a strong correlation between obesity and hypertension, and there are several proposed mechanisms that link the two conditions. This includes adipocytes increasing free fatty acid and angiotensinogen levels. Additionally, it causes stimulation of the renin angiotensin system leading to retention of salt and water, which increases the blood pressure [26]. As such, decreasing obesity will in turn reverse these effects.

Bariatric surgery has been demonstrated to be both effective and safe in patients who are clinically hypertensive. Studies suggest approximately 78.5% who undergo SG will see improvements in hypertension, whilst 67.1% will report resolution [27]. The literature on the effects of SG on hypertension suggests that SG does improve blood pressure levels. However, many studies don't define the values that they classify as hypertensive, and there is heterogeneity in those that do define their values which makes it difficult to combine data, and fully analyse the outcomes [28].

5   Impact on Dyslipidaemia

As with hypertension, the link with obesity and dyslipidaemia is well established, with between 50–80% of obese patients also presenting with dyslipidaemia [29]. Obese patients tend to have lower amounts of high-density lipoprotein (HDL) levels, but greater amounts of low-density lipoproteins (LDL) and triglyceride levels. This may be as a result of the insulin resistance that obese patients also tend to have, which contributes to increased levels of free fatty acids being transported to the liver. The liver, in turn, produces very low-density lipoprotein (VLDL), which promotes the circulation of triglycerides and LDL levels [30]. Dyslipidaemia has significant consequences for patients, causing increased atherogenesis as well as adversely influencing cardiovascular disorders.

For the majority of patients (83.5%), SG will improve hyperlipidaemia, and a significant proportion of patients (54%) will experience complete resolution, perhaps as a result of the reversal of insulin resistance [31]. Patients will see a greater level of HDL, and lower LDL and triglyceride levels after the operation, with the effects lasting for over a year [32]. Removal of the fundus also leads to reduced gastric lipase and ghrelin secretion, hormones that contribute to dyslipidaemia [33–35]. Additionally, reduced caloric intake and changes in gastrointestinal transit time means that patients absorb less food which will all lead to improvements in hyperlipidaemia.

6   Complications

Whilst a SG is a routine procedure that produces significant benefits for patients, there are numerous complications that, although uncommon, should be considered. The SG operation has a mortality of close to less than 0.01%, with morbidity typically associated in cases involving inexperienced surgeons [36]. As an example, mid-gastric stenosis, which occurs in less than 1% of cases, occurs as a result of over-sewing of the staple line or if the SG is calibrated on a tube that is too narrow [37, 38]. Complications can be categorised dependent on their expected duration of occurrence following the operation (Table 2). However, as will all operations, there are also non-surgical complications that are attributed to SG.

7   Non-Surgical Complications of Sleeve Gastrectomy

The non-surgical complications of SG include an increased incidence of pulmonary embolism, which is expected in up to 0.6% of bariatric patients. However, mortality remains low at up to 0.4% with appropriate anticoagulation [39–42]. Additional respiratory complications including pneumopathies, pleural effusion, and atelectasis, although these are rare affecting approximately 1% of bariatric patients [43, 44]. As with all surgeries, prognosis tend to be worse with increasing

Table 2 Complications associated with sleeve gastrectomy

Complications	Chronicity
Haemorrhage	Acute
Pulmonary embolism	Acute
Nutritional deficiency	Chronic
GERD	Chronic
Abscess	Chronic
Stricture	Chronic
Leak	Acute/chronic
Alteration to bile flow	Chronic
Anatomical changes	Chronic
Hormonal changes	Chronic
Impact on metabolism	Acute/chronic
Cardiovascular effects	Acute/chronic
Changes to the microbiota	Chronic

age, BMI, pre-existing cardiovascular risk factors, and intra-operative complications. However, bariatric operations will specifically lead to nutritional deficiencies, as a direct consequence of anatomical manipulation or indeed following the procedure for example due to vomiting and reduced food intake. Five years following a SG, patients report a deficiency of zinc (14.3% of patients), vitamin D (42% of patients), vitamin B1 (30.8% of patients), along with hypoalbuminaemia (5.5% of patients), and low serum haemoglobin (28.6% of patients) [45].

8 Nutritional Deficiency After Sleeve Gastrectomy

The severity of disease as a result of nutritional deficiency would likely depend on the length of duration without correction. As an example, those with vitamin D deficiency can develop osteoporosis from secondary hyperparathyroidism. Additionally, deficiency of thiamine, a water-soluble B-complex vitamin, is necessary for cerebral metabolism. Deficiency, therefore, can damage regions of the brain including the cerebellum, mamillary bodies, superior and inferior colliculi, medial thalamus, periventricular region of the third ventricle, as well as the periaqueductal area. Whilst Wernicke encephalopathy is classically defined as a triad of ophthalmoplegia, ataxia, and reduced consciousness, many patients will not exhibit all these symptoms and so the condition may often go unreported [46]. As a side note, this condition is more likely to occur following a Roux-en-Y bypass because the jejunum is involved in maximal absorption of thiamine. Thiamine deficiency can also result in beriberi, a condition characterised by sensory and motor impairment [47].

Following a SG, vomiting is a prominent risk factor for vitamin deficiency. This can be due to the formation of strictures, leakage, or bleeding from the staple-line. Additionally, reduced energy intake, rapid weight loss, and non-compliance of supplements can all contribute to vitamin deficiency [48–50].

9   Early Complications of Sleeve Gastrectomy

Early complications of SG include the formation of a fistula which is likely to affect approximately 2% of patients. Fistulae typically arise at the upper edge of the staple line and may be produced as a result of increased intragastric pressure, ischaemia on the staple lines, or indeed by poor technique. Other complications include formation of strictures (0.7–4% in patients), haemorrhage (1.5% of patients), and leakage (1.5–2.4%) [51–53]. It is important to recognise that complication rates increase if revision surgery is required or if patients require conversion of other bariatric surgical procedures into a SG [54]. Leakage typically occurs near the gastro-oesophageal junction at the top of the suture lines, but the post-operative time onset varies widely. Most cases will occur between 3–14 days following the operation with a median onset at 7 days [55].

These complications are largely driven by operative skill and the risk can be diminished with an experienced surgeon, and a compliant patient. However, the physiological changes that occur following a bariatric operation can sometimes be unpredictable and the effects of bariatric operations go beyond simply reducing weight. These effects can be split into 5 distinct categories through the so-called BRAVE effects of bypass surgery, that is: alteration to bile flow; restriction of the stomach; anatomical changes; effects on vagus nerve function; and entero-humoral modulation.

10   Alteration to Bile Flow After Sleeve Gastrectomy

SG can disrupt enterohepatic circulation resulting in elevated plasma bile acid [56–58]. Bile acid salts bind to farnesoid X nuclear receptor (FXR), which in turn lead to downstream metabolic sequences that ultimately reduce bile acid biosynthesis from cholesterol [59–63]. Additionally, FXR induces the secretion of fibroblastic growth factor-19 (FGF-19) from enterocytes. In addition to decreasing cholesterol biosynthesis, FGF-19 also increases the basal metabolic rate [64]. The increased basal metabolic rate can be measured through reduced TSH levels and a greater conversion of T4 to T3 following bariatric operations [65]. As expected, this disruption to the lipid metabolism results in a reduction in low-density lipoprotein (LDL), an increase in high-density lipoprotein (HDL) levels, and a significant improvement in total cholesterol and triglyceride levels. These changes are measurable up to 10 years following the bariatric operation [66, 67]. The improvement in lipid profiles is likely polymodal but the influence of bile acids in regulating transcription of several genes associated with lipolysis alongside fatty acid and triglyceride synthesis is well established [68]. Moreover, bile acids lead to reduced endoplasmic reticulum stress, which can improve glucose tolerance and beta-cell mass [69].

11   Anatomical Changes After Sleeve Gastrectomy

Anatomical changes that occur during a SG can result in complications. The majority (more than 85%) of leaks following SG occur in the upper part of the gastric tube [70] perhaps owing to the reduction in vascular supply of that region [71], and increased pressure in the gastric tube following the operation [72]. Additionally, anatomical changes clearly lead to a reduced stomach capacity and resultant decreased digestion which accelerates weight loss. Removal of the fundus during a SG results in significant hormonal effects as well. This isn't surprising, with the gastrointestinal tract being the largest endocrine organ in the body. The gastric fundus produces ghrelin, a hormone best known for its orexigenic properties. However, this 28 amino acid peptide also has many more important roles including inhibition of insulin secretion as well as upregulation of gluconeogenesis and glycogenolysis leading to greater levels of glucose in the bloodstream [73]. However, the removal of the gastric fundus through a SG means that there are reduced ghrelin levels [74], which reverses the effects associated with ghrelin. In these patients, the insulinostatic activity is overturned and the islet cells can secrete more insulin to meet with the increased demand in obese patients. This may be aided in part by increased levels of Glucagon-like Peptide-1 (GLP-1) and peptide YY, both released from L cells in the small intestine as a result of the increased passage of undigested nutrients. GLP-1 can stimulate the pancreas to release insulin and additionally also preserves the beta cells involved in releasing insulin. On the other hand, peptide YY binds to Y2 receptors that are highly expressed in the arcuate nucleus, and acutely suppresses appetite but may also ameliorate insulin resistance [75].

12   Vagus Nerve Modulation After Sleeve Gastrectomy

The role of the vagus nerve is important in modulating energy metabolism, food intake, and glycaemic control. The afferent fibres of the vagus nerve is known to be sensitive to mechanical stretch following ingestion of food. The visceral sensory information is relayed to the nucleus of tractus solitarius, where converging signals from hormonal, metabolic, and cortical centres are processed to influence satiety [76, 77]. The vagus nerve is however perhaps more important in other bariatric operations such as the Roux-en-Y gastric bypass where the ventral and dorsal gastric branches of the vagus nerve are transected when forming the gastric pouch. Disruption of normal vagal activity can lead to early satiety and weight loss. Interestingly, patients who experienced SG plus truncal vagotomy did not experience an improvement in diabetes, when compared with SG alone [78–80].

13   Cardiovascular Effects of Sleeve Gastrectomy

There are several mechanisms that link obesity with hypertension and, as with diabetes, they involve intricate biochemical pathways, although it is still an evolving area of research. Atherosclerotic plaques in patient's arteries can impair the baroreflex sensitivity leading to impaired parasympathetic cardiac modulation, as a result of affected arteries becoming stiffer. This therefore leads to the sympathetic system dominating arterial resistance thereby inducing hypertension [81]. Furthermore, it appears that free fatty acids (FFAs) are critical to inducing hypertension in obese patients. They inhibit Na+/K+ATPase enzymes leading to greater vascular smooth muscle contraction and resistance. However, they can also have a more direct effect on ion channels causing activation of the smooth muscles and again leading to greater vascular resistance [82]. In the early phases of obesity, there is increased renal tubular reabsorption which causes primary retention. However, this is short lived and compensation through renal vasodilation and increased glomerular filtration rate tends to normalise the blood pressure. However, incomplete compensation can result in expansion of the extracellular fluid and, over time, resetting of the kidney-fluid balance. This can be aided by compression of the renal medulla causing compression of the vasa recta and loop of Henle [83, 84]. However, the process causing hypertension is much more complex and research suggests hormones such as insulin and leptin, as well as endothelial dysfunction that can result from the pro-inflammatory state in obesity all have a role in causing hypertension [85–87]. The reduction in the level of adipocytes following SG would diminish these effects and over 80% of patients reportedly see lasting improvements to their blood pressure [6].

Whilst bariatric surgery is highly effective for treating the comorbidities mentioned, the results on triglycerides aren't as successful. The total cholesterol levels don't change significantly but there is an improvement in the HDL and triglyceride levels. These changes appear to be long-lasting [88, 89].

14   Effects on Microbiota After Sleeve Gastrectomy

Additionally, the microbiota composition changes following a SG surgery. Obese patients have already been shown to have increased Firmicutes and decreased Bacteroidetes [90, 91]. However, following SG, there appears to be an increase in the level of Verrunomicrobia bacteria, and significant increases in the level of Akkermansia muciniphila. Studies suggest Akkermansia muciniphila can reduce weight and adipocyte levels, as well as improve metabolic outcomes [92, 93]. The changes in microbiota composition are gradual when compared to Roux-en-Y gastric bypass, perhaps because Roux-en-Y leads to a much greater reduction in pH of the gut environment [94].

15   Impact on Metabolism After Bariatric Surgery

There is also a significant effect on patients' metabolic state. This is important considering the substantial comorbidities that obese patients present with. These include dyslipidaemia, hypertension, heart failure, type 2 diabetes. Furthermore, obesity can also lead to renal failure and, as our understanding about obesity evolves, it is evident that the harmful biochemical processes involving fatty acids and triglycerides can produce far more significant pathology than previously thought.

Fatty acids can activate several serine kinase pathways, notably IkK kinase (IKK) and c-Jun N-terminal kinase (JNK) that are involved in particularly potent proinflammatory cascades. This can act to inhibit insulin function leading to insulin resistance and contributing to a greater risk of developing type 2 diabetes [95]. Further studies have demonstrated the involvement of the immune system which becomes activated by the action of fatty acids on toll-like receptors in adipocytes and macrophages. The downstream inflammatory cascade can lead to further insulin resistance and a greater cardiovascular risk [96, 97]. It is clear therefore that obesity is a highly complex process. As such, bariatric procedures should be given greater consideration for their ability to alleviate many of these harmful comorbidities affiliated with obesity.

16   Conclusion

Since the introduction of SG, the outcomes of surgery are durable with weight recidivism and success comparable to other stapled/bypass bariatric procedures. Complications from SG are uncommon but can be severe, and the involved mechanisms are only partially revealed. However, optimisation of risk factors in the months leading up to the operation can significantly improve outcomes in patients. This involves an early implementation of a healthy lifestyle including advising patients to exercise more regularly and adopt a low fat, low salt diet. Additionally, cessation of smoking and limiting alcohol consumption along with optimisation of cardiovascular disease and diabetes will not only aid in improving weight-loss outcomes but will also lead to a reduction in complications.

References

1. Pedroso FE, Angriman F, Endo A, et al. Weight loss after bariatric surgery in obese adolescents: a systematic review and meta-analysis. Surg Obes Relat Dis Off J Am Soc Bariatr Surg. 2018;14(3).
2. Committee ACI. Updated position statement on sleeve gastrectomy as a bariatric procedure. Surg Obes Relat Dis. 2012;8(3):e21–26.
3. Sjostrom L, Lindroos AK, Peltonen M, et al. Lifestyle, diabetes, and cardiovascular risk factors 10 years after bariatric surgery. N Engl J Med. 2004;351(26):2683–93.

4. Sarkhosh K, Birch DW, Shi X, Gill RS, Karmali S. The impact of sleeve gastrectomy on hypertension: a systematic review. Obes Surg. 2012;22(5):832–7.
5. Gill RS, Birch DW, Shi X, Sharma AM, Karmali S. Sleeve gastrectomy and type 2 diabetes mellitus: a systematic review. Surg Obes Relat Dis. 2010;6(6):707–13.
6. Al Khalifa K, Al Ansari A, Alsayed AR, Violato C. The impact of sleeve gastrectomy on hyperlipidemia: a systematic review. J Obes. 2013;2013:643530.
7. van Rutte PW, Smulders JF, de Zoete JP, Nienhuijs SW. Outcome of sleeve gastrectomy as a primary bariatric procedure. Br J Surg. 2014;101(6):661–8.
8. Sieber P, Gass M, Kern B, Peters T, Slawik M, Peterli R. Five-year results of laparoscopic sleeve gastrectomy. Surg Obes Relat Dis. 2014;10(2):243–9.
9. Rawlins L, Rawlins MP, Brown CC, Schumacher DL. Sleeve gastrectomy: 5-year outcomes of a single institution. Surg Obes Relat Dis. 2013;9(1):21–5.
10. Himpens J, Dobbeleir J, Peeters G. Long-term results of laparoscopic sleeve gastrectomy for obesity. Ann Surg. 2010;252(2):319–24.
11. Eid GM, Brethauer S, Mattar SG, Titchner RL, Gourash W, Schauer PR. Laparoscopic sleeve gastrectomy for super obese patients: forty-eight percent excess weight loss after 6 to 8 years with 93% follow-up. Ann Surg. 2012;256(2):262–5.
12. Diamantis T, Apostolou KG, Alexandrou A, Griniatsos J, Felekouras E, Tsigris C. Review of long-term weight loss results after laparoscopic sleeve gastrectomy. Surg Obes Relat Dis. 2014;10(1):177–83.
13. D'Hondt M, Vanneste S, Pottel H, Devriendt D, Van Rooy F, Vansteenkiste F. Laparoscopic sleeve gastrectomy as a single-stage procedure for the treatment of morbid obesity and the resulting quality of life, resolution of comorbidities, food tolerance, and 6-year weight loss. Surg Endosc. 2011;25(8):2498–504.
14. Abd Ellatif ME, Abdallah E, Askar W, et al. Long term predictors of success after laparoscopic sleeve gastrectomy. Int J Surg. 2014;12(5):504–8.
15. Shi X, Karmali S, Sharma AM, Birch DW. A review of laparoscopic sleeve gastrectomy for morbid obesity. Obes Surg. 2010;20(8):1171–7.
16. Chang S-H, Stoll CRT, Song J, Esteban Varela J, Eagon CJ, Colditz GA. The effectiveness and risks of bariatric surgery: an updated systematic review and meta-analysis, 2003–2012. JAMA Surg. 2014;149(3).
17. Schauer PR, Bhatt DL, Kirwan JP, et al. Bariatric surgery versus intensive medical therapy for diabetes - 5-year outcomes. The New Engl J Med. 2017;376(7).
18. Adams TD, Arterburn DE, Nathan DM, Eckel RH. Clinical outcomes of metabolic surgery: microvascular and macrovascular complications. Diabetes Care. 2016;39(6).
19. Arterburn D, et al. Comparing the outcomes of sleeve gastrectomy and Roux-en-Y gastric bypass for severe obesity. JAMA. 2018;319(3).
20. Coleman KJ, Haneuse S, Johnson E, et al. Long-term microvascular disease outcomes in patients with type 2 diabetes after bariatric surgery: evidence for the legacy effect of surgery. Diabetes Care. 2016;39(8).
21. McTigue KM, Wellman R, Nauman E, et al. Comparing the 5-year diabetes outcomes of sleeve gastrectomy and gastric bypass: the national patient-centered clinical research network (PCORNet) bariatric study. JAMA Surg. 2020.
22. Salminen P, Helmiö M, Ovaska J, et al. Effect of laparoscopic sleeve gastrectomy vs laparoscopic Roux-en-Y gastric bypass on weight loss at 5 years among patients with morbid obesity: the SLEEVEPASS randomized clinical trial. JAMA. 2018;319(3).
23. Li J, Lai D, Wu D. Laparoscopic Roux-en-Y gastric bypass versus laparoscopic sleeve gastrectomy to treat morbid obesity-related comorbidities: a systematic review and meta-analysis. Obes Surg. 2016;26(2).
24. Peterli R, Wolnerhanssen BK, Peters T, et al. Effect of laparoscopic sleeve gastrectomy vs laparoscopic Roux-en-Y gastric bypass on weight loss in patients with morbid obesity: the SM-BOSS randomized clinical trial. JAMA. 2018;319(3):255–65.

25. Abbasi J. Unveiling the "Magic" of diabetes remission after weight-loss surgery. JAMA. 2017;317(6).
26. Deitel M, Gagner M, Erickson AL, Crosby RD. Third international summit: current status of sleeve gastrectomy. Surg Obes Relat Dis Off J Am Soc Bariatr Surg. 2011;7(6).
27. Buchwald H, Avidor Y, Braunwald E, et al. Bariatric surgery: a systematic review and meta-analysis. JAMA. 2004;292(14).
28. Graham C, Switzer N, Reso A, et al. Sleeve gastrectomy and hypertension: a systematic review of long-term outcomes. Surg Endosc. 2019;33(9).
29. Catapano AL, Graham I, De Backer G, et al. 2016 ESC/EAS guidelines for the management of dyslipidaemias. Eur Heart J. 2016;37(39).
30. Bays HE, Toth PP, Kris-Etherton PM, et al. Obesity, adiposity, and dyslipidemia: a consensus statement from the national lipid association. J Clin Lipidol. 2013;7(4).
31. Omana JJ, Nguyen SQ, Herron D, Kini S. Comparison of comorbidity resolution and improvement between laparoscopic sleeve gastrectomy and laparoscopic adjustable gastric banding. Surg Endosc. 2010;24(10).
32. Raffaelli M, Guidone C, Callari C, Iaconelli A, Bellantone R, Mingrone G. Effect of gastric bypass versus diet on cardiovascular risk factors. Ann Surg. 2014;259(4).
33. Auclair N, Patey N, Melbouci L, et al. Acylated ghrelin and the regulation of lipid metabolism in the intestine. Sci Rep. 2019;9(1).
34. Pafumi Y, Lairon D, de la Porte PL, Juhel C, Storch J, Hamosh M, Armand M. Mechanisms of inhibition of triacylglycerol hydrolysis by human gastric lipase. J Biol Chem. 2002;277(31).
35. Romo Vaquero M, Yáñez-Gascón MJ, García Villalba R, et al. Inhibition of gastric lipase as a mechanism for body weight and plasma lipids reduction in zucker rats fed a rosemary extract rich in carnosic acid. PLoS One. 2012;7.
36. Chang SH, Stoll CR, Song J, Varela JE, Eagon CJ, Colditz GA. The effectiveness and risks of bariatric surgery: an updated systematic review and meta-analysis, 2003–2012. JAMA Surg. 2014;149(3):275–87.
37. Rosenthal RJ, Diaz AA, Arvidsson D, et al. International sleeve gastrectomy expert panel consensus statement: best practice guidelines based on experience of >12,000 cases. Surg Obes Relat Dis Off J Am Soc Bariatr Surg. 2012;8(1).
38. Dapri G, Cadière GB, Himpens J. Laparoscopic seromyotomy for long stenosis after sleeve gastrectomy with or without duodenal switch. Obes Surg. 2009;19(4).
39. Finks JF, English WJ, Carlin AM, et al. Predicting risk for venous thromboembolism with bariatric surgery: results from the Michigan bariatric surgery collaborative. Ann Surg. 2012;255(6).
40. Biertho L, Lebel S, Marceau S, et al. Perioperative complications in a consecutive series of 1000 duodenal switches. Surg Obes Relat Dis Off J Am Soc Bariatr Surg. 2013;9(1).
41. Kakarla VR, Nandipati K, Lalla M, Castro A, Merola S. Are laparoscopic bariatric procedures safe in superobese (BMI $\geq$50 kg/m^2) patients? An NSQIP data analysis. Surg Obes Relat Dis Off J Am Soc Bariatr Surg. 2011;7(4).
42. Magee CJ, Barry J, Javed S, Macadam R, Kerrigan D. Extended thromboprophylaxis reduces incidence of postoperative venous thromboembolism in laparoscopic bariatric surgery. Surg Obes Relat Dis Off J Am Soc Bariatr Surg. 2010;6(3).
43. Nguyen NT, Lee SL, Goldman C, et al. Comparison of pulmonary function and postoperative pain after laparoscopic versus open gastric bypass: a randomized trial. J Am Coll Surg. 2001;192(4).
44. van Huisstede A, et al. Pulmonary function testing and complications of laparoscopic bariatric surgery. Obes Surg. 2013;23(10).
45. Saif T, Strain GW, Dakin G, Gagner M, Costa R, Pomp A. Evaluation of nutrient status after laparoscopic sleeve gastrectomy 1, 3, and 5 years after surgery. Surg Obes Relat Dis Off J Am Soc Bariatr Surg. 2012;8(5).

46. Harper CG, Giles M, Finlay-Jones R. Clinical signs in the Wernicke-Korsakoff complex: a retrospective analysis of 131 cases diagnosed at necropsy. J Neurol Neurosurg Psychiatry. 1986;49(4).
47. Durán B, de Angulo DR, Parrilla P. Beriberi: an uncommon complication of sleeve gastrectomy. Surg Obes Relat Dis Off J Am Soc Bariatr Surg. 2015;11(6).
48. Clements RH, Katasani VG, Palepu R, et al. Incidence of vitamin deficiency after laparoscopic Roux-en-Y gastric bypass in a university hospital setting. Am Surg. 2006;72(12).
49. Watson WD, Verma A, Lenart MJ, et al. MRI in acute Wernicke's encephalopathy. Neurology. 2003;61(4).
50. Aasheim ET. Wernicke encephalopathy after bariatric surgery: a systematic review. Ann Surg. 2008;248(5).
51. Aurora AR, Khaitan L, Saber AA. Sleeve gastrectomy and the risk of leak: a systematic analysis of 4,888 patients. Surg Endosc. 2012;26(6).
52. Parikh M, Issa R, McCrillis A, Saunders JK, Ude-Welcome A, Gagner M. Surgical strategies that may decrease leak after laparoscopic sleeve gastrectomy: a systematic review and meta-analysis of 9991 cases. Ann Surg. 2013;257(2).
53. Zellmer JD, Mathiason MA, Kallies KJ, Kothari SN. Is laparoscopic sleeve gastrectomy a lower risk bariatric procedure compared with laparoscopic Roux-en-Y gastric bypass? A meta-analysis. Am J Surg. 2014;208(6).
54. Tan JT, Kariyawasam S, Wijeratne T, Chandraratna HS. Diagnosis and management of gastric leaks after laparoscopic sleeve gastrectomy for morbid obesity. Obes Surg. 2010;20(4).
55. Sakran N, Goitein D, Raziel A, et al. Gastric leaks after sleeve gastrectomy: a multicenter experience with 2,834 patients. Surg Endosc. 2013;27(1).
56. Haluzíková D, Lacinová Z, Kaválková P, et al. Laparoscopic sleeve gastrectomy differentially affects serum concentrations of FGF-19 and FGF-21 in morbidly obese subjects. Obesity (Silver Spring, Md). 2013;21(7).
57. Steinert RE, Peterli R, Keller S, et al. Bile acids and gut peptide secretion after bariatric surgery: a 1-year prospective randomized pilot trial. Obesity (Silver Spring, Md). 2013;21(12).
58. Ryan KK, Tremaroli V, Clemmensen C, et al. FXR is a molecular target for the effects of vertical sleeve gastrectomy. Nature. 2014;509(7499).
59. Brendel C, Schoonjans K, Botrugno OA, Treuter E, Auwerx J. The small heterodimer partner interacts with the liver X receptor alpha and represses its transcriptional activity. Mol Endocrinol (Baltimore, Md). 2002;16(9).
60. Goodwin B, Jones SA, Price RR, et al. A regulatory cascade of the nuclear receptors FXR, SHP-1, and LRH-1 represses bile acid biosynthesis. Mol Cell. 2000;6(3).
61. Makishima M, Okamoto AY, Repa JJ, et al. Identification of a nuclear receptor for bile acids. Science (New York, NY). 1999;284(5418).
62. Parks DJ, Blanchard SG, Bledsoe RK, et al. Bile acids: natural ligands for an orphan nuclear receptor. Science (New York, NY). 1999;284(5418).
63. Resnekov L, Chediak J, Hirsh J, Lewis HD Jr. Antithrombotic agents in coronary artery disease. Chest. 1986;89(2 Suppl).
64. Fu L, John LM, Adams SH, et al. Fibroblast growth factor 19 increases metabolic rate and reverses dietary and leptin-deficient diabetes. Endocrinology. 2004;145(6).
65. Watanabe M, Houten SM, Mataki C, et al. Bile acids induce energy expenditure by promoting intracellular thyroid hormone activation. Nature. 2006;439(7075).
66. Milone M, Lupoli R, Maietta P, et al. Lipid profile changes in patients undergoing bariatric surgery: a comparative study between sleeve gastrectomy and mini-gastric bypass. Int J Surg. (London, England). 2015;14.
67. Corradini SG, Eramo A, Lubrano C, et al. Comparison of changes in lipid profile after bilio-intestinal bypass and gastric banding in patients with morbid obesity. Obes Surg. 2005;15(3).

68. Lee J, Seok S, Yu P, et al. Genomic analysis of hepatic Farnesoid X receptor binding sites reveals altered binding in obesity and direct gene repression by Farnesoid X receptor in mice. Hepatology (Baltimore, Md). 2012;56(1).
69. Cummings BP, Bettaieb A, Graham JL, et al. Bile-acid-mediated decrease in endoplasmic reticulum stress: a potential contributor to the metabolic benefits of ileal interposition surgery in UCD-T2DM rats. Dis Models Mech. 2013;6(2).
70. Burgos AM, Braghetto I, Csendes A, et al. Gastric leak after laparoscopic-sleeve gastrectomy for obesity. Obes Surg. 2009;19(12).
71. Baker RS, Foote J, Kemmeter P, Brady R, Vroegop T, Serveld M. The science of stapling and leaks. Obes Surg. 2004;14(10).
72. Yehoshua RT, Eidelman LA, Stein M, et al. Laparoscopic sleeve gastrectomy-volume and pressure assessment. Obes Surg. 2008;18(9).
73. Pradhan G, Samson SL, Sun Y. Ghrelin: much more than a hunger hormone. Curr Opin Clin Nutr Metab Care. 2013;16(6):619–24.
74. Karamanakos SN, Vagenas K, Kalfarentzos F, Alexandrides TK. Weight loss, appetite suppression, and changes in fasting and postprandial ghrelin and peptide-YY levels after Roux-en-Y gastric bypass and sleeve gastrectomy: a prospective, double blind study. Ann Surg. 2008;247(3):401–7.
75. Murphy KG, Bloom SR. Gut hormones and the regulation of energy homeostasis. Nature. 2006;444(7121):854–9.
76. Berthoud HR. Vagal and hormonal gut-brain communication: from satiation to satisfaction. Neurogastroenterol Motil Off J Eur Gastrointest Motil Soc. 2008;20 Suppl 1(01).
77. Schwartz MW, Woods SC, Porte D Jr, Seeley RJ, Baskin DG. Central nervous system control of food intake. Nature. 2000;404(6778).
78. Hao Z, Townsend RL, Mumphrey MB, Patterson LM, Ye J, Berthoud HR. Vagal innervation of intestine contributes to weight loss after Roux-en-Y gastric bypass surgery in rats. Obes Surg. 2014;24(12).
79. Goligher JC, Pulvertaft CN, Irvin TT, et al. Five-to eight-year results of truncal vagotomy and pyloroplasty for duodenal ulcer. Br Med J. 1972;1(5791).
80. Liu T, Zhong MW, Liu Y, et al. Effects of sleeve gastrectomy plus trunk vagotomy compared with sleeve gastrectomy on glucose metabolism in diabetic rats. World J Gastroenterol. 2017;23(18).
81. Kotsis VT, Stabouli SV, Papamichael CM, Zakopoulos NA. Impact of obesity in intima media thickness of carotid arteries. Obesity (Silver Spring). 2006;14(10):1708–15.
82. Ordway RW, Singer JJ, Walsh JV Jr. Direct regulation of ion channels by fatty acids. Trends Neurosci. 1991;14(3):96–100.
83. Hall JE. Mechanisms of abnormal renal sodium handling in obesity hypertension. Am J Hypertens. 1997;10(5 Pt 2):49s–55s.
84. Hall JE, Brands MW, Hildebrandt DA, Kuo J, Fitzgerald S. Role of sympathetic nervous system and neuropeptides in obesity hypertension. Braz J Med Biol Res. 2000;33(6):605–18.
85. Kuo JJ, Jones OB, Hall JE. Inhibition of NO synthesis enhances chronic cardiovascular and renal actions of leptin. Hypertension. 2001;37(2 Pt 2):670–6.
86. Kim F, Pham M, Maloney E, et al. Vascular inflammation, insulin resistance and reduced nitric oxide production precede the onset of peripheral insulin resistance. Arterioscler Thromb Vasc Biol. 2008;28(11):1982–8.
87. Sechi LA. Mechanisms of insulin resistance in rat models of hypertension and their relationships with salt sensitivity. J Hypertens. 1999;17(9):1229–37.
88. Zhang F, Strain GW, Lei W, Dakin GF, Gagner M, Pomp A. Changes in lipid profiles in morbidly obese patients after laparoscopic sleeve gastrectomy (LSG). Obes Surg. 2011;21(3):305–9.
89. Golomb I, Ben David M, Glass A, Kolitz T, Keidar A. Long-term metabolic effects of laparoscopic sleeve gastrectomy. JAMA Surg. 2015;150(11):1051–7.

90. Turnbaugh PJ, Hamady M, Yatsunenko T, et al. A core gut microbiome in obese and lean twins. Nature. 2009;457(7228).
91. Armougom F, Henry M, Vialettes B, Raccah D, Raoult D. Monitoring bacterial community of human gut microbiota reveals an increase in lactobacillus in obese patients and methanogens in anorexic patients. PloS one. 2009;4(9).
92. Dao MC, Everard A, Aron-Wisnewsky J, et al. Akkermansia muciniphila and improved metabolic health during a dietary intervention in obesity: relationship with gut microbiome richness and ecology. Gut. 2016;65(3).
93. Furet JP, Kong LC, Tap J, et al. Differential adaptation of human gut microbiota to bariatric surgery-induced weight loss: links with metabolic and low-grade inflammation markers. Diabetes. 2010;59(12).
94. Sánchez-Alcoholado L, Gutiérrez-Repiso C, Gómez-Pérez AM, García-Fuentes E, Tinahones FJ, Moreno-Indias I. Gut microbiota adaptation after weight loss by Roux-en-Y gastric bypass or sleeve gastrectomy bariatric surgeries. Surg Obes Relat Dis Off J Am Soc Bariatr Surg. 2019;15(11).
95. Schenk S, Saberi M, Olefsky JM. Insulin sensitivity: modulation by nutrients and inflammation. J Clin Invest. 2008;118(9):2992–3002.
96. Shi H, Kokoeva MV, Inouye K, Tzameli I, Yin H, Flier JS. TLR4 links innate immunity and fatty acid-induced insulin resistance. J Clin Invest. 2006;116(11):3015–25.
97. Rocha VZ, Libby P. Obesity, inflammation, and atherosclerosis. Nat Rev Cardiol. 2009;6(6):399–409.

How to Manage Sleeve Complications: Hemorrhage

Karl A. Miller

1   Background

Laparoscopic Sleeve Gastrectomy (LSG) has gained popularity among surgeons and patients alike, due to its multiple benefits, which include: maintaining gastro-intestinal continuity, absence of foreign body, lack of malabsorption, and a good option of conversion to multiple bariatric procedures [1]. The stomach has an enriched blood supply via a network of submucous plexus which is derived from the left and right gastric arteries, gastroepiploic vessels and short gastric arteries. Multiple modalities in the management of bleeding situations are available (Table 1).

The most significant operative complications of LSG are staple line leak and bleeding, with reported total complication incidence of up to 13.7% [2–5]. However, hemorrhage, both intra-abdominal and intra-peritoneal, can be more challenging not only because of their rare occurrence, but also because of their life-threatening postoperative complication impact following bariatric surgery. The reported incidence of staple line hemorrhage is up to 3% [2, 3]. However according to the MBSQIB data base, unplanned readmission of patients who had postoperative bleeding within 30 days was up to 21.7% [6]. There is concern that the actual percentage of patients who experience bleeding is much higher than those undergoing re-operation which could lead to possible late complications of bleeding, specifically leaks that appear late due to infected hematomas [7].

K. A. Miller (✉)
Diakonissen Private Hospital, Salzburg, Austria
e-mail: karl@miller.co.at

K. A. Miller
Kings College Hospital London, Dubai, UAE

S. Al-Sabah et al. (eds.), *Laparoscopic Sleeve Gastrectomy*,
https://doi.org/10.1007/978-3-030-57373-7_42

Table 1 Modalities in hemostasis

Mechanical techniques
• Direct pressure
• Sutures
• Staples
• Ligating clips
• Fabric pads
• Gauzes
• Sponges
• Blood component/replacement therapy
Thermal techniques
• Electrocautery
• Hemostatic scalpel
• Laser
• Radiofrequency
Chemical techniques
• Pharmacotherapy
• Hypotensive anesthesia
• Epinephrine
• Vitamin K
• Protamine
• Desmopressin
• Aminocaproic acid
• Tranexamic acid
Topical hemostats
• Collagen
• Cellulose
• Gelatins
• Thrombins
Topical sealants and adhesives
• Fibrin sealants
• Synthetic glues

Multiple attempts to reduce the incidence of these complications have been done by staple line reinforcement (SLR) with synthetic or biologic material or suturing, but the evidence is equivocal; hence, there is no consensus with respect to the best method for SLR or its necessity [8–10]. Having mentioned that, it is important to emphasize that postoperative bleeding does not only occur at the staple line even though such bleeding has a reported incidence between 55 and 57%. The occurrence of post-operative bleeding that require re-operation, varies from 20 to 69% [11, 12].

Postoperative hemoglobin and heart rate are associated with bleeding but not systolic blood pressure or patient characteristics. Further research would be needed to develop a robust predictive model [13]. Multiple factors that could affect hemostasis during surgery are summarized in Table 1. Computed tomography

(CT) scan can be used in the stable patient and can be important in differentiating between the locations. In the case of the intraperitoneal bleeding, the CT can visualize a fluid collection in an extra luminal location; whereas, in the intralumenal bleeding there may be clot seen in the lumen of the bowel or distention of the remnant stomach. Patients who are hemodynamically unstable as well as those with an important intraperitoneal hematoma are candidates for surgery. Surgical exploration allows blood clots evacuation and eventually the identification and treatment of the bleeding source. Evacuation of the hematoma simplifies the postoperative course because spontaneous resorption is longer and needs monitoring. Furthermore, the hematoma can open into the stomach through the staple line and/or get infected secondarily. In case of intraluminal bleeding at the staple line that persists after conservative treatment, endoscopy can achieve hemostasis. In case of endoscopic failure or impossibility to perform endoscopy, hemostasis can be achieved by oversewing the entire staple line with sutures.

2   Bleeding Cascade, Patient and Surgeon Factor

Hemorrhage after LSG is multifactorial and therefore bleeding cascade and patient factors should be addressed briefly. A simplified major pathway version of the clotting cascade, emphasizing two mechanisms for initiating blood clotting is shown in Fig. 1. These are the contact activation pathway (also known as the intrinsic pathway), and the tissue factor pathway (also known as the extrinsic pathway), which both lead to the reactions that produce fibrin. The primary pathway for the initiation of blood coagulation is the tissue factor or extrinsic pathway. Various substances are required for the proper functioning of the coagulation cascade such as Calcium and Phospholipid, Vitamin K, and several Regulators.

Medications may interfere with the platelet clot and fibrin clot formation (Fig. 1). In addition, pathogenic bacteria may secrete agents that alter the coagulation system, such as coagulase and streptokinase which use this enzyme to break up blood clots [14].

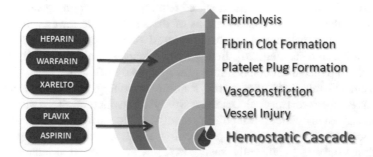

Fig. 1 The hemostatic cascade and antithrombotic medications that disrupt the ability to form a clot

Aminian et al. analyzed the data of 5871 cases of primary LSG extracted from the American College of Surgeons National Surgical Quality Improvement Program (ACS-NSQIP) database. Several factors that contributed to the risk of serious adverse events were identified as follows: diabetes, body mass index, male sex, congestive heart failure, steroid use, bilirubin level, and hematocrit level [15]. Janik et al. showed in a retrospective multivariate regression analysis several independent risk factors for postoperative hemorrhagic complications, in particular history for hypertension, obstructive sleep apnea, low surgeons experience in bariatric surgery and no staple line reinforcement use [11]. In that observational study the surgeon's level of expertise in bariatric surgery is essential, demonstrating significantly less hemorrhagic complications among experienced surgeons. According to the literature, the technical skill of practicing bariatric surgeons varies widely, and greater skill is associated with fewer postoperative complications and lower rates of reoperation, readmission, and less visits to the emergency department [16]. However in the Michigan Bariatric Collaborative, surgical skill did not affect the bleeding rate in the early postoperative period, nor the postoperative weight loss or resolution of medical comorbidities.[17].

Recently an observation was made that routine elevation of systolic blood pressure (SBP) to 140 mmHg at the end of stomach resection to identify bleeding and oversewing the staple line minimized hemorrhagic complications [7, 12].

3   Surgical Stapler Technology

Stapler technology has aided in advancing surgical techniques and have shortened operative time and improved perioperative safety [18]. The development and improvement of stapling devices in which cartridges are manufactured with a variety of different staple heights, correspond to the thickness of the intended tissue and allows a perfect staple formation to the relevant tissue [19]. Kimura and Terashita demonstrated in an experimental study the superiority of the shapes of the formed staples with powered stapling devices. The intestine is not fixed completely with the stapler after the squeezing motion. Deviation of the intestine occurs even when the stapling is being performed. In addition to this, tremors of the hands and staplers plus suspension and resumption of stapling result in further deviation of the intestine. Malformations of the staples were fewer with powered stapling devices. They concluded that powered staplers possibly result in more reliable and secure stapling [20]. Better formed staples could potentially produce fewer leaks and bleeding complications postoperatively [21–24].

The clinical relevance of powered stapling technology is demonstrated in a "Premier Perspective Hospital Database Study", in which 31.409 Patients were identified as having either powered or manual stapling performed during the bariatric procedure. The adjusted rate of bleeding and/or transfusion during the hospital admission was significantly lower (24%) in the powered vs manual stapler group. In addition the adjusted mean total hospital costs and supply costs were statistically significantly lower in the powered vs manual stapler group [25].

Additional innovation was developed in the Gripping Surface Technology (GST) of the cartridge deck. Fegelman et at. could demonstrate, that in the use of the GST stapling system a reduced need for staple line interventions as non-prophylactic actions taken in response to bleeding along the staple line following tissue transection, was necessary. The use of the GST stapling system reduces the need for staple line interventions in LSG [26].

4 Management and Prevention

High costs are an additional argument to reduce complication rate such as leak and bleeding. Prolonged hospitalization in the ward and intensive care unit will account for the costs of bleeding, 50% and 35% respectively [27]. Bleeding can occur during the division of the greater curvature vessels or during gastric stapling. The division of the short gastric vessels during the mobilization of the gastric fundus in proximity to the splenic upper pole particularly exposes to the risk of hemorrhage. In case of bleeding, the injured vessel can retract, making any attempts to achieve hemostasis very difficult. If bleeding occurs, mechanical compression should be attempted first followed by the placement of hemostatic gauze. Mechanical hemostats, adhesives with patch or sealants should always be available in anticipation of potential bleeding with anatomical difficult access and situations with potential rebleeding risk [28].

The bleeding on the staple line can be controlled by stitches, metallic clips or bipolar coagulation which has been a controversial practice. The rebleeding risk can be treated with hemostats. All these techniques are generally very effective and conversion to laparotomy due to bleeding is unusual. Appropriate staple size (height) for the tissue is recommended. Using longer staple height for thin tissues may cause bleeding from stapler line or intraluminal bleeding at the site. These may lead to early postoperative intra-abdominal or upper gastrointestinal (GI) hemorrhage. On the other hand, using short height cartridges on a thick tissue can be a risk factor for leakage from the anastomosis or staple line, or can create serosal tearing and bleeding. These differing staple heights are designed to ensure that, when closed, the staples provide secure apposition of the edges of the bowel [29]. Shipping safety cover should not be removed until the cartridge is loaded into the Stapler. Handling of the instrument must be motion free while firing, avoiding tension on the stapling tissue. Usually, waiting at least 15 s before firing allows adequate compression time before cutting the tissue by staplers [30–32].

The author's recommended checklist before, during and after linear stapling is shown in Table 2.

4.1 Buttressing, Oversewing

Buttressing material has been shown to ensure more even distribution of the staple pressure over a wider surface area thus resulting in higher burst pressures and

Table 2 Factors that could affect hemostasis during surgery

Surgical
• Disease state—certain conditions lead to increased bleeding from compromised tissue
• Medications may interfere with clot formation
• Patient factors such as bmi, age, vitamin deficiencies and smoking obstructive sleep apnea
• Blood pressure
• Anesthesia routine (e.g. amount of infusions)
• Surgeons expertise
Mechanical
• Buttressing • Oversewing
• Clips
• Prophylactic use of hemostats
• Surgical technique in the use of the stapling device (dissection, tissue compression, tissue tension, staple height)
• Stapler technology

lower bleed rates [29]. Although gastric wall thickness has been reported to vary, it is thick in the antrum (3.1 mm), moderate in the body (2.4 mm), and thin in the fundus (1.7 mm), the choice of staple height is very important when a buttressing material is added. The height of the buttress decreases the actual height of the staple, and a longer staple height should be considered for safe and proper closure [29, 33]. A number of materials have been studied in staple-line reinforcement, including porcine small intestinal submucosa strips [34], absorbable polyglycolic acid [35] and bovine pericardial strips [36, 37]. The use of integrated absorbable synthetic polymers has proved feasible and well tolerated [38], and glycolide copolymer reinforcement sleeves have been shown to reduce staple-line bleeding and may reduce gastrointestinal hemorrhaging [24, 39]. However in literature reviews Knapps reported that mortality, bleeding, and reintervention rates were not affected by reinforcement and that there is no statistical difference in the pooled rate of bleeding, or reintervention [10]. Shikora analyzed out of 253 primary included studies and abstracts 215 bleed study arms the two most commonly used buttresses, bovine pericardium and a biocompatible glycolide copolymer buttress [23]. In this meta analyzes the total bleed rate was 3.45%. Overall, reinforcing with bovine pericardium had the lowest bleed rate of 1.23%. Buttressing with a biocompatible glycolide copolymer resulted in a bleed rate of 2.48% but had significantly lower bleed rates than no reinforcement. However inconsistency is seen in systematic reviews and meta analyses, where the incidence of bleeding is 0–6.7% without reinforcement and 0–8% with reinforcement [10], and comparative studies which did not find a statistically significant decrease in staple line hemorrhage [21]. Stapler with preloaded buttress material could potentially provide ease of use, might have less staple line bleeding and reduced waste in the operating room [48, 49]. Conflicting results make it difficult to generally justify the use of buttressing materials to reduce staple line bleeding most probably also because of a lack of a consistent definition of post-operative staple line bleeding [38, 40–45].

Oversewing the staple line with a continuous suture has been used widely to reduce postoperative complications after LSG [45]. However, Choi et al. suggested that oversewing could reduce the frequency of leak but that it might increase the risk of bleeding after LSG although the results were not statistically significant [21]. Oversewing itself could be potentially dangerous. Tearing at the point of suture penetration may increase bleeding and leak, and the running suture could cause sleeve stricture and tissue ischemia [29, 46]. On one hand, studies have shown that the rates of sleeve stenosis and hematoma formation respectively were significantly higher in the oversewing group [30, 47]. In a meta-analysis of 7 prospective randomized studies, Wang et al. found no significant difference in staple line bleeding between oversewing and no staple line treatment but it does prolong the operative time [8]. In addition omentopexy technique have shown no significant difference in bleeding, thrombosis, gastric reflux or gastric stenosis but increased operating time as well, compared to no omentopexy [50].

Despite the disagreement observed when reviewing the recent literature, staple line reinforcement might play a role in high risk patients in prevention of postoperative bleeding and rebleeding.

5 Hemostats

A wide variety of hemostatic agents (Table 4) are available as adjunctive measures to improve hemostasis during surgical procedures if residual bleeding persists despite correct standard surgical technique (eg, electrocautery, sutures) for hemorrhage control. Topical and tissue adhesives are particularly useful for diffuse nonanatomic bleeding, bleeding associated with sensitive structures, and bleeding in patients with hemostatic abnormalities. Active Hemostatic agents are considered active agents, since containing fibrinogen and thrombin, actively participating at the end of the coagulation cascade to form a fibrin clot [51]. Hemostats can be used effectively in different scenarios in patients with spontaneous oozing or drug-induced coagulation disorders in LSG [Table 3]. The most important factors are the ability of a product to achieve and maintain hemostasis and the speed in which bleeding is controlled [52]. Adhesives (Liquid fibrin adhesives, Fibrin patch), mechanical hemostats, sealants can be used either in different bleeding situations or to apply it in reducing the rebleeding risk.

Adhesives are active agents which participate at the final step of the coagulation cascade to form a fibrin clot (Fig. 1). They are made of two components: human purified fibrinogen and/or thrombin [53]. Sroka et al. have shown in a prospective randomized study that the routine use of fibrin sealant in LSG has little benefit to reduce hemorrhagic complications [54]. Bülbüller et al. conducted a four-arm randomized trial with a total of 65 patients. They had no bleeding complications, but severe complications in the barbed oversewing group [54]. Musella et al. has so

Table 3 Checklist in linear gastric stapling (K. Miller)

Closing of the device
• No bunching at crotch √
• Crotch staple removed √
• Staple height appropriate √
• Device parallel to the tissue √
• Tension on the stomach released √
Before firing
• Tissue compression 15 s √
• Interrupted firing if indicated (e.g. thick tissue) √
After firing check staple line
• Check staple line of B-formed staples √
• Leak proof test √
• Hemostasis if indicated or necessary √

Table 4 Addressing surgical bleeding situations with adjunctive hemostats

Bleeding situation	Problem definition	Possible use of hemostats
Continuous quzing	• Will not stop with compression or simple packing • Is more time consuming than difficult	Oxidized regenerated cellulose (ORC)
Problematic bleeding	• Is accessible but could be difficult to expose • Is more than routine bleeding • Requires immediate attention • Disruptive to the normal progression of surgery	Fibrin/thrombin matrix (patch)
Difficult to access	• Occurs in tight and irregular spaces • Can not be precisely visualized • Raises concerns that accessing the space will cause more harm	Flowable gelatin
Rebleeding risk	• Is addressed intraoperatively • Could later develop into more serious complications especially in high risk patients	Fibrin sealant

far shown also in a prospective randomized trial the use of fibrin sealant in LSG to significantly reduce postoperative bleeding [55].

Mechanical hemostats provide platelet activation and aggregation and form a matrix at the site of bleeding, which allows clotting to occur. Oxidized cellulose regenerated or non-regenerated [56, 57], porcine gelatin [58], bovine collagen [59], and plant-derived polysaccharides spheres [60], are known as mechanical hemostats, by providing platelet activation and aggregation. Mechanical hemostats are not biologically active, they rely on patient's own fibrin production, considered as passive hemostats and are only appropriate for patients who have an intact coagulation system. Cellulose can be either regenerated to form organized fibers or non-regenerated with unorganized fibers prior to oxidation. When cellulose fibers are oxidized, conversion of hydroxyl groups to carboxylic acid groups occurs, yielding to polyuronic acid [61, 62]. The low pH of the carboxylic acid groups is responsible for several actions: primary local hemostyptic action, secondary platelet activation to form a temporary platelet plug [61, 62], and proven bactericidal against a broad range of gram-positive and gram-negative organisms [63–65]. Recently developed oxygenized regenerated cellulose (ORC) hemostat with structured non-woven fabric, needle punched with interlocking fibers are faster in hemostasis compared to loose knit structured. The scientific evidence of the use in bariatric and metabolic surgery is very limited. In gastric bypass surgery Moon et al. reported excellent experience in stapler buttressing with loose knit structured ORC versus bovine pericardial strips. With the use of absorbable hemostat as buttress material, the study has shown significant less acute postoperative bleeding at a lower cost [66]. The use of ORC as a staple line reinforcement is off label, therefore I prefer to use it as a hemostat on the staple line in LSG to prevent bleeding and rebleeding (Fig. 2). Recently ORC has also been made available as powder. The structure of the powder penetrates the surface of the blood which saturates the material, providing a surface for platelet adhesion and aggregation, and initiating clot formation.

Sealants are low viscosity liquids that polymerize forming a solid film that connects the tissue surfaces [67–71]. This characteristic makes these agents effective both as sealants and as hemostats. They can be divided in synthetic (cyanoacrylate and polyethylene glycol-PEG) and semisynthetic (glutaraldhyde albumin-derived) sealants.

The use of a porous collagen matrix would provide greater hemostatic effectiveness than oxidized cellulose. The protein-binding layer adheres to the collagen pad more rapidly than a fibrinogen–thrombin-coated collagen pad. Hemostatic

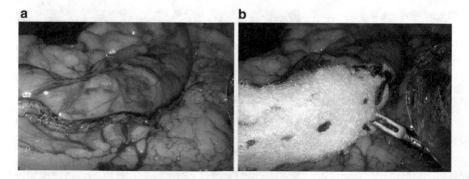

Fig. 2 **a** Oozing staple line **b** oxygenized regenerated cellulose (structured non-woven fabric, needle punched with interlocking fibers

pads consist of a sheet-like backing and a self-adhering surface. The various backings include collagen, neutralized oxidized cellulose, or an oxidized cellulose–polyglactin composite; while the active surfaces include fibrinogen and thrombin or a synthetic, protein-reactive monomer [71, 72].

In bleeding situations where it is difficult to access and visibility is limited, gelatin matrix sealants might have a great value (Fig. 3). Gelatin-based foam that flows into the bleeding area serves as a scaffold for platelet adhesion and can be combined with thrombin to expedite clot formation. The mixture of a flowable gelatin matrix (bovine or porcine) and a human-derived thrombin component are typically prepared immediately before use and directly injected to the site of bleeding [73–75].

6   Summary

Tissue healing is a dynamic process consisting of continuous, overlapping, and precisely programmed phases. This includes prompt hemostasis and blood perfusion of the tissue. The right staple height in LSG will find the right balance between hemostasis without compromising the blood supply and microvascular invasion. Restricted circulation could be noticed in hand-sewn anastomoses whilst such lack of vascular supply was not seen in stapled anastomoses. The intramural arteries passed through the B-shaped staples without hindrance [76, 77].

The versatility and utility of hemostats might replace traditional hemostatic methods on the staple line (eg, electrocautery, sutures, clips) which might affect the blood supply and healing process, to improve surgical outcomes with less bleeding.

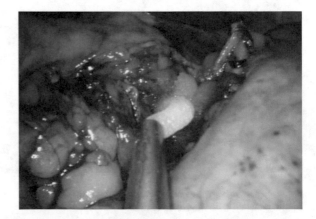

Fig. 3 Flowable gelatin matrix with or without thrombin in difficult to access and visibility bleeding situations

References

1. Shoar S, Saber AA. Long-term and midterm outcomes of laparoscopic sleeve gastrectomy versus Roux-en-Y gastric bypass: a systematic review and meta-analysis of comparative studies. Surg Obes Relat Dis. 2017;13(2):170–80.
2. Deitel M, Gagner M, Erickson AL, Crosby RD. Third international summit: current status of sleeve gastrectomy. Surg Obes Relat Dis. 2011;7:749–59.
3. Chen B, Kiriakopoulos A, Tsakayannis D, Wachtel MS, Linos D, Frezza EE. Reinforcement oes not necessarily reduce the rate of staple line leaks after sleeve gastrectomy. A review of the literature and clinical experiences. Obes Surg. 2009;19:166–172.
4. Brethauer SA, Hammel JP, Schauer PR. Systematic review of sleeve gastrectomy as staging and primary bariatric procedure. Surg Obes Relat Dis. 2009;5:469–75.
5. Gentileschi P, Camperchioli I, D'Ugo S, et al. Staple-line reinforcement during laparoscopic sleeve gastrectomy using three different techniques: a randomized trial. Surg Endosc. 2012;26:2623–9.
6. Zafar SN, Felton J, Miller K, Wise ES, Kligman M. Staple line treatment and bleeding after laparoscopic sleeve gastrectomy. JSLS. 2018;22(4).
7. Sroka G. Hemorrhagic complications in laparoscopic sleeve gastrectomy. Obes Surg. 2016;26:379–80.
8. Wang H, Lu J, Feng J, Wang Z. Staple line oversewing during laparoscopic sleeve Gastrectomy. Ann R Coll Surg Engl. 2017;99:509–14.
9. Gagner M, Buchwald JN. Comparison of laparoscopic sleeve gastrectomy leak rates in four staple-line reinforcement options: a systematic review. Surg Obes Relat Dis. 2014;10(4):713–23.
10. Knapps J, Ghanem M, Clements J, Merchant AM. A systematic review of staple-line reinforcement in laparoscopic sleeve gastrectomy. JSLS. 2013;17(3):390–9.
11. Janik MR, Walędziak M, Brągoszewski J, Kwiatkowski A, Paśnik K. Prediction model for hemorrhagic complications after laparoscopic sleeve gastrectomy: devclopment of SLEEVE BLEED calculator. Obes Surg. 2017;27(4):968–72.
12. Banescu B, Balescu I, Copaescu C. Postoperative bleeding risk after sleeve gastrectomy. a two techniques of stapled line reinforcement comparative study in 4996 patients. Chirurgia (Bucur). 2019;114(6):693–703.
13. Fecso AB, Samuel T, Elnahas A, et al. Clinical indicators of postoperative bleeding in bariatric surgery. Surg Laparosc Endosc Percutan Tech. 2018;28(1):52–5.
14. Babashamsi M, Razavian MH, Nejadmoghaddam MR. Production and purification of streptokinase by protected affinity chromatography. Avicenna J Med Biotechnol. 2009;1(1):47–51.
15. Aminian A, Brethauer SA, Sharafkhah M, et al. Development of a sleeve gastrectomy risk calculator. Surg Obes Relat Dis. 2015;11(4):758–64.
16. Birkmeyer JD, Finks JF, O'Reilly A, et al. Surgical skill and complication rates after bariatric surgery. N Engl J Med. 2013;369(15):1434–42.
17. Scally CP, Varban OA, Carlin AM, Birkmeyer JD, Dimick JB; Michigan Bariatric Surgery Collaborative. Video ratings of surgical skill and late outcomes of bariatric surgery. JAMA Surg. 2016;151(6):e160428.
18. Simper SC, Erzinger JM, Smith SC. Comparison of laparoscopic linear staplers in clinical practice. Surg Obes Relat Dis. 2007;3(4):446–51.
19. Mery CM, Shafi BM, Binyamin G, et al. Profiling surgical staplers: effect of staple height, buttress, and overlap on stapleline failure. Surg Obes Relat Dis. 2008;4(3):416–22.
20. Kimura M, Terashita Y. Superior staple formation with powered stapling devices. Surg Obes Relat Dis. 2016;12(3):668–72.
21. Choi YY, Bae J, Hur KY, Choi D, Kim YJ. Reinforcing the staple line during laparoscopic sleeve gastrectomy: does it have advantages? A meta analysis. Obes Surg. 2012;8:1206–13.

22. Consten EC, Gagner M, Pomp A, Inabnet WB. Decreased bleeding after laparoscopic sleeve gastrectomy with or without duodenal switch for morbid obesity using a stapled buttressed absorbable polymer membrane. Obes Surg. 2004;14:1360–6.
23. Shikora SA, Mahoney CB. Clinical benefit of gastric staple line reinforcement (SLR) in gastrointestinal surgery: a meta-analysis. Obes Surg. 2015;25:1133–41.
24. Dapri G, Cadière GB, Himpens J. Reinforcing the staple line during laparoscopic sleeve gastrectomy: prospective randomized clinical study comparing three different techniques. Obes Surg. 2010;20:462–467.
25. Roy S, Yoo A, Yadalam S, Fegelman EJ, Kalsekar I, Johnston SS. Comparison of economic and clinical outcomes between patients undergoing laparoscopic bariatric surgery with powered versus manual endoscopic surgical staplers. J Med Econ. 2017;20(4):423–33.
26. Fegelman E, Knippenberg S, Schwiers M, et al. Evaluation of a powered stapler system with gripping surface technology on surgical interventions required during laparoscopic sleeve gastrectomy. J Laparoendosc Adv Surg Tech A. 2017;27(5):489–94.
27. Bransen J, Gilissen LP, van Rutte PW, Nienhuijs SW. Costs of leaks and bleeding after sleeve gastrectomies. Obes Surg. 2015;25(10):1767–71.
28. Chiara O, Cimbanassi S, Bellanova G, et al. A systematic review on the use of topical hemostats in trauma and emergency surgery. BMC Surg. 2018;18(1):68.
29. Baker RS, Foote J, Kemmeter P, Brady R, Vroegop T, Serveld M, et al. The science of stapling and leaks. Obes Surg. 2004;14:1290–8.
30. Musella M, Susa A, Manno E, De Luca M, Greco F, Raffaelli M, et al. Complications following the mini/one anastomosis gastric bypass (MGB/OAGB): a multi-institutional survey on 2678 patients with a mid-term (5 Years) follow-up. Obes Surg. 2017;27:2956–67.
31. Silecchia G, Iossa A. Complications of staple line and anastomoses following laparoscopic bariatric surgery. Ann Gastroenterol. 2018;31:56–64.
32. Parikh M, Issa R, McCrillis A, Saunders JK, Ude-Welcome A, Gagner M, et al. Surgical strategies that may decrease leak after laparoscopic sleeve gastrectomy: a systematic review and meta-analysis of 9991 cases. Ann Surg. 2013;257:231–7.
33. Causey MW, Fitzpatrick E, Carter P. Pressure tolerance of newly constructed staple lines in sleeve gastrectomy and duodenal switch. Am J Surg. 2013;205:571–4.
34. Pinheiro JS, Correa JL, Cohen RV, Novaes JA, Schiavon CA. Staple line reinforcement with new biomaterial increased burst strength pressure: an animal study. Surg Obes Relat Dis. 2006;2(3):397–9.
35. Kawamura M, Kase K, Sawafuji M, Watanabe M, Horinouchi H, Kobayashi K. Staple-line reinforcement with a new type of polyglycolic acid felt. Surg Laparosc Endosc Percutan Tech. 2001;11(1):43–4.
36. Shikora S. The use of staple-line reinforcement during laparoscopic gastric bypass. Obes Surg. 2004;14(10):1313–20.
37. Stamou K, Menenakos E, Dardamanis D, et al. Prospective comparative study of the efficacy of staple-line reinforcement in laparoscopic sleeve gastrectomy. Surg Endosc. 2011;25(11):3526–3530.
38. Alley J, Fenton S, Harnisch M, Angeletti M, Peterson R. Integrated bioabsorbable tissue reinforcement in laparoscopic sleeve gastrectomy. Obes Surg. 2011;21(8):1311–5.
39. Nguyen NT, Longoria M, Welbourne S, Sabio A, Wilson SE. Glycolide copolymer staple-line reinforcement reduces staple site bleeding during laparoscopic gastric bypass: a prospective randomized trial. Arch Surg. 2005;140(8):773–8.
40. Consten EC, Gagner M, Pomp A, InabnetWB. Decreased bleeding after laparoscopic sleeve gastrectomy with or without duodenal switch for morbid obesity using a stapled buttressed absorbable polymer membrane. Obes Surg. 2004;14(10):1360–6.
41. Daskalakis M, Berdan Y, Theodoridou S, Weigand G, Weiner R. Impact of surgeon experience and buttress material on postoperative complications after laparoscopic sleeve gastrectomy. Surg Endosc. 2011;25(1):88–97. English.

42. Sanchez-Santos R, Masdevall C, Baltasar A, Martinez-Blazquez C, Garcia Ruiz de Gordejuela A, Ponsi E. Short- and mid-term outcomes of sleeve gastrectomy for morbid obesity: the experience of the Spanish National Registry. Obes Surg. 2009;19(9):1203–10.

43. Ser KH, Lee WJ, Lee YC, Chen JC, Su YH, Chen SC. Experience in laparoscopic sleeve gastrectomy for morbidly obese Taiwanese: staple-line reinforcement is important for preventing leakage. Surg Endosc. 2010;24(9):2253–9.

44. Stamou KM, Menenakos E, Dardamanis D, Arabatzi C, Alevizos L, Albanopoulos K, et al. Prospective comparative study of the efficacy of staple-line reinforcement in laparoscopic sleeve gastrectomy. Surg Endosc. 2011;25(11):3526–30.

45. D'Ugo S, Gentileschi P, Benavoli D, Cerci M, Gaspari A, Berta RD, et al. Comparative use of different techniques for leak and bleeding prevention during laparoscopic sleeve gastrectomy: a multicenter study. Surg Obes Relat Dis: Off J Am Soc Bariatric Surg. 2014;10(3):450–4.

46. Barreto TW, Kemmeter PR, Paletta MP, Davis AT. A comparison of a single center's experience with three staple line reinforcement techniques in 1,502 laparoscopic sleeve gastrectomy patients. Obes Surg. 2015;25:418–22.

47. Albanopoulos K, Tsamis D, Arapaki A et al. Staple line reinforcement with stitch in laparoscopic sleeve gastrectomies. Is it useful or harmful? J Laparoendosc Adv Surg Tech A 2015; 25: 561–565.

48. Rosenthal RJ, International Sleeve Gastrectomy Expert Panel, Diaz AA, et al. International sleeve gastrectomy expert panel consensus statement: best practice guidelines based on experience of >12,000 cases. Surg Obes Relat Dis. 2012;8(1):8–19.

49. El Moussaoui I, Limbga A, Mehdi A. Staple line reinforcement during sleeve gastrectomy with a new type of reinforced stapler. Minerva Chir. 2018;73(2):127-32.

50. Sharma N, Chau WY. Remodifying omentopexy technique used with laparoscopic sleeve gastrectomy: does it change any outcomes? Obes Surg. 2020;30(4):1527–35.

51. Dhillon S. Fibrin sealants (Evicel®, [Quixil®/Crosseal™]) a review of its use as supportive treatment for haemostasis in surgery. Drugs. 2011;71:1893–915.

52. Msezane LP, Katz MH, Gofrit ON, Shalhav AL, Zorn KC: Hemostatic agents and instruments in laparoscopic renal surgery. J Endourol. 2008, 22(3):403–408.

53. Spotnitz WD. Fibrin sealant: the only approved hemostat, sealant, and adhesive-a laboratory and clinical perspective. Surgery. 2014;1:1–29.

54. Bülbüller N, Aslaner A, Oner OZ, et al. Comparison of four different methods in staple line reinforcement during laparascopic sleeve gastrectomy. Int J Clin Exp Med. 2013;6(10):985–90.

55. Musella M, Milone M, Maietta P, Bianco P, Pisapia A, Gaudioso D. Laparoscopic sleeve gastrectomy: efficacy of fibrin sealant in reducing postoperative bleeding. A randomized controlled trial. Updates Surg. 2014;66(3):197–201.

56. Wagenhauser MU, Mulorz J, Simon F, Spin JM, Schelzig H, Oberhuber A. Oxidized (non)-regenerated cellulose affects fundamental cellular processes of wound healing. Sci Rep. 2016;6:32238. https://doi.org/10.1038/srep32238.

57. Lewis KM, Spazierer D, Urban MD, Lin L, Redl H, Goppelt A. Comparison of regenerated and non-regenerated oxidized cellulose hemostatic agents. Eur Surg. 2013;45:213–20.

58. Ragusa R, Faggian G, Rungatscher A, Cugola D, Macron A, Mazzucco A. Use of gelatin powder added to rifamycin versus bone wax in sternal wound hemostasis after cardiac surgery. Interact Cardiovasc Thorac Surg. 2007;6:52–5.

59. Sabino L, Andreoni C, Faria EF, Ferreira PSVS, Paz AR, Kalil W, et al. Evaluation of renal defect healing, hemostasis, and urinary fistula after laparoscopic partial nephrectomy with oxidized cellulose. J Endourol. 2007;21(5):551–6.

60. Emmez H, Tonge M, Tokgoz N, Durdag N, Gonul I, Ceviker N. Radiological and Histopathological comparison of microporous polysaccharide hemospheres and oxidized regenerated cellulose in the rabbit brain: a study of efficacy and safety. Turkish Neurosurg. 2010;20(4):485–91.

61. Pierce AM, Wiebkin OW, Wilson DF: Surgicel: its fate following implantation. J Oral Pathol. 1984;13(6):661–707.
62. Miller JM, Jackson DA, Collier CS. An investigation of the chemical reactions of oxidized regenerated cellulose. Exp Med Surg. 1961;19(196–201):8.
63. Dineen P. Antibacterial activity of oxidized regenerated cellulose. Surg Gynecol Obstet. 1976;142(4):481–6.
64. Dineen P. The effect of oxidized regenerated cellulose on experimental infected splenotomies. J Surg Res. 1977;23:114–6.
65. Spangler D, Rothenburger S, Nguyen K, Jampani H, Weiss S, Bhende S. In vitro antimicrobial activity of oxidized regenerated cellulose against antibiotic-resistant microorganisms. Surg Infect. 2003;4(3):255–62.
66. Moon R, Teixeira A, Varnadore S, Potenza K, Jawad MA. Reinforcing the staple line with Surgicel® Nu-knit® in Roux-en-Y gastric bypass: comparison with bovine pericardial strips. Obes Surg. 2013;23(6):788–93.
67. Lewis KM, Kuntze CE, Gulle H. Control of bleeding in surgical procedures: critical appraisal of HEMOPATCH (sealing hemostat). Med Devices: Evid Res. 2016;9:1–10.
68. Ollinger R, Mihaljevic AL, Schuhmacher C, Bektas H, Vondran F, Kleine M, et al. A multicenter, randomized clinical trial comparing Veriset™ haemostatic patch with fibrin sealant for the management of bleeding during hepatic surgery. HPB. 2013;15:548–58.
69. Allen MS, Wood DE, Hawkinson RW. Prospective randomized study evaluating a biodegradable polymeric sealant for sealing intraoperative air leaks that occur during pulmonary resection. Ann Thorac Surg. 2004;77:1792–801.
70. Miscusi M, Polli FM, Forcato S, Coman SA, Ricciardi L, Ramieri A, et al. The use of surgical sealants in the repair of dural tears during non-instrumented spinal surgery. Eur Spine J. 2014;23(8):1761–6.
71. Lewis KM, McKee J, Schiviz A, Bauer A, Wolfsegger M, Goppelt A. Randomized, controlled comparison of advanced hemostatic pads in hepatic surgical models. ISRN Surg. 2014;2014:930803.
72. Fischer CP, Bochicchio G, Shen J, et al. A prospective, randomized controlled trial of the efficacy and safety of fibrin pad as an adjunct to control soft tissue bleeding during abdominal retroperitoneal, pelvic, and thoracic surgery. J Am Coll Surg. 2013;217(3):385–93.
73. Obermair H, Janda M, Obermair A. Real-world surgical outcomes of a gelatin-hemostatic matrix in women requiring a hysterectomy: a matched case-control study. Acta Obstet Gynecol Scand. 2016;95(9):1008–14.
74. Echave M, Oyaguez I, Casado MA. Use of Floseal®, a human gelatinthrombin matrix sealant, in surgery: a systematic review. BMC Surg. 2014;14:111–24.
75. Mayol JM, Zapata C. Gelatin-thrombin matrix for intraoperative hemostasis in abdomino-pelvic surgery: a systematic review. Surg Technol Int. 2013;23:23–8.
76. Hansen H, Sommer HJ, Eichelkraut W. The blood supply of manually sutured and stapled colonic anastomoses. Langenbecks Arch Chir. 1987;370(2):141–51. https://doi.org/10.1007/bf01254091.
77. Ballantyne GH, Burke JB, Rogers G, Lampert EG, Boccia J (1985) Accelerated wound healing with stapled enteric suture lines. Ann Surg. 1985;201:360–4.

Endoscopic Management of Leak and Abscess Following Laparoscopic Sleeve Gastrectomy

Iqbal Siddique⊙

1 Introduction

Laparoscopic sleeve gastrectomy (SG) is currently the most popular primary bari-atric surgical procedure for morbid obesity [1, 2]. Approximately 10 to 13% of patients undergoing this surgery have complications such as bleeding, stenosis, and leaks [3]. Leaks after SG are typically found at the upper end of the staple line, near the angle of His, where the staple line meets the gastroesophageal junction because of staple line-height mismatch, ischemia, and unfavorable pressure gradients secondary to distal intraluminal narrowing of the sleeve [4, 5]. The incidence of leaks or fistulas after SG is approximately 2 to 5% of the cases, and it is the second most common cause of death after bariatric surgery with an overall mortality rate of 0.4% [6].

The management of post SG leaks is challenging, resource-intensive and invari-ably requires a multidisciplinary team approach involving surgery, gastrointestinal endoscopy, and interventional radiology. The optimum management of leaks and subsequent intra-abdominal collections following SG is still controversial despite several reported techniques. The American Society for Metabolic and Bariatric Surgery position statement on prevention, detection, and treatment of gastrointes-tinal leak after gastric bypass and sleeve gastrectomy, including the roles of imag-ing, surgical exploration, and non-operative management was published in 2015 [7]. It states that the initial step in the management of an acute leak is to con-trol the infection secondary to the leak. Thus, surgical washout with drain place-ment is mandatory in a patient whose condition is unstable, with an acute leak

I. Siddique (✉)
Department of Medicine, Faculty of Medicine, Kuwait University, Jabriya, Kuwait
e-mail: iqbal.siddique@ku.edu.kw

© The Editor(s) (if applicable) and The Author(s), under exclusive license to Springer
Nature Switzerland AG 2021
S. Al-Sabah et al. (eds.), *Laparoscopic Sleeve Gastrectomy*,
https://doi.org/10.1007/978-3-030-57373-7_43

443

and systemic inflammatory response syndrome or peritonitis, and should not be delayed. In a more stable patient, any collection should be drained whether surgically, radiologically or endoscopically. In addition to adequate drainage, nutritional support and antibiotics are the mainstays of the treatment.

Leaks after SG may be difficult to seal despite adequate drainage because of the higher pressures within the sleeve conduit. Because surgical re-intervention is associated with increased morbidity, non-operative management should be favored whenever possible [7]. Revision surgery before endoscopic management may also delay treatment success [8]. Thus, the role of endoscopy in the management of leaks is usually preferred, and, is being performed more frequently [5].

2 Definitions and Technical Principles of Endoscopic Management

The role of endoscopy in the scenario of leaks is constantly evolving. Endoscopic treatment options of leaks vary widely and currently, there is no consensus on the optimum endoscopic approach to managing SG leaks. In addition, there is an absence of prospective and randomized trials comparing different endoscopic techniques. Primary endoscopic closure is rarely successful or feasible for chronic leak and fistula management. The endoscopic therapeutic strategies have evolved and have increasingly standardized along two lines of management. The first of these is closure of the leak site, which generally includes the use of a covered self-expanding metallic stent (SEMS) to cover the leak [9, 10]. The second strategy is internal drainage, which aims to guide the drainage of the perigastric collection towards the lumen of the gastrointestinal tract and eventually closure of the fistula tract. When using any of the endoscopic methods to treat a post SG leak, it is important to manage any downstream stenosis, twist, or kink within the sleeve that creates an unfavorable pressure gradient to enhance drainage and resolution. Optimizing the pressure gradient allows closure of the cavity by secondary intention, through granulation tissue formation and fibrosis [11].

2.1 Definition of Post SG Leak

The clinical presentation of post SG leak is defined according to the modified UK Surgical Infection Study Group classification [12]. The presence of a leak is confirmed by upper gastrointestinal swallow study or abdominal computed tomography. Leaks are classified as acute (≤1 week), early (1–6 weeks), late (6–12 weeks), and chronic (>12 weeks) according to the Rosenthal classification [1].

2.2 Definition of Post SG Leak Healing

Healing of post SG leak is usually defined as resumption of oral feeding and the absence of (1) percutaneous drainage; (2) leakage of contrast agent seen on upper gastrointestinal swallow study or abdominal computed tomography; (3) intra-abdominal collections; and (4) flow through a previous surgical path (such as gastro-cutaneous fistula).

3 Closure of the Leak Site

The first principle of management of post SG leaks is closure of the leak site, which generally includes the use of a covered SEMS to cover the leak [9, 10] but may also include the use of through-the scope or over-the-scope and clips (OTSC) [13], and endoscopic suturing [14]. Endoscopic treatment of post SG leak with the placement of a covered SEMS or clips should only be done after abdominal collections have been drained either surgically or percutaneously before stent placement. In cases involving inaccessible, especially large, collections, the stenting should be postponed or abandoned.

3.1 Self-Expanding Metal Stents

SEMS have been the most widely studied devices for endoscopic management of SG leaks. SEMS have been used for the palliation of dysphagia in esophageal cancer since the early 1990s [15]. Although primarily used to palliate malignant strictures, other indications for SEMS placement now include strictures from extrinsic compression, malignant perforations and fistulas, and, more recently, benign conditions such as recalcitrant esophageal strictures, perforations, fistulas, post-surgical leaks and bleeding esophageal varices [16].

SEMSs are relatively easy to place and are widely available in most endoscopy units. One benefit to their use, compared to other endoscopic modalities for SG leaks, such as OTSC, suture, and internal drainage, is that SEMS placement does not require endoscopic navigation and identification of the leak or fistula orifice, which can be often difficult to locate. The SEMS coating isolates the leak orifice from gastric contents and allows re-feeding during the healing process (Fig. 1). There is evidence that high intragastric pressure from either mechanical or functional stenosis in the SG may contribute to persistent leak and delayed healing, which can be also be successfully managed by SEMS placement [17, 18]. However, covered SEMS placement for the treatment of post SG leaks should be performed in patients with adequate external drainage of the perigastric collection. It should be mentioned that the use of SEMS for the management of leaks after SG is currently not Food and Drug Administration approved, and is an off-label use of the device.

3.2 Types of SEMS

Commercially available stents are usually made of a shape-retaining nickel and titanium alloy (nitinol) and covered with polyurethane or silicone. Partially

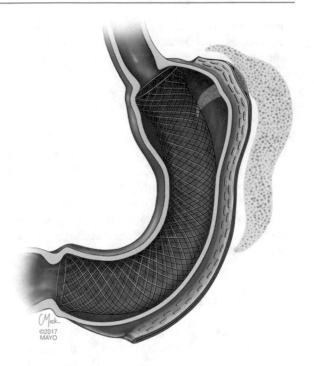

covered SEMSs have a portion of the exposed bare metal at the proximal and distal ends, which allows for ingrowth of surrounding tissue and could increase watertightness. Fully covered SEMSs do not have any exposed bare metal at either end. Partially covered stents have less risk of migration because of hyperplasia and ingrowth of tissue into the uncovered ends [19]. However, tissue ingrowth into the uncovered end also makes their removal more difficult resulting in tissue trauma and limits placement for a longer period. Fully covered stents, on the other hand, are more prone to migration but are easier to remove. New, extra-long, fully covered SEMSs have been developed especially for post SG leaks, such as the MEGA esophageal stent (Taewoong Medical, Gyeonggi-do, South Korea) and the Hanarostent (MITECH, Seoul, South Korea). These SEMS are available in lengths up to 23 cm and 24 cm, respectively, and are associated with less incidence of stent-specific complications such as migration and difficulty with removal [20, 21]. These stents are currently not available in the United States.

3.3   SEMS Insertion Procedure

All endoscopic procedures for placement of SEMSs for post SG leaks should be performed under fluoroscopic guidance with patients under general anesthesia. Once the site of the leak is identified, it should be marked with an external radio-opaque marker taped to the patient's skin (Fig. 2). A stiff guidewire is then

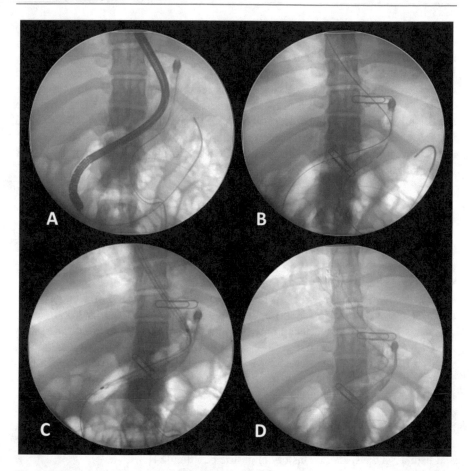

Fig. 2 Fluoroscopic images of a fully covered SEMS insertion for a post SG leak. **A** A guidewire has been passed through the endoscope into the duodenum. **B** External markers are placed on the skin marking the location of the pylorus and the site of the leak. **C** A fully covered SEMS is passed over the guidewire. **D** The fully covered SEMS is deployed, coving the leak site

passed through the endoscope all the way to the third part of the duodenum. The SEMS is then deployed over the guidewire to cover the leak orifice with the covered part of the SEMS. The longest available stent should be used to provide adequate coverage above and below the leak. In some cases, placement of a second SEMS may be necessary because of liquid reflux from the distal end between the gastric wall and the SEMS, or because of lack of watertightness at the proximal end due to the angle between the proximal end of the stent and the esophagus. If one of the new fully covered, extra-long SEMS, specifically designed for post-SG leaks is used, then it should be placed such that the proximal end is in the mid esophagus and the distal end in the proximal duodenal bulb, just distal to the pylorus. The SEMS are usually left in place from 3 to 4 weeks [19, 20].

SEMS extraction is usually done by pulling gently but firmly on the proximal end of the stent with a rat−tooth forceps. In case of a partially covered SEMS, argon plasma coagulation may be used to help destroy hyperplasia that develops between the SEMS meshes. This technique is used mainly in patients who had only proximal and mild hyperplasia. For this reason, another extraction technique can be employed, in which a Self-Expanding Plastic Stent (SEPS) is placed into the SEMS in order to induce necrosis of the hyperplastic proliferation. Extraction is then easily performed in a second endoscopic session [19]. In some cases, relapse or persistence of leakage after SEMS extraction justifies another SEMS implantation.

3.4   Outcome of SEMS Placement

The reported overall success rate of SEMS, with percutaneous drainage, in the closure of SG leaks, ranges from 65 to 95% [22, 23]. Table 1 shows the comparison of nine reported series of SEMSs in the management of laparoscopic sleeve gastrectomy leaks. However, these success rates are usually seen after multiple endoscopies (mean 4.7 procedures per patient) until fistula closure is achieved [24]. Permanent closure is usually obtained using only one stent in about 40%, and multiple stents in 20% of patients. In another 20% of patients presenting with a large fistula tract, stenting has to be complemented by another modality, such as insertion of a bio-prosthetic plug into the fistula or use of an OTSC. The success rates of SEMS placement correlates with the duration of treatment with a diminishing chance of fistula closure as the treatment period lengths. Multivariate analysis identified four predictive factors of healing following endoscopic treatment: interval <21 days between fistula diagnosis and first endoscopy, small fistula size (<1 cm), interval between SG and fistula ≤3 days, and, no history of gastric banding [24].

Tolerance to the placement of SEMSs is variable but usually fair. The reported symptoms such as nausea, dysphagia, and retrosternal discomfort are mild and transient, usually resolving within a few days [19]. The adverse events related to SEMS placement for SG leaks include migration, impaction and ulceration, digestive perforation, and incarceration. Stent migration is the most common complication of SEMS placement and is highly dependent on the type of stent used. A large meta-analysis revealed an overall stent migration rate of 16.94% [25]. The migration rate of fully covered SEMS is between 25 and 58% [26, 27]. The SEMSs have been reported to migrate even when they are clipped in position [28, 29]. The migration may require endoscopic stent repositioning, retrieval, or replacement. There have been reports of a number of patients who passed the stent via the rectum without incident [19, 26], but there have also been cases of stents which had to be removed surgically because of migration into the small intestine with subsequent failure to pass the stent through the rectum [26]. When stents migrate, they may become impacted into the wall of the digestive tract, creating a contact ulcer. Gastrointestinal bleeding and intestinal perforations have also been reported, and are due to migration and subsequent impaction of a metallic stent [24].

Table 1 Comparison of reported series of self-expanding metallic stents in the management of laparoscopic sleeve gastrectomy leaks

Author (reference)	No. of patients	Bariatric surgery	Type of SEMS	Duration of SEMS placement (days)	Success rate (%)	Complications (n)
Eisendrath et al. (2007) [19]	21	SG: 12 RYGB: 8 BPD: 1	Partially covered	21	81	Stricture: 2 Migration: 1
Bège et al. (2011) [58]	27 (22 treated with SEMS)	SG: 25 RYGB: 2	Covered	64	70	Migration: 13
El Mourad et al. (2013) [9]	47	SG: 24 RYGB: 14 Others: 12	Partially covered	45	87	Migration: 7 Stricture: 1 Perforation: 1 Bleeding: 1
Alazmi et al. (2014) [59]	17	SG: 17	Partially covered	42	76	Dysphagia: 3 Bleeding: 2 Migration: 1
Murino et al. (2015) [43]	91	SG: 55 RYGB: 36	Partially covered	70	81	Stricture: 13 Migration: 7 Bleeding: 5 Perforation: 2
Fishman et al. (2015) [22]	26	SG: 26	Fully covered	28	65	Migration: 7 Severe intolerance: 4 Severe bleeding: 1
Southwell et al. (2016) [23]	20	SG: 20	Fully covered: 16 Partially covered: 4	75	95	Migration: 10 Severe intolerance: 5 Perforation: 2 Stricture: 2
Martin Del Campo et al. (2018) [60]	24	SG: 24	Fully covered	29	67	Migration: 9
Smith et al. (2019) [61]	85 (61 treated with SEMS)	SG: 85	Fully covered: 59 Partially covered: 2	NA	73	Migration: 21 Bleeding: 7 Embedded SEMS: 2

SG Laparoscopic sleeve gastrectomy
RYGB Roux-en-Y gastric bypass
SEMS Self-expanding metallic stent

The other major complication of SEMS placement is incarceration. This is again dependent on the type of stent used and has been reported to occur up 90% of partially covered and about 7% of fully covered SEMS [24]. Removal of an incarcerated partially covered SEMS can even be associated with complications, such as esophageal wall striping and perforation, when not managed properly [30]. Incarcerated SEMS extraction is usually obtained by careful traction, with the help of a SEPS left in place for 1–2 weeks (stent-in-stent technique), or by surgical extraction. The use of a SEPS is an effective technique for the removal of an incarceration SEMS [31]. However, tissue hyperplasia into partially covered SEMS is sometimes responsible for stricture development attributed to a fibrotic healing process after removal in up to 14% of patients and may require endoscopic dilation [31].

3.5 Over-The Scope Clip System

Over-the Scope Clip (OTSC) is a system for endoscopic closure of gastrointestinal leaks and defects after endoscopic or surgical procedures and is a promising option for treatment of leaks and fistula after bariatric surgery. The system is designed to secure larger tissue volume, provide higher stability at the site of leak or perforation, and decrease the strain on the surrounding tissue [32]. It has a very strong grasp to include full wall thickness and can allow closure of defects up to 30 mm [33]. However, simply putting an OTSC at the site of a leak is not usually successful in permanently sealing a leak. Reasons for clip failure include friability of tissue, tissue ischemia, presence of infection, and presence of distal stenosis forming a high-pressure zone at the site of leakage. For this reason, OTSCs are usually placed in combination with a SEMS or just after their removal [34]. A recent systemic review looking at the efficacy and safety of the OTSC system in the management of post SG leaks showed an overall success rate of 86% [32] but success rates are much lower in cases of chronic leaks due to difficulty approximating fibrous tissue [32]. Predictive criteria for fistula closure success using OTSC are as follows: very early fistula (<7 days); fistulas with less fibrosis, leak size 10–30 mm; and leakages after LSG [33].

4 Internal Drainage

Internal drainage is the second principle for management of post SG leaks and aims to guide the drainage of the perigastric collection towards the lumen of the gastrointestinal tract and eventually closure of the fistula tract. This is usually achieved by either endoscopic internal drainage (EID) with biliary double pigtail stents (DPS) [35], or placement of a naso-cystic drain [5] Other, less-often used therapies include endo-luminal vacuum therapy [36].

4.1 Endoscopic Internal Drainage

First described in 2012, EID is a relatively recent strategy in the management of SG leaks [37]. EID is usually performed by the deployment of biliary DPSs across the leak orifice, positioning one end inside the collection and the other end in the lumen of the stomach (Fig. 3a). Alternatively, a naso-cystic tube is placed through the fistula and connected to suction (Fig. 3b). The principle of EID is similar to that of endoscopic cystogastrostomy in pancreatic pseudocyst drainage. The DPS keep the fistula tract between the stomach lumen and the infected para-gastric space open, allowing the para-gastric space to drain and heal by secondary intention progressively reducing it to a "virtual" cavity that is only occupied by pigtail loops.

EID is effective both clinically and from a cost perspective, especially for subacute or chronic leaks with an organized walled-off collection [5, 38–40]. Another advantage of EID is that concurrent endoscopic necrosectomy may be performed to remove necrotic infected material from within the cavity and enhance drainage and healing. As experience with EID increases, there is an apparent trend in many centers to move towards early EID, especially in stable patients with a localized perigastric collection and no or minimal signs of sepsis [8, 18]. In some patients, percutaneous drainage may not be possible because of the interposition of spleen or bowel. In these situations, EID offers a viable alternative and may be the only therapy required, precluding the need for external drainage. In those patients who already have external drainage, EID may facilitate its early removal with concomitant capping and slow withdrawal of the percutaneous drain [11]. EID can also be used as a rescue method in cases of failed SEMS-based treatment, with no statistical difference in terms of clinical success between these two groups [41].

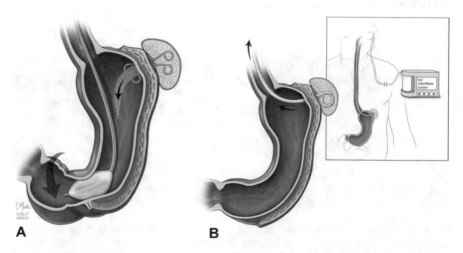

Fig. 3 **A** An organized post SG leak treated by endoscopic internal drainage with two pigtail drains and pneumatic dilation device dilating a twisted and tight distal stomach, facilitating drainage. **B** An organized post SG leak treated by endoscopic internal drainage with nasocystic drain on low intermittent suction, facilitating drainage. Reprinted from Vargas EJ, Abu Dayyeh BK. Keep calm under pressure: a paradigm shift in managing postsurgical leaks. Gastrointest Endosc. 2018;87:438–441 [11], with permission from Elsevier

4.2   EID Procedure

All endoscopic procedures for EID for post SG leaks should be performed under fluoroscopic guidance with patients under general anesthesia. In the majority of the patients, the fistulous opening is identified in the upper end of the staple line, between the gastric fold, by careful examination. The opening is then cannulated with an ERCP cannula and the leak confirmed by injection of water-soluble contrast into the fistula and extravasation into the para-gastric cavity. A guidewire is passed, through the ERCP cannula, until it looped in the cavity. A double pigtail biliary stent (7–10 Fr, 4–7 cm) is then placed into the cavity, through the fistula, leaving the proximal end of the stent in the stomach or distal esophagus. The process was repeated and a second pigtail stent was placed alongside the first one (Figs. 4 and 5).

If the fistulous opening is not initially identified during endoscopy then placement of a Savary guidewire or a nasogastric tube may help to open up the gastroesophageal junction and facilitate the identification of the fistula. Sometimes flushing radiographic contrast material through the endoscope in the lower esophagus, under fluoroscopy may show the leak site on fluoroscopy, which can then be identified on endoscopic vision. The leak site may also be identified on endoscopy after methylene blue dye is injected through a percutaneous drain, if available. If the fistulous opening is tight and does not allow passage of the DPS into the cavity, then, biliary dilatation balloon or Soehendra biliary dilation catheter may be used to dilate the track to facilitate the insertion of the stents. Removal of the DPS is performed endoscopically by grasping the proximal end of the stent with a snare and removing it with gentle traction of the endoscope.

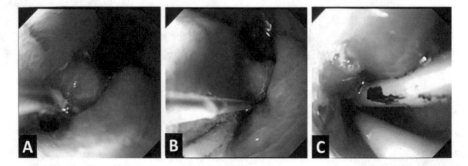

Fig. 4 Endoscopic images of internal drainage procedure. **A** A guidewire has been passed into the perigastric collection, through the leak site. **B** A double pigtail stent deployed in the perigastric collection. The guidewire is reinserted into the perigastric collection. **C** Two double pigtail stents deployed in the perigastric collection

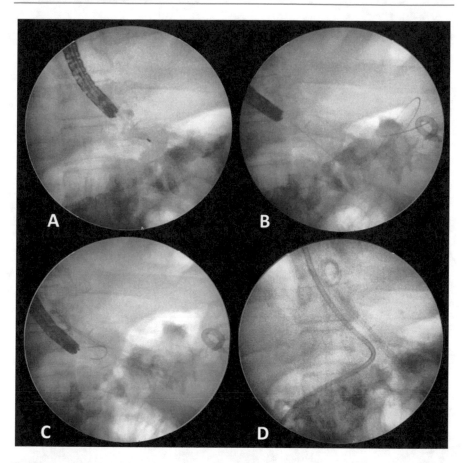

Fig. 5 Fluoroscopic images of endoscopic internal drainage procedure. **A** Injection of contrast into the perigastric collection, through the leak site. **B** A guidewire has been passed and looped into the perigastric collection. **C** Two double pigtail stents deployed in the perigastric collection. **D** Two pigtail stents deployed along with a naso-jejunal feeding tube

4.3   Outcome of EID Procedure

The overall success of EID in healing a post SG leak ranges from 78 to 95% [5, 35, 37, 38, 41, 42], with one small series of nine patients even reporting a 100% success rate [17]. Table 2 shows the comparison of eight reported series of EID in the management of laparoscopic sleeve gastrectomy leaks. This is better with the reported healing rates of 62 to 87% achieved with placement of SEMS with percutaneous drainage [9, 19, 43, 44]. EID has also been shown to be successful in

Table 2 Comparison of reported series of endoscopic internal drainage by double pigtail biliary stents in the management of laparoscopic sleeve gastrectomy leaks

Author (reference)	No. of patients	Management prior to EID (n)	Mean duration of EID (days)	EID success rate (%)	EID complications (%)
Pequignot et al. (2012) [37]	25	Surgery: 14 SEMS: 13	62	84	8
Donatelli et al. (2014) [42]	21	Laparoscopic drainage: 15	55 (26–180)	95	10
Nedelcu et al. (2015) [17]	9	Laparoscopic drainage: 9	2.8 months	100	11
Donatelli et al. (2015) [38]	67	External drainage: 42	57 (10–206)	78	4
Bouchard et al. (2016) [41]	33[a]	SEMS:19	47	79	15
Lorenzo et al. (2018) [5]	44	SEMS: 22	12.2 ± 15.8 months	84	–
Gonzalez et al. (2018) [35]	44	SEMS: 61% Surgical drain: 33%	226 days	84	5
Siddique et al. (2020) [62]	20	Laparoscopic drainage: 11 Surgical drainage: 4 SEMS: 8	83 days	85	10

[a]28 Laparoscopic sleeve gastrectomy; 5 Gastric bypass
EID Endoscopic internal drainage
SG Laparoscopic sleeve gastrectomy
SEMS Self-expanding metallic stent

healing post SG leak in patients who have previously failed to respond to covered SEMS placement [35, 37, 41]. Additionally, EID is better tolerated by the patient compared to SEMS, which usually causes symptoms such as pain, nausea, vomiting, and bleeding.

The rate of complications of EID ranges from 4 to 15% [38, 41]. Most of these adverse events are mild and easily tolerated, such as ulceration at the tip of the DPS and bleeding [38]. Migration of the DPS is rare, and if occurs, is usually towards the gastric lumen and spontaneous passage through the rectum. There are reports of distal migration of the DPS. Four of these caused serious complications such as massive upper gastrointestinal bleeding from a pseudoaneurysm of the splenic artery [45] and splenic injury [46–48]. The other distal migrations included two patients with the migration of the DPS into the abdominal wall and the other with DPS migrating completely into the perigastric collection. All of these were easily removed endoscopically [41, 49, 50].

The presence of a gastrobronchial fistula is a recognized factor associated with the failure of EID in healing post SG leaks [5]. A statistical analysis evaluating whether other factors such as the type of bariatric surgery, treatment or diagnostic delays, or the use of EID as a primary or secondary treatment demonstrated no significant predictor of success [34, 41, 51]. Success rates were also not influenced by the type of leak according to the Rosenthal classification [1].

A recent study looking at the cost-effectiveness of SEMS placement vs. EID in the endoscopic management of post SG leaks found that EID with DPSs is more effective and reduces the cost by making management easier and shortening hospital stay [40]. The authors recommended that EID should be proposed as standard management for patients with post SG leak.

4.4 Endoscopic Vacuum Therapy

Endoscopic vacuum therapy (EVT), also known as endoscopic negative pressure therapy, involves endoscopic placement of a sponge connected to a nasogastric tube into the defect cavity or gastrointestinal lumen. This promotes healing, which is similar to the mechanisms in which skin wounds are treated with commonly employed wound vacuums [52]. One of the disadvantages of EVT is the need for repeated endoscopic procedures because the sponge needs to be changed every 3 to 5 days.

A recent study, evaluated the use of EVT in patients with early infradiaphragmatic leakage after bariatric surgery, including SG and gastric bypass. In some patients, EVT was performed alone, while others had EVT with a SEMS (stent-over-sponge). In 80% of patients, the leak was connected to abscess cavities. Clinical success, defined as no signs of persistent leakage, was achieved in all patients studied [53]. In another study including patients with acute, early, late, and chronic leaks after SG, the use of EVT was associated with 100% resolution of leaks confirmed by upper GI series, with an average of 10 sponge exchanges over an average of 50 days [36].

In general, EVT is a safe procedure with a low complication rate. The most frequent adverse events are sponge dislocation, minor bleeding after sponge exchange due to ingrowth of granulation tissue into the sponge, and anastomotic strictures. However, major bleeding events have also been reported due to the risk of development of a fistula between the cavity and surrounding major blood vessels and structures due to the ongoing inflammatory process of EVT [54].

5 Septotomy and Pneumatic Balloon Dilatation

Intraluminal pressure in the stomach increases after SG [55] and can lead to a pressure gradient that favors flow through the fistula or leak into the abscess cavity, thus preventing closure. Endoscopic septotomy has been described as a resolution technique that could be useful in the setting of late and chronic leaks. It

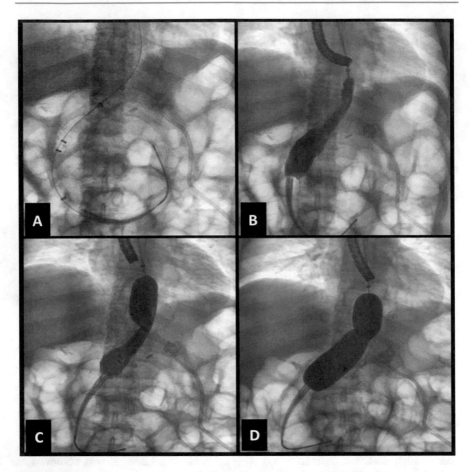

Fig. 6 Fluoroscopic images of balloon dilatation procedure for post SG gastric stenosis. **A** A guide wire is passed into the duodenum and a balloon is seen going over the guide wire. **B** The balloon inflation is started by filling it with radiographic contrast. **C** The balloon is gradually filled with radiologic contrast the stenosis becomes evident in the middle part of the sleeved stomach. **D** The balloon is gradually filled until the gastric stenosis is dilated

allows for fluid drainage from the abscess cavity into the stomach by dividing the septum that separates the abscess from the gastric lumen [56], which when combined with aggressive sleeve dilatation, equalizes cavity pressures and promotes secretion flow into the gastrointestinal tract.

Endoscopic septotomy is performed by dividing the septum separating the gastric lumen and the abscess cavity. This is done with a needle knife or a Triangle Tip Knife and electrosurgical energy. The division of the septum is considered complete when the entire abscess cavity communicates with the gastric lumen, thus allowing drainage of secretion into the lumen of the stomach.

When a downstream stenosis is present, the patient may require pneumatic balloon dilation. This can be combined with a septotomy or performed by itself [57]. The dilatation is performed with a large achalasia balloon, usually with a 30 mm diameter balloon, but it may gradually be increased up to 40 mm in case of suboptimal response (Fig. 6).

6 Conclusion

As bariatric surgery becomes more prevalent, so will the complications associated with this procedure. Thus, gastroenterologists and endoscopists must become familiar with the types of bariatric surgery, the main complications, and the various endoscopic ways to safely and effectively manage these complications. The optimal approach to managing these patients is through the development of multi-disciplinary teams (MDT) consisting of bariatric surgeons, therapeutic gastroenterologists, interventional radiologist, and intensivists. It is only through following these best practice guidelines that we will be able to provide the best care for these patients.

References

1. Rosenthal RJ, Diaz AA, Arvidsson D, Baker RS, Basso N, Bellanger D, Boza C, El Mourad H, France M, Gagner M, International Sleeve Gastrectomy Expert Panel, et al. International sleeve gastrectomy expert panel consensus statement: best practice guidelines based on experience of >12,000 cases. Surg Obes Relat Dis. 2012;8(1):8–19.
2. Parikh M, Issa R, McCrillis A, Saunders JK, Ude-Welcome A, Gagner M. Surgical strategies that may decrease leak after laparoscopic sleeve gastrectomy: a systematic review and meta-analysis of 9991 cases. Ann Surg. 2013;257(2):231–7.
3. Trastulli S, Desiderio J, Guarino S, Cirocchi R, Scalercio V, Noya G, Parisi A. Laparoscopic sleeve gastrectomy compared with other bariatric surgical procedures: a systematic review of randomized trials. Surg Obes Relat Dis. 2013;9(5):816–29.
4. Heymsfield SB, Wadden TA. Mechanisms, pathophysiology, and management of obesity. N Eng J Med. 2017;376:254–66.
5. Lorenzo D, Guilbaud T, Gonzalez JM, Benezech A, Dutour A, Boullu S, Berdah S, Bège T, Barthet M. Endoscopic treatment of fistulas after sleeve gastrectomy: a comparison of internal drainage versus closure. Gastrointest Endosc. 2018;87(2):429–37.
6. Benedix F, Poranzke O, Adolf D, Wolff S, Lippert H, Arend J, Manger T, Stroh C. Staple line leak after primary sleeve gastrectomy-risk factors and mid-term results: do patients still benefit from the weight loss procedure? Obes Surg. 2017;27:1780–8.
7. Kim J, Azagury D, Eisenberg D, DeMaria E, Campos GM. ASMBS position statement on prevention, detection, and treatment of gastrointestinal leak after gastric bypass and sleeve gastrectomy, including the roles of imaging, surgical exploration, and nonoperative management. Surg Obes Relat Dis. 2015;11:739–48.
8. Brethauer SA, Kothari S, Sudan R, Williams B, English WJ, Brengman M, Kurian M, Hutter M, Stegemann L, Kallies K, Nguyen NT, Ponce J, Morton JM. Systematic review on reoperative bariatric surgery: American Society for Metabolic and Bariatric Surgery Revision Task Force. Surg Obes Relat Dis. 2014;10(5):952–72.

9. El Mourad H, Himpens J, Verhofstadt J. Stent treatment for fistula after obesity surgery: results in 47 consecutive patients. Surg Endosc. 2013;27(3):808–16.

10. Simon F, Siciliano I, Gillet A, Castel B, Coffin B, Msika S. Gastric leak after laparoscopic sleeve gastrectomy: early covered self-expandable stent reduces healing time. Obes Surg. 2013;23:687–92.

11. Vargas EJ, Abu Dayyeh BK. Keep calm under pressure: a paradigm shift in managing post-surgical leaks. Gastrointest Endosc. 2018;87:438–41.

12. Surgical Infection Study Group. Peel AL, Taylor EW. Proposed definitions for the audit of postoperative infection: a discussion paper. Ann R Coll Surg Engl. 1991;73(6):385–8.

13. Zacharoulis D, Perivoliotis K, Sioka E, Zachari E, Kapsoritakis A, Manolakis A, Tzovaras G. The use of over-the-scope clip in the treatment of persistent staple line leak after re-sleeve gastrectomy: review of the literature. J Minim Access Surg. 2017;13:228–30.

14. Schweitzer M, Steele K, Mitchell M, Okolo P. Transoral endoscopic closure of gastric fistula. Surg Obes Relat Dis. 2009;5:283–4.

15. Lindberg CG, Cwikiel W, Ivancev K, Lundstedt C, Stridbeck H, Tranberg KG. Laser therapy and insertion of Wallstents for palliative treatment of esophageal carcinoma. Acta Radiol. 1991;32:345–8.

16. Irani S, Kozarek R. Esophageal stents: past, present, and future. Tech Gastrointest Endosc. 2010;12:178–90.

17. Nedelcu M, Manos T, Cotirlet A, Noel P, Gagner M. Outcome of leaks after sleeve gastrectomy based on a new algorithm adressing leak size and gastric stenosis. Obes Surg. 2015;25(3):559–63.

18. Manos T, Nedelcu M, Cotirlet A, Eddbali I, Gagner M, Noel P. How to treat stenosis after sleeve gastrectomy? Surg Obes Relat Dis. 2017;13:150–4.

19. Eisendrath P, Cremer M, Himpens J, Cadière GB, Le Moine O, Devière J. Endotherapy including temporary stenting of fistulas of the upper gastrointestinal tract after laparoscopic bariatric surgery. Endoscopy. 2007;39(7):625–30.

20. Galloro G, Magno L, Musella M, Manta R, Zullo A, Forestieri P. A novel dedicated endoscopic stent for staple-line leaks after laparoscopic sleeve gastrectomy: a case series. Surg Obes Relat Dis. 2014;10:607–11.

21. Bezerra Silva L, Galvão Neto M, Marchesini JC, S N Godoy E, Campos J. Sleeve gastrectomy leak: endoscopic management through a customized long bariatric stent. Gastrointest Endosc. 2017;85:865–6.

22. Fishman S, Shnell M, Gluck N, Meirsdorf S, Abu-Abeid S, Santo E. Use of sleeve-customized self-expandable metal stents for the treatment of staple-line leakage after laparoscopic sleeve gastrectomy. Gastrointest Endosc. 2015;81:1291–4.

23. Southwell T, Lim TH, Ogra R. Endoscopic therapy for treatment of staple line leaks post-laparoscopic sleeve gastrectomy (LSG): experience from a large bariatric surgery centre in New Zealand. Obes Surg. 2016;26:1155–62.

24. Christophorou D, Valats JC, Funakoshi N, Duflos C, Picot MC, Vedrenne B, Prat F, Bulois P, Branche J, Decoster S, Coron E, Charachon A, Pineton De Chambrun G, Nocca D, Bauret P, Blanc P. Endoscopic treatment of fistula after sleeve gastrectomy: results of a multicenter retrospective study. Endoscopy. 2015;47:988–96.

25. Puli SR, Spofford IS, Thompson CC. Use of self-expandable stents in the treatment of bariatric surgery leaks: a systematic review and meta-analysis. Gastrointest Endosc. 2012;75:287–93.

26. Eubanks S, Edwards CA, Fearing NM, Ramaswamy A, de la Torre RA, Thaler KJ, Miedema BW, Scott JS. Use of endoscopic stents to treat anastomotic complications after bariatric surgery. J Am Coll Surg. 2008;206:935–8.

27. Leenders BJ, Stronkhorst A, Smulders FJ, Nieuwenhuijzen GA, Gilissen LP. Removable and repositionable covered metal self-expandable stents for leaks after upper gastrointestinal surgery: experiences in a tertiary referral hospital. Surg Endosc. 2013;27:2751–9.

28. Babor R, Talbot M, Tyndal A. Treatment of upper gastrointestinal leaks with a removable, covered, self-expanding metallic stent. Surg Laparosc Endosc Percutan Tech. 2009;19:e1–e4.

29. Fukumoto R, Orlina J, McGinty J, Teixeira J. Use of polyflex stents in treatment of acute esophageal and gastric leaks after bariatric surgery. Surg Obes Relat Dis. 2007;3:68–71.

30. Hirdes MM, Vleggaar FP, Van der Linde K, Willems M, Totté ER, Siersema PD. Esophageal perforation due to removal of partially covered self-expanding metal stents placed for a benign perforation or leak. Endoscopy. 2011;43:156–9.

31. Eisendrath P, Jacques D. Major complications of bariatric surgery: endoscopy as first-line treatment. J Nat Rev Gastroenterol Hepatol. 2015;12:701–10.

32. Shoar S, Poliakin L, Khorgami Z, Rubenstein R, El-Matbouly M, Levin JL, Saber AA. Efficacy and safety of the over-the-scope clip (OTSC) system in the management of leak and Fistula after laparoscopic sleeve gastrectomy: a systematic review. Obes Surg. 2017;27:2410–8.

33. Mercky P, Gonzalez JM, Aimore Bonin E, Emungania O, Brunet J, Grimaud JC, Barthet M. Usefulness of over-the-scope clipping system for closing digestive fistulas. Dig Endosc. 2015;27:18–24.

34. Shehab HM, Hakky SM, Gawdat KA. An endoscopic strategy combining mega stents and over-the-scope clips for the management of post-bariatric surgery leaks and fistulas. Obes Surg. 2016;26(5):941–8.

35. Gonzalez JM, Lorenzo D, Guilbaud T, Bège T, Barthet M. Internal endoscopic drainage as first line or second line treatment in case of postsleeve gastrectomy fistulas. Endosc Int Open. 2018;6(6):E745–50.

36. Leeds SG, Burdick JS. Management of gastric leaks after sleeve gastrectomy with endoluminal vacuum (E-Vac) therapy. Surg Obes Relat Dis. 2016;12:1278–85.

37. Pequignot A, Fuks D, Verhaeghe P, Dhahri A, Brehant O, Bartoli E, Delcenserie R, Yzet T, Regimbeau JM. Is there a place for pigtail drains in the management of gastric leaks after laparoscopic sleeve gastrectomy? Obes Surg. 2012;22(5):712–20.

38. Donatelli G, Dumont JL, Cereatti F, Ferretti S, Vergeau BM, Tuszynski T, Pourcher G, Tranchart H, Mariani P, Meduri A, Catheline JM, Dagher I, Fiocca F, Marmuse JP, Meduri B. Treatment of leaks following sleeve gastrectomy by endoscopic internal drainage (EID). Obes Surg 2015;25(7):1293–301.

39. Donatelli G, Fuks D, Tabchouri N, Pourcher G. Seal or drain? Endoscopic management of leaks following sleeve gastrectomy. Surg Innov. 2018;25(1):5–6.

40. Cosse C, Rebibo L, Brazier F, Hakim S, Delcenserie R, Regimbeau JM. Cost-effectiveness analysis of stent type in endoscopic treatment of gastric leak after laparoscopic sleeve gastrectomy. Br J Surg. 2018;105(5):570–7.

41. Bouchard S, Eisendrath P, Toussaint E, Le Moine O, Lemmers A, Arvanitakis M, Devière J. Trans-fistulary endoscopic drainage for post-bariatric abdominal collections communicating with the upper gastrointestinal tract. Endoscopy. 2016;48(9):809–16.

42. Donatelli G, Ferretti S, Vergeau BM, Dhumane P, Dumont JL, Derhy S, Tuszynski T, Dritsas S, Carloni A, Catheline JM, Pourcher G, Dagher I, Meduri B. Endoscopic internal drainage with enteral nutrition (EDEN) for treatment of leaks following sleeve gastrectomy. Obes Surg. 2014;24(8):1400–7.

43. Murino A, Arvanitakis M, Le Moine O, Blero D, Devière J, Eisendrath P. Effectiveness of endoscopic management using self-expandable metal stents in a large cohort of patients with post-bariatric leaks. Obes Surg. 2015;25(9):1569–76.

44. Swinnen J, Eisendrath P, Rigaux J, Kahegeshe L, Lemmers A, Le Moine O, Devière J. Self-expandable metal stents for the treatment of benign upper GI leaks and perforations. Gastrointest Endosc. 2011;73(5):890–9.

45. Chahine E, D'Alessandro A, Elhajjam M, Moryoussef F, Vitte RL, Carlier R, Alsabah S, Chouillard E. Massive gastrointestinal bleeding due to splenic artery erosion by a pigtail drain in a post sleeve gastrectomy leak: a case report. Obes Surg. 2019;29(5):1653–6.

46. Marchese M, Romano L, Giuliani A, Cianca G, Di Sibio A, Carlei F, Amicucci G, Schietroma M. A case of intrasplenic displacement of an endoscopic double-pigtail stent as a treatment for laparoscopic sleeve gastrectomy leak. Int J Surg Case Rep. 2018;53:367–9.
47. Donatelli G, Airinei G, Poupardin E, Tuszynski T, Wind P, Benamouzig R, Meduri B. Double-pigtail stent migration invading the spleen: rare potentially fatal complication of endoscopic internal drainage for sleeve gastrectomy leak. Endoscopy. 2016;48(Suppl 1):E74–5.
48. Genser L, Pattou F, Caiazzo R. Splenic abscess with portal venous gas caused by intrasplenic migration of an endoscopic double pigtail drain as a treatment of post-sleeve gastrectomy fistula. Surg Obes Relat Dis. 2016;12:e1–3.
49. Debs T, Petrucciani N, Kassir R, Vanbiervliet G, Ben Amor I, Staccini AM, Sejor E, Gugenheim J. Migration of an endoscopic double pigtail drain into the abdominal wall placed as a treatment of a fistula post revisional bariatric surgery. Obes Surg. 2017;27:1335–7.
50. AlAtwan AA, AlJewaied A, AlKhadher T, AlHaddad M, Siddique I. A complication of an endoscopic pigtail stent migration into the cavity during deployment as a treatment for gastric leak. Case Rep Surg. 2019;6974527.
51. Guillaud A, Moszkowicz D, Nedelcu M, Caballero-Caballero A, Rebibo L, Reche F, Abba J, Arvieux C. Gastrobronchial fistula: a serious complication of sleeve gastrectomy. Results of a French multicentric study. Obes Surg. 2015;25(12):2352–9.
52. de Moura DTH, de Moura BFBH, Manfredi MA, Hathorn KE, Bazarbashi AN, Ribeiro IB, de Moura EGH, Thompson CC. Role of endoscopic vacuum therapy in the management of gastrointestinal transmural defects. World J Gastrointest Endosc. 2019;16:329–44.
53. Morell B, Murray F, Vetter D, Bueter M, Gubler C. Endoscopic vacuum therapy (EVT) for early infradiaphragmal leakage after bariatric surgery-outcomes of six consecutive cases in a single institution. Langenbecks Arch Surg. 2019;404:115–21.
54. Laukoetter MG, Mennigen R, Neumann PA, Dhayat S, Horst G, Palmes D, Senninger N, Vowinkel T. Successful closure of defects in the upper gastrointestinal tract by endoscopic vacuum therapy (EVT): a prospective cohort study. Surg Endosc. 2017;31:2687–96.
55. Yehoshua RT, Eidelman LA, Stein M, Fichman S, Mazor A, Chen J, Bernstine H, Singer P, Dickman R, Beglaibter N, Shikora SA, Rosenthal RJ, Rubin M. Laparoscopic sleeve gastrectomy—volume and pressure assessment. Obes Surg. 2008;18:1083–8.
56. Guerron AD, Ortega CB, Portenier D. Endoscopic abscess septotomy for management of sleeve gastrectomy leak. Obes Surg. 2017;27:2672–4.
57. Campos JM, Ferreira FC, Teixeira AF, Lima JS, Moon RC, D'Assunção MA, Neto MG. Septotomy and balloon dilation to treat chronic leak. Obes Surg. 2016;26:1992–3.
58. Bège T, Emungania O, Vitton V, Ah-Soune P, Nocca D, Noël P, Bradjanian S, Berdah SV, Brunet C, Grimaud JC, Barthet M. An endoscopic strategy for management of anastomotic complications from bariatric surgery: a prospective study. Gastrointest Endosc. 2011;73(2):238–44.
59. Alazmi W, Al-Sabah S, Ali DA, Almazeedi S. Treating sleeve gastrectomy leak with endoscopic stenting: the Kuwaiti experience and review of recent literature. Surg Endosc. 2014;28:3425–8.
60. Martin Del Campo SE, Mikami DJ, Needleman BJ, Noria SF. Endoscopic stent placement for treatment of sleeve gastrectomy leak: a single institution experience with fully covered stents. Surg Obes Relat Dis. 2018;14:453–61.
61. Smith ZL, Park KH, Llano EM, Donboli K, Fayad L, Han S, Kang L, Simril RT, Patel R Hollander T, Rogers MC, Elmunzer BJ, Siddiqui UD, Aadam AA, Mullady DK, Lang GD, Das KK, Jamil LH, Lo SK, Gaddam S, Chapman C, Keswani R, Cote G, Kumbhari V, Kushir V. Outcomes of endoscopic treatment of leaks and fistulae after sleeve gastrectomy: results from a large multicenter U.S. cohort. Surg Obes Relat Dis. 2019;15:850–5.
62. Siddique I, Al-Sabah S, Alazmi W. Endoscopic internal drainage by double pigtail stents in the management of laparoscopic sleeve gastrectomy leaks. Surg Obes Relat Dis. 2020;S1550–7289(20):30169–6. doi: https://doi.org/10.1016/j.soard.2020.03.028.

How to Manage Sleeve Complications: Surgical Leak and Abscess

Elie Chouillard ⓘ

1   Introduction

Laparoscopic sleeve gastrectomy (SG) has become the most commonly performed primary bariatric procedure worldwide [1, 2]. However, the staple-line leak (SGL) remains the most serious concern averaging 2% and ranging from less than 1% to nearly 5% [3]. Over the past 10 years, numerous studies [4–7] addressed risk factors linked to SGL, including bougie size, distance from the pylorus, surgeon's experience, and reinforcement of the staple line. Next to the surgeon's learning curve [8], the later may be the most important risk factor of the occurrence of SGL. Recently, Gagner et al. [3] performed a systematic review of nearly 150 studies representing 40,653 patients, demonstrating an overall SGL rate of 1.5%. Reinforcement of the staple line with an absorbable polymer membrane had the lowest statistically significant SGL rate of 0.7%. This was lower than oversewing, other subtypes of reinforcement, or no reinforcement at all. A recent randomized study [9] comparing the use of owersewing with invagination to no reinforcement demonstrated a reduction in SGL rates for the suturing approach, although longer the operative time was. Previously, a metaanalysis of published studies did not show any significant benefit of oversewing, either on the rate of SGL itself or on the overall rate of complications after SG [10].

Among others [3, 7, 8], we believe that the reduction in SGL is most likely related to accomplished surgical experience. Progressively, the fields of improvements in surgical techniques included better dissection with preservation of well vascularized tissue, reduction of thermal injury and tissue trauma, selection of

E. Chouillard (✉)
Université Saint-Joseph, Chef de Service de Chirurgie Générale et Digestive Centre
Hospitalier de Poissy/Saint-Germain-en-Laye, Saint-Germain-en-Laye, France
e-mail: chouillard@yahoo.com

© The Editor(s) (if applicable) and The Author(s), under exclusive license to Springer   461
Nature Switzerland AG 2021
S. Al-Sabah et al. (eds.), *Laparoscopic Sleeve Gastrectomy*,
https://doi.org/10.1007/978-3-030-57373-7_44

appropriate staple thickness, avoidance of narrowing the incisura angularis, choice of adequate bougie sizes, and avoidance of stapling along the esophagus.

Mortality of a patient with SGL could reach up to 3% or ten times that of the SG itself [11]. A French study showed that the mean cost of a SGL could reach more than 75,000 euros [12].

Theoretically, a digestive leak could be defined as the spilling of luminal contents from a surgical join between two hollow viscera [13]. By extrapolation, SGL could be considered as an effluent of gastrointestinal content through the gastric staple line, which may collect near the stomach, or exit through the abdominal wall, the pleural cavity, or a drain. SGL can be classified based either on the time of onset, clinical presentation, site of dehiscence, radiological appearance, or mix of these factors.

Early, intermediate, and late SGLs are those appearing 1 to 4, 5 to 9, and 10 or more days following surgery, respectively [14]. By clinical relevance and extent of dissemination, one may define *type I or subclinical* SGLs as those that are well localized, infra-clinical, and without dissemination (i.e., peritoneal or pleural cavities). On the opposite, *type II* are SGLs with dissemination into the abdominal or pleural cavity, with consequent severe and systemic clinical manifestations. Based on both clinical and radiological findings, *type A* SGLs are microperforations without clinical or radiographic signs, while *type B* are macroperforations detected by radiological studies but without any clinical finding, and finally, *type C* SGLs present with both radiological and clinical evidence [15].

2 Principles of Management

Despite the absence of a standardized algorithm, the treatment of SGL may involve surgical, endoscopic, or radiological procedures. The purpose of the present chapter is to define the place of surgical treatment of the SGL and its complications.

Surgery should no more be considered as a secondary option after failure of endoscopy but as another dimension of a treatment targeting definite healing of SGL and not only long remission.

The management of the patient with a SGL, either surgical or non surgical should target the following:

- Treat the *endoluminal* or *exoluminal* complications
- Control the *site* of the dehiscence
- Optimize the *nutritional status* of the patient

The healing of a SGL is defined as a combination of two conditions:

- Disappearance of clinical, biological, endoscopic and radiological features of the leak
- Absence of recurrence

All endoscopic measures and some of the surgical procedures fall short from fulfilling the second component of the previous definition. Consequently, we prefer to use the term remission, as opposed to the healing (i.e., remission plus absence of recurrence).

Endoscopy is still a major tool in the current dogmatic treatment of SGL. In the most optimistic scenarios, it could lead to high rates of control of the SGL. Otherwise, it represents a *bridging measure* that controls the complications, builds-up the nutritional status, allowing upcoming definite surgical treatment.

3   Endoscopy

Over the last years, endoscopic management evolved with the development and improvement of several techniques including self-expanding metal and plastic stents, clips, tissue sealants, suturing systems, and internal drainage devices [16]. The use of endoscopic therapies has gained popularity over time, mainly due to the presumed complexity and high-risk of surgical options, and not to an inherent better outcome per se.

The median interval between implantation and removal of a stent or an endoscopic device could vary between 15 and more than 120 days. The overall proportion of successful control of the SGL could be as high as 90%, but usually averages 70%. However, the overall proportion of stent-related complications including dysphagia, migration, ulcers, stenosis, perforation, or bleeding could reach as high as 25% [17–21]. Many of these techniques require repeated, additional, or combined sessions.

The use of endoscopic therapies demands precise visualization of the internal fistula orifice, which can be a great challenge, especially in *Type A* microperforations. Proper selection of patients seems to be critical for favorable outcomes. Patients qualified to endoscopic therapy should be hemodynamically stable, otherwise surgery should be immediately indicated. Patients with uncontrolled sepsis with peritonitis should be treated surgically. The success of endoscopic therapies in the management of SGL also depends on the defect's size. However, this observation lacks clear evidence in the literature. Other unclear items include the optimal time to start endoscopic therapy, the length of endoscopic treatment, and the weaning chances of control with time.

In recent years, the endoscopic treatment has become more sophisticated using surgical endoscopy and natural orifice transluminal endoscopic surgery (NOTES) techniques with combined, simultaneous, or sequential use of several endoscopic methods. Internal endoscopic drainage (IED) using pigtail drains (PTD) may reduce the need for more invasive, trans-cutaneous, radiology-guided drainage of para-gastric collections.

Our approach to SGL is based on conservative treatment initially unless the septic condition of the patient mandates explorative surgery. Besides antibiotics and artificial nutrition, either enteral or parenteral, our preferred approach is the use of one or more PTDs with or without naso-cavity drainage if the fistula is more than 1 cm diameter. Rarely, an over-the-scope clip is used if the fistula is very recent (i.e., less than 10 days), and large (more than 20-mm diameter). Usually, gastro-pleural SGL should be considered as contra-indications to the insertion of PTDs since the negative intra-thoracic pressure may disturb the flow of fluids from the lumen towards the pleura. Therefore, future research should focus on assessing the effectiveness of complex therapies rather than individual endoscopic methods.

Some believe that the use of endoscopic methods could contribute to reducing the costs associated with reoperation and the patient's hospital stay [16]. However, this does not seem to be easy to prove. Many factors contribute to the overall cost of a SGL, including hospital stay, number of endoscopic attempts, return to normal oral feeding, and resuming of normal activities.

4   Surgery

Surgery of the SGL addresses also the 3 components of the targeted management, including control of *early complications*, the patient's *nutritional status*, and the *leak site* itself.

4.1   Control of Early Complications and Nutritional Status

In case of suspicion of sepsis (i.e., early tachycardia), peritonitis, purulent pleural effusion, or profound abscess (either abdominal, pelvic, or thoracic), prompt laparoscopic surgery is mandatory. Usually, these complications occur within 3 weeks after the primary SG. Consequently, tenacious adhesions should not be a limiting factor. Laparoscopy provides better visualization of the surgical field, permits pressurized, high-volume (i.e., more than 20 liters) lavage, and preserves the patient's abdominal wall allowing smoother post-operative outcome.

During this acute phase, we do not recommend to attempt surgical control of the leak site itself (i.e., suture, patching, resleeve, etc.). This is almost certainly vowed to failure, while hindering residual vascularization and future preservation of the sleeved stomach itself. However, a combination of interventional endoscopy and surgery seems interesting. As an example, inserting a PTD in order to drain the peri-gastric area may obviate the need for trans-abdominal, surgical or radiological drainage. These later options may eventually create an epithelialized tract, synonymous of future delayed complications.

During this early surgery, one must not forget to insert a naso-jejunal, feeding tube, preferentially guided by endoscopy, and reaching beyond the duodeno-jejunal angle. This low-profile tube allows better enteral feeding while generating less adhesions as compared to surgical jejunostomy.

In case of pleural contamination, large trans-thoracic drains should be used. We recommend to avoid PTDs since associated to inversion of intraluminal flow which may entertain thoracic sepsis.

In the acute phase of the SGL, no surgical attempt should be made on correction of associated anomalies (i.e., stenosis at the incisura angularis, fundic stenosis, twist). This is to be addressed later when the patient's condition is stabilized and the nutritional status optimized. However, adding an expandable metallic stent in order to bypass a narrowed stomach may be of some help.

4.2   The Leak Site

If SGL remains patent for more than 3 months despite conservative therapeutic attempts, surgical control of the leak site may be indicated. The 3 most commonly proposed procedures for SGL include Roux en Y Fistulo-Jenunostomy [22, 23] (RYFJ) or Roux en Y Gastro-jejunostomy [24], Roux-en-Y Gastric Bypass [25] (RYGB), and Total Gastrectomy [26] (TG). Other options, either nowadays abandoned or very rarely used, include serosa or omentum patching, re-SG, direct suturing, or the use of sealants.

The choice of the specific surgical approach depends on the team's experience, the specificities of each SGL, and the patient's expectations. The later is very important to take in consideration since many of the patients prefer keeping eventually their "sleeve". For example, a mid gastric SGL could be treated with a RYGB, if the patient accepts the proposition. Moreover, non resectional solutions should be preferred (i.e., RYFJ or RYGB) as compared to more radical solutions (i.e., TG).

4.3   Roux en Y Fistulo-Jejunostomy

In 2007, we performed our first RYFJ, as a salvage procedure for SGL reluctant to non-operative treatment. We defined this procedure as being a RYFJ, including a side-to-side fistula-jejunostomy and a side-to-side jejuno-jejunostomy, respectively. Figure 1 represents the first drawing of the procedure back in 2007 in order to explain it to the first patient.

In 2020, we are about to report the long-term results of the largest ever series of a single surgical treatment of SGL, including 82 patients who had RYFJ. We always attempted primary laparoscopy, even in patients with previous laparotomy.

The RYFJ is standardized in 7 steps including:

- Control of distant adhesions (small bowel/omentum)
- Anterior approach: Left liver lobe separation
- Right lateral approach: Right crux to be reached (*Danger points: spiegelian lobe/retro hepatic inferior vena cava*)
- Left lateral approach: Left crux to be reached (*Danger points: spleen/left pleura/splenic flexure*)
- Posterior approach: Through the lesser sac (*Danger points: pancreas/splenic vein/transverse colon*)

Fig. 1 The first
representation of the RYFJ as
a drawing used to explain the
procedure to the first operated
patient back in 2007

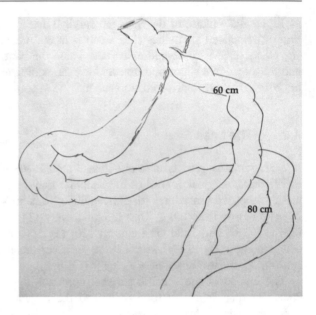

- Revitalization of the leak site: previous endoscopic material removal/
  debridement
- Reconstruction: Hand sewn side-to side Fistulo-Jejunostomy, stapled side-to
  side Jejuno-Jejunostomy.

The left liver lobe is usually intimately affected by the neighboring inflammatory
process (Fig. 2).

Complete dissection of the sleeved stomach is performed. In case of previous
percutaneous drainage, the drain tract could be used as a guide to reach the leak
site, avoiding inadvertent tissue damage. It is recommended to preferentially use
previously non dissected planes, including the pars flaccida, the right crux, and the
lesser sac (Fig. 3).

Every effort should be made in order to avoid damaging the remaining gastric blood supply (i.e., the right and left gastric arteries). Complete dissection of
the esophagogastric junction with some mobilization of the lower third of the
esophagus is mandatory (Fig. 4). This enables, tension-free anastomosis between
the leak site and the jejunum, especially in very high fistulas. In case of associated diaphragmatic defects, closure with interrupted non absorbable sutures is
recommended.

Debridement of the fistula margins is an important step in order to perform the
fistula-jejunostomy on a well vascularized, healthy tissue (Fig. 5).

The jejunum is then divided 60–80 cm from the Treitz angle and mobilized
through the transverse mesocolon. Side to side, fistulo-jejunostomy is performed
using absorbable running sutures (Fig. 6). Stapled, side-to-side jejunojejunostomy
is the performed 60 cm more distally.

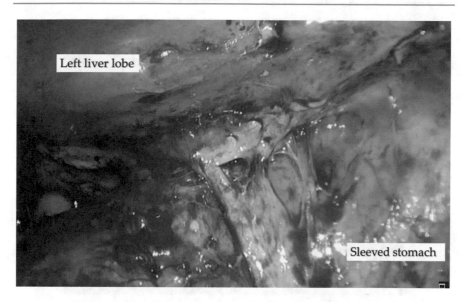

Fig. 2 Anterior approach to the RYFJ: Adhesions between the left liver lobe and the sleeved stomach are divided

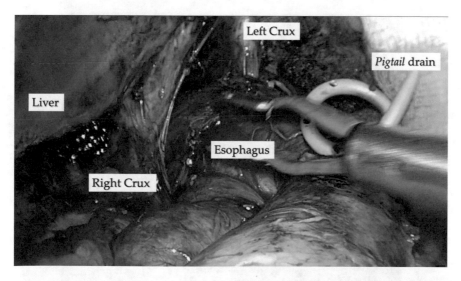

Fig. 3 Mobilization of the esophagogastric junction: Both the left and the right arms of the diaphragmatic crura are identifible as well as a previously inserted pigtail drain (PTD)

It is not mandatory to close the mesocolon defect around the Roux limb. Percutaneous closed drainage of the hiatal area is optional. No naso-gastric tube is required.

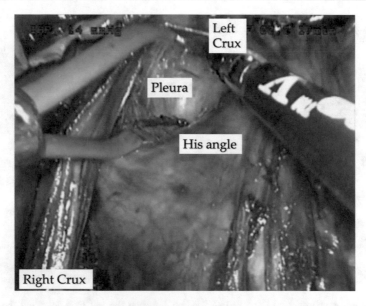

Fig. 4 Mobilization of the esophagogastric junction: The Angle of His is to be detached from the left arm of the crura while making sure the left pleura is not teared

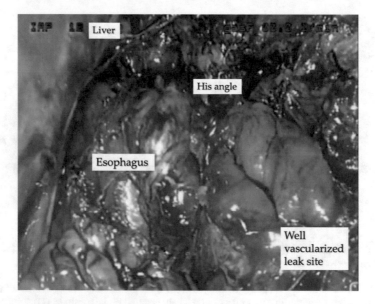

Fig. 5 The fistula site is now completely debrided with well-vascularized, healthy edges, ready to be anastomosed to the jejunum

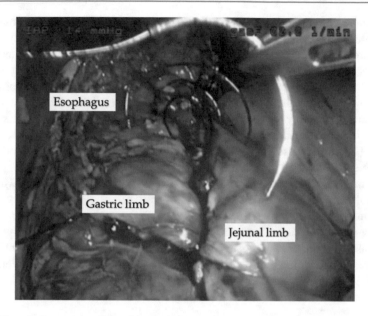

Fig. 6 The closing stages of the side-to-side fistulo-jejunostomy using an absorbable runing suture

In the postoperative period, patients had control CT scan with oral contrast fluid at POD3 before resuming oral intake.

Between January 2007 and December 2018, we managed 221 patients with SGL. Remission is defined as the absence of clinical or radiological expression of the SGL site itself or by its consequences (i.e., collection, extravasation, air bubbles). Healing is nothing by a definite remission (i.e., apparent remission + absence of recurrence). We made this distinction after noticing that apparently "healed" SGL may recur even many years later (i.e., pregnancy, pancreatitis, malnutrition, chronic illness) [27]. We could easily understand the situation if we compare a SGL to type 2 diabetes mellitus. Its remission after bariatric surgery and weight loss must not be confound with healing.

Of the initial 221 patients, 82 (37.1%) underwent eventually RYFJ. The median age of SGL in the entire population of patients presenting for RYFJ was 5 months (range, 0–133). The longest interval between the primary SG and the declaration of the SGL (during a pregnancy) was more than 10 years. In the subgroup of patients who presented with less than 3-months SGL, the median interval was 16 days (range, 1–88).

Endoscopic treatment was attempted in almost all of the patients, including stenting, IED, clips, glue, sponge, or septotomy. The success rate of the first attempt at endoscopic treatment was 66.4%. In patients with more than one cycle of endoscopic treatment, the remission rate rose eventually to 79.1%.

Laparoscopy was attempted in 96.4% of the patients, while 3 patients had open surgery (i.e., the first 3 patients of the series in 2007). Secondary conversion to laparotomy occurred in only 2 patients (2.5%). The causes of conversion were poor exposure and bleeding in both cases. The left lobe of the liver was the major cause of poor exposure. The splenic vessels were the most common cause of bleeding. The mean operative time was 200 minutes (100–450). Besides two limited bleedings, no major operative incident was encountered. No splenectomy had to be performed.

The mortality rate was nil. The post-operative rate of complications was 6.1% with Only 2 patients had persistent post operative leak (24%). Both eventually healed in less than 10 days with conservative management.

Long-term analysis of this series revealed that the 10-years control rate of the SGL was 100% either endoscopic wise (Fig. 7) or as defined by radiology (Fig. 8).

Interestingly, the long-term analysis of the results revealed that the patients who had RYFJ obtained better long-term weight loss results as compared to those who had primary SG with no complications (Fig. 9).

4.4 Literature Review of the Remaining Surgical Options

Excluding our experience, less than 20 studies in the literature addressed series with more than 5 patients who had some form of surgical treatment for patients with SGL [28]. Almost 60% of these reported patients who had TG (inreality, these were mainly open Total Degastro-Gastrectomy with Roux en Y Eso-Jejunal anastomosis). Surprisingly, nearly 10% of authors performed Roux En Y Gastric Bypass, even for high SGL.

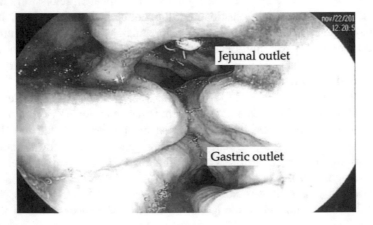

Fig. 7 Illustrative endoscopic endoscopic view of the esophagogastirc junction in a patient who had previous RYFJ, showing a double oulet pattern (i.e., jejunal and gastric) with no residual fistula

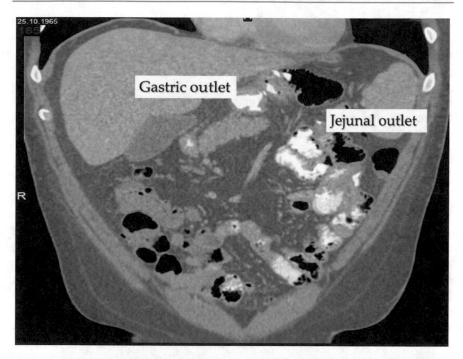

Fig. 8 Illustrative radiological, CT, coronal view of the upper abdomen in a patient who had previous RYFJ, showing a double oulet pattern (i.e., jejunal and gastroduodenal) with no residual fistula

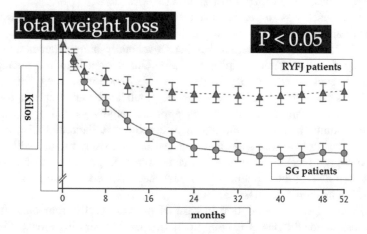

Fig. 9 5-year, total weight loss pattern in patients who had RYFJ for leak after SG as compared to matched patients who had non-complicated SG at the same period

The laparoscopic approach succeeded in less than 70% of cases with a conversion rate of 6.4% [28]. The most common complication reported for all types of definitive reconstructive surgeries was another leak (15%), including 37.5% following RYGB, 30% other forms of fistula-jejunostomy, and 8% after TG. The healing time for a leak following definitive reconstructive surgeries varied between 10 and 165 days. Other complications were reported in 12.3% of patients, including included intra-abdominal abscesses, wound infection, pulmonary embolism, intestinal obstruction, and miscellaneous other entities.

Mortality was reported in 1% of cases. However, we believe this is under-estimated since patients may die from complications linked to the SGL before surgery or more than 30 days after surgery, without being accounted for in the overall rate.

4.5 Discussion of the Surgical Approach

SGL are more likely to occur in SG patients with distal stenosis, resulting in difficulties in gastric emptying [29]. High intraluminal pressure and low compliance of the gastric tube may be entertaining causes of SGL [30]. This is why RYFJ seems to be a pathophysiologically relevant solution since it bypasses both difficulties (i.e., gastric lack of compliance and endo-luminal high pressure). Additionally, RYFJ is a surgically conservative option requiring no organ removal (as compared to TG) while not leaving in situ the leak site (as compared to the majority of RYGBs). However, additional factors are most probably implicated in the occurrence of SGL, including impaired suture line healing, poor blood flow, infection, and poor oxygenation with subsequent ischemia. All of these items are addressed either by the preoperative optimization of the patient's nutritional status or the peroperative surgical debridement during the RYFJ.

Our experience was forged from a heterogeneous panel of techniques used in SG since patients came from 8 different countries with as many different techniques. However, the management has been eventually homogeneous and implemented by the same multidisciplinary team. Our approach to the management of SGL has evolved after nearly 15 years of experience with this technique. Our first SG was performed in 2002 as a part of a duodenal switch and in 2004 as a stand-alone procedure. Multidisciplinary approach is always indicated with decisions taken jointly by the surgeon, the gastroenterologist, the radiologist, the nutritionist, and the critical care specialist. The patient is closely monitored by a team of psychologists specialized in obesity management. Depression and suicide ideas are common among these patients who have been treated, for some of them, for years with long cumulated hospital stays.

RYGB could still be an option in case of possible gastric remnant. However, limitations include the risk of leaving the fistula tract in very high localization and the metabolic consequences of the procedure. Moreover, numerous patients are reluctant to the idea of having a RYGB. TG is associated to a relatively high risk of complications related to both the esophagojejunal anastomosis and the duodenal stump. Moreover, the long term nutritional consequences are cumbersome with malnutrition, weight loss, anemia and the need to readjust the volume and frequencies of meals.

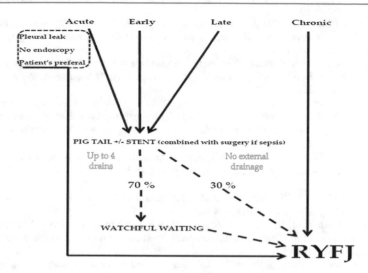

Fig. 10 A proposed algorithm for the management of leak after SG

We believe that RYFJ is the most adequate option since it controls the fistula site in all cases, may preserve the chance of maintaining the SG preferential pathway in the future and avoid the complications of an anastomosis performed on an ill-vascularized esophagus. The use of a Roux limb type for the anastomosis aims to allow less tension on the gastrojejunal anastomosis while avoiding the risk of biliary reflux. Finally, our recent results on long term control of weight loss in patients with RYFJ are very encouraging.

5   Conclusion

In conclusion, we believe that RYFJ is a safe and confirmed treatment for patients with persistent SGL. It may even be used as a first option in some patients with acute SGL.

Figure 10 summarizes our algorithm of management of SGL.

References

1. Varela JE, Nguyen NT. Laparoscopic sleeve gastrectomy leads the US utilization of bariatric surgery at academic medical centers. Surg Obes Relat Dis. 2015;11:987–90.
2. International Federation for the Surgery of Obesity and Metabolic Disorders website; https://www.ifso.com/sleeve-gastrectomy/.
3. Gagner M, Kemmeter P. Comparison of laparoscopic sleeve gastrectomy leak rates in five staple-line reinforcement options: a systematic review. Surg Endosc. 2020;34:396–407.

4. Cesana G, Cioffi S, Giorgia R, et al. Proximal leakage after laparoscopic sleeve gastrectomy: an analysis of preoperative and operative predictors on 1738 consecutive procedures. Obes Surg. 2018;28:627–35.

5. D'Ugo S, Gentileschi P, Benavoli D, et al. Comparative use of different techniques for leak and bleeding prevention during laparoscopic sleeve gastrectomy: a multicenter study. Surg Obes Relat Dis. 2014;10:450–4.

6. Berger ER, Clements RH, Morton JM, et al. The impact of different surgical techniques on outcomes in laparoscopic sleeve gastrectomies: the first report from the metabolic and bariatric surgery accreditation and quality improvement program (MBSAQIP). Ann Surg. 2016;264:464–73.

7. Varban OA, Sheetz KH, Cassidy RB, et al. Evaluating the effect of operative technique on leaks after laparoscopic sleeve gastrectomy: a case-control study. Surg Obes Relat Dis. 2017;13:560–7.

8. Birkmeyer JD, Finks JF, O'Reilly A, et al. Surgical skill and complication rates after bariatric surgery. N Engl J Med. 2013;369:1434–42.

9. Hany M, Ibrahim M. Comparison between stable line reinforcement by barbed suture and non-reinforcement in sleeve gastrectomy: a randomized prospective controlled study. Obes Surg. 2018;28:2157–64.

10. Wang H, Lu J, JFeng J, Z Wang Z. Staple line oversewing during laparoscopic sleeve gastrectomy. Ann R Coll Surg Engl. 2017;99:509–14.

11. Hughes D, Hughes I, Khanna A. Management of staple line leaks following sleeve gastrectomy: a systemic review. Obes Surg. 2019;29:2759–72.

12. Nedelcu M, Manos T, Gagner M, Eddbali I, Ahmed A, Noel P. Cost analysis of leak after sleeve gastrectomy. Surg Endosc. 2017;31:4446–50.

13. Peel AL, Taylor EW. Proposed definitions for the audit of 26 postopérative infections: a discussion paper. Surgical Infection Study Group. Ann R Coll Surg Engl. 1991;73:385–8.

14. Csendes A, Burdiles P, Burgos AM, Maluenda F, Diaz JC. Conservative management of anastomotic leaks after 557 open gastric bypasses. Obes Surg. 2005;15:1252–6.

15. Welsch T, von Frankenberg M, Schmidt J, Büchler MW. Diagnosis and definition of anastomotic leakage from the surgeon's perspective. Chirurg. 2011;82:48–55.

16. Rogalski P, Swidnicka-Siergiejko A, Wasielica-Berger J, et al. Endoscopic management of leaks and fistulas after bariatric surgery: a systematic review and meta-analysis. Surg Endosc. 2020. https://doi.org/10.1007/s00464-020-07471-1. Epub ahead of print. PMID: 32107632.

17. Chahine E, D'Alessandro A, Elhajjam M, et al. Massive gastrointestinal bleeding due to splenic artery erosion by a pigtail drain in a post sleeve gastrectomy leak: a case report. Obes Surg. 2019;29:1653–6.

18. Siddique I, Alazmi W, Al-Sabah SK. Endoscopic internal drainage by double pigtail stents in the management of laparoscopic sleeve gastrectomy leaks. Surg Obes Relat Dis. 2020. https://doi.org/10.1016/j.soard.2020.03.028.

19. El Kary N, Chahine E, Moryoussef F, et al. Esophageal stricture due to a self-expandable metal stent (SEMS) placement for post sleeve gastrectomy leak: a case report. Obes Surg. 2019;29:1943–5.

20. Puli SR, Spofford IS, Thompson CC. Use of self-expandable stents in the treatment of bariatric surgery leaks: a systematic review and meta-analysis. Gastrointest Endosc. 2012;75:287–93.

21. Okazaki O, Bernardo WM, Brunaldi VO, et al. Efficacy and safety of stents in the treatment of fistula after bariatric surgery: a systematic review and meta-analysis. Obes Surg. 2018;28:1788–96.

22. Chouillard E, Younan A, Alkandari M, et al. Roux-en-Y Fistulo-Jejunostomy as a salvage procedure in patients with post-sleeve gastrectomy fistula: mid-term results. Surg Endosc. 2016;304200–4.

23. Chouillard E, Chahine E, Schoucair N, et al. Roux-En-Y Fistulo-Jejunostomy as a salvage procedure in patients with post-sleeve gastrectomy fistula. Surg Endosc. 2014;28:1954–60.

24. Chouillard E, Chahine E, D'Alessandro A, Vitte RL, Gumbs A, Kassir R. Roux-en-Y Gastro-Jejunostomy for complex leak after the "Nissen" variant of sleeve gastrectomy. Obes Surg. 2020. https://doi.org/10.1007/s11695-020-04731-w.
25. Chour M, Alami RS, Sleilaty F, Wakim R. The early use of Roux limb as surgical treatment for proximal postsleeve gastrectomy leaks. Surg Obes Relat Dis. 2014;10:106–10.
26. Bruzzi M, Douard R, Voron T, Berger A, Zinzindohoue F, Chevallier JM. Open total gastrectomy with Roux-en-Y reconstruction for a chronic fistula after sleeve gastrectomy. Surg Obes Relat Dis. 2016;12:1803–8.
27. Zanotti D, Elkalaawy M, Mohammadi B, Hashemi M, Jenkinson A, Adamo M. Gastro-cutaneous fistula 4 years after a fully resolved staple line leak in sleeve gastrectomy. J Surg Case Rep. 2015;12:rjv152. https://doi.org/10.1093/jscr/rjv152. PMID: 26654903; PMCID: PMC4674533.
28. Nedelcu M, Danan M, Noel P, Gagner M, Nedelcu A, Carandina S. Surgical management for chronic leak following sleeve gastrectomy: review of literature. Surg Obes Relat Dis. 2019;15:1844–9.
29. Yehoshua RT, Eidelman LA, Stein M, et al. Laparoscopic sleeve gastrectomy–volume and pressure assessment. Obes Surg. 2008;18:1083–8.
30. Baltasar A, Bou R, Bengochea M, Serra C, Cipagauta L. Use of a Roux Limb to correct esophagogastric junction fistulas after sleeve gastrectomy. Obes Surg. 2007;17:1408–10.

How to Manage Sleeve Complications Through Endoscopy: Strictures

Thomas R. McCarty⊙ and Christopher C. Thompson⊙

1   Introduction

As the total number of individuals within the United States and worldwide with obesity has continued to increase over the past several decades, so too has the use of bariatric surgery [1–3]. As of 2013, laparoscopic sleeve gastrectomy has become the most common type of bariatric surgery performed in the United States, accounting for more than 50% of all bariatric procedures at this time [4–7]. Although this increase in the number of laparoscopic sleeve gastrectomy procedures reflects several advantages over alternative bariatric surgeries, namely a reduced number of complications with lower morbidity compared to traditional Roux-en-Y gastric bypass, sleeve-related leaks, de novo gastroesophageal reflux disease (GERD), and sleeve-associated stenosis may occur [8–10]. In this review, we will discuss proper identification, classification, and endoscopic management of sleeve stenosis.

2   Timing, Classification, and Rate of Sleeve Stenosis

While sleeve gastrectomy-related leaks and GERD typically occur early and late in the post-operative course, respectively, sleeve stenosis and stricture formation may occur are any time post-surgery. After sleeve leaks, stenosis is the most

T. R. McCarty · C. C. Thompson (✉)
Brigham and Women's Hospital, Boston, USA
e-mail: CCTHOMPSON@bwh.harvard.edu

T. R. McCarty
e-mail: trmccarty@bwh.harvard.edu

© The Editor(s) (if applicable) and The Author(s), under exclusive license to Springer Nature Switzerland AG 2021
S. Al-Sabah et al. (eds.), *Laparoscopic Sleeve Gastrectomy*,
https://doi.org/10.1007/978-3-030-57373-7_45

common complication associated with laparoscopic sleeve gastrectomy. Sleeve stenosis may occur early in the post-operative course (even days after the surgery) or years post-sleeve gastrectomy [8, 11]. Broadly speaking, laparoscopic sleeve gastrectomy associated stenosis may be classically classified into two categories: acute and chronic [12]. Acute stenoses may be a result by mucosal edema and acute angulation of the sleeve while chronic stenoses are considered to be related to ischemia of the pouch and angulation or retraction due to fibrosis or scarring. Current literature estimates that sleeve gastrectomy associated strictures occur in 0.2–4.0% of laparoscopic sleeve operations [8, 13–15]. Despite this number being as high as 4%, typically less than 1% of stenoses require endoscopic revision or surgical reintervention [16].

3   Mechanisms, Location, and Classification of Stricture

Sleeve stenosis typically develops as a result of luminal narrowing or torsional scarring—Fig. 1 [12]. Although multiple etiologies and mechanisms exist to potentially explain stricture formation, risk factors for stricture formation are

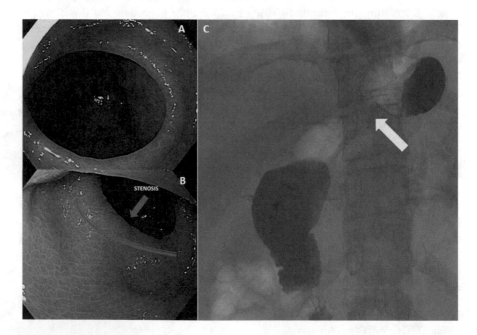

Fig. 1 a and **b** Endoscopic images of sleeve stenosis at the level of the incisuria angularis **c** Upper gastrointestinal series image demonstrating a stricture after laparoscopic sleeve gastrectomy. Permission obtained from de Moura DTH, Jirapinyo P, Aihara H, Thompson CC. Endoscopic tunneled stricturotomy in the treatment of stenosis after sleeve gastrectomy. VideoGIE. 2019;4(2):68–71

mainly related to the surgical technique—most commonly improper alignment of the staple line along the greater curvature is believed to be the main driver of sleeve stenosis [17, 18]. Alternative mechanisms to explain sleeve stenosis include narrowing of the gastric sleeve as a result of using thin, small bougies, over-aggressive imbrication of the staple-line, stapling too close to the bougie, or unintentional progressive rotation of the staple-line in an anterior to posterior fashion, potentially causing a functional helix-like stenosis of the sleeve [10, 18–20].

Although these mechanisms are mostly structural in nature, functional sleeve stenosis as a result of axis deviation has also been demonstrated. These type of functional sleeve stenoses develop as a result of edema or hematomas at the staple line, and typically do not require treatment and resolve spontaneously—unlike mechanical etiologies. The most common location for stricture formation includes the incisura angularis or more proximally at the gastroesophageal junction [20, 21]. Previous data by Deslauriers and others has shown that proximal strictures may have a more symmetric appearance, potentially due to mechanical narrowing [22]. Distal stenoses, which are classically located at the incisura angularis, are typically due to axial deviation with a twisting-like stricture formation and may be more difficult to treat endoscopically.

4   Signs and Symptoms

It is important to first underscore that there are two types of stenosis following sleeve gastrectomy: a clinical (symptomatic) and subclinical (asymptomatic) stenosis [23]. Clinical or symptomatic stenosis is by far the most relevant to clinicians as it warrants timely investigation and treatment. Classic symptoms of sleeve stenosis include nausea, vomiting, abdominal pain, and typically dysphagia. These manifestations present with obstructive symptoms and inability to tolerate oral intake though severity of symptoms largely depends upon the degree of sleeve narrowing. Given these non-specific symptoms, it is also critical to evaluate for potential motility disorders as well as other causes.

5   Diagnosis and Management

Although an upper gastrointestinal series with fluoroscopy may be used to confirm the diagnosis of sleeve stenosis, endoscopic management provides an ideal first diagnostic and therapeutic approach for short-segment sleeve stenoses. Additionally, while upper gastrointestinal series may be selected for some patients, it remains vital to underscore these tests may miss leaks and to consider cross-sectional imaging if a high clinical suspicion remains. While current sleeve stenosis treatments range from endoscopic treatment and revisional surgical interventions, seromyotomy, or conversion to Roux-en-Y gastric bypass, endoscopic management remains a first-line strategy when conservative management fails. This is mostly due to high initial success rates with balloon or pneumatic dilation as well as providing the least minimally invasive approach [24]. Given the excellent safety profile of endoscopy, an approach using balloon dilation has emerged as a promising initial treatment option and alternative to revisional surgery with laparoscopic seromyotomy [19, 25]. A summary table for sleeve stenosis is highlighted in Table 1.

6   Bougie Dilation

At present, there is limited evidence to recommend endoscopic bougienage as a first-line strategy for the treatment of short-segment sleeve stenosis. Published data is largely limited to a small case series by Burgos et al., where the authors describe successful dilation with various sized Savary bougies [24]. In this series, a single endoscopic dilation with a Savary 48F bougie was successful at improving a sleeve-related stricture at the incisura angularis that developed 7 months post-operatively. While this patient with a late occurring stenosis remained asymptomatic at follow-up 11 months post-dilation, another patient included in this study developed a sleeve leak and distal stenosis 2 weeks post-surgery and required progressive bougienage (using Savary dilators 45F, 51F, and 54F). Another patient in this study developed stenosis at the middle-third portion of the sleeve within the first month following the surgery and required Savary dilation with a 36F bougie. The final patient included in this case series developed an early stricture at the incisura angularis within 2 weeks of the surgery; however, did not respond to multiple endoscopic dilations with the Savary bougie. Based on this one series, it is impossible to draw strong conclusions regarding a role for Savary dilation of sleeve stenosis. Additionally, concerns have been raised regarding the blind dilation of early sleeve stenosis with a Savary dilator, especially within the first 2 weeks of post-operation, as the wound is still healing and the risk of perforation is high [23]. Given the paradigm shift towards controlled radial expansion (CRE) balloons for the treatment of esophageal stenosis, it is likely balloon dilation will be a much more common first-line treatment for sleeve stenosis.

7   Controlled Radial Expansion (CRE) Balloon and Pneumatic Dilation

In a recent systematic review by Brunaldi and colleagues, 9 studies have evaluated the role of CRE balloon dilation in the management of sleeve stenosis [17]. Among these 9 studies, including 129 cases, CRE balloon dilation was successful for 108 cases (non-pooled success rate of 83.7%). Of note, most of these studies were small in number and case series, potentially allowing for selection bias. A representative image of CRE balloon dilation of sleeve stenosis is shown in Fig. 2. In this same systematic review, the success rate for studies evaluating pneumatic dilation was reported to be 88.7%—including 7 studies with 115 patients [17]. In another recent meta-analysis by Chang et al. data was combined for multiple

Table 1 Summary table for endoscopic management of stenosis following sleeve gastrectomy

Complication of sleeve gastrectomy	Classic symptom presentation	Time course to develop	Diagnosis	Treatment strategy
Stenosis	Dysphagia; nausea/vomiting; abdominal pain	Anytime (early and late development)	Fluoroscopy, endoscopy, or cross-sectional imaging	Endoscopic balloon or pneumatic dilation; consider SEMS placement or surgical intervention if failure

Adapted from: Schulman AR, Thompson CC. Complications of Bariatric Surgery: What You Can Expect to See in Your GI Practice. Am J Gastroenterol 2017;112:1640–55

Fig. 2 Successful dilation of sleeve gastrectomy stricture using a through-the-scope (TTS) using a controlled radial expansion (CRE) balloon

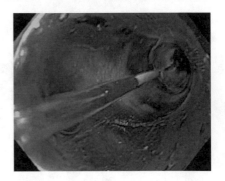

types of balloon dilators (including CRE and Rigiflex II pneumatic dilation balloons) [19]. This study provided key data including an overall pooled success rate of 76%. More importantly, these authors also stratified success rates for sleeve stenosis by stricture location. Proximal strictures were successfully dilated with endoscopic balloon dilators in 90% of cases while dilation was only effective in 70% of cases for distal stenoses. Furthermore, stratification by early and late stenosis was also performed for studies reporting these characteristics and demonstrated success rates of 59% and 61%, respectively. Additionally, on meta-regression analyses, balloon type (CRE versus pneumatic) as well as balloon size, did not affect rates of clinical success [19]. Step-by-step instructions for use of balloon dilation is highlighted in Fig. 3. Overall, for severe stenoses, we recommend a graded or step-up approach, involving first treatment with CRE balloon dilation, and then consideration for pneumatic dilation for refractory strictures.

8 Self-Expanding Metal Stent (SEMS) Placement

For patients that fail to respond to endoscopic balloon dilation, placement of a self-expanding metal stent (SEMS) may also be a viable option for many. This may be especially helpful in the setting of concomitant sleeve leak and offers a safe and effective alternative, obviating the need for repeat surgical intervention. While an effective treatment for leaks, these stents should be removed after 6–8 weeks as stent migration has been noted to occur in up to 15% of cases [26]. Importantly, use of a dumbbell shaped, lumen apposing metal stent (LAMS) with a bi-flanged design may reduce the migration rate [10, 27]. Although limited literature exists from cases series, the non-pooled success rate of SEMS as a first-line strategy for the management of sleeve stenosis is 95.5% [17]. When used after balloon dilation for refractory strictures, SEMS placement has a success rate of approximately 78% to 83%, though a significant risk of migration has been reported [17, 19]. Reported adverse events and stent migration with SEMS placement have ranged widely from 5% to >50% in some studies [17, 19, 28]. Although suturing of the stent in place has been described, similar to what is performed for

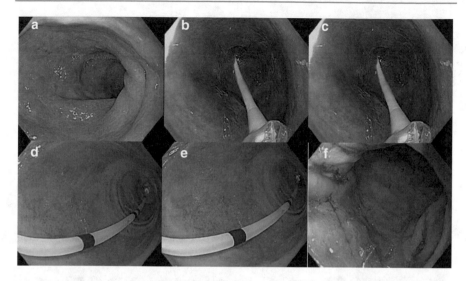

Fig. 3 In this case, **a** sleeve stenosis was noted at the incisura angularis. Next, a Savary guide-wire was placed deep in the second portion of the duodenum, then the scope was exchanged over the wire. **b** and **c** The pneumatic balloon was advanced over the wire and the endoscope was advanced adjacent to the balloon. **d** Dilation with a 40 mm pneumatic balloon was then performed under fluoroscopic and endoscopic guidance. The balloon was inflated to 18 PSI with complete effacement of the balloon waist. **e** Pressure was held for 5 minutes before balloon deflation and withdrawal. **f** Final appearance of incisura angularis post-sleeve dilation

some esophageal stents, the location of stenosis as well as the limited maneuverability within the sleeve may make this challenging for the endoscopist [29]. Figure 4 demonstrates successful placement of a SEMS on endoscopic and fluoroscopic imaging [30]. We advocate SEMS placement only in the setting of a severe stricture refractory to first-line balloon dilation or in the setting of a distal stenosis with length >3 cm. Most importantly, this should ideally be performed in centers with significant expertise and after consultation with the patient and surgical colleagues.

9 Alternative Endoscopic Treatments for Sleeve Stenosis

Several other novel or alternative endoscopic treatments have been described in the literature to date. It should be noted, however, that these are limited to case reports and small case series and likely only possible at centers with significant expertise. As such, we will highlight a few of these novel strategies but do not feel they should be rapidly adopted in clinical practice at this time. One such treatment that our group has previously described includes use of a novel endoscopic tunneled stricturotomy technique [12]. The steps involved for this technique include submucosal injection proximal to the area of the stricture followed by submucosal

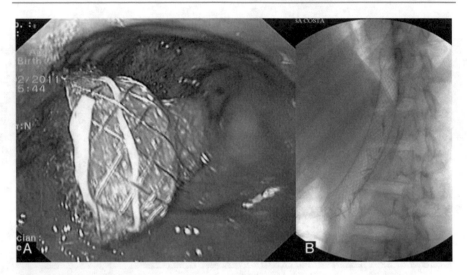

Fig. 4 Placement of a fully covered self-expandable metal stent (SEMS) for sleeve stenosis. **a** Endoscopic image. **b** Fluoroscopic image. Images and permission obtained from Costa MN, Capela T, Seves I, Ribeiro R, Rio-Tinto R. Endoscopic Treatment of Early Gastric Obstruction After Sleeve Gastrectomy: Report of Two Cases. GE Port J Gastroenterol. 2016;23(1):46–9

tunneling to disrupt the muscle layer and perform stricturotomy, and then closure—Fig. 5 [12]. In another case report by the Hopkins group, led by Vivek Kumbhari, these authors described successful gastric peroral endoscopic myotomy (G-POEM) for the treatment of sleeve stenosis [31]. While more recently developed as a treatment for delayed gastric emptying, G-POEM was performed after the patient had previously not responded to endoscopic balloon dilation—Fig. 6 [31]. The procedure was highly successful with with resolution of the tortuosity. While these case reports of novel techniques and treatments demonstrate these methods to be feasible and may provide an alternative for patients unable to undergo or refractory to balloon dilation and not amenable to surgical revision, additional studies are needed to measure their efficacy and safety.

10   Strategies for Endoscopic Success

Currently, there are no data driven or consensus guidelines to suggest which balloon type or methodology offers the best outcomes for the endoscopic management of sleeve stenosis. Additionally, there are a lack of randomized trials or well-designed case-controlled studies to compare balloon versus pneumatic dilation as well as to other treatment modalities such as seromyotomy. Ultimately, these types of studies, along with cost-effectiveness analyses, are needed to guide future therapy and identify optimal algorithms to ensure the best patient care.

Despite the current lack of evidence, the meta-analysis by Chang and colleagues perhaps provides the best current estimate or strategy for adoption to clinical practice [19]. Endoscopic balloon dilation was more successful for proximal

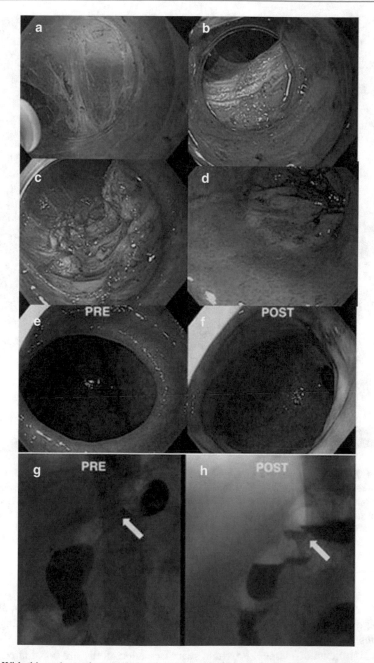

Fig. 5 With this endoscopic tunneled stricturotomy technique, first submucosal injection is performed approximately 3 to 5 cm proximal the area of stenosis. **a** Next, submucosal tunneling dissection is performed, **b** with careful attention to identify muscle fibers during submucosal tunneling. **c** Demonstrates submucosal tunneled stricturotomy with **d** final appearance after endoscopic suturing to close the defect. **e** and **f** Endoscopic and **g** and **h** fluoroscopic images are shown to illustrate the area of stenosis pre- and post-intervention. Permission obtained from de Moura DTH, Jirapinyo P, Aihara H, Thompson CC. Endoscopic tunneled stricturotomy in the treatment of stenosis after sleeve gastrectomy. VideoGIE. 2019;4(2):68–71

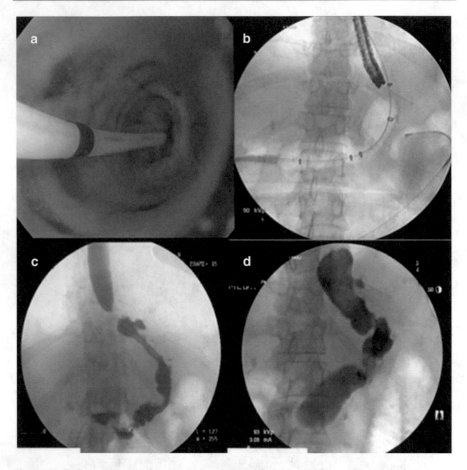

Fig. 6 **a** Balloon dilation image demonstrating sleeve stenosis—entire stomach becomes ischemic as opposed to simply seeing a single ring-like ischemic area (high risk of perforation). **b** Fluoroscopic image highlights sleeve stricture. **c** Upper gastrointestinal series demonstrating stenosis at the incisura angularis. **d** Upper gastrointestinal series demonstrating improved stricture after gastric peroral endoscopic myotomy (G-POEM) has been performed. Permission obtained from Farha J, Fayad L, Kadhim A, Simsek C, Badurdeen DS, Ichkhanian Y, et al. Gastric Per-Oral Endoscopic Myotomy (G-POEM) for the Treatment of Gastric Stenosis Post-Laparoscopic Sleeve Gastrectomy (LSG). Obes Surg. 2019;29(7):2350–4

stenoses when compared to more distal strictures; however, this was not statistically significant (90% versus 70%; P=0.28). Due to limited study reporting (only 3 studies including a total of 68 patients), this may be underpowered to detect a true or significant difference. Proximal strictures anecdotally are considered easier to treat given improved visibility, ease of maneuverability, and potential underlying pathophysiology of stricture formation.

Based upon these results, Chang and colleagues (including an author of this review) have proposed an algorithm for endoscopic management of sleeve stenosis—Fig. 7. This strategy recommends CRE balloon dilation as a first-line strategy for all proximal strictures as well as short (defined as <3 cm) distal stenoses. For long strictures in the distal sleeve, we recommend starting with pneumatic dilation at 30 mm. From there, the pneumatic dilation balloon may be progressively increased and reattempted at a maximum 40 mm for a total of 3 times prior to consideration of SEMS placement or surgical reintervention. It should be emphasized that these recommendations do not relate to the immediate post-operative period where fresh staple lines may have a high risk of perforation.

11 Conclusions

In summary, we have reviewed the pathophysiology and characteristics of sleeve stenosis as well as discussed how to endoscopically manage stricture complications from laparoscopic sleeve gastrectomy. It remains critical for the endoscopist to be in close communication with the patient and surgical colleagues, understand bariatric surgery anatomy, and evaluate for alternative complications such as leaks or GERD during the endoscopic examination. While balloon dilation, either via

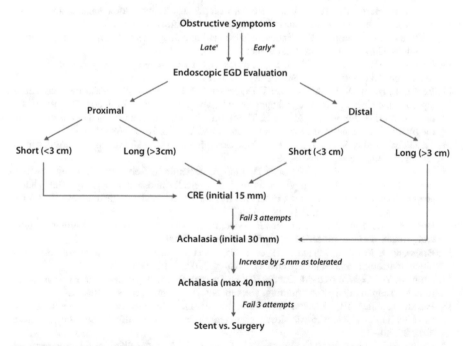

Fig. 7 Proposed algorithm for endoscopic management of sleeve stenosis Permission obtained from Chang SH, Popov VB, Thompson CC. Endoscopic balloon dilation for treatment of sleeve gastrectomy stenosis: a systematic review and meta-analysis. Gastrointest Endosc. 2020;91(5):989–1002 e4

CRE balloon dilation or pneumatic dilation, remains a first-line strategy based upon stricture length and location, it is critical to individualize treatment based on timing of stenosis formation, mechanism of stricture formation, patient reported symptoms, and ability to achieve successful dilation.

References

1. Collaborators GBDO, Afshin A, Forouzanfar MH, et al. Health effects of overweight and obesity in 195 countries over 25 years. N Engl J Med. 2017;377:13–27.
2. Obesity and Overweight. World Health Organization. Available from: https://www.who.int/news-room/fact-sheets/detail/obesity-and-overweight. Accessed: 16 April 2020.
3. Caballero B. The global epidemic of obesity: an overview. Epidemiol Rev. 2007;29:1–5.
4. Bariatric Surgery Procedures. American Society for Metabolic and Bariatric Surgery (ASMBS). Available at: https://asmbs.org/patients/bariatric-surgery-procedures. Accessed 3 May 2020.
5. Gagner M, Hutchinson C, Rosenthal R. Fifth international consensus conference: current status of sleeve gastrectomy. Surg Obes Relat Dis. 2016;12:750–6.
6. Varela JE, Nguyen NT. Laparoscopic sleeve gastrectomy leads the U.S. utilization of bariatric surgery at academic medical centers. Surg Obes Relat Dis. 2015;11:987–90.
7. Estimate of Bariatric Surgery Numbers. American Society for Metabolic and Bariatric Surgery (ASMBS). https://asmbs.org/resources/estimate-of-bariatric-surgery-numbers. Accessed 19 April 2020.
8. Zundel N, Hernandez JD, Galvao Neto M, Campos J. Strictures after laparoscopic sleeve gastrectomy. Surg Laparosc Endosc Percutan Tech. 2010;20:154–8.
9. Schulman AR, Thompson CC. Endoscopic evaluation/management of bariatric surgery complications. Curr Treat Options Gastroenterol. 2017a;15:701–16.
10. Schulman AR, Thompson CC. Complications of bariatric surgery: what you can expect to see in your GI practice. Am J Gastroenterol. 2017b;112:1640–55.
11. Rebibo L, Hakim S, Dhahri A, Yzet T, Delcenserie R, Regimbeau JM. Gastric stenosis after laparoscopic sleeve gastrectomy: diagnosis and management. Obes Surg. 2016;26:995–1001.
12. de Moura DTH, Jirapinyo P, Aihara H, Thompson CC. Endoscopic tunneled stricturotomy in the treatment of stenosis after sleeve gastrectomy. VideoGIE. 2019;4:68–71.
13. Frezza EE, Reddy S, Gee LL, Wachtel MS. Complications after sleeve gastrectomy for morbid obesity. Obes Surg. 2009;19:684–7.
14. Javanainen M, Penttila A, Mustonen H, Juuti A, Scheinin T, Leivonen M. A retrospective 2-year follow-up of late complications treated surgically and endoscopically after laparoscopic Roux-en-Y gastric bypass (LRYGB) and laparoscopic sleeve gastrectomy (LSG) for morbid obesity. Obes Surg. 2018;28:1055–62.
15. Brethauer SA, Hammel JP, Schauer PR. Systematic review of sleeve gastrectomy as staging and primary bariatric procedure. Surg Obes Relat Dis. 2009;5:469–75.
16. Braghetto I, Korn O, Valladares H, et al. Laparoscopic sleeve gastrectomy: surgical technique, indications and clinical results. Obes Surg. 2007;17:1442–50.
17. Brunaldi VO, Galvao Neto M, Zundel N, Abu Dayyeh BK. Isolated sleeve gastrectomy stricture: a systematic review on reporting, workup, and treatment. Surg Obes Relat Dis. 2020.
18. Parikh A, Alley JB, Peterson RM, et al. Management options for symptomatic stenosis after laparoscopic vertical sleeve gastrectomy in the morbidly obese. Surg Endosc. 2012;26:738–46.
19. Chang SH, Popov VB, Thompson CC. Endoscopic balloon dilation for treatment of sleeve gastrectomy stenosis: a systematic review and meta-analysis. Gastrointest Endosc. 2020;91(989–1002):e4.

20. Rosenthal RJ, International Sleeve Gastrectomy Expert Panel, Diaz AA, et al. International Sleeve Gastrectomy Expert Panel Consensus Statement: best practice guidelines based on experience of >12,000 cases. Surg Obes Relat Dis. 2012;8:8–19.
21. Dapri G, Cadiere GB, Himpens J. Laparoscopic seromyotomy for long stenosis after sleeve gastrectomy with or without duodenal switch. Obes Surg. 2009;19:495–9.
22. Deslauriers V, Beauchamp A, Garofalo F, et al. Endoscopic management of post-laparoscopic sleeve gastrectomy stenosis. Surg Endosc. 2018;32:601–9.
23. Hussain A, El-Hasani S. Gastric stenosis after laparoscopic sleeve gastrectomy in morbidly obese patients. Obes Surg. 2014;24:820–1.
24. Burgos AM, Csendes A, Braghetto I. Gastric stenosis after laparoscopic sleeve gastrectomy in morbidly obese patients. Obes Surg. 2013;23:1481–6.
25. Ogra R, Kini GP. Evolving endoscopic management options for symptomatic stenosis post-laparoscopic sleeve gastrectomy for morbid obesity: experience at a large bariatric surgery unit in New Zealand. Obes Surg. 2015;25:242–8.
26. McCarty TR, Thompson CC. Bariatric endoscopy. Yamada' s Textbook of Gastroenterology. 7th Edn. Accepted.
27. Sharma P, McCarty TR, Chhoda A, et al. Alternative uses of lumen apposing metal stents. World J Gastroenterol. 2020. Accepted.
28. Joo MK. Endoscopic approach for major complications of bariatric surgery. Clin Endosc. 2017;50:31–41.
29. Agnihotri A, Barola S, Hill C, et al. An algorithmic approach to the management of gastric stenosis following laparoscopic sleeve gastrectomy. Obes Surg. 2017;27:2628–36.
30. Costa MN, Capela T, Seves I, Ribeiro R, Rio-Tinto R. Endoscopic treatment of early gastric obstruction after sleeve gastrectomy: report of two cases. GE Port J Gastroenterol. 2016;23:46–9.
31. Farha J, Fayad L, Kadhim A, et al. Gastric per-oral endoscopic myotomy (G-POEM) for the treatment of gastric stenosis post-laparoscopic sleeve gastrectomy (LSG). Obes Surg. 2019;29:2350–4.

Sleeve Gastrectomy Stenosis: Surgical Treatment

Jacques M. Himpens

1 Introduction

According to the latest literature data, laparoscopic sleeve gastrectomy (LSG) has become the most popular bariatric-metabolic procedure across the world [1]. One of the obvious explanations for this rather unexpected situation is the relative technical ease of the laparoscopic sleeve gastrectomy operation, but also the fact that, according to most publications, LSG appears to cause fewer short- and mid-term complications than Roux-en-Y gastric bypass (RYGB) procedure, which was considered the "champion" bariatric-metabolic technique up until recently. In addition, the metabolic activity of LSG appears to closely match the clinical outcomes of RYGB [2].

In terms of mid- to long-term LSG-linked complications, the most frequently reported is stenosis. This condition is usually described either at the mid-gastric body level (incisura angularis) or, less frequently, at the level of the cardia [3].

2 Diagnosis

Until recently, the diagnosis of sleeve stenosis typically was achieved by conventional radiology (contrast swallow) but this approach has been widely abandoned to the benefit of upper gastro-intestinal endoscopy [4]. Conversely, however,

J. M. Himpens (✉)
Delta CHIREC Hospitals, Brussels, Belgium
e-mail: jacques_himpens@hotmail.com

J. M. Himpens
St Pierre University Hospital, Brussels, Belgium

© The Editor(s) (if applicable) and The Author(s), under exclusive license to Springer Nature Switzerland AG 2021
S. Al-Sabah et al. (eds.), *Laparoscopic Sleeve Gastrectomy*,
https://doi.org/10.1007/978-3-030-57373-7_46

endoscopy may generate a false negative diagnosis because often stenosis are functional and allow passage of the endoscope [5], which is the criterion usually used by endoscopists for ruling out stenosis. Nowadays the most accurate diagnosis relies in three-dimensional CT reconstruction of the sleeved stomach [6].

Three-dimensional CT- reconstructions allow to accurately locate the possible stricture (i.e. actual significant diameter reduction of the stomach), but at the same time to detect axial aberrations such as torsions (the so-called corkscrew deformity) and kinks, that are significant contributors to functional stenosis [7].

3   Incidence

Stenosis after LSG, is quite rare a condition (occurring in between 0.1 and 4% of the cases according to a recent meta-analysis [8]. Post-LSG stenosis symptoms usually include gastro-esophageal reflux (GERD), sometimes accompanied by significant dysphagia, regurgitation and vomiting of thick, white slime. Most stenosis, located at the level of the angulus, are due either to technical factors (such as overstretching the tissues causing the stapler to staple closer to the endoluminal bougie), or oversewing the staple line, or to scarring issues [9].

4   Prevention

Post-sleeve stenosis may be avoided by the judicious use of peroperative endoscopy. Nimeri et al. [10] demonstrated that with this strategy the incidence of stenosis may drop from 3.2 to 0%. Possible mechanisms resulting in better outcomes—as mentioned by the authors—included the ability to detect and remove ill placed sutures covering the staple line, or to address stapling errors such as staples placed too close to the incisura, Of note, Nimeri et al. mentioned that short stenosis created by stapling flaws may be addressed by an immediate short seromyotomy, a technique that will be described later. In one Italian study, it appeared that oversewing the staple line was accompanied by a significant increase of stenosis rate, while it did not improve bleeding and fistula prevalence [10]. This experience has recently been duplicated [9].

Along the same lines, smaller bougie sizes may negatively affect the stenosis rate after sleeve gastrectomy, as concluded during the fifth consensus conference on sleeve gastrectomy [11]. More recent data, however, do not confirm this assumption [12].

5   Treatment

First line treatment of sleeve stenosis nowadays is undoubtedly endoscopic, and consists of balloon dilation, preferably with high pressure balloons dilations, kept dilated for a substantial length of time [8, 13]. The balloon treatment may be complemented by placement of self-expandable fully or partly covered metallic stents. Of note, the endoscopic insertion of fully covered self-expanding metallic stents, usually requires endoscopic fastening to avoid migration [14].

The surgical options usually are kept for the failure cases of repeated balloon dilation treatment. Nath et al. [5] found that, while close to 10% of the individuals submitted to sleeve gastrectomy had developed stenosis or symptomatic angulation, 69% of those were successfully treated by one or more sessions of balloon dilation. Chang et al. [15] reported a success rate of the endoscopic approach of 37%, but 50% of the patients still required conversion to Roux-en-Y gastric bypass. Burgos et al. [16] reported a success rate of 80% in a small group of patients, the remaining failures being addressed by conversion to Roux-en-Y gastric bypass.

A recently described "minimally invasive" technique consists of endoscopic tunneled stricturotomy, but the numbers are small [17].

Considering the abundance of endoscopic techniques, nowadays, surgery is mostly saved for recalcitrant post-sleeve stenosis. There are still several surgical options to address the stenosis of the gastric body after sleeve gastrectomy. The theoretically most appealing technique (briefly mentioned above to address peroperatively diagnosed stenosis induced by ill stapling) is probably laparoscopic seromyotomy [18] (Fig. 1). The laparoscopic technique is quite similar to proximal gastric seromyotomy used in achalasia (Heller's procedure). In brief, in gasric seromyotomy, the serosal and muscular layers of the anterior stomach are incised by cautery or harmonic scissors, leaving the mucosa intact. Burning lesions must be avoided at all cost and simple mechanical disruption of the deepest layers may be a good and safe technique to this regard. It is essential to extend the incision far

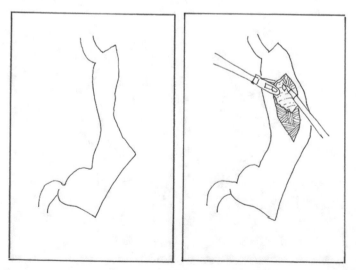

Fig. 1 Artist impression of seromyotomy in sleeve stenosis. The magnified view provided by the laparoscopy facilitates the identification of the different layers of the gastric wall, authorizing the safe severance of the muscular fibers, and the preservation of the mucosa

beyond the stenosis, both proximally and distally to tackle the entire stenotic area. However, the drawbacks of this approach appeared to be many and included a high leak rate, a substantial stenosis recurrence rate, and weight regain [18]. This is the reason why many teams have looked for surgical alternatives. Our group reported on a small group of patients who had their stenotic sleeve gastrectomy treated by resecting the stenotic area, followed by an end to end manual reanastomosis [19] (Fig. 2). A similar approach was described by Kalaseilvan et al. [20]. Unfortunately, attempts at resecting the stenosis appeared to be unsatisfactory because of the recurrence of the condition, as reported both by our team and by the team of Kalaseilvan who experienced a stenosis recurrence in one of their two patients.

Another theoretical option to deal with gastric stenosis after LSG consists of stricturoplasty, in analogy with the technique used in small bowel strictures linked with Crohn's disease [21]. Despite the elegance of this approach we could find only one report on this technique [22].

Because of the drawbacks and possible complications of the "direct" treatment technique of post-LSG stenosis, conversion to Roux-en-Y gastric bypass (RYGB) (Fig. 3) remains the most frequently described strategy in addressing the side-effects of an ill-fated sleeve gastrectomy, ranging from chronic leaks to highly symptomatic stenosis, recurrence of the condition despite other treatment modes, and, quite frequently, invalidating gastro-esophageal reflux (GERD).

Laparoscopic conversion of the stenotic sleeve to RYGB must comprise transection of the stomach proximal to the stenosis in order to avoid possible recurrence of stenosis symptoms [23]. Of note, whereas conversion from sleeve

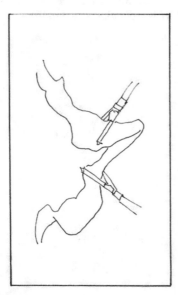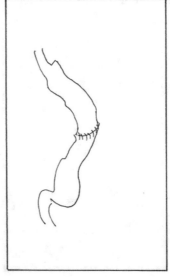

Fig. 2 Artist impression of the "wedge" or "segmental resection" dealing with the "corkscrew deformity" of a stenotic sleeve. The redundant part is being resected and the continuity restored by a manual end-to-end anastomosis

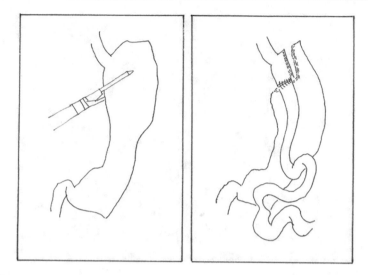

Fig. 3 Conversion of sleeve gastrectomy to Roux-en-Y Gastric Bypass for sleeve stenosis. The small gastric pouch is constructed well proximal to the stenotic area

to RYGB does not appear to offer a sound solution in case of associated insufficient weight loss or weight recovery after initial acceptable weight loss the consequences of gastric corpus stenosis appear to be adequately addressed [24]. Consequently, some consensus exists as to the efficacy of converting sleeve gastrectomy stenosis to RYGB, with reported good clinical outcomes, but at the cost of more complications than primary RYGB [25, 26].

A more recently reported solution for sleeve gastrectomy stenosis is conversion to One Anastomosis (or mini-) Gastric Bypass [27] (OAGB) (Fig. 4). This technique that involves just one anastomosis is obviously simpler than conversion to RYGB and is accompanied by fewer complications.

In our department we are however reluctant to use this solution because constructing a correct OAGB implies a long pouch that extends beyond the crow's foot, hence more often than not the stenotic area will not be excluded. In addition, theoretical long-term side effects such as bile reflux must still be assessed.

6   Conclusion

The treatment of post-LSG stenosis is endoscopic in the majority of cases. In case of failure of endoscopic treatment, surgical options are available, including seromyotomy, segmental resection and, theoretically, stricturoplasty. The high incidence of complications after seromyotomy and other "targeted treatment mode" make these technique less desirable for the indication of (late) post-sleeve stenosis. Consequently, the preferred solution remains conversion to Roux-en-Y gastric bypass. Conversions to single anastomosis gastric bypass are at risk of leaving the stenosis in place.

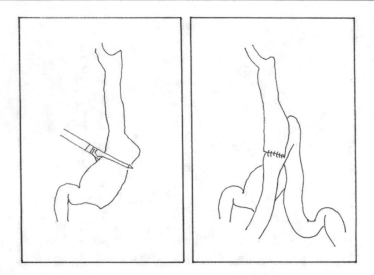

Fig. 4 Conversion of sleeve gastrectomy to One Anastomosis Gastric Bypass. Because the gastric pouch must be quite long it is often difficult to avoid the stenotic part of the sleeve while constructing the pouch

Treatment Algorithm

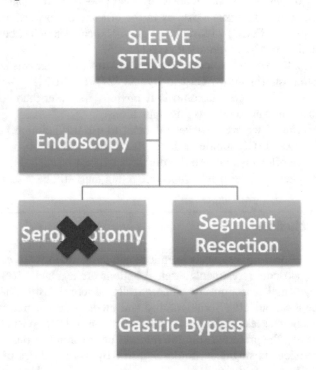

References

1. Angrisani L, Santonicola A, Iovino P, Vitiello A, Higa K, Himpens J, Buchwald H, Scopinaro N. IFSO worldwide survey 2016: primary, endoluminal, and revisional procedures. Obes Surg. 2018;28(12):3783–94.
2. Peterli R, Wölnerhanssen BK, Peters T, Vetter D, Kröll D, Borbély Y, Schultes B, Beglinger C, Drewe J, Schiesser M, Nett P, Bueter M. Effect of laparoscopic sleeve gastrectomy vs laparoscopic Roux-en-Y gastric bypass on weight loss in patients with morbid obesity: the SM-BOSS randomized clinical trial. JAMA. 2018;319(3):255–65.
3. Iannelli A, Treacy P, Sebastianelli L, Schiavo L, Martini F. Perioperative complications of sleeve gastrectomy: review of the literature. J Minim Access Surg. 2019;15(1):1–7.
4. Bhalla S, Yu JX, Varban OA, Schulman AR. Upper gastrointestinal series after sleeve gastrectomy is unnecessary to evaluate for gastric sleeve stenosis. Surg Endosc. 2020.
5. Nath A, Yewale S, Tran T, Brebbia JS, Shope TR. Koch TR Dysphagia after vertical sleeve gastrectomy: evaluation of risk factors and assessment of endoscopic intervention. World J Gastroenterol. 2016;22(47):10371–9.
6. Blanchet MC, Mesmann C, Yanes M, Lepage S, Marion D, Galas P, Gouillat C. 3D gastric computed tomography as a new imaging in patients with failure or complication after bariatric surgery. Obes Surg. 2010;20:1727–33.
7. Hanssen A, Plotnikov S, Acosta G, Nuñez JT, Haddad J, Rodriguez C, Petrucci C, Hanssen D, Hanssen R. 3D volumetry and its correlation between postoperative gastric volume and excess weight loss after sleeve gastrectomy. Obes Surg. 2018;28(3):775–80.
8. Chang S, Popov V, Thompson CC. Endoscopic balloon dilation for treatment of sleeve gastrectomy stenosis: a systematic review and meta-analysis. Gastrointest Endosc. 2019.
9. Guerrier JB, Mehaffey JH, Schirmer BD, Hallowell PT. Reinforcement of the Staple Line during gastric sleeve: a comparison of buttressing or oversewing, *versus* no reinforcement: a single-institution study. Am Surg. 2018;84(5):690–4.
10. Nimeri A, Maasher A, Salim E, Ibrahim M, El Hadad M. The use of intraoperative endoscopy may decrease postoperative stenosis in laparoscopic sleeve gastrectomy. Obes Surg. 2016;26(7):1398–401.
11. Gagner M, Hutchinson C, Rosenthal R. Fifth international consensus conference: current status of sleeve gastrectomy. Surg Obes Relat Dis. 2016;12(4):750–6.
12. Guetta O, Ovnat A, Czeiger D, Vakhrushev A, Tsaban G, Sebbag G. The impact of technical surgical aspects on morbidity of 984 patients after sleeve gastrectomy for morbid obesity. Obes Surg. 2017.
13. Sabah SA, Haddad EA, Siddique I. Endoscopic management of post-laparoscopic sleeve gastrectomy stenosis. Surg Endosc. 2016;31(9):3559–63. https://doi.org/10.1007/s00464-016-5385-9.
14. Fayad L, Simsek C, Oleas R, Ichkhanian Y, Fayad GE, Ngamreungphong S, Schweitzer M, Oberbach A, Kalloo AN, Khashab MA, Kumbhari V. Safety and efficacy of endoscopically secured fully covered self-expandable metallic stents (FCSEMS) for post-bariatric complex stenosis. Obes Surg. 2019;29(11):3484–92.
15. Chang J, Sharma G, Boulis M, Brethauer S, Rodriguez J, Kroh M. Endoscopic stents in the management of anastomotic complications after foregut surgery: new applications and techniques. Surg Obes Relat Dis. 2016;12(7):1373–81.
16. Burgos AM, Csendes A, Braghetto I. Gastric stenosis after laparoscopic sleeve gastrectomy in morbidly obese patients. Obes Surg. 2013;23(9):1481–6.
17. De Moura EGH, de Moura DTH, Sakai CM, Sagae V, Neto ACM, Thompson CC. Endoscopic tunneled stricturotomy with full-thickness dissection in the management of a sleeve gastrectomy stenosis. Obes Surg. 2019;29(8):2711–2.
18. Dapri G, Cadière GB, Himpens J. Laparoscopic seromyotomy for long stenosis after sleeve gastrectomy with or without duodenal switch. Obes Surg. 2009;19(4):495–932.

19. Vilallonga R, Himpens J, van de Vrande S. Laparoscopic management of persistent structures after laparoscopic sleeve gastrectomy. Obes Surg. 2013;23(10):1655–61.
20. Kalaiselvan R. Ammori BJ Laparoscopic median gastrectomy for stenosis following sleeve gastrectomy. Surg Obes Relat Dis. 2015;11(2):474–722.
21. Thienpont C, Van Assche G. Endoscopic and medical management of fibrostenotic Crohn's disease. Dig Dis. 2014;32(Suppl 1):35–8.
22. Chang PC, Tai CM, Hsin MC, Hung CM, Huang IY, Huang CK. Surgical standardization to prevent gastric stenosis after laparoscopic sleeve gastrectomy: a case series. Surg Obes Relat Dis. 2017;13(3):385–90.
23. Lacy A, Ibarzabal A, Pando E, Adelsdorfer C, Delitala A, Corcelles R, Delgado S, Vidal J. Revisional surgery after sleeve gastrectomy. Surg Laparosc Endosc Percutan Tech. 2010;20(5):351–6.
24. Parmar CD, Mahawar KK, Boyle M, Schroeder N, Balupuri S, Small PK. Conversion of sleeve gastrectomy to Roux-en-Y gastric bypass is effective for gastro-oesophageal reflux disease but not for further weight loss. Obes Surg. 2017;27(7):1651–8.
25. Cheung D, Switzer NJ, Gill RS, Shi X, Karmali S. Revisional bariatric surgery following failed primary laparoscopic sleeve gastrectomy: a systematic review. Obes Surg. 2014;24(10):1757–63. https://doi.org/10.1007/s11695-014-1332-9.
26. Landreneau JP, Strong AT, Rodriguez JH, Aleassa EM, Aminian A, Brethauer S, Schauer PR, Kroh MD. Conversion of sleeve gastrectomy to Roux-en-Y gastric bypass. Obes Surg. 2018;28(12):3843–50.
27. Musella M, Bruni V, Greco F, Raffaelli M, Lucchese M, Susa A, De Luca M, Vuolo G, Manno E, Vitiello A, Velotti N, D'Alessio R, Facchiano E, Tirone A, Iovino G, Veroux G, Piazza L. Conversion from laparoscopic adjustable gastric banding (LAGB) and laparoscopic sleeve gastrectomy (LSG) to one anastomosis gastric bypass (OAGB): preliminary data from a multicenter retrospective study. Surg Obes Relat Dis. 2019;15(8):1332–9.

How to Manage Sleeve Complications Through Endoscopy: Gastroesophageal Reflux Disease

Thomas R. McCarty⑩ and Christopher C. Thompson⑩

1 Introduction

The development of gastroesophageal reflux disease (GERD) and heartburn associated symptoms is quite common among patients following sleeve gastrectomy. New-onset GERD or worsening GERD among individuals with pre-existing heartburn symptoms is a well-known complication of laparoscopic sleeve gastrectomy. Although GERD symptoms improve for the vast majority of patients (87–100%) following Roux-en-Y gastric bypass, sleeve gastrectomy has been shown to result in an increase in GERD for patients post-procedure [1–5]. As such, less invasive endoscopic treatments are needed to target this specific population. In this chapter, we will review the mechanisms that predispose to GERD after sleeve gastrectomy, incidence of GERD post-procedure, screening recommendations, as well as proper diagnosis and treatment. Additionally, we review three endoscopic interventions that may provide improvement for patients with GERD after sleeve gastrectomy.

2 Mechanisms of GERD Post-Sleeve Gastrectomy

Many potential theories for the development of GERD after sleeve gastrectomy have been proposed [6]. Given the nature of the gastric sleeve, there is a decrease in gastric compliance, resulting in a rigid stiff stomach with little ability for accommodation [7]. This likely leads to an increased intraluminal pressure,

T. R. McCarty · C. C. Thompson (✉)
Brigham and Women's Hospital, Boston, USA
e-mail: CCTHOMPSON@bwh.harvard.edu

T. R. McCarty
e-mail: trmccarty@bwh.harvard.edu

© The Editor(s) (if applicable) and The Author(s), under exclusive license to Springer   499
Nature Switzerland AG 2021
S. Al-Sabah et al. (eds.), *Laparoscopic Sleeve Gastrectomy*,
https://doi.org/10.1007/978-3-030-57373-7_47

thereby increasing regurgitation or reflux of stomach contents into the esophagus with an intact pylorus. Additionally, laparoscopic sleeve gastrectomy results in a lower esophageal sphincter (LES) pressure and shortens the abdominal length of the esophagus [8]. Other potential causes may be iatrogenic in nature and are related to overlooking the presence of hiatal hernias and general shape of the sleeve, including over-dilation of the proximal part of the sleeve to create a reservoir which may increase GERD [9, 10].

3 Incidence of GERD After Sleeve Gastrectomy

A landmark study by Genco et al. found that sleeve gastrectomy was associated with a significant increase in erosive esophagitis and non-dysplastic Barrett's esophagus with no correlation between patient-reported symptoms and endoscopic findings [11]. This key finding that symptoms may not correlate with endoscopic findings was critical to the realization that a large majority of post-sleeve gastrectomy patients may develop GERD-related sequalae even without overt symptoms. In a recent systematic review and meta-analysis of 46 studies and over 10,000 patients, 19% of patients developed worsening GERD post-sleeve gastrectomy with another 23% reporting de novo symptoms [12]. Similar to the previous study, the long-term prevalence of esophagitis and Barrett's esophagus after sleeve gastrectomy was 28% and 8%, respectively.

4 Screening Recommendations

This increased risk of new onset Barrett's esophagus has been estimated to be 15–17% by the International Federation for the Surgery of Obesity and Metabolic Disorders (IFSO). As such, this society currently recommends a surveillance endoscopy after sleeve gastrectomy at 1, 3, and 5 years, then subsequently every 10 years—with more frequent surveillance needed and consideration of conversion to Roux-en-Y gastric bypass should patients develop non-dysplastic Barrett's esophagus [13]. Yet, despite this recommendation, significant variability remains among surgeons and gastroenterologists with respect to screening for GERD and de novo Barrett's esophagus post-sleeve gastrectomy. Furthermore, beyond traditional pharmacologic therapies, including proton pump inhibitors (PPIs), few endoscopic treatment options are available for symptomatic and asymptomatic patients post-sleeve gastrectomy. In this review, we will highlight the important role of endoscopy in the management of GERD after sleeve gastrectomy and discuss several potential endoscopic treatments.

5 Role of Pharmacotherapy, Diagnosis, and Testing

For all patients with symptomatic GERD or evidence of esophagitis on upper endoscopy, standard PPI therapy (typically with starting dose of omeprazole 20 mg daily) is recommended. Although far less common compared to patients with Roux-en-Y anatomy, heartburn symptoms that fail to response to traditional PPI therapy (classically higher dose PPI twice daily) should prompt investigation for non-acid reflux. Due to the anatomy of Roux-en-Y gastric bypass, proper recognition of bile acid reflux with gastropathy or non-acid reflux as an alternative to GERD is important [14]. While the clinical diagnosis of GERD is based upon typical symptoms that respond to treatment with a PPI, more objective measures including via 24 hour esophageal pH monitoring (diagnosed by having a pH < 4.0 and the length of time the esophagus is exposed to acid) may be helpful—especially for patients that may have no symptoms. Motility testing with pH and impedance testing along with manometry may also help to identify acid and non-acid reflux etiologies. Impedance testing is critical to differentiate acid versus non-acid reflux, thereby allowing proper identification of the underlying etiology. Esophageal manometry (i.e., motility testing) is also key as this may identify underlying functional disorders or explain difficult to control symptoms. Gastroenterologists and surgeons should collaborate in the care of these patients.

6 Anti-Reflux Mucosectomy (ARMS)

Given the significantly increased rate of de novo GERD and downstream consequences of possible Barrett's esophagus, a need has been created for effective, sleeve-specific endoscopic GERD treatments. One such treatment for patients with refractory disease, and utilized as a potential alternative to surgical conversion to Roux-en-Y gastric bypass is the endoscopy procedure called anti-reflux mucosectomy (ARMS). This procedure involves endoscopic mucosal resection (EMR) or endoscopic submucosal dissection (ESD) of the gastroesophageal junction (GEJ) at the level of the gastric cardia from a retroflexed view [15]. Although this is a newer technique, this endoscopic procedure has really come to the forefront of endoscopic therapies in recent years. By performing EMR or ESD of the GEJ, this creates an area of fibrosis or scar formation potentially tightening the GEJ to reduce esophageal acid exposure and improve symptoms—similar to documented improvement in previous studies examining GERD symptoms after mucosal resection for short-segment Barrett's esophagus [16–18].

The first case of the ARMS procedure was reported in a pilot study of 10 patients with normal gastric anatomy by Inoue and colleagues in 2014 [16]. In this study, importantly among patients without sleeve gastrectomy, DeMeester score, Hill classification (hiatal hernia), and time of esophageal acid exposure (pH < 4), all significantly improved post-ARMS procedure. Perhaps most importantly, symptoms improved across the board with PPI therapy completely discontinued for all 10 patients. Notably, stenosis did develop in 10 patients requiring endoscopy balloon dilation with control of symptoms. A subsequent case report by our group demonstrated application of this novel ARMS technique in a sleeve gastrectomy patient with a relatively narrow stomach with altered blood supply [15]. In this case, a 71-year-old woman with sleeve gastrectomy approximately 5 years prior developed worsening GERD post-procedure despite twice daily PPI therapy. Step-by-step procedure details are shown in Fig. 1 with significant resolution of

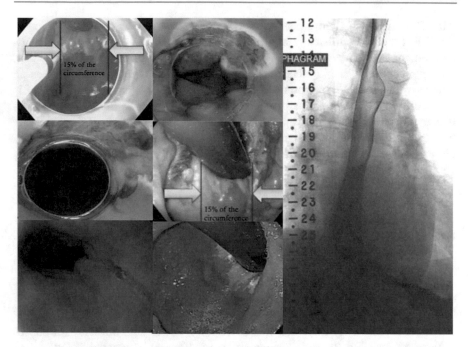

Fig. 1 Antireflux mucosectomy (ARMS) procedure. (**A**) Pulsed argon plasma coagulation marks the 85% circumferential area of mucosa to be treated and the 15% of the circumference to be left untreated. (**B** and **C**) Gastroesophageal junction after 2 EMR procedures and after 8 EMR procedures. (**D**) Retroflexed view after the completion of 10 resections, highlighting partial circumferential resection. (**E** and **F**) Follow-up EGD at 3 months, with the gastroesophageal junction in forward view and retroflexed view. (**G**) Timed barium swallow performed 3 months after ARMS with normal esophageal caliber, contour, distensibility, and prompt passage of contrast material

symptoms at 12 month follow-up. While more data among a population of patients with prior bariatric surgery is needed, ARMS may provide an alternative to surgical conversion to Roux-en-Y gastric bypass. At this time, use of ARMS is limited to tertiary academic centers with high volume endobariatric expertise.

7 Radiofrequency Ablation

Use of radiofrequency ablation to the LES has been well studied as an effective treatment for GERD refractory to medical therapy [19]. Applied through a procedure call Stretta (Mederi Therapeutics, Greenwich, CT, United States), which is a minimally invasive endoscopic procedure for the treatment of GERD, radiofrequency energy is applied to the LES and gastric cardia which results in local inflammation, collagen deposition, and muscular thickening to disrupt nerve fibers [20, 21]. This was approved by the United States Food and Drug Administration (FDA) in 2000. The device is a soft, flexible, bougie tip (20 French) that includes a balloon/basket with four 5.5 mm NiTi electrodes along with temperature and impedance monitoring—Fig. 2. The radiofrequency ablation procedure involves a balloon assembly with needle electrodes that are positioned

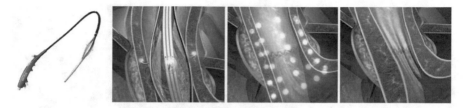

Fig. 2 Representative images of Stretta device and procedure. Available at: https://www.restech.com/solutions/stretta/

approximately one cm above the GEJ and deliver radiofrequency energy waves directly to the submucosa [22].

While effective, the vast majority of data is limited to non-sleeve gastrectomy patients. However, within the last few years, some literature has emerged regarding the safety and efficacy of radiofrequency ablation among a population of patients with sleeve gastrectomy. In a retrospective analysis of 15 patients at a single-center, Khidir and colleagues found that Stretta did not improve GERD symptoms in patients post-sleeve gastrectomy at follow-up of 6 months. Furthermore, adverse events occurred in 6.7% of patients and ranged from mild to severe and refractory symptoms. Overall, two-thirds of patients (n = 10) were not satisfied with the therapy despite 20% of patients being able to completely discontinue PPI therapy. Another small case series of a two patients undergoing Stretta after sleeve gastrectomy revealed positive results [24]. Given this limited data among patients with a history of sleeve gastrectomy, a multi-center clinical trial was underway (NCT02637713); however, this was terminated and results have not been released [25].

8 Transoral Incisionless Fundoplication (TIF)

The transoral incisionless fundoplication (TIF) procedure was first introduced in 2005 and later approved by the United States FDA in 2007. The procedure is performed using the the EsophyX device (EndoGastric Solutions, Redmond, Washington, USA) to reconfigure the GEJ to obtain a full-thickness esophageal valve from inside the gastric body, using serosa-to-serosa plications that include the muscle layers. The EsophyX device constructs an omega-shaped valve approximately 3–5 cm long, in a 250°–300° circumferential pattern around the GEJ, by deploying non-absorbable polypropylene fasteners through the two layers (esophagus and stomach) under endoscopic visualization—Fig. 3 [23, 26].

In a systematic review and meta-analysis by the lead author of this review, TIF was associated with a high success rate of 99% and adverse event rate of only 2% [23]. Subjective data based upon the GERD Health-Related Quality of Life (HRQL) score, Gastroesophageal Reflux Symptom Score (GERSS), and Reflux Symptom Index (RSI) as well as objective measures such as DeMeester scores improved significantly post-TIF. Furthermore, PPI therapy was discontinued in 89% of patients. Importantly, none of the 32 studies (n = 1475 patients) included in this meta-analysis study included patients with a history of sleeve gastrectomy. Currently, the role of TIF among patients post–sleeve gastrectomy who

Fig. 3 Representative images of transoral incisionless fundoplication (TIF) device and procedure. Available at: https://www.endogastricsolutions.com/tif-procedure/

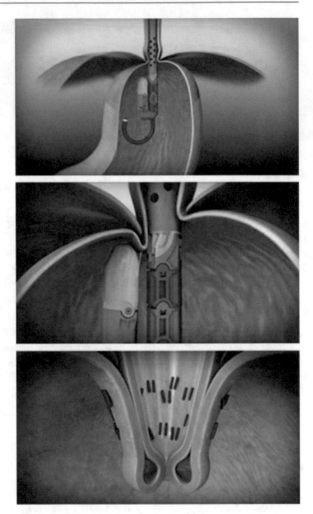

report severe GERD-related symptoms remains unclear and an area of needed research. However, given the size of the device, TIF may only be a viable treatment for patients with significantly dilated sleeves. While promising results have been shown for non-bariatric surgery patients, more data is needed for patients with a history of sleeve gastrectomy.

9   Conclusion

At this time, there is poor evidence to support the use of any endoscopic modalities for the treatment of GERD post-sleeve gastrectomy. We acknowledge there is limited data at this time for endoscopic therapies as a whole. Procedures like

ARMS, Stretta, and TIF require more data before increased adoption to patients with sleeve gastrectomy. Furthermore, given the paucity of data, future studies are needed to specifically examine this uniquely at-risk population. Given limited data, the use of endoscopic therapy for post-sleeve GERD is driven largely by expert opinion, and limited to centers with expertise. Other laparoscopic procedures, such as the LINX Reflux Management System (Torax Medical, St. Paul, MN, USA) and conversion to Roux-en-Y gastric bypass, should be strongly considered in this patient population. It is important to underscore the mechanisms that contribute to reflux and role of proper surveillance of GERD and Barrett's esophagus post-sleeve gastrectomy.

References

1. Chiu S, Birch DW, Shi X, Sharma AM, Karmali S. Effect of sleeve gastrectomy on gastroesophageal reflux disease: a systematic review. Surg Obes Relat Dis. 2011;7:510–5.
2. de Jong JR, Besselink MG, van Ramshorst B, Gooszen HG, Smout AJ. Effects of adjustable gastric banding on gastroesophageal reflux and esophageal motility: a systematic review. Obes Rev. 2010;11:297–305.
3. Frezza EE, Ikramuddin S, Gourash W, et al. Symptomatic improvement in gastroesophageal reflux disease (GERD) following laparoscopic Roux-en-Y gastric bypass. Surg Endosc. 2002;16:1027–31.
4. Perry Y, Courcoulas AP, Fernando HC, Buenaventura PO, McCaughan JS, Luketich JD. Laparoscopic Roux-en-Y gastric bypass for recalcitrant gastroesophageal reflux disease in morbidly obese patients. JSLS. 2004;8:19–23.
5. Woodman G, Cywes R, Billy H, et al. Effect of adjustable gastric banding on changes in gastroesophageal reflux disease (GERD) and quality of life. Curr Med Res Opin. 2012;28:581–9.
6. Torquati A. Treatment for severe GERD after Sleeve Gastrectomy: conversion to gastric bypass or endoluminal radiofrequency. https://web.duke.edu/surgery/2015BariatricMasters/session6_gerd_after_sleeve_torquati.pdf. Accessed 24 May 2020.
7. Braghetto I, Korn O, Valladares H, et al. Laparoscopic sleeve gastrectomy: surgical technique, indications and clinical results. Obes Surg. 2007;17:1442–50.
8. Braghetto I, Lanzarini E, Korn O, Valladares H, Molina JC, Henriquez A. Manometric changes of the lower esophageal sphincter after sleeve gastrectomy in obese patients. Obes Surg. 2010;20:357–62.
9. Lazoura O, Zacharoulis D, Triantafyllidis G, et al. Symptoms of gastroesophageal reflux following laparoscopic sleeve gastrectomy are related to the final shape of the sleeve as depicted by radiology. Obes Surg. 2011;21:295–9.
10. Michalsky D, Dvorak P, Belacek J, Kasalicky M. Radical resection of the pyloric antrum and its effect on gastric emptying after sleeve gastrectomy. Obes Surg. 2013;23:567–73.
11. Genco A, Soricelli E, Casella G, et al. Gastroesophageal reflux disease and Barrett's esophagus after laparoscopic sleeve gastrectomy: a possible, underestimated long-term complication. Surg Obes Relat Dis. 2017;13:568–74.
12. Yeung KTD, Penney N, Ashrafian L, Darzi A, Ashrafian H. Does sleeve gastrectomy expose the distal esophagus to severe reflux?: A systematic review and meta-analysis. Ann Surg. 2020;271:257–65.
13. Gagner M, Hutchinson C, Rosenthal R. Fifth international consensus conference: current status of sleeve gastrectomy. Surg Obes Relat Dis. 2016;12:750–6.

14. Kumar N, Thompson CC. Remnant gastropathy due to bile reflux after Roux-en-Y gastric bypass: a unique cause of abdominal pain and successful treatment with ursodiol. Surg Endosc. 2017;31:5399–402.
15. Hathorn KE, Jirapinyo P, Thompson CC. Endoscopic management of gastroesophageal reflux disease after sleeve gastrectomy by use of the antireflux mucosectomy procedure. VideoGIE. 2019;4:251–3.
16. Inoue H, Ito H, Ikeda H, et al. Anti-reflux mucosectomy for gastroesophageal reflux disease in the absence of hiatus hernia: a pilot study. Ann Gastroenterol. 2014;27:346–51.
17. Satodate H, Inoue H, Fukami N, Shiokawa A, Kudo SE. Squamous reepithelialization after circumferential endoscopic mucosal resection of superficial carcinoma arising in Barrett's esophagus. Endoscopy. 2004;36:909–12.
18. Satodate H, Inoue H, Yoshida T, et al. Circumferential EMR of carcinoma arising in Barrett's esophagus: case report. Gastrointest Endosc. 2003;58:288–92.
19. Fass R, Cahn F, Scotti DJ, Gregory DA. Systematic review and meta-analysis of controlled and prospective cohort efficacy studies of endoscopic radiofrequency for treatment of gastroesophageal reflux disease. Surg Endosc. 2017;31:4865–82.
20. Hopkins J, Switzer NJ, Karmali S. Update on novel endoscopic therapies to treat gastroesophageal reflux disease: a review. World J Gastrointest Endosc. 2015;7:1039–44.
21. Torquati A, Houston HL, Kaiser J, Holzman MD, Richards WO. Long-term follow-up study of the Stretta procedure for the treatment of gastroesophageal reflux disease. Surg Endosc. 2004;18:1475–9.
22. Crawford C, Gibbens K, Lomelin D, Krause C, Simorov A, Oleynikov D. Sleeve gastrectomy and anti-reflux procedures. Surg Endosc. 2017;31:1012–21.
23. McCarty TR, Itidiare M, Njei B, Rustagi T. Efficacy of transoral incisionless fundoplication for refractory gastroesophageal reflux disease: a systematic review and meta-analysis. Endoscopy. 2018;50:708–25.
24. Guerron D, Portenier D. A case series on gastroesophageal reflux disease and the bariatric patient: stretta therapy as a non-surgical option. Bariatric Times. 2016;13(11):18–20.
25. Management of Reflux After Sleeve Using Stretta (MaRSS). U.S. National Library of Medicine: ClinicalTrials.gov Identifier: NCT02637713. https://clinicaltrials.gov/ct2/show/NCT02637713. Accessed 24 May 2020.
26. Testoni PA, Mazzoleni G, Testoni SG. Transoral incisionless fundoplication for gastro-esophageal reflux disease: Techniques and outcomes. World J Gastrointest Pharmacol Ther. 2016;7:179–89.

How to Manage Sleeve Gastrectomy Complications Through Surgery: Gastroesophageal Reflux Disease

Shujhat Khan and Hutan Ashrafian [ORCID]

1   Background

The sleeve gastrectomy (SG) procedure was evolved from the biliopancreatic diversion- duodenal switch procedure in order to reduce complication rates and improve outcomes for patients. The complications can be categorised as early, medium, and long-term. Early complications include gastric leak, bleeding, obstruction, formation of abscess, and infection. Mid-late complications typically include fistula development, stenosis, neofundus, regain of weight, nutritional deficiencies and gastro-oesophageal reflux disease (GERD) [1–3]. GERD is a prominent complication that patients will often complain about, and symptoms include chest pain, dysphagia, heartburn, regurgitation, chronic cough, and laryngitis. With the rise in obesity, and the already high prevalence of GERD in these populations, this is a significant cause of morbidity in western populations and is likely set to worsen.

2   Pathophysiology

GERD can be categorised as non-erosive or erosive based on the endoscopic appearance of the oesophageal mucosa. It is particularly important considering the high prevalence particularly in the western countries. Approximately 20%

S. Khan
Milton Keynes University Hospital, London, UK
e-mail: shujhat.khan15@imperial.ac.uk

H. Ashrafian (✉)
Institute of Global Health Innovation, Imperial College London, London, UK
e-mail: h.ashrafian@imperial.ac.uk

© The Editor(s) (if applicable) and The Author(s), under exclusive license to Springer Nature Switzerland AG 2021
S. Al-Sabah et al. (eds.), *Laparoscopic Sleeve Gastrectomy*,
https://doi.org/10.1007/978-3-030-57373-7_48

of individuals in USA alone are effected by GERD [4] and, if left untreated, can subsequently lead to the formation of Barret's oesophagus and adenocarcinoma. There are several mechanisms for the formation of GERD (Table 1). Removal of the gastric fundus and body has consequences on both acid secretion and gastric accommodation and shifts the balance between these protective and exacerbating factors leading to GERD. However, another peak is seen after 6 years, likely caused by incomplete resection of the gastric tissue, thereby leading to a neo-fundus years later [5–7].

The exact mechanism of GERD in both obesity and post-operatively following SG is unclear [8]. However, one method that has been suggested involves transient relaxation of the lower oesophageal sphincter, which is seen more often in obese patients. This typically occurs following distention of the fundus after a large meal. As a result, these patients experience greater amounts of acid exposure to the distal oesophagus [9, 10].

Additionally, it has been demonstrated that severely obese patients are more likely to present with a motility disorder. This includes a low lower oesophageal sphincter resting pressure, nonspecific motility disorders, and nutcracker oesophagus, a diagnosis given to those patients who have a mean contraction amplitude of the lower oesophagus of greater than 180 mmHg. Whilst these features would likely increase the risk of GERD, the majority of these patients were found to be asymptomatic [11–13]. Importantly, SG itself can also lead to the development of GERD in patients following the operation through a separate mechanism. However, it is likely that GERD occurs as a result of a combination of pre-, intra- and post-operative factors.

Our studies suggest approximately 20% of patients who undergo this procedure will develop de-novo GERD following a SG whereas approximately 19% of patients will have an increase in reflux symptoms [8]. However, this is likely to be lower than the true value. Indeed, many patients will have GERD but not experience any of the symptoms. In patients who underwent SG, active monitoring through upper gastrointestinal endoscopy and pH manometry revealed a much higher rate of de novo GERD as well as worsening GERD in those who had pre-existing symptoms [14–17]. In addition, patients were found to have a higher rate of oesophagitis, hiatus hernia, as well as Barrett's oesophagus [18–21]. Measuring such complications is difficult simply because many patients won't

Table 1 Mechanisms for gastro-oesophageal reflux disease in sleeve gastrectomy

Intraoperative causes	Postoperative causes
Poor surgical technique causing strictures	Hiatus hernia
Opening of the angle of His	Smoking
Resection of the fundus reducing stomach compliance	Dietary factors
Damage to vagus nerve	Regain of weight
Dissection of sling of Helvetius	Alcohol

complain of symptoms, and therefore using the obvious symptomology of patients as a screening tool is unreliable and likely to disregard a large group of patients. As such, we recommend routine post-operative follow-up in these patients to monitor for changes to mucosal tissue.

Many patients who need to be re-operated on following SG do so after developing severe, medically resistant oesophageal reflux. It is therefore clearly a major problem in patients who undergo this operation, but the complex pathophysiology behind this has led to discrepancy amongst surgeons. Whilst approximately 23.3% of surgeons questioned in a survey felt that GERD was an absolute contraindication, 52.6% felt that the pathological presentation of Barrett's oesophagus was an absolute contraindication [22]. Understanding the exact pathophysiology and the effect of environmental factors may help determine the subset of patients who should be investigated further, or who require post-operative screening.

There are several mechanisms that contribute to patients experiencing GERD following a SG operation. These can be separated into intra-operative and post-operative complications. Poor surgical technique leads to an increased number of complications as a result of the formation of strictures. This is infrequently seen, however, but the remnant stomach is intentionally constructed as a narrow tube and can subsequently stenose or obstruct, increasing the risk of reflux [23].

Competence of anatomical structures have a vital role in preventing anti-reflux. The obvious structure would be the lower oesophageal sphincter but others such as the diaphragmatic crus, the gastric sling fibres, the phrenic-oesophageal and cardiac-phrenic ligaments all have an important role in preventing reflux. The cardia of the stomach can also act as a weak mechanical valve through constriction on the oesophagogastric junction, partly aided by the oblique direction in which the oesophagus enters the stomach, commonly known as the angle of His. The importance of this angle has been studied extensively for decades within literature [24–26]. The flap of mucous membrane that extends from the greater curvature of the cardia is maintained by the movement of the muscularis mucosae, which moves the mucosa forming a barrier in the orifice. In this instance, SG can open the angle of His, weakening the barrier and leading to reflux.

Additionally, SG leads to an increase in gastric pressure because of the resection of the fundus, the most expandable portion of the stomach. However, if the gastro-oesophageal pressure gradient is exceedingly high, it can lead to reflux. Conversely, a reduction in gastro-oesophageal pressure reduces the risk of GERD. This can occur following a reduction in BMI, which reduces gastro-oesophageal pressures and accelerates gastric emptying following a SG [27]. Moreover, the deepest muscles of the stomach wall arrange to form oblique fibres which maintain the angle of His by forming a sling around the lateral portion of the cardia. This is known as the sling of Helvetius and has an important role in maintaining competence of the cardia. During a SG however, dissection of the sling muscle fibres can impair the lower oesophageal sphincter and lead to reflux. Furthermore, intra-operative damage to the vagus nerve can also lead to reflux and is a well-known complication of anti-reflux surgery. During a SG, gastric branches of the vagus nerve can be divided leading to preganglionic afferent and efferent fibre damage. This is usually performed by splitting the stomach longitudinally, damaging the distal portions of the gastric vagal branches [28, 29]. However, it is difficult to determine the extent to which the nerve has been damaged and as such, surgeons must rely on clinical symptoms including nausea, vomiting, and diarrhoea [30–32].

Post-operatively, the stomach may slip into the thoracic cavity leading to a hiatus hernia. Because of the increased esophago-gastric pressure gradient, obese patients are already at an increased risk of developing a hiatus hernia [33]. The increased pressure likely results from the high levels of adipose tissue which provides greater gravitational force on the abdominal cavity. On the other hand, the mechanism for hiatus hernia following SG appears complicated and may be due to a multitude of factors. During creation of the gastric tube, dissection of the angle of His and the left·pillar can increase the risk of herniation. Furthermore, there is an increased risk of herniation in patients who regain weight after SG due to an increased intra-gastric pressure. Notably, the amount of weight that is regained varies substantially, with studies reporting a range of weight gain from between 5.7% at 2 years to 75.6% at 6 years after the operation [34]. Interestingly, studies also suggest that there is no significant difference in the level of ghrelin and leptin in post-operative patients who reported change in appetite and those without any change in their appetite, suggesting hormones may not have a major role in this process [35]. Additionally, in patients who had a retained fundus following a SG, there was no significant difference in the level of weight loss in comparison to those with complete resection of gastric fundus [36]. Nonetheless larger prospective studies will need to be done to conclusively determine the significance of ghrelin in long term weight regain. In the acute phase following the operation however, the rapid weight loss can lead to enlargement of the hiatus orifice and hypotonia of the diaphragm due to muscular depletion, also increasing the risk of a hiatus hernia. However, de novo hiatus hernia following a SG is rarely discussed in literature and understanding more about the pathophysiology of this complication may help us to understand and better manage patients in the future [37].

There is no clear consensus on treatment options for patients who develop symptomatic GERD following bariatric surgery, and a multitude of treatment options are available.

Modification of timing, quantity, and quality of patient's diets, as well as a reduction in smoking and alcohol consumption are well known to reduce the risk of GERD. Items such as coffee, alcohol, chocolate, and mint can reduce lower oesophageal sphincter tone, whereas acidic foods and beverages and spicy foods can cause direct oesophageal mucosal irritation. Large meals and carbonated drinks in particular can lead to increased gastric distention and a greater gastro-oesophageal pressure gradient [38]. On the other hand, smoking decreases the lower oesophageal sphincter pressure and also reduces salivary bicarbonate secretion leading to prolonged acid secretion [39, 40]. Evidence suggests that patients may report a significant decrease in acid reflux, after only 48 hours of not smoking [41].

Reflux tends to occur more frequently in the postprandial state and is largely composed of non-acidic ingested food. This is perhaps the reason for the absence of symptoms and lack of PPI efficacy for managing GERD-related complications [42]. It is clear therefore that the mechanisms underpinning GERD are complex, and the intricate pathophysiology leading to GERD in both obesity as well as a complication of SG can complicate the picture making it difficult to manage these patients. However, use of acid-reducing medications such as proton pump inhibitors or H2-receptor blockers can still be extremely beneficial to patients. Many patients are already likely to be on such medication prior to the surgery because of the association of GERD and obesity. Evidence suggests that less patients will need to continue these medications, although this is dependent on bariatric procedure type. SG appears to have a higher association of post-operative GERD than other bariatric operations [43, 44]. In those who continue to experience GERD symptoms or alternatively experience de-novo GERD symptoms, these medications can be useful in the short term.

3   Management

If symptoms of GERD are present despite maximal medical therapy, invasive therapy options can be considered.

These include converting the SG to a Roux-en-Y gastric bypass. Multiple studies suggest the high success rate with this operation for intractable GERD symptoms after a failed SG [45, 46]. There is evidence suggesting that conversion to Roux-en-Y gastric bypass is superior than conversion to other bariatric operations for managing intractable GERD following a failed SG. Patients can experience further weight-loss with an estimated weight loss of greater than 50% after 2 years when compared with baseline weight [47]. However, this operation carries greater risk than the other options. There is a slightly increased risk of developing a gastro-jejunal anastomotic leak compared to a primary Roux-en-Y bypass (3% vs. 1%) [48]. The increased risk could be due to several reasons including fibrous scar created from the previous SG, fistula development from the first operation, and possible devascularisation to the gastric pouch whilst performing the revision surgery. A late complication of the revision surgery is the formation of a marginal ulcer, although this is a rare occurrence [49]. Because the gastric bypass is a more malabsorptive procedure in comparison to the SG, it can lead to nutritional deficiencies. These can occur despite supplemental nutrition. The extent to the deficiency varies within literature and depends somewhat on the length of the bypass. Nonetheless, patients can be deficient in vitamin B12, Iron, folic acid, vitamin D, vitamin B1 and B6, magnesium, and zinc [50].

The concerning side-effect profile of this revision surgery has led surgeons to proactively seek more innovative solutions to prophylactically prevent reflux symptoms from occurring. Studies have shown that addition of hiatoplasty and 180° cardioplication as an anti-reflux procedure demonstrated improvement in

GERD symptoms. Whilst transient lower oesophageal relaxations is associated with symptoms of GERD, many individuals who are asymptomatic will also experience the relaxations as well [51, 52]. As discussed earlier, they occur primarily as a result of gastric distention, but can also occur following relaxation of the diaphragmatic crura. Vagally stimulated receptors in the fundus in association with oral and pharyngeal contractions can additionally relax the lower oesophagus sphincter [51] and as such the SG in particular can be helpful to prevent this because dissection of the fundus can remove the basis of transient lower oesophageal relaxations. In patients who have their short gastric vessels and associated nerves cut, there are lower rates of relaxation of the lower oesophagus sphincter. However, to obtain the best outcome, the stapling line has to be as close as possible to the oesophageal gastric junction, which has an adverse effect of increasing the risk of fistula development, and also risks damage to the sling fibres of the lower oesophageal sphincter [53]. In this operation, the addition of hiatoplasty, fat pad removal, fixation of the stomach, and cardioplication sufficiently reduced GERD symptoms, and led to a reduction in the number of patients who required the use of PPI medication [54].

Alternatively, another team performed a Nissen SG alongside a SG as a prophylactic measure to prevent GERD [55]. In these patients, an N-sleeve also has an added benefit of lowering leak rate that is achieved by covering the angle of His with the anti-reflux valve and moving the staple line to a region that is more vascularised. The result would lead to a sleeved stomach with an appropriate Nissen valve. Whilst these techniques serve to add to SG procedure, others have tried to modify the gastrectomy itself. Examples include the laparoscopic sleeve-Collis-Nissen gastroplasty [56], a procedure involving a 4 cm gastrotomy of the anterior section of the stomach followed by a gastrogastrostomy and subsequent Nissen fundoplication. The advantages to this include a reduction in the sectors of stomach removed, and because the operation is simpler, it also leads to a reduction in cost, whilst the fundoplication provides additional protection. Other procedures are more creative in their approach including the use of the ligamentum teres. This ordinarily forms the superior border of the suprahepatic ligament, running from the liver to the umbilicus, whilst the hepatic artery provides it with a rich blood supply through small arterial branches. By manipulating the ligamentum teres such that it connects the gastro-oesophageal junction to the left lobe of the liver, it pushes the gastro-oesophageal junction anteriorly, inferiorly and to the right, thus maintaining the angle of His [57].

4   Conclusion

The SG can be viewed as more of an evolution of procedures. It originally began as an open duodenal switch procedure before being modified to an open sleeve gastrectomy and subsequently to a laparoscopic sleeve gastrectomy, taking inspiration from the Magenstrasse and Mill operation along the way [58–61]. However, in its current status, because of the post-operative risk of GERD in SG, there is a need to consent patients about the risk of developing GERD. Additionally, more evidence and international collaborations would help determine which patient groups require counselling and will benefit from novel management to minimise complications.

References

1. Damms-Machado A, Friedrich A, Kramer KM, et al. Pre-and postoperative nutritional deficiencies in obese patients undergoing laparoscopic sleeve gastrectomy. Obes Surg. 2012;22(6).
2. Gagner M, Deitel M, Erickson AL, Crosby RD. Survey on laparoscopic sleeve gastrectomy (LSG) at the fourth international consensus summit on sleeve gastrectomy. Obes Surg. 2013;23(12).
3. Ferrer-Márquez M, Belda-Lozano R, Ferrer-Ayza M. Technical controversies in laparoscopic sleeve gastrectomy. Obes Surg. 2012;22(1).
4. El-Serag HB, Sweet S, Winchester CC, Dent J. Update on the epidemiology of gastro-oesophageal reflux disease: a systematic review. Gut. 2014;63(6):871–80.
5. Himpens J, Dapri G, Cadière GB. A prospective randomized study between laparoscopic gastric banding and laparoscopic isolated sleeve gastrectomy: results after 1 and 3 years. Obes Surg. 2006;16(11).
6. Weiner RA, Weiner S, Pomhoff I, Jacobi C, Makarewicz W, Weigand G. Laparoscopic sleeve gastrectomy-influence of sleeve size and resected gastric volume. Obes Surg. 2007;17(10).
7. Gadiot RP, Biter LU, van Mil S, Zengerink HF, Apers J, Mannaerts GH. Long-term results of laparoscopic sleeve gastrectomy for morbid obesity: 5 to 8-year results. Obes Surg. 2017;27(1):59–63.
8. Yeung KTD, Penney N, Ashrafian L, Darzi A, Ashrafian H. Does sleeve gastrectomy expose the distal esophagus to severe reflux?: A systematic review and meta-analysis. Ann Surg. 2020;271(2):257–65.
9. Wu JC, Mui LM, Cheung CM, Chan Y, Sung JJ. Obesity is associated with increased transient lower esophageal sphincter relaxation. Gastroenterology. 2007;132(3):883–9.
10. Kahrilas PJ, Shi G, Manka M, Joehl RJ. Increased frequency of transient lower esophageal sphincter relaxation induced by gastric distention in reflux patients with hiatal hernia. Gastroenterology. 2000;118(4):688–95.
11. Jaffin BW, Knoepflmacher P, Greenstein R. High prevalence of asymptomatic esophageal motility disorders among morbidly obese patients. Obes Surg. 1999;9(4):390–5.
12. Suter M, Dorta G, Giusti V, Calmes JM. Gastro-esophageal reflux and esophageal motility disorders in morbidly obese patients. Obes Surg. 2004;14(7):959–66.
13. Koppman JS, Poggi L, Szomstein S, Ukleja A, Botoman A, Rosenthal R. Esophageal motility disorders in the morbidly obese population. Surg Endosc. 2007;21(5):761–4.
14. Althuwaini S, Bamehriz F, Aldohayan A, et al. Prevalence and predictors of gastroesophageal reflux disease after laparoscopic sleeve gastrectomy. Obes Surg. 2018;28(4):916–22.
15. Borbely Y, Schaffner E, Zimmermann L, et al. De novo gastroesophageal reflux disease after sleeve gastrectomy: role of preoperative silent reflux. Surg Endosc. 2019;33(3):789–93.
16. Georgia D, Stamatina T, Maria N, et al. 24-h multichannel intraluminal impedance PH-metry 1 year after laparocopic sleeve gastrectomy: an objective assessment of gastroesophageal reflux disease. Obes Surg. 2017;27(3):749–53.
17. Sheppard CE, Sadowski DC, de Gara CJ, Karmali S, Birch DW. Rates of reflux before and after laparoscopic sleeve gastrectomy for severe obesity. Obes Surg. 2015;25(5):763–8.
18. Carabotti M, Silecchia G, Greco F, et al. Impact of laparoscopic sleeve gastrectomy on upper gastrointestinal symptoms. Obes Surg. 2013;23(10):1551–7.

19. Felsenreich DM, Ladinig LM, Beckerhinn P, et al. Update: 10 years of sleeve gastrectomy-the first 103 patients. Obes Surg. 2018;28(11):3586–94.
20. Genco A, Soricelli E, Casella G, et al. Gastroesophageal reflux disease and Barrett's esophagus after laparoscopic sleeve gastrectomy: a possible, underestimated long-term complication. Surg Obes Relat Dis. 2017;13(4):568–74.
21. Soricelli E, Casella G, Baglio G, Maselli R, Ernesti I, Genco A. Lack of correlation between gastroesophageal reflux disease symptoms and esophageal lesions after sleeve gastrectomy. Surg Obes Relat Dis. 2018;14(6):751–6.
22. Gagner M, Hutchinson C, Rosenthal R. Fifth international consensus conference: current status of sleeve gastrectomy. Surg Obes Relat Dis. 2016;12(4):750–6.
23. Zundel N, Hernandez JD, Galvao Neto M, Campos J. Strictures after laparoscopic sleeve gastrectomy. Surg Laparosc Endosc Percutan Tech. 2010;20(3):154–8.
24. Barrett NR. Hiatus hernia. Proc R Soc Med. 1952;45(5):279–86.
25. Barrett NR. Hiatus hernia: a review of some controversial points. Br J Surg. 1954;42(173):231–43.
26. Dick RCS, Hurst A. Chronic peptic ulcer of the oesophagus and its association with congenitally short oesophagus and diaphragmatic hernia. QJM Int J Med. 1942;11(2):105–20.
27. Garay M, Balague C, Rodriguez-Otero C, et al. Influence of antrum size on gastric emptying and weight-loss outcomes after laparoscopic sleeve gastrectomy (preliminary analysis of a randomized trial). Surg Endosc. 2018;32(6):2739–45.
28. Chambers AP, Wilson-Perez HE, McGrath S, et al. Effect of vertical sleeve gastrectomy on food selection and satiation in rats. Am J Physiol Endocrinol Metab. 2012;303(8):E1076–1084.
29. Grayson BE, Fitzgerald MF, Hakala-Finch AP, et al. Improvements in hippocampal-dependent memory and microglial infiltration with calorie restriction and gastric bypass surgery, but not with vertical sleeve gastrectomy. Int J Obes (Lond). 2014;38(3):349–56.
30. Papasavas P. Functional problems following esophageal surgery. Surg Clin North Am. 2005;85(3):525–38.
31. Kozarek RA, Low DE, Raltz SL. Complications associated with laparoscopic anti-reflux surgery: one multispecialty clinic's experience. Gastrointest Endosc. 1997;46(6):527–31.
32. Trus TL, Bax T, Richardson WS, et al. Complications of laparoscopic paraesophageal hernia repair. J Gastrointest Surg. 1997;1(3):221–227; discussion 228.
33. Pandolfino JE, El-Serag HB, Zhang Q, Shah N, Ghosh SK, Kahrilas PJ. Obesity: a challenge to esophagogastric junction integrity. Gastroenterology. 2006;130(3):639–49.
34. Lauti M, Kularatna M, Hill AG, MacCormick AD. Weight regain following sleeve gastrectomy-a systematic review. Obes Surg. 2016;26(6):1326–34.
35. Buzga M, Zavadilova V, Holeczy P, et al. Dietary intake and ghrelin and leptin changes after sleeve gastrectomy. Wideochir Inne Tech Maloinwazyjne. 2014;9(4):554–61.
36. Salamat A, Afrasiabi MR, Lutfi RE. Is a "retained fundus" seen on postoperative upper gastrointestinal series after laparoscopic sleeve gastrectomy predictive of inferior weight loss? Surg Obes Relat Dis. 2017;13(7):1145–51.
37. Amor IB, Debs T, Kassir R, Anty R, Amor VB, Gugenheim J. De novo hiatal hernia of the gastric tube after sleeve gastrectomy. Int J Surg Case Rep. 2015;15:78–80.
38. Newberry C, Lynch K. The role of diet in the development and management of gastroesophageal reflux disease: why we feel the burn. J Thorac Dis. 2019;11(Suppl 12):S1594-s1601.
39. Dennish GW, Castell DO. Inhibitory effect of smoking on the lower esophageal sphincter. N Engl J Med. 1971;284(20):1136–7.
40. Trudgill NJ, Smith LF, Kershaw J, Riley SA. Impact of smoking cessation on salivary function in healthy volunteers. Scand J Gastroenterol. 1998;33(6):568–71.
41. Kadakia SC, Kikendall JW, Maydonovitch C, Johnson LF. Effect of cigarette smoking on gastroesophageal reflux measured by 24-h ambulatory esophageal pH monitoring. Am J Gastroenterol. 1995;90(10):1785–90.

42. Del Genio G, Tolone S, Limongelli P, et al. Sleeve gastrectomy and development of "de novo" gastroesophageal reflux. Obes Surg. 2014;24(1):71–7.
43. Varban OA, Hawasli AA, Carlin AM, et al. Variation in utilization of acid-reducing medication at 1 year following bariatric surgery: results from the Michigan Bariatric Surgery Collaborative. Surg Obes Relat Dis. 2015;11(1):222–8.
44. Barr AC, Frelich MJ, Bosler ME, Goldblatt MI, Gould JC. GERD and acid reduction medication use following gastric bypass and sleeve gastrectomy. Surg Endosc. 2017;31(1):410–5.
45. Poghosyan T, Lazzati A, Moszkowicz D, et al. Conversion of sleeve gastrectomy to Roux-en-Y gastric bypass: an audit of 34 patients. Surg Obes Relat Dis. 2016;12(9):1646–51.
46. Cheung D, Switzer NJ, Gill RS, Shi X, Karmali S. Revisional bariatric surgery following failed primary laparoscopic sleeve gastrectomy: a systematic review. Obes Surg. 2014;24(10):1757–63.
47. Gautier T, Sarcher T, Contival N, Le Roux Y, Alves A. Indications and mid-term results of conversion from sleeve gastrectomy to Roux-en-Y gastric bypass. Obes Surg. 2013;23(2):212–5.
48. Thereaux J, Veyrie N, Barsamian C, et al. Similar postoperative safety between primary and revisional gastric bypass for failed gastric banding. JAMA Surg. 2014;149(8):780–6.
49. Ribeiro-Parenti L, Arapis K, Chosidow D, Marmuse JP. Comparison of marginal ulcer rates between antecolic and retrocolic laparoscopic Roux-en-Y gastric bypass. Obes Surg. 2015;25(2):215–21.
50. Gasteyger C, Suter M, Gaillard RC, Giusti V. Nutritional deficiencies after Roux-en-Y gastric bypass for morbid obesity often cannot be prevented by standard multivitamin supplementation. Am J Clin Nutr. 2008;87(5):1128–33.
51. Mittal RK, Holloway RH, Penagini R, Blackshaw LA, Dent J. Transient lower esophageal sphincter relaxation. Gastroenterology. 1995;109(2):601–10.
52. Dent J, Dodds WJ, Friedman RH, et al. Mechanism of gastroesophageal reflux in recumbent asymptomatic human subjects. J Clin Invest. 1980;65(2):256–67.
53. Braghetto I, Lanzarini E, Korn O, Valladares H, Molina JC, Henriquez A. Manometric changes of the lower esophageal sphincter after sleeve gastrectomy in obese patients. Obes Surg. 2010;20(3):357–62.
54. Santoro S, Lacombe A, Aquino CG, Malzoni CE. Sleeve gastrectomy with anti-reflux procedures. Einstein (Sao Paulo). 2014;12(3):287–94.
55. Nocca D, Skalli EM, Boulay E, Nedelcu M, Michel Fabre J, Loureiro M. Nissen Sleeve (N-Sleeve) operation: preliminary results of a pilot study. Surg Obes Relat Dis. 2016;12(10):1832–7.
56. da Silva LE, Alves MM, El-Ajouz TK, Ribeiro PC, Cruz RJ Jr. Laparoscopic sleeve-Collis-Nissen gastroplasty: a safe alternative for morbidly obese patients with gastroesophageal reflux disease. Obes Surg. 2015;25(7):1217–22.
57. Galvez-Valdovinos R, Cruz-Vigo JL, Marin-Santillan E, Funes-Rodriguez JF, Lopez-Ambriz G, Dominguez-Carrillo LG. Cardiopexy with ligamentum teres in patients with hiatal hernia and previous sleeve gastrectomy: an alternative treatment for gastroesophageal reflux disease. Obes Surg. 2015;25(8):1539–43.
58. Hess DS, Hess DW. Biliopancreatic diversion with a duodenal switch. Obes Surg. 1998;8(3).
59. Johnston D, Dachtler J, Sue-Ling HM, King RFGJ, Martin IG. The magenstrasse and mill operation for morbid obesity. Obes Surg. 2003;13(1).
60. Almogy G, Crookes PF, Anthone GJ. Longitudinal gastrectomy as a treatment for the high-risk super-obese patient. Obes Surg. 2004;14(4).
61. Hamoui N, Anthone GJ, Kaufman HS, Crookes PF. Sleeve gastrectomy in the high-risk patient. Obes Surg. 2006;16(11).

How to Manage Sleeve Complications: Portal/Mesenteric Vein Thrombosis

Noe Rodriguez and Ali Aminian

Porto-mesenteric and splenic vein thrombosis (PMSVT) is a complication that can result in bowel ischemia with subsequent infarction [1], and liver failure that may lead to liver transplantation [2]. PMSVT most commonly involves the main portal vein, superior mesenteric vein, and a splenic vein.

Although as a surgical complication PMSVT has been reported across all spectrums of laparoscopic surgery [3], it has also been notoriously reported after bariatric procedures. Early descriptions followed procedures that distinctly involved ligation and surgical manipulation of major portal tributaries, such as splenectomy, liver transplantation, and portal shunts, suggesting the prominence of local factors. However, it has also been described after surgical procedures that do not inflict injury to the portal system highlighting the role of other factors.

This section reviews the available literature about PMSVT after laparoscopic sleeve gastrectomy. A summary of this complication is provided presenting its incidence and possible etiology, with the description of common clinical presentations and options for diagnosis and treatment, as well as outcomes.

1   Etiology and Risk Factors

The literature recognizes incidence rates of PMSVT after sleeve gastrectomy of 0.3–1% [4–6]. Unfortunately, no systematic analysis has yet elucidated the definitive risk factors for post-sleeve PMSVT, its etiology is deemed

N. Rodriguez · A. Aminian (✉)
Department of General Surgery, Bariatric and Metabolic Institute, Clevland Clinic, Clevland, OH, USA
e-mail: AMINIAA@ccf.org

N. Rodriguez
e-mail: rodriguez.noe@gmail.com

S. Al-Sabah et al. (eds.), *Laparoscopic Sleeve Gastrectomy*,
https://doi.org/10.1007/978-3-030-57373-7_49

multi-factorial. Laparoscopic operative conditions including pneumoperitoneum pressures >15 mm Hg, prolonged reverse Trendelenburg position, and hypercapnia may cause mesenteric vasospasm and subsequently reduce portal blood flow. Tan and coauthors [1] reported intraoperative factors in laparoscopic sleeve gastrectomy noting that prolonged liver retraction, and both mechanical and thermal effects inflicted by electrosurgical devices during takedown of gastroepiploic and short gastric vessels may cause thrombosis and affect venous return from the stomach. Similar local factors are deemed responsible of PMSVT after fundoplication. However, obesity itself is a well-accepted predisposing factor to venous thrombosis by reduction of fibrinolysis, elevation of clotting factor levels, and release of proinflammatory mediators [7]. It is known that surgical interventions and hospitalizations are prothrombotic events. Nevertheless, PMSVT may present even in bariatric patients whose procedures require <35 minutes of operative time and short hospitalizations <2 days. In a cohort of 40 patients undergoing laparoscopic sleeve gastrectomy [8], factor VIII elevation has been described as the most common (76%) hypercoagulable abnormality. Shoar and coauthors [9] assessed systemic risk factors from a meta-analysis of 41 studies including 110 patients with post bariatric PMSVT. Overall, 43% of patients had a known hypercoagulable disorder. The other most commonly inherited risk factors were identified as prothrombin 20210 mutation (10%), protein C deficiency (10%), and protein S deficiency (8%). Other risk factors included factor V Leiden mutation, increased fibrinogen level, Methylenetetrahydrofolate deficiency, the JAK2 mutation, and lupus anticoagulants. Smoking and oral contraceptive pills are established risk factors for development of deep vein thrombosis. Perioperative exposure to them may also increase the risk of PMSVT.

2   Diagnosis

Early diagnosis of PMSVT is an important task for any surgeon participating in the care of bariatric surgery patients. At present, the most valuable tool for diagnosis remains a high index of clinical suspicion. The majority of patients with PMSVT only present vague symptoms with median time to diagnosis of 13 days (interquartile range, 5–25) following bariatric surgery, although some patients may present several years after surgery.

PMSVT most common symptoms are abdominal pain (83%), nausea and vomiting (38%). Other, less common symptoms include fever (13%), sepsis (8%), GI bleeding, shoulder tip pain, and diarrhea (Fig. 1).

Laboratory results are of limited diagnostic utility. For example, leukocytosis is present in 20%, and elevated erythrocyte sedimentation rate and C-reactive protein in 10% of patients.

In most patients, the diagnosis of acute PMSVT can be established using noninvasive imaging. Ultrasonography can show hyperechoic material in the vessel lumen with distention of the portal vein and its tributaries. Doppler imaging shows partial or complete absence of flow. A CT scan without contrast can show hyperattenuating material in the portal vein. However, the first line diagnostic entity with

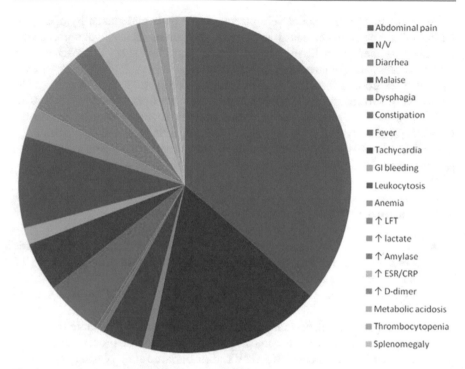

Fig. 1 Presentations of PMSVT after bariatric surgery. Adapted from [9]

a sensitivity of 90% is a CT scan with intravenous contrast that reveals lack of intraluminal enhancement and a pattern that may involve thrombosis of the main portal vein, superior mesenteric vein, and splenic vein vessels [10]. Thrombosis commonly occludes the involved vessels, rarely causing changes in the intestinal wall or lack of mucosal enhancement of a thickened intestinal wall suggestive of intestinal infarction. This involvement pattern can be attributed to the proximity of the affected vessels to the anatomic region of the procedure.

3   Management

Anticoagulation therapy is the first treatment option at present. The current guidelines suggest that anticoagulation therapy should be started promptly after the diagnosis of PMSVT [11, 12]. When possible, any predisposing conditions should also be treated to ensure the persistence of recanalization and to avoid future recurrence. A metanalysis of 41 included studies [9] points out that in practice, treatment ranges from the use of unfractionated heparin to bowel resection and liver transplantation in rare cases. Unfractionated heparin (59%), vitamin K antagonists (51%), and low-molecular weight heparin (39%) were the most common treatment options for PMSVT. Other antithrombotic modalities including factor Xa inhibitors (6%) and thrombolysis (4%) are less often used.

Attempts to establish portal vein patency have been undertaken by open portal thrombectomy, percutaneous transhepatic, and percutaneous jugular portal vein thrombolytic therapy with AngioJet suction of the clot. These approaches have limited success and are now rarely attempted.

Bowel resection and splenectomy may be required in 20% and 2% of patients, respectively. Orthotopic liver transplantation has also been reported in 3% of patients as the final treatment option for refractory ascites secondary to chronic PMSVT [2]. The types and invasiveness of therapeutic interventions depends on the timing of PMSVT after bariatric surgery, the extent of the thrombosis, and the severity of the ischemic damage to the gastrointestinal organs (Fig. 2).

4   Summary

- As more patients are successfully treated for severe obesity through bariatric surgery and especially laparoscopic sleeve gastrectomy, we can expect PMSVT cases to occur in the coming years.
- PMSVT is a rare complication but increases the mortality of bariatric surgery 40 times higher.
- Similar to gastroesophageal reflux disease (GERD), PMSVT is more frequently seen after sleeve gastrectomy compared with other bariatric procedures.
- About half of reported cases of PMSVT after bariatric surgery had hypercoagulable state. In patients with congenital or acquired hypercoagulable state, bariatric procedures other than sleeve gastrectomy can be suggested.
- The current incidence of PMSVT is similar to the incidence of gastric leak after sleeve gastrectomy. While we always think about the leak, we usually do not consider PMSVT in our differential diagnosis in patients who develop adverse events after sleeve gastrectomy.
- In any patient who develops abdominal pain, fever, prolonged vomiting, GI bleeding, tachycardia, leukocytosis, abnormal liver function tests, or elevated pancreatic enzymes in days or weeks after sleeve gastrectomy, we should perform CT scan to rule out PMSVT.
- In most cases with early diagnosis, anticoagulation for 3–6 months is the appropriate treatment.
- Preventive measures to decrease the risk of PMSVT would include:
  - Stop smoking 2–3 months before sleeve gastrectomy
  - Stop oral contraceptive pills 4-weeks before and after sleeve gastrectomy
  - Perioperative thromboprophylaxis
  - Hydration
  - Suppress nausea and vomiting
  - Liberal use of extended thromboprophylaxis after hospital discharge (in high risk patients or patients with hypercoagulable state) [13]

- Patient and physician education may assist in screening, treating, and thus avoiding PMSVT.

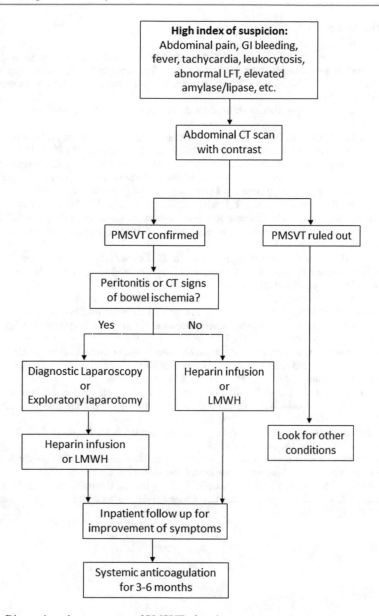

Fig. 2 Diagnosis and management of PMSVT after sleeve gastrectomy

References

1. Tan SBM, Greenslade J, Martin D, Talbot M, Loi K, Hopkins G. Portomesenteric vein thrombosis in sleeve gastrectomy: a 10-year review. Surg Obes Relat Dis. 2018;14(3):271–5.
2. Danion J, Genser L, Scatton O. Sleeve gastrectomy: you might lose your liver! Obes Surg. 2019;29(1):350–2.
3. James AW. Portomesenteric venous thrombosis after laparoscopic surgery. Arch Surg. 2009;144(6):520.
4. Goitein D, Matter I, Raziel A, Keidar A, Hazzan D, Rimon U, Sakran N. Portomesenteric thrombosis following laparoscopic bariatric surgery. JAMA Surg. 2013;148(4):340.
5. Alsina E, Ruiz-Tovar J, Alpera MR, Ruiz-Garcia JG, Lopez-Perez ME, Ramon-Sanchez JF, Ardoy F. Incidence of deep vein thrombosis and thrombosis of the portal-mesenteric axis after laparoscopic sleeve gastrectomy. J Laparoendosc Adv Surg Tech A. 2014;24(9):601–5.
6. Berger ER, Huffman KM, Fraker T, Petrick AT, Brethauer SA, Hall BL, Ko CY, Morton JM. Prevalence and risk factors for bariatric surgery readmissions: findings from 130,007 admissions in the metabolic and bariatric surgery accreditation and quality improvement program. Ann Surg. 2018;267(1):122–31.
7. Cottam DR, Mattar SG, Barinas-Mitchell E, Eid G, Kuller L, Kelley DE, Schauer PR. The chronic inflammatory hypothesis for the morbidity associated with morbid obesity: implications and effects of weight loss. Obes Surg. 2004;14(5):589–600.
8. Parikh M, Adelsheimer A, Somoza E, Saunders JK, Ude Welcome A, Chui P, Ren-Fielding C, Kurian M, Fielding G, Chopra A, et al. Factor VIII elevation may contribute to portomesenteric vein thrombosis after laparoscopic sleeve gastrectomy: a multicenter review of 40 patients. Surg Obes Relat Dis. 2017;13(11):1835–9.
9. Shoar S, Saber AA, Rubenstein R, Safari S, Brethauer SA, Al-Thani H, Asarian AP, Aminian A. Portomesentric and splenic vein thrombosis (PMSVT) after bariatric surgery: a systematic review of 110 patients. Surg Obes Relat Dis. 2018;14(1):47–59.
10. Dane B, Clark J, Megibow A. Multidetector computed tomography evaluation of mesenteric venous thrombosis following laparoscopic bariatric surgery. J Comput Assist Tomogr. 2017;41(1):56–60.
11. DeLeve LD, Valla DC, Garcia-Tsao G. American association for the study liver D: vascular disorders of the liver. Hepatology. 2009;49(5):1729–64.
12. European Association for the Study of the Liver. Electronic address eee: EASL clinical practice guidelines: vascular diseases of the liver. J Hepatol. 2016;64(1):179–202.
13. Aminian A, Andalib A, Khorgami Z, Cetin D, Burguera B, Bartholomew J, Brethauer SA, Schauer PR. Who should get extended thromboprophylaxis after bariatric surgery? Ann Surg. 2017;265(1):143–50.

How to Manage Sleeve Complications: Neuropathy

Jasem Yousef AL-Hashel and Ismail Ibrahim Ismail

1   Introduction

Obesity rates has nearly tripled since the 1970s reaching pandemic proportions. According to the World Health Organization (WHO) estimates in 2016, more than 1.9 billion adults, 18 years and older, were overweight of which over 650 million were obese [1].

Obesity, if untreated, is associated with higher rates of numerous comorbidities, including hypertension, diabetes mellitus, osteoarthritis, obstructive sleep apnea, intracranial hypertension, infertility, certain types of cancers, as well as associated nutritional deficiencies [2].

One of the most effective treatments for obesity is bariatric surgery, because of its efficient and sustained results. There is a growing evidence to support its effectiveness in reducing morbidity and mortality for patients with BMI >40 and for those with BMI >35 and obesity- related complications [3].

Bariatric restrictive surgeries, such as sleeve gastrectomy (SG) and gastric banding, have been widely used to manage morbid obesity. SG has recently gained popularity as the leading bariatric procedure for the treatment of morbid obesity. It generates weight loss solely through restriction of stomach size. Although these surgeries are known to cause less metabolic derangements than malabsorptive surgeries (e.g. gastric bypass), it was also associated with a rise in the incidence of neurological complications [4].

J. Y. AL-Hashel (✉)
Faculty of Medicine, Department of Medicine, Kuwait University, Kuwait City, Kuwait
e-mail: jasemkumsa@hotmail.com

J. Y. AL-Hashel · I. I. Ismail
Department of Neurology, Ibn Sina Hospital, Safat, Kuwait
e-mail: dr.ismail.ibrahim2012@gmail.com

© The Editor(s) (if applicable) and The Author(s), under exclusive license to Springer   523
Nature Switzerland AG 2021
S. Al-Sabah et al. (eds.), *Laparoscopic Sleeve Gastrectomy*,
https://doi.org/10.1007/978-3-030-57373-7_50

Peripheral neuropathy is a one of the common complications following any type of bariatric surgery affecting 5–16% of patients. It is a collection of disorders arising from damage in the somatosensory system. It usually presents years later and progress insidiously but may be seen early in the course following SG. Symptoms involve distal, painful paresthesias "burning feet syndrome" and loss of pinprick and temperature sensation. Patterns have included sensory-predominant polyneuropa- thy, motor-predominant polyneuropathy, sensory motor polyneuropathy, mononeuropathy, and radiculoneuropathy. The polyneuropathies typically described are length dependent with an axonal pathophysiology. Mononeuropathy is also a documented after bariatric surgery with carpal tunnel syndrome being the most common. Less common are ulnar neuropathy at the elbow, radial mononeuropathy and peroneal neuropathy and lateral femoral cutaneous neuropathy have also been reported [5, 6].

However, despite the fact that most cases of neuropathy post-gastric bypass procedures are nutritional, this is not the case with SG. It is not commonly associated with malabsorption and it is important for physicians dealing with bariatric surgery patients to differentiate between those two types of surgeries as they have different mechanisms for neuropathy [7].

Available data in literature addressing peripheral neuropathy following SG are limited and consists mainly of case series and case reports. A wide spectrum of clinical presentations can ensue, with both acute and chronic neuropathies. Tabbara et al. reported only 1.18% of 592 SG cases to present with neurological complications. Symptoms included motor and sensory deficits with absence of deep tendon reflexes of the lower limbs and in some cases. All patients had uneventful post-operative course, but all had feeding difficulties, accompanied by severe dysphagia, and rapid weight loss, with a mean weight loss of 35 kg (30–40 kg) 3 months after SG. All patients were treated for neuropathy secondary to vitamin B1 deficiency and had a significant improvement and resolution of their symptoms [8]. Abarbanel et al. described neurological complications after gastric restrictive surgery in 4.6% of their 500 patients in 3–20 months period. Their symptoms included chronic or subacute symmetric polyneuropathy, acute severe polyneuropathy, burning feet syndrome, myotonic syndrome, myelopathy, and Wernicke-Korsakoff encephalopathy [9].

Another study reported that seven out of 635 SG patients developed foot drop as a result of peroneal nerve entrapment neuropathy (PNEN). It was attributed to rapid weight loss as patients had no nutritional deficiencies [10].

Peripheral neuropathy following SG can be attributed to several factors. First, obese patients tend to have a presurgical baseline deficiencies of several micronutrients. Second, gastrointestinal symptoms postoperatively including dysphagia, gastro-esophageal reflux and recurrent vomiting. Third, rapid and excessive weight loss within the first 3 months after SG. Fourth, postoperatively they tend to have poor nutritional habits including inadequate vitamin supplementation, poor food choices, limited portion sizes or food intolerance [11].

In several case series, the neurological complications after SG were attributed to vitamin storage depletion. In a study of 112 SG patients, vitamin and nutritional deficiencies appeared to be a common phenomenon and was corrected with the deficiencies before surgery, insufficient supplementation immediately after the procedure, and lack of routine long follow-up [12]. Another study of 32 patients from Kuwait, post-SG neuropathy was associated with older age, low levels of vitamin B1, B2, and copper and high vitamin B6 levels, which at toxic levels, can be associated with neuropathy [13]. SG limits the production of intrinsic factor by removing part of the stomach, therefore, can also lead to vitamin B12 deficiency [13].

2   Management

Education is of utmost importance to patients undergoing bariatric surgery and should be done regularly. The potential risks of each SG should be clearly explained to the patients before undergoing this type of surgery. Early identification of neurological symptoms after the surgery and early intervention may help reduce the occurrence of these complications. A multidisciplinary approach (surgery, endocrinology, neurology, nutrition and physiotherapy) with careful nutritional monitoring at regular intervals is crucial in all patients for early diagnosis and management of these complications [14, 15].

The American Society for Metabolic and Bariatric Surgery (ASMBS) recommends presurgical screening for levels of vitamins B1, B12, folate, iron, calcium, zinc, copper and fat-soluble vitamins (A, D, E, K). It also further recommends nutrient assessment every 3–6 months in the first postoperative year. ASMBS recommends micronutrient supplementation for all patients following bariatric surgery [15, 16].

All patients with neurological complications should be readmitted to the hospital for evaluation. They should undergo full gastrointestinal work-up to rule out functional stenosis. All patients should do vitamin measurements (vitamins B1, B6, B9, B12, and D) at the time of presentation with neurological complications and before beginning vitamin supplementation. All patients should be evaluated by a neurologist. A thorough clinical examination must be performed. Electrophysiological studies (nerve conduction study and electromyography) are needed to confirm the presence of axonal peripheral polyneuropathy [17].

Treatment consists of aggressive multivitamin and mineral replacement therapy. Treatment is usually achieved by parenteral administration of vitamin B1, B6, B12, fat-soluble vitamins (A, D, E and K), folate, iron, copper, zinc and selenium. Several regimens and guidelines are available but the information is mostly empiric rather than evidence-based.

Vitamin B1 standard dose of 100 mg intravenously daily may not improve thiamine status or the clinical picture and a more aggressive dose of 500 mg IV three times a day for 2–3 days can be given, then 250 mg IV daily until improvement is seen, followed by an oral dose of 50–100 mg three times a day thereafter [Class IV]. Vitamin B12 dose is 1,000 μg per day for a week (either intramuscularly or deeply subcutaneous), followed by 1,000 μg weekly for 1 month then every month is suggested [Class IV]. Copper replacement is 6 mg per day for a week, 4 mg per day the next week, and 2 mg daily thereafter. If oral replacement fails to increase copper levels, then IV replacement at a dose of 2 mg per day for 5 days (repeated as necessary) is suggested [Class IV]. Vitamin D dose is 3000–6000 IU of D3 daily (preferred), or 50,000 IU of D2 1–3 times per week. Vitamin E dose is 90–300 mg (100–400 IU) daily. Folate is given in a 1000 mcg dose daily until the level is normalized, then maintenance dose (400–800 mcg daily) is resumed.

Iron can be given orally in a dose of 150–300 mg 2–3 times a day. Parenteral iron can be given to those who do not respond to oral supplementation. Zinc optimal repletion dose is unknown. Caution must be taken from overdose as it can be associated with toxicity or copper deficiency. Calcium dose is 1200–1500 mg daily in divided doses. Selenium role is unclear but can be in patients who develop cardiomyopathy rather than neuropathy in a dose of 2 mcg/kg/day. Patients should continue on oral multivitamin supplementations after discharge from the hospital [18–20].

In conclusion, peripheral neuropathy after SG is not uncommon and can be prevented by avoiding rapid and/or excessive weight loss, regular counseling and follow-ups with a nutritionist, adequately treating recurrent vomiting and oral multivitamin and mineral supplementations.

References

1. Arroyo-Johnson C, Mincey KD. Obesity epidemiology worldwide. Gastroenterol Clin North Am. 2016;45:571–9. https://doi.org/10.1016/j.gtc.2016.07.012.
2. WHO. Obesity: preventing and managing the global epidemic. Report of a WHO Consultation. WHO Technical Report Series 894. Geneva: World Health Organization; 2000.
3. Chang SH. The effectiveness and risks of bariatric surgery: an updated systematic review and meta-analysis, 2003–2012. JAMA Surg. 2014;149:275–87.
4. Ismail II, Yassin OM, Foad SS. Copper deficiency myeloneuropathy mimicking subacute combined degeneration following bariatric surgery. J Neurol Neurol Disord. 2014;1(1):104. https://doi.org/10.15744/2454-4981.1.104.
5. Thaisetthawatkul P, Collazo-Clavell ML, Sarr MG, Norell JE, Dyck PJB. A controlled study of peripheral neuropathy after bariatric surgery. Neurology. 2004;63(8):1462–70.
6. Clark N. Neuropathy following bariatric surgery. Semin Neurol. 2010;30(4):433–5.
7. Skroubis G, Sakellaropoulos G, Pouggouras K, et al. Comparison of nutritional deficiencies after Roux-en-Y gastric bypass and after biliopancreatic diversion with Roux-en-Y gastric bypass. Obes Surg. 2002;12:12551–8.
8. Tabbara M, Carandina S, Bossi M, et al. Rare neurological complications after sleeve gastrectomy. Obes Surg. 2016;26(12):2843–8.
9. Abarbanel JM, Berginer VM, Osimani A, et al. Neurologic complications after gastric restriction surgery for morbid obesity. Neurology. 1987;37(2):196–200.
10. Şen O, Karaca FC, Türkçapar A. Neurological complication after laparoscopic sleeve gastrectomy: foot drop. Obes Surg. 2019. https://doi.org/10.1007/s11695-019-04285-6.
11. Kröll D, Laimer M, Borbély YM, Laederach K, Candinas D, Nett PC. Wernicke encephalopathy: a future problem even after sleeve gastrectomy? A systematic literature review. Obes Surg. 2015.
12. Al-Mulhim AS. Laparoscopic sleeve gastrectomy and nutrient deficiencies: a prospective study. Surg Laparosc Endosc Percutan Tech. 2016;26(3):208–11.

13. Alsabah A, Al Sabah S, Al-Sabah S, et al. Investigating factors involved in post laparoscopic sleeve gastrectomy (LSG) neuropathy. Obes Surg. 2016;26(10):23027. https://doi.org/10.1007/s11695-016-2119-y.

14. Algahtani HA, Khan AS, Khan MA, Aldarmahi AA, Lodhi Y. Neurological complications of bariatric surgery. Neurosciences (Riyadh). 2016;21(3):241–5. https://doi.org/10.17712/nsj.2016.3.20160039.

15. Parrott J, Frank L, Rabena R, Craggs-Dino L, Isom KA, Greiman L. American society for metabolic and bariatric surgery integrated health nutritional guidelines for the surgical weight loss patient 2016 Update: micronutrients. Surg Obes Relat Dis. 2017;13:727–41.

16. English WJ, DeMaria EJ, Brethauer SA, et al. American society for metabolic and bariatric surgery estimation of metabolic and bariatric procedures performed in the United States in 2016. Surg Obes Relat Dis. 2018;14(3):259–63.

17. van Rutte PW, Aarts EO, Smulders JF, et al. Nutrient deficiencies before and after sleeve gastrectomy. Obes Surg. 2014;24(10):1639–46.

18. Stein J, Stier C, Raab H, Weiner R. Review article: The nutritional and pharmacological consequences of obesity surgery. Aliment Pharmacol Ther. 2014;40:582.

19. Juhasz-Pocsine K, Rudnicki SA, Archer RL, Harik SI. Neurologic complications of gastric bypass surgery for morbid obesity. Neurology. 2007;68(21):1843–50.

20. Rashad HM, Youssry D, Mansour DF, et al. Post-bariatric surgery peripheral neuropathies: Kuwaiti experience. Egypt J Neurol Psychiatry Neurosurg. 2019;55:22. https://doi.org/10.1186/s41983-019-0064-0.

Revisional Surgery

Revisional Surgery: Sleeve to SADI

C. Sanchez-del-Pueblo, A. Ruano, A. Sánchez-Pernaute
and A. Torres

1   Introduction

Sleeve gastrectomy (SG) is a highly effective stand-alone surgical procedure for morbidly obese patients and an adequate operation as a first step for super-obese patients or high-risk patients. However, long-term results indicate that up to 70% of patients present with insufficient weight loss despite proper preoperative management [1].

If weight loss after SG is inadequate, or the patient regains weight, there are different surgical options available as a revisional surgery, such as re-sleeve, sleeve plication, banding of the sleeve, gastric bypass (GB), or duodenal switch (BPD-DS) [2, 3]. For insufficient weight loss in a patient with a correct sleeve anatomy, in our department we normally opt for a malabsorptive procedure, especially if the patient was initially super-obese, as it offers the best weight loss for this subset of patients. Laparoscopic single-anastomosis duodeno-ileal bypass with sleeve gastrectomy (SADI-S) was first described in our department in 2007 as a simplified BPD-DS that has achieved satisfactory short and long-term results [4]. This was carried out by practicing a vertical gastrectomy as a restrictive procedure with pyloric preservation, followed by an end-to-side duodeno-ileal anastomosis in the first duodenal portion, beyond the pylorus (Fig. 1). Since its development, SADI-S procedure has offered good results for the treatment of both morbid obesity and its metabolic complications [5–7]. Initially, the procedure was performed with a 200 cm common limb. The initial series of 50 patients achieved excellent weight loss results after 3 years of follow-up. However, nearly 5% of the patients

C. Sanchez-del-Pueblo · A. Ruano · A. Sánchez-Pernaute · A. Torres (✉)
Department of Surgery, Complutense University of Madrid. Hospital Clinico San Carlos.
IdISSC, Madrid, Spain
e-mail: ajtorresgarcia@gmail.com

S. Al-Sabah et al. (eds.), *Laparoscopic Sleeve Gastrectomy*,
https://doi.org/10.1007/978-3-030-57373-7_51

Fig. 1 SADI-S

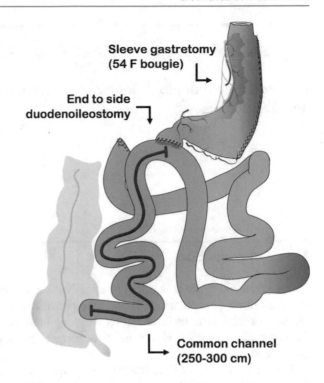

had to be submitted to reoperation for persistent diarrhoea or malabsorption, and so in 2009 the length of the common limb was modified to 250 cm.

Two years later, after demonstrating outstanding results as a primary restrictive and metabolic procedure, we decided to introduce single-anastomosis duodeno-ileal bypass (SADI) as a second step after SG for insufficient weight loss or as a scheduled second-step surgery in super-obese patients, regardless of satisfactory weight loss at 12 months from SG. SADI was performed as a revisional surgery in those patients without problems derived from the SG and without any accompanying conditions contraindicating a malabsorptive procedure.

2   Patient Preparation

Patients are thoroughly evaluated before surgery by a team of specialized endocrinologists, surgeons and anesthetists, and they undergo a number of tests including an upper gastrointestinal endoscopy, barium swallow, chest X-ray, electrocardiogram, and blood tests. Respiratory function tests and psychiatric evaluation is also performed. Before the intervention, endocrinologists recommend a healthy, low-calorie diet. Patients are encouraged to lose as much weight as possible and to start a healthy lifestyle, as this will not only reduce the possibility of postoperative complications, but it will also improve results.

3 Surgical Technique

3.1 Position of the Patient and the Surgical Team

For SG the operating table is placed in anti-Trendelenburg position. The surgeon is positioned between the legs of the patient, the first assistant on the patient´s left side, holding the camera, and the second assistant on the patient´s right side, holding the liver retractor (Fig. 2).

For the second part of the surgery, the duodeno-ileal by-pass, the position is changed. The patient is placed horizontally and the surgeon moves from the initial position between the legs towards the left side of the patient, as well as the camera assistant, who will introduce the laparoscope through the left subcostal trocar, leaving the supraumbilical and right midline trocars as working trocars (Fig. 3).

3.2 Trocar Position

The standard laparoscopic approach for both procedures is performed by placing the same four trocars. A 10–12 mm optical trocar (Optiview) is inserted above the umbilicus, slightly left from the midline, and pneumoperitoneum is applied. A 10–12 mm left subcostal trocar and a 5 mm trocar in a subxiphoid position are placed. Also, a 10–12 mm trocar is placed right from the midline position.

Fig. 2 SG trocar and surgical team positioning

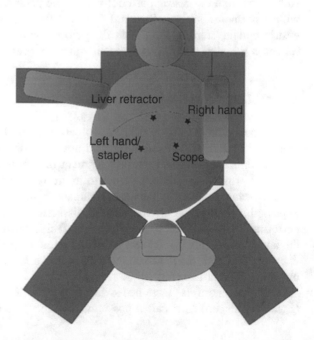

Fig. 3 SADI surgical team
positioning

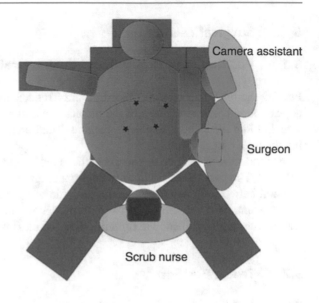

Camera assistant

Surgeon

Scrub nurse

4   Procedures

4.1   Sleeve Gastrectomy

Complete devascularization of the greater gastric curvature is performed.
Adhesions from the gastric posterior wall to the pancreatic surface are also divided
with a harmonic scalpel. Standard SG is then performed over a 42–54-French
gastric bougie, starting 5 cm from the pylorus, with a black plated linear stapler
(Echelon Ethicon), reinforced with Seamguard (Gore) sheets.

4.2   Duodeno-Ileal Bypass

After a complete evaluation of the abdomen, the distal end of the previous sleeve
is identified, and with the stomach held upwards, dissection of the greater curvature is completed down to the first segment of the duodenum. The duodenum is
dissected proximally, taking care not to injure the right gastric artery. The peritoneum overlying the hepatoduodenal ligament is slightly opened and a vessel loop
is passed posteriorly. A circumferential dissection of the first duodenal portion is
performed, 3–4 cm distal to the pylorus, to facilitate an adequate mobilization and
the anastomosis (Fig. 4). Dissection of the duodenum from the pancreatic surface
is carried out until the pancreatoduodenal groove is reached and the gastroduodenal artery is identified (Fig. 5).

The duodenum is sectioned with a 60 mm blue cartridge linear stapler
(Echelon Ethicon) as distal as possible from the pylorus. The ileo-cecal valve is

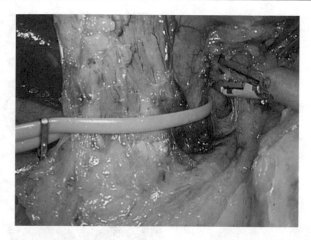

Fig. 4 Verticalized duodenum and circumferential dissection of the first portion

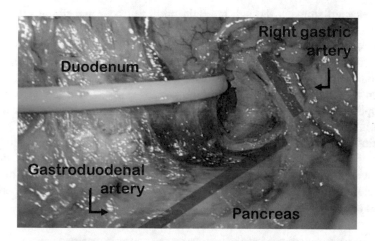

Fig. 5 Gastroduodenal and right gastric arteries

identified and 250–300 cm are measured upwards. In special situations, such as aged patients, patients with low BMI or liver or bowel diseases, 300 cm is the preferred length of the common limb to avoid important nutritional complications. Measurement of the bowel is performed, stretching the loops at 10 cm intervals and after infusion of hyoscine butylbromide (Buscapin) to completely relax the bowel wall and obtain the maximum possible length. The selected loop is ascended in an ante-colic fashion, and an end-to-side, double-layer, hand-sewn anastomosis to the proximal duodenal stump is carried out with running sutures of V-Loc 3/0 (Covidien) and PDS 3/0 (Johnson & Johnson) (Fig. 6).

Both SG staple line and duodeno-ileal anastomosis are checked for leaks by oral introduction of methylene blue. The surgery is completed with the removal

Fig. 6 Duodeno-ileal
anastomosis

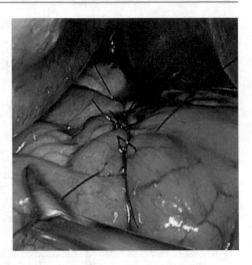

of the resected stomach through the right midline trocar and the placement of a vacuum drain.

The patient is taken to a post-anaesthesia recovery unit for immediate postoperative care. Six to eight hours postoperatively the patient begins oral intakes of water on the surgical ward, starting with a low caloric liquid diet the following day. On the second day after surgery the patient starts with a low-caloric shake diet (Optifast). The abdominal drain is removed on the third postoperative day and patient is discharged the next day if postoperative course is uneventful.

During follow-up, for the first postoperative month, patients follow a low-caloric diet based on self-prepared shakes. Multivitamin supplements, calcium and iron are initially prescribed and maintained depending on the results of subsequent blood tests. The patient will continue with periodical visits to the endocrinologist and the surgeon.

5 Results

Torres et al. have recently published their results with SADI as a revisional procedure [8]. Over the last 10 years, 49 patients (34 women and 15 men, mean age 42 years) have been submitted to SADI as a revisional surgery after a SG in our department. Their mean initial weight was 141 kg (99–216) and their mean initial BMI was 52 kg/m^2 (36–71); 75% of patients were initially super-obese patients. Mean maximum excess weight loss (EWL) following SG was 63% (34–113) in the first postoperative year (4–24 months). Mean time between the first and second surgery was 34 months (11–111). Mean EWL was 43% (20–70) when performing SADI. In 70% of patients the common limb was 250 cm long, and in

Fig. 7 EWL% after SG and after SADI as a revisional surgery

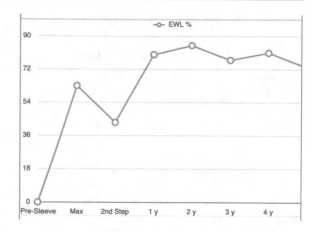

Table 1 Evolution of type 2 diabetes after SG and SADI

	Pre-sleeve	After sleeve	After SADI
Glycemia (mg/dl)	171	140	92,7
HbA1c (%)	8,15	7,2	5,2
Off therapy (%)	26	60	92

the other 30% its length was 300 cm. In three cases, re-sleeve over a 54-French bougie was also performed during revisional surgery. No postoperative complications were encountered and mean hospital stay was 4 days long.

EWL was 80% at one year after revisional surgery, 85% at two years, 77% at three years, 81% at four years, and 73% at 5 years (Fig. 7). During follow-up, one patient was reoperated on to undergo reversion of the procedure due to liver failure; she had an underlying liver cirrhosis due to HVC infection. Two patients were submitted to trimming of previous sleeve in a third procedure due to insufficient weight loss.

Forty-five percent of our patients had type-2 diabetes mellitus (DM2), 30% of them were under insulin therapy. Diabetes improved considerably following SG with an important reduction in mean glycemia and HbA1c of patients. Moreover, outstanding results were observed after revisional surgery, with normalization of mean levels of HbA1c and glycemia (Table 1).

All patients after SADI received different postoperative supplements *to* meet their daily requisite of vitamins after surgery and to prevent nutritional deficiencies from occurring. I is important to take this into account in an adequate follow-up. Blood tests during follow-up demonstrated deficiencies in the red series, iron, vitamin D, and some micronutrients (Table 2). Many of these parameters worsen after SADI in spite of correct supplementation.

Table 2 Comparison between blood test parameters preoperatively, after SG and after SADI

	Preoperative		After sleeve		After SADI	
	Mean	Abnormal (%)	Mean	Abnormal (%)	Mean	Abnormal (%)
Hemoglobin	13,8	18	14,3	3	12,5	39
Hematocrit	41,9	9	41,7	0	38,1	35
Iron	67,7	5,5	89,3	11	65	32
Calcium	9,5	5	9,5	0	8,9	0
Parathormone	74,6	50	62,4	39	95,7	57
Vitamin D	16,8	73	21,4	52	24,9	62
Copper	140	0	129	0	99	20
Zinc	85	0	83	0	59	52
Selenium	83	0	78	0	99	20
Proteins	7,2	5	7,08	0	6,4	9
Albumin	4,1	9	4,1	3	3,8	41

6   Conclusions

In our series, outstanding weight loss results after the second-step procedure were seen, ranging from SADI as a revisional procedure after Sleeve Gastrectomy gets an outstanding weight loss, ranging from an initial 43% EWL after SG to a final 73% EWL after SADI. Comorbidities were successfully controlled after revisional surgery. These results are similar to those published in other series such as the one studied by Balibrea et al. [9], where an %EWL and a BMI at 24 months of 78.93% and 28.64 kg/m^2, respectively, were encountered.

SG was born as the first step of BPD-DS. BPD-DS has been the recommendation of many surgeons because most of the patients submitted to a second-step procedure after SG had initially been super-obese, and so BPD-like operations, such as SADI, exhibit better long-term metabolic results in this subset of patients.

This weight loss is comparable to that obtained 1–2 years after re-sleeve or Roux-en-Y gastric bypass (RYGBP) in the literature. In fact, as stated in Dijkhorst's study, 72% of RYGB patients regained part of their lost weight 2 years after revisional surgery; as opposed to SADI patients, who seemed to progressively keep losing weight during this time span [10]. Another important finding in this study was the comparable rate of complications following SADI and RYGB.

The rates of comorbidity resolution, especially DM2, were more than satisfactory. This has been studied by Balibrea et al., where 71.4% patients showed complete remission of DM2. Dyslipidemia disappeared in 31.2% and improved in 25% of patients. High blood pressure remission and improvement rates were 27.7 and 22.2%, respectively.

An important concern associated with malabsorptive procedures, such as a SADI, is an increase in the occurrence of nutritional deficiencies. In Ceha's study, it appeared that SADI leads to an equal remission of comorbidities, fewer vitamin deficiencies and fewer complications [11]. Moreover, Dijkhort found similar amount of nutritional deficiencies between the two procedures, likely related to sufficient supplementation.

SADI offers satisfactory metabolic results for those patients submitted previously to a SG. It is a simplified technique with satisfactory weight loss, low postoperative complication rates and acceptable nutritional deficiency parameters, and should be considered as an adequate revisional technique after SG.

References

1. Himpens J, Dobbeleir J, Peeters G. Long-term results of laparoscopic sleeve gastrectomy for obesity. Ann Surg. 2010;252:319–24.
2. Deitel M, Gagner M, Erickson AL, Crosby RD. Third International Summit: current status of sleeve gastrectomy. Surg Obes Relat Dis. 2011;7:749–59.
3. Magee CJ, Barry J, Arumugasamy M, et al. Laparoscopic sleeve gastrectomy for high-risk patients: weight loss and comorbidity improvement—short-term results. Obes Surg. 2011;21(5):547–605.
4. Sanchez-Pernaute A, et al. Proximal duodenal-ileal end-to-side bypass with sleeve gastrectomy: proposed technique. Obes Surg. 2007;17(15):1614–8.
5. Sanchez-Pernaute A, et al. Single Anastomosis Duodeno–Ileal Bypass with Sleeve Gastrectomy (SADI-S). One to three-year follow-up. Obes Surg. 2010;20:1720–26.
6. Sanchez-Pernaute A, et al. Single- anastomosis duodenoileal bypass with sleeve gas- trectomy: metabolic improvement and weight loss in first 100 patients. Surg Obes Relat Dis. 2013;9(5):731–5.
7. Sanchez-Pernaute A, et al. Single- anastomosis duodenoileal by- pass with sleeve gastrectomy (SADI-S) for obese diabetic patients. Surg Obes Relat Dis. 2015;11(5):1092–8.
8. Josa Martinez BM, et al. Single anastomosis duodenoileal bypass (SADI-S) as a second step procedure after a sleeve gastrectomy. Bariátrica & Metabólica Ibero-Americana. 2017;7.4.11:1941–45.
9. Balibrea JM, Vilallonga R, Hidalgo M, Ciudin A, González Ó, Caubet E, et al. Mid-term results and responsiveness predictors after two-step single-anastomosis duodeno-ileal bypass with sleeve gastrectomy. Obes Surg. 2016;27(5):1302–8.
10. Dijkhorst PJ, Boerboom AB, Janssen IMC. Failed sleeve gastrectomy: single anastomosis duodenoileal bypass or Roux-en-Y gastric bypass? A multicenter cohort study. Obes Surg. 2018;28:3834–42.
11. Ceha CMM, et al. Matched short-term results of SADI versus GBP after sleeve gastrectomy. Obes Surg. 2018;28:3809–14.

Revisional Surgery: LSG to OAGB

Michael Courtney and Kamal Mahawar

1 Introduction

Laparoscopic Sleeve Gastrectomy (LSG) is the most commonly performed bariatric operation worldwide [1], this is not surprising given its shorter operating time and relative safety. Patients may experience early or late complications, de novo symptoms, worsening of pre-operative symptoms, inadequate weight loss, weight regain or unsatisfactory improvement in comorbidities after any bariatric procedure. Some patients do not achieve a satisfactory response following primary bariatric surgery, and a significant other group experience a gradual waning of satisfactory initial response [2]. It is inevitable that many of these patients will seek Revisional Bariatric Surgery (RBS) for further weight loss or co-morbidity resolution.

Data suggests that a number of patients undergoing primary LSG will need consideration of RBS in later life [3]. These numbers are not small: Clapp et al. [4] describe a failure rate due to weight gain following LSG of 33.6% at 11yrs [4], likewise at 11 years Arman et al. [5] found that 32% undergoing LSG in their study had required RBS (22% for weight regain) and Felsenreich et al. [6] 36% at ten years (21% for weight regain) [5–6]. It is therefore important for bariatric surgeons performing LSG to understand the various options available for RBS following LSG.

M. Courtney (✉)
Specialty Trainee in Upper GI/Bariatric Surgery, Sunderland Royal Hospital, Sunderland, UK
e-mail: mjcourtney01@doctors.org.uk

K. Mahawar
Consultant General and Bariatric Surgeon, Sunderland Royal Hospital, Sunderland, UK
e-mail: kmahawar@gmail.com

S. Al-Sabah et al. (eds.), *Laparoscopic Sleeve Gastrectomy*,
https://doi.org/10.1007/978-3-030-57373-7_52

Presently there is no consensus on the best RBS following LSG [7]. In a worldwide survey of practicing revisional surgeons, we found widespread variation in practices for all RBS, explained by a lack of high-quality studies and almost absence of randomised trials [8]. The results from the same survey showed that Roux-en-Y gastric bypass (RYGB), One-anastomosis gastric bypass (OAGB), Biliopancreatic diversion/duodenal switch (BPD-DS) and Single Anastomosis Duodeno-Ileal Bypass with Sleeve Gastrectomy (SADI-S) are options used by surgeons around the world after LSG for further weight loss or metabolic benefit. Interestingly, in spite of OAGB's relatively recent mainstream utilisation as a primary procedure, it was the second most commonly utilised RBS option after RYGB for these patients. This chapter will explore outcomes with conversion of LSG to OAGB.

2   OAGB as a Primary Procedure

In 1997 Rutledge coined the term "mini gastric bypass" after crucially modifying the previously described (and disregarded) Mason's loop gastric bypass by anastomosing an ante-colic Billroth II gastrojejunostomy to a long narrow gastric pouch [9]. In 2001, he published his initial experience and excellent results after performing over 1000 procedures, concluding that the MGB *"appears to meet many of the criteria of an ideal weight loss operation"* [10]. A number of variations to the originally described procedure have since been reported (most notably the OAGB technique of Carbajo), and so to avoid confusion the International Federation for the Surgery of Obesity and Metabolic Disorders (IFSO) agreed in 2018 that the standard term mini gastric bypass-one anastomosis gastric bypass (MGB-OAGB) should be used to incorporate all the variations of this procedure [11]. For the purposes of this book, the term OAGB refers to the antecolic, isoperistaltic anastomosis of a Billroth II type gastrojejunostomy to a long, narrow gastric pouch.

Following Rutledge's series, many surgeons from all over the world have reported their experience with OAGB for both primary and revisional surgery, and it is now considered a mainstream surgical option in the treatment of obesity [12–13]. This rapid uptake of OAGB is understandable,compared to LSG and RYGB, OAGB has been shown to have superior mid- and long-term weight loss outcomes and improvements in comorbidities [14]. OAGB also has fewer short-term complications than RYGB and has a shorter learning-curve [12, 15–16].

In the longer term, internal hernias seem very rare, as does dumping and post-prandial hyperinsulinaemic hypoglycaemia (PHH) [12]. Similarly, the creation of a long gastric tube does not seem to be associated with a higher marginal ulcer rate compared to RYGB [17–18]. Whilst OAGB is associated with a higher rate of diarrhoea and steatorrhoea than RYGB, Lee et al. [15] did not find that this translated into a worse quality of life [15]. Concerns regarding a high frequency of gastro-oesophageal reflux (GORD) post-OAGB have not been supported by conclusive literature, with studies reporting a prevalence of approximately 0.5% [12, 19–21]. At the same time, we feel that the true number of patients who need further revisional surgery for persistent symptoms of GORD despite best medical management after OAGB is likely higher and probably in the range of 3.0–4.0%.

Earlier concerns that that OAGB would be associated with a high oesophagogastric cancer rate has also not materialised. A recent narrative review of all published literature [22] found that, since the advent of the MGB in 1997 there were only five reported gastric cancers (four of which were in the gastric remnant and so not linked to reflux), and two oesophageal-type cancers (AEG 1 of the gastric cardia) [22].

3   The Rationale for Conversion from LSG to OAGB

Many of the reasons that make OAGB an appealing primary bariatric procedure are applicable to OAGB as a revisional procedure for further weight loss or metabolic benefit after a gastric band or sleeve gastrectomy. As previously discussed, compared to RYGB, the OAGB is faster to perform, safer and results in fewer complications whilst producing (at least) equal improvements in weight and comorbidity [12, 14–16]. Furthermore, OAGB is a safer and carries a lower risk of nutritional complications than BPD or DS [23–24]. OAGB as a revisional procedure is consequently growing in popularity throughout the world [11, 25–26]. In a recent study, approximately 42% of revisional bariatric surgery experts reported that they would perform OAGB after a LSG, with OAGB being the preferred revisional option for 21% [8].

At the same time, it is widely recognised that revisional bariatric surgery carries higher risks than primary bariatric surgery and is associated with lower weight loss and metabolic benefits [27]. Noun et al. [19] in their series of 1000 OAGBs of which 77 were revisional (after gastric band or vertical banded gastroplasty) found that there was a significantly higher rate of short term complications (11.6%) and long-term bile reflux (5.2%) in the revisional cases than primary OAGBs [19].

We further know that conversion of LSG to RYGB improves reflux symptoms but does not yield clinically significant weight loss [28]. Though head to head comparisons are lacking available data seems to suggest that conversion to OAGB might offer superior benefits at lower risk.

4   OAGB as a Revisional Procedure

The available literature on conversion from LSG to OAGB is sparse. To the best of our knowledge, there are only six published studies reporting on the outcomes of LSG to OAGB Table 1 [3, 7, 25, 29–31]. In total 348 patient outcomes were reported, with median follow-ups ranging from one- to five-years. There is wide variability between the numbers of patients, the post-operative follow-up, and reported measures between studies. Operative techniques are quite similar but with subtle variations. In the following few paragraphs we will summarise these findings. Where available, outcomes are compared to those achieved with primary OAGB.

Table 1 Studies reporting outcomes of conversion from LSG to OAGB

Authors	Date	Country	Method	Number of patients	Indication for OAGB	Follow-up	Percentage excess weight loss	Complications
AlSabah et al. [25]	2018	Kuwait	Case series	29	Weight regain / inadequate weight loss	1 year	59% since OAGB	7% early 3% late
Bhandari et al. [29]	2019	India	Case series	32	Weight regain / inadequate weight loss	3 years	36% EWL in addition to LSG	Nil
Chiappetta et al. [3]	2019	Germany	Retrospective cohort	34	Weight regain / inadequate weight loss (29) Reflux with BMI >50 (5)	1 year	40% in addition to LSG	0% early 18% late
Debs et al. [7]	2020	France	Case series	77	Weight regain / inadequate weight loss	5 years	77% since OAGB	4% early 3% late
Musella et al. [30]	2019	Italy	Case series, multicentre	104	Weight regain / inadequate weight loss (87) Reflux (17)	2 years	50% EWL in addition to LSG	1% early 1% late
Poghosyan et al. [31]	2019	France	Case series	72	Weight regain / inadequate weight loss	5 years	45% EWL in addition to LSG	4.2% early 15.2% late

5   Indications for Surgery

In 4/6 papers the indication for conversion from LSG to OAGB was either defined by inadequate weight loss following LSG or weight regain [7, 25, 29–30]. Two papers also included patients converted for gastro-oesophageal reflux (GORD) following LSG (N = 22) [3, 30]. The median time between LSG and OAGB ranged from 1–5 years.

6   Weight Loss

Weight loss reporting between studies varies according to whether it is percentage excess weight loss including that lost with LSG, or since conversion to OAGB (see Table 1). The indication for conversion for almost all patients was inadequate weight loss or weight regain. In summary, all but one study reported significant further weight loss following conversion. In the two largest studies reporting excess weight loss since LSG (with 72 and 104 patients respectively), percentage excess weight loss changed from 21 and 23% post-LSG/pre-OAGB to 66% and 73% respectively [30–31]. Those commenting on percentage excess weight loss after OAGB report 59% and 77% [7, 25]. A recent meta-analysis of twenty articles and over 4000 OAGB patients reported a range of percentage excess weight loss of 31 to 85% at 12 months, and 51 to 98% at five years [32]. The results of the 5/6 studies reporting significant weight loss post-OAGB imply that conversion from LSG to OAGB is effective for weight loss, and may be comparable to primary OAGB (in contrast with Parmar et als' findings following LSG to RYGB conversion) [28]. One study, however, reported no significant weight loss following conversion to OAGB at three year follow-up [29]. The study design and operative technique appears similar to the others and so the reason for this discrepancy is unclear. The authors rightly conclude that more studies with larger numbers at multiple centres are required.

7   Comorbidity Resolution

Five out of the six studies commented on the outcomes of patients with Type 2 diabetes mellitus (T2DM) undergoing LSG to OAGB conversion [3, 7, 29–31]. In all of these T2DM improved post surgery with resolution rates ranging from 50 to 100%.

All studies reported outcomes for patients with hypertension post-OAGB. In one study there was no improvement of hypertension [31], with the other five reporting improvement, with remission rates ranging from 50 to 83%.

Three studies commented on obstructive sleep apnoea (OSA), all showing improvements with resolution in 70% to 82% of cases [3, 7, 31].

Two studies reported outcomes for patients with dyslipidaemia, one of which showed no improvement and the other showing 60% remission [25, 30].

8   Complications

There were no reported mortalities in any study. Overall there were eight early complications related to OAGB and 18 late (excluding de novo reflux) (see Table 2), equating to 2.3% and 5.2% respectively. For comparison, in Noun et als' [19] series of a thousand OAGBs, the early complication rate for primary OAGB was 2.7% and late 4.1% [19].

One of the main concerns following OAGB is the development of troublesome reflux. In the studies that reported on this (3/6), incidence ranged from 8 to 12%, totalling 19 patients. In one study 4/6 (67%) patients with post-OAGB reflux required conversion to RYGB [31], another 2/7 (29%) [7] and the other not converting any [3]. This incidence of reflux seems high compared to primary OAGB [12].

In two studies the indication for conversion from LSG to OAGB included gastro-oesophageal reflux (N=22) [3, 30]. Musella at el found that 60% of patients with de novo reflux after LSG were cured by OAGB, whereas Chiappetta found no significant difference between reflux symptoms pre- and post-OAGB (although in their series the patients also had weight regain and BMI >50, and so reflux was not the sole indication for surgery) [3].

Table 2   - **Complications**

Early	Late
Anastomotic leak (n=3) [7, 25]	Anastomotic stenosis (n=2) [25, 31]
Gastrointestinal bleed (n=1) [7]	Anastomotic ulcer (n=6) [3]
Pleural effusion (n=1) [31]	Chronic diarrhoea (n=3) [7, 31]
Pneumonia (n=1) [7]	Dumping (n=2) [7]
Post-operative haemorrhage (n=1) [31]	Incisional hernia (n=3) [31]
Strangulated port site hernia (n=1) [31]	Marginal ulcer (n=2) [31]
	Gastro-oesophageal reflux (inc bile reflux) (n=19) [3, 7, 31]
	– 6 converted to RYGB

9   Operative Technique

All studies clearly described their surgical technique. In all cases division of the stomach as done at the level of the lesser curve crow's foot or distal to it. In 5/6 studies the pouch was then calibrated with an orogastric tube and re-sleeve performed if required; the calibre of the tube varied from 32 to 42Fr [3, 7, 29–31]. Authors prefer an orogastric tube of 36 Fr for calibration of the OAGB pouch for these patients. A gastrojejunostomy was then performed using an antecolic biliopancreatic (BP) loop between 150 and 250 cm in these studies. We recommend using a Biliopancreatic limb of 150 cm for both our primary and revisional OAGB patients. Interestingly the study that reported no significant weight loss after OAGB used a 250 cm BP limb, which was the longest of all of the studies [29]. We do not routinely approximate crura for patients with hiatus hernia but recommend routine closure of Petersen's defect using either clips or non-absorbable sutures in both primary and revisional OAGB patients,whilst the incidence of internal hernia after OAGB is lower than after RYGB there are several reported cases, including one resulting in gastric remnant perforation [33–34].

10 Summary

There is relative scarcity of published data on LSG conversion to OAGB. Given the current popularity of sleeve, it is inevitable that many of these patients will seek further metabolic intervention in the course of their lifetime. Given that RYGB does not yield clinically meaningful further weight loss in these patients and that Duodenal Switch or even Single Anastomosis Duodeno-Ileal Bypass with Sleeve Gastrectomy (SADI-S) may be associated with higher complication rates, OAGB is an attractive option for these patients.

There is need for high quality data comparing the safety and efficacy of OAGB with RYGB , DS, and SADI-S in these patients. Early results with LSG conversion to OAGB seem satisfactory. The procedure is technically simple and is associated with a low complication rate. It further appears that conversion from LSG to OAGB is safe and likely to provide short- to medium- term improvements in terms of weight and comorbidities. The incidence of troublesome reflux however appears higher than with primary surgery and merits further investigation.

11 Conclusion

Primary OAGB is an increasingly performed procedure worldwide and is viewed by many experts as a valid option for revision after sleeve gastrectomy for patients seeking further weight loss or metabolic benefit. The relative technical ease, safety and outcomes of primary OAGB make it an attractive revisional options for these patients. Longer term, and comparative data are needed.

References

1. Angrisani L, Santonicola A, Lovino P, et al. IFSO Worldwide Survey 2016: primary, endoluminal, and revisional procedures. Obes Surg. 2018;28:3783–94.
2. Mahawar KK, Himpens JM, Shikora SA, et al. The first consensus statement on revisional bariatric surgery using a modified Delphi approach. Surg Endosc. 2019.
3. Chiappetta S, Stier C, Scheffel O, et al. Mini/one anastomosis gastric bypass versus Roux-en-Y Gastric bypass as a second step procedure after sleeve gastrectomy—a retrospective cohort study. Obes Surg. 2019;29:819–27.

4. Clapp B, Wynn M, Martyn C, et al. Long term (7 or more years) outcomes of the sleeve gastrectomy: a meta-analysis. Surg Obes Relat Dis. 2018;14(6):741–7.
5. Arman GA, Himpens J, Dhaenens J, Ballet T, Vilallonga R, Leman G. Long-term (11+years) outcomes in weight, patient satisfaction, comorbidities, and gastroesophageal reflux treatment after laparoscopic sleeve gastrectomy. Surg Obes Relat Dis. 2016;12(10):1778–86.
6. Felsenreich D, Langer F, Kefurt R, et al. Weight loss, weight regain, and conversions to Rou-en-Y gastric bypass: 10-year results of laparoscopic sleeve gastrectomy. Surg Obes Relat Dis. 2016;12(9):1655–62.
7. Debs T, Petrucciani N, Kassir R, et al. Laparoscopic conversion of sleeve gastrectomy to one anastomosis gastric bypass for weight loss failure: mid-term results. Obes Surg. 2020.
8. Mahawar KK, Nimeri A, Adamo M, et al. Practices concerning revisional bariatric surgery: a survey of 460 surgeons. Obes Surg. 2018;28:2650–60.
9. Haskins O. Dr. Robert Rutledge and the 'Mini-Gastric Bypass' (Part 1). https://www.bariatricnews.net/?q=news/112385/dr-robert-rutledge-and-%E2%80%98mini-gastric-bypass%E2%80%99-part-1. Accessed 25 Feb 2020.
10. Rutledge R. The mini-gastric bypass: experience with the first 1,274 cases. Obes Surg. 2001;11:276–80.
11. De Luca M, Tie T, Ooi G, et al. Mini Gastric Bypass-One Anastomosis Gastric Bypass (MGB-OAGB)-IFSO position statement. Obes Surg. 2018;28:1188–206.
12. Mahawar KK, Kumar P, Carr WR, et al. Current status of mini-gastric bypass. J Minim Access Surg. 2016;12(4):305–10. https://doi.org/10.4103/0972-9941.181352.
13. Mahawar KK, Himpens J, Shikora SA, et al. The First consensus statement on One Anastomosis/Mini Gastric Bypass (OAGB/MGB) using a modified Delphi approach. Obes Surg. 2018;28:303–12.
14. Ruiz-Tovar J, Carbajo MA, Jimenez JM, et al. Long-term follow-up after sleeve gastrectomy versus Roux-en-Y gastric bypass versus one-anastomosis gastric bypass: a prospective randomized comparative study of weight loss and remission of comorbidities. Surg Endosc. 2019;33:401–10.
15. Lee W, Ser K, Lee Y, et al. Laparoscopic Roux-en-Y versus Mini-gastric Bypass for the treatment of morbid obesity: a 10-year experience. Obes Surg. 2012;22:1827–34.
16. Musella M, Susa A, Manno E, et al. Complications following the Mini/One Anastomosis Gastric Bypass (MGB/OAGB): a multi-institutional survey on 2678 patients with a mid-term (5 years) follow-up. Obes Surg. 2017;27:2956–67.
17. Lee WJ, Yu PJ, Wang W, Chen TC, Wei PL, Huang MT. Laparoscopic Roux-en-Y versus mini-gastric bypass for the treatment of morbid obesity: a prospective randomized controlled clinical trial. Ann Surg. 2005;242(1):20–8. https://doi.org/10.1097/01.sla.0000167762.46568.98.
18. Bennett J, Small P, Parmar C, et al. Is marginal ulceration more common after mini gastric bypass? Obes Surg. 2015;25(Suppl 1):S1–S364.
19. Noun R, Skaff J, Riachi E, et al. One thousand consecutive mini-gastric bypass: short- and long-term outcome. Obes Surg. 2012;22:697–703.
20. Kular KS, Manchanda N, Rutledge R. A 6-year experience with 1,054 mini-gastric bypasses—first study from indian subcontinent. Obes Surg. 2014;24:1430–5.
21. Chevallier JM, Arman GA, Guenzi M, et al. One thousand single anastomosis (omega loop) gastric bypasses to treat morbid obesity in a 7-year period: outcomes show few complications and good efficacy. Obes Surg. 2015;25:951–8.
22. Runkel M, Runkel N. Esophago-gastric cancer after One Anastomosis Gastric Bypass (OAGB). Chirurgia (Bucur). 2019;114(6):686–92.
23. Disse E, Pasquer A, Espalieu P, et al. Greater weight loss with the omega loop bypass compared to the Roux-en-Y gastric bypass: a comparative study. Obes Surg. 2014;24:841–6.
24. Cavin JB, Voitellier E, Cluzeaud F, et al. Malabsorption and intestinal adaptation after one anastomosis gastric bypass compared with Roux-en-Y gastric bypass in rats. Am J Physiol Gastrointest Liver Physiol. 2016;311(3):G492–500.

25. AlSabah S, Al Haddad E, Al-Subaie S, et al. Short-term results of revisional single-anastomosis gastric bypass after sleeve gastrectomy for weight regain. Obes Surg. 2018;28(8):2197–202.
26. Jammu GS, Sharma R. A 7-year clinical audit of 1107 cases comparing sleeve gastrectomy, roux-en-y gastric bypass, and mini-gastric bypass, to determine an effective and safe bariatric and metabolic procedure. Obes Surg. 2016;26(5):926–32.
27. Mahawar KK, Graham Y, Carr WR, et al. Revisional Roux-en-Y gastric bypass and sleeve gastrectomy: a systematic review of comparative outcomes with respective primary procedures. Obes Surg. 2015;25(7):1271–80. https://doi.org/10.1007/s11695-015-1670-2.
28. Parmar CD, Mahawar KK, Boyle M, Schroeder N, Balupuri S, Small PK. Conversion of sleeve gastrectomy to roux-en-y gastric bypass is effective for gastro-oesophageal reflux disease but not for further weight loss. Obes Surg. 2017;27(7):1651–8.
29. Bhandari M, Humes T, Kosta S, et al. Revision operation to one-anastomosis gastric bypass for failed sleeve gastrectomy. Surg Obes Relat Dis. 2019;15(12):2033–7.
30. Musella M, Bruni V, Greco F, et al. Conversion from laparoscopic adjustable gastric banding (LAGB) and laparoscopic sleeve gastrectomy (LSG) to one anastomosis gastric bypass (OAGB): preliminary data from a multicenter retrospective study.
31. Poghosyan T, Alameh A, Bruzzi M, et al. Conversion of sleeve gastrectomy to one anastomosis gastric bypass for weight loss failure. Obes Surg. 2019;29:2436–41.
32. Wu C, Bai R, Yan W, Yan M, Song M. Clinical outcomes of one anastomosis gastric bypass versus sleeve gastrectomy for morbid obesity. Obes Surg. 2020;30(3):1021–31.
33. Magouliotis DE, Tasiopoulou VS, Tzovaras G. One anastomosis gastric bypass versus Roux-en-Y gastric bypass for morbid obesity: an updated meta-analysis. Obes Surg. 2019;29(9):2721–30.
34. AlZarooni N, Abou Hussein B, Al Marzouqi O, Khammas A. Gastric remnant perforation caused by peterson's hernia following one anastomosis gastric bypass: a rare complication [published online ahead of print, 2020 Mar 6]. Obes Surg. 2020. doi:https://doi.org/10.1007/s11695-020-04524-1

Revisional Surgery: Sleeve to ReSleeve

Patrick Noel, Imane Ed dbali and Marius Nedelcu

1 Introduction

The laparoscopic sleeve gastrectomy (LSG) was introduced in the early 2000s as the first step of a bariatric procedure for super-obese and high-risk patients, to reduce the high morbidity rate of laparoscopic biliopancreatic diversion/duodenal switch [1]. Because of the excellent weight loss, LSG has been validated as a sole bariatric procedure. Today, the LSG has become the most common bariatric procedure in the world with almost 2 of 3 patients operated.

This growth can be explained by several advantages that LSG has over more complex bariatric procedures that involve the small bowel like RYGBP or duodenal switch (DS) with a lower morbidity rate of dumping syndrome and malnutrition and without specific complications like small bowel obstruction, internal hernia, or marginal ulcers.

Comparable results with other techniques were achieved at 5 years in randomized studies [2, 3].

With an increasing number of LSG performed, the significant issue of weight regain is becoming more prevalent and it will represent a major issue that revisional bariatric surgery will need to address in the upcoming years. The long-term

P. Noel (✉) · I. E. dbali
Emirates Specialty Hospital, Dubai, United Arab Emirates
e-mail: casanoel@gmail.com

I. E. dbali
e-mail: imane.eddbali@gmail.com

M. Nedelcu
Bouchard Private Hospital, ELSAN, Clinique Saint Michel, ELSAN, MarseilleToulon, France
e-mail: nedelcu.marius@gmail.com

© The Editor(s) (if applicable) and The Author(s), under exclusive license to Springer Nature Switzerland AG 2021
S. Al-Sabah et al. (eds.), *Laparoscopic Sleeve Gastrectomy*,
https://doi.org/10.1007/978-3-030-57373-7_53

weight loss results following LSG are extremely variable, ranging between 40 and 86% Excess Weight Loss (EWL) [4, 5]. Some authors incriminate the learning curve as one of the favorable factors for weight loss failure. Even without a clear definition, the percentage of weight regain following LSG must be discussed and it has been reported to be up to 35% at 5 years [6].

A second intervention, such as revisional sleeve gastrectomy (ReSG) [7–9], RYGB [10], OAGB, or biliopancreatic diversion with DS [11] or its variant SADI [12] can be proposed. It is also necessary to know the frequency and causes of failures of LSG as well as the indications and outcomes of revision after LSG. Each team should use a specific algorithm in order to evaluate their results. We have previously proposed an algorithm to use for failed LSG [7].

The results of the revisional surgery after LSG may be expected to be inferior compared to the primary surgery.

2 Surgical Methods

The posterior approach with the 3-port technique should remain constant [7]. Any intraperitoneal attachment between the left lobe of the liver and the anterior gastric surface should be carefully dissected. The greater curvature would be dissected next, to expose the previous staple line. All adhesions between the stomach and the pancreas should be taken down carefully not to injure the splenic artery or the pancreas. Once the mobilization of the stomach is completed, the anesthesiologist would insert a 36F orogastric bougie to reach the pylorus, and different applications of a linear stapler Echelon 60–4.1 mm (Ethicon Endo-Surgery Inc., Cincinnati, OH) would be fired.

All patients should be followed up on an outpatient basis, regularly over the entire period. The follow-up should consist of a careful documentation of changes in weight and comorbidities. The radiological studies of the patients should be reviewed, and the dilatation would be classified as primary or secondary. A primary or localized dilation is defined as an upper posterior gastric pouch incompletely dissected during the initial procedure due to learning curve or difficult cases (super-super-obesity) with poor posterior exposure and incomplete visualization of the left crus of the diaphragm. A secondary or diffuse dilation is defined as a homogeneous dilated gastric tube of more than 300 mL in volume at CT scan volumetry, seen later during follow-up.

3 Discussion

The surgical technique of the LSG is one of the major determinants of the success of this procedure in term of complications and long-term results. Removal of the entire gastric fundus is a key point. The left crus of the diaphragm must be systematically visualized. Our technique includes the following: the posterior part of the fundus is grasped repeatedly with forceps operated by the right hand, while the left hand releases the stapler and pulls laterally before the stapler is definitively clamped and fired [13].

Revisional bariatric surgery after LSG is becoming more common due to the rapid increase of number of patients undergoing this procedure as treatment for morbid obesity. The problem of the inadequate weight loss and weight regain after LSG is an issue as for other bariatric procedures. Some of the existing data in the literature is summarized in Table 1. Weight regain after gastric bypass is equally prevalent, but the procedure is less performed today due to lack of successful options, except for conversion to DS. Hence, LSG is more frequently revised, giving the impression that this procedure fails more frequently. Also, it is often performed as a two-stage procedure and when the second stage is performed it is often considered as a failure, when it is not.

A systematic review of weight regain following bariatric surgery identified five principal etiologies: nutritional non-compliance, hormonal/metabolic imbalance, mental health, physical inactivity and anatomical/surgical factors [14]. For the latter one, Deguines et al. [15] have demonstrated a correlation between residual gastric volume and LSG success as defined by %EWL > 50%, BAROS > 3, BMI < 35 kg/m^2, and/or the Biron criteria. They have proved that with a residual gastric volume > 225 cc, the probability of weight loss failure after LSG was higher. Possible explanations for other anatomical LSG failures include the following: dilatation of the residual stomach, calibration of the stomach with an excessively large gastric bougie, [16] and incomplete section of the gastric fundus (from where ghrelin is secreted) [17]. In an experience we had with 39 patients followed up for 5 years, the best results were achieved for the 28 patients (71.8% of patients) with >50% EBMIL. Analyzing this group of patients, there were 26 out of 28 patients with primary/localized dilatation and only two patients with secondary dilatation. Hence, the primary/localized dilatation represents a positive prognostic factor to achieve satisfactory weight loss results following ReSG at long term follow up.

Table 1 Literature review of long-term results following LSG

Study	Journal/year	Number of patients	Follow up	EWL
D'Hondt et al. [15]	Surg. Endos/2011	23	26.5% (6 yrs)	55.9
Rawlins et al. [5]	SOARD/2013	49	100% (5 yrs)	86
Peterli et al. [16]	SOARD/2014	68	91% (5 yrs)	57.4
Boza et al. [17]	SOARD/2014	161	70% (5 yrs)	62.9
Lemanu et al. [6]	SOARD/2015	96	57% (5 yrs)	40
Himpens et al. [18]	SOARD/2016	110	59.1% (11 yrs)	62.5
Noel et al. [19]	SOARD/2017	168	69% (8 yrs)	67

LSGLaparoscopic Sleeve Gastrectomy; RYGBPRoux en Y Gastric Bypass; DSDuodenal Switch; SADISingle Anastomosis Duodeno–Ileal bypass; ReSGResleeve gastretomy; BMI – Body Mass Index; EWLExcess weight loss; Yrsyears

For the LSG, the risk of dilatation in time, with weight loss failure, was a constant source of debate. In a current study 35 patients were isolated with primary or localized dilatation (upper gastric pouch), thus a question came up rapidly among the authors: has this part of the stomach undergone dilatation or was it incompletely dissected from the beginning? The answer remains unknown; a prospective randomized study based on CT scan volumetry would be needed. With the development of CT scan gastric volumetry, it will be easier to differentiate between secondary and primary dilation.

A short literature review on significant data for alternative revisional surgeries following LSG is summarized in Table 2. In the setting of weight loss failure following LSG, many bariatric centers have advocated the LRYGBP as the standard revisional procedure, especially in patients with postoperative GERD. In our experience, for 5 out of 9 patients who underwent LRYGBP additional revisional surgery following ReSG, the main indication was invalidating gastroesophageal reflux with no or minimal weight regain. In patients with important weight regain or insufficient weight loss following ReSG with minimal reflux, the procedure of choice was SADI. Today we have added the possibility to do OAGB

Table 2 Literature review of revisional surgery following LSG

Study	Journal/year	Number of patients	Revisional procedure	Weight loss results
Birch et al. [20]	Am J Surg./2017	18	RYGBP	Mean BMI dropped from 40.5 to 36.4
Kim et al. [21]	SOARD/2016	48	RYGBP	Percentage total weight loss at 36 Mo was 6.5%
Crovari et al. [22]	SOARD/2016	28	RYGBP	Percentage total weight loss at 36 Mo was 19.3%
Prager et al. [23]	SOARD/2016	11	RYGBP	Mean BMI dropped from 40.6 to 34.7
Berends et al. [24]	SOARD/2015	43	25 DS vs 18 RYGBP	EWL greater for DS (59%) compared to LRYGB (23%)
Keidar et al. [25]	SOARD/2015	19	9 DS vs 10 RYGBP	EWL greater for DS (80%) compared to LRYGB (65%)
Torres et al. [12]	SOARD/2015	16	SADI	mean EWL was 72%
AlSabah et al. [26]	Obes Surg/2016	36	12 RYGBP vs 24 ReSG	at 1 year, EWL was 61,3% for RYGBP and 57% ReSG
Noel et al.	Current series	31	ReSG	58% achieved > 50%EWL at 5 years follow up

LSG—Laparoscopic Sleeve Gastrectomy; RYGBP—Roux en Y Gastric Bypass; DSDuodenal Switch; SADI—Single Anastomosis Duodeno–Ileal bypass; ReSGResleeve gastretomy; BMI—Body Mass Index; EWL—Excess weight loss; Mo—Months;

for these patients without major acid reflux. The long-term results of LRYGBP as a revisional procedure following LSG, are disappointing in term of weight loss. The reported percentage of total weight loss at 36 months following revisional LRYGBP varies between 6.5 and 19.3% [18, 19]. There is only one comparative study between LRYGBP and ReSG as revisional surgery following LSG. Al Sabah et al. [21] have reported similar weight loss results one year after revisional surgery with an EWL of 61.3% for LRYGBP and 57% for ReSG.

Consensual opinion exists concerning the superior weight loss obtained with the DS compared with LRYGBP, as revisional surgery following LSG. Berends et al. [22] reported 25 patients with revisional DS with an EWL of 59%, 3 years after the surgery, compared with 23% EWL following revisional LRYGBP. Similarly, Keidar et al. [23] reported an EWL of 80% following DS and 65% following LRYGBP. The interest in using this approach in the treatment of recurrent morbid obesity following LSG has grown with the widespread of SADI. Torres et al. [12] have reported the first 16 patients with revisional SADI with an EWL of 72%.

4 Conclusions

At 5 years postoperative, the ReSG as a definitive bariatric procedure remains effective in the majority of patients. For the patients who did not require an additional procedure after resleeve, the success rate of EBMIL >50% is usually high. The results appear to be more favorable especially for the non-super-obese patients and for primary or localized dilatation. For patients with a global dilatation of the SG the procedure of ReSG should be avoided. ReSG remains a pathway rescue after a technical mistake during the first LSG and is an acceptable bariatric procedure with low long-term complication rates. Further prospective clinical trials are required to compare the outcomes of ReSG with those of RYGB, OAGB or SADI for weight loss failure after LSG.

References

1. Ponce J, DeMaria EJ, Nguyen NT, Hutter M, Sudan R, Morton JM. American Society for Metabolic and Bariatric Surgery estimation of bariatric surgery procedures in 2015 and surgeon workforce in the United States. Surg Obes Relat Dis. 2016.
2. Salminen P, Helmiö M, Ovaska J, et al. Effect of laparoscopic sleeve gastrectomy versus laparoscopic Roux-en-Y gastric bypass on weight loss at 5 years among patients with morbid obesity: the SLEEVEPASS randomized clinical trial. JAMA. 2018;319(3):241–54.
3. Peterli R, Wölnerhanssen BK, Peters T, et al. Effect of laparoscopic sleeve gastrectomy versus laparoscopic Roux-en-Y gastric bypass on weight loss in patients with morbid obesity: the SM-BOSS randomized clinical trial. JAMA. 2018;319(3):255–65.
4. Rawlins L, Rawlins MP, Brown CC, Schumacher DL. Sleeve gastrectomy: 5-year outcomes of a single institution. Surg Obes Relat Dis. 2013;9:21–5.

5. Lemanu DP, Singh PP, Rahman H, Hill AG, Babor R, MacCormick AD. Five-year results after laparoscopic sleeve gastrectomy: a prospective study. Surg Obes Relat Dis. 2015;11(3):518–24.

6. Baig SJ, Priya P, Mahawar KK, Shah S; Indian Bariatric Surgery Outcome Reporting (IBSOR) Group. Weight regain after bariatric surgery-a multicentre study of 9617 patients from Indian bariatric surgery outcome reporting group. Obes Surg. 2019;29(5):1583–92.

7. Nedelcu M, Noel P, Iannelli A, Gagner M. Revised sleeve gastrectomy (re-sleeve). Surg Obes Relat Dis. 2015;11(6):1282–8.

8. Gagner M, Rogula T. Laparoscopic reoperative sleeve gastrectomy for poor weight loss after biliopancreatic diversion with duodenal switch. Obes Surg. 2003;13:649–54.

9. Rebibo L, Fuks D, Verhaeghe P, Deguines JB, Dhahri A, Regimbeau JM. Repeat sleeve gastrectomy compared with primary sleeve gastrectomy: a single-center, matched case study. Obes Surg. 2012;22(12):1909–15.

10. Regan JP, Inabnet WB, Gagner M, Pomp A. Early experience with two-staged laparoscopic Roux-en-Y gastric bypass as an alternative in the super-super obese patient. Obes. Surg. 2003;13:861–4.

11. Dapri G, Cadière GB, Himpens J. Laparoscopic repeat sleeve gastrectomy versus duodenal switch after isolated sleeve gastrectomy for obesity. Surg Obes Relat Dis. 2011;7(1):38–43.

12. Sánchez-Pernaute A, Rubio MÁ, Conde M, Arrue E, Pérez-Aguirre E, Torres A. Single-anastomosis duodenoileal bypass as a second step after sleeve gastrectomy. Surg Obes Relat Dis. 2015;11(2):351–5.

13. Nedelcu M, Eddbali I, Noel P. Three-port sleeve gastrectomy: complete posterior approach. Surg Obes Relat Dis. 2016;12(4):925–7.

14. Karmali S, Brar B, Shi X, Sharma AM, de Gara C, Birch DW. Weight recidivism post-bariatric surgery: a systematic review. Obes Surg. 2013;23(11):1922–33.

15. Deguines JB, Verhaeghe P, Yzet T, Robert B, Cosse C, Regimbeau JM. Is the residual gastric volume after laparoscopic sleeve gastrectomy an objective criterion for adapting the treatment strategy after failure? Surg Obes Relat Dis. 2013;9(5):660–6.

16. Weiner RA, Weiner S, Pomhoff I, et al. Laparoscopic sleeve gastrectomy—influence of sleeve size and 120 resected gastric volume. Obes Surg. 2007;17:1297–305.

17. Lin E, Gletsu N, Fugate K, et al. The effects of gastric surgery on systemic ghrelin levels in the morbidly obese. Arch Surg. 2004;139:780–4.

18. Yorke E, Sheppard C, Switzer NJ, et al. Revision of sleeve gastrectomy to Roux-en-Y gastric bypass: a Canadian experience. Am J Surg. 2017;213(5):970–4.

19. Casillas RA, Um SS, Zelada Getty JL, Sachs S, Kim BB. Revision of primary sleeve gastrectomy to Roux-en-Y gastric bypass: indications and outcomes from a high-volume center. Surg Obes Relat Dis. 2016;12(10):1817–25.

20. Felsenreich DM, Langer FB, Kefurt R, et al. Weight loss, weight regain, and conversions to Roux-en-Y gastric bypass: 10-year results of laparoscopic sleeve gastrectomy. Surg Obes Relat Dis. 2016;12:1655–62.

21. AlSabah S, Alsharqawi N, Almulla A, Akrof S, Alenezi K, Buhaimed W, Al-Subaie S, Al Haddad M. Approach to poor weight loss after laparoscopic sleeve gastrectomy: re-sleeve versus gastric bypass. Obes Surg. 2016;26(10):2302–7.

22. Homan J, Betzel B, Aarts EO, van Laarhoven KJ, Janssen IM, Berends FJ. Secondary surgery after sleeve gastrectomy: Roux-en-Y gastric bypass or biliopancreatic diversion with duodenal switch. Surg Obes Relat Dis. 2015;11(4):771–7.

23. Carmeli I, Golomb I, Sadot E, Kashtan H, Keidar A Laparoscopic conversion of sleeve gastrectomy to a biliopancreatic diversion with duodenal switch or a Roux-en-Y gastric bypass due to weight loss failure: our algorithm. Surg Obes Relat Dis. 2015;11(1):79–85.

24. Homan J, Betzel B, Aarts EO, van Laarhoven KJ, Janssen IM, Berends FJ (2015) Secondary surgery after sleeve gastrectomy: Roux-en-Y gastric bypass or biliopancreatic diversion with duodenal switch. Surg Obes Relat Dis 11(4):771–777

25. Carmeli I, Golomb I, Sadot E, Kashtan H, Keidar A (2015) Laparoscopic conversion of sleeve gastrectomy to a biliopancreatic diversion with duodenal switch or a Roux-en-Y gastric bypass due to weight loss failure: our algorithm. Surg Obes Relat Dis 11(1):79–85
26. AlSabah S, Alsharqawi N, Almulla A, Akrof S, Alenezi K, Buhaimed W, Al-Subaie S, Al Haddad M (2016) Approach to Poor Weight Loss After Laparoscopic Sleeve Gastrectomy: Re-sleeve Vs. Gastric Bypass. Obes Surg 26(10):2302–2307
27. Quezada N, Hernández J, Pérez G, Gabrielli M, Raddatz A, Crovari F. Laparoscopic sleeve gastrectomy conversion to Roux-en-Y gastric bypass: experience in 50 patients after 1 to 3 years of follow-up. Surg Obes Relat Dis. 2016;12(8):1611–15.

Revisional Surgery: Sleeve Gastrectomy to Roux-En-Y Gastric Bypass

Meshka Kamal Anderson and Abdelrahman Nimeri

1 Introduction

Laparoscopic Sleeve Gastrectomy's (SG) is the most common weight loss procedure performed in the United States (US), Europe, Asia, Middle East and North Africa [1]. In the US, as of 2018, over 61% of bariatric procedures performed are SG [1]. Despite similar mid-term effectiveness of primary SG and lower rates of complications compared to Roux-en-Y gastric bypass (RYGB), long term outcomes show that many patients may need revisional surgery after SG mainly for weight regain or gastroesophageal reflux disease (GERD) [2, 3]. In this chapter we will review the indications, preoperative workup, operative technique and outcomes of conversion of SG to RYGB.

2 Indications for Conversion of SG to RYGB

There are no randomized controlled trials, systematic reviews or meta analyses comparing conversion of SG to RYGB to other procedures. In addition, most of the series comparing conversion of SG to RYGB are small series (18–77 patients); with the exception of few matched controlled studies or multi center studies.

M. K. Anderson
Surgery Residency Program, Department of Surgery, Carolinas Medical Center, Atrium Health, Charlotte, NC, USA
e-mail: meshka.anderson@atriumhealth.org

A. Nimeri (✉)
Atrium Health Weight Management, Section of Bariatric & Metabolic Surgery, Department of Surgery, Carolinas Medical Center, Atrium Health, Charlotte, NC, USA
e-mail: nimeri@gmail.com

© The Editor(s) (if applicable) and The Author(s), under exclusive license to Springer Nature Switzerland AG 2021
S. Al-Sabah et al. (eds.), *Laparoscopic Sleeve Gastrectomy*,
https://doi.org/10.1007/978-3-030-57373-7_54

The most common reason to covert SG to RYGB is due to the development of GERD because RYGB is more effective in treating GERD than biliopancreatic diversion (BPD), BPD-duodenal switch (BPD-DS), single anastomosis duodeno-ileostomy (SADI) or one anastomosis gastric bypass (OAGB) [2, 3]. In contrast, several studies report that conversion of SG to RYGB is not as effective for weight regain as described in a study by Parmar et al. [4]. Similarly, a multi-center study from the Netherlands by Dijkhorst et al. compared conversion of SG to RYGB or SADI [5]. It was able to demonstrate that RYGB was very effective for the resolution of GERD. However, SADI was more effective than RYGB for conversion from SG for weight regain, with a similar complication rate and higher rate of nutritional deficiencies after SADI (34%) compared to RYGB (26%) [5].

The high incidence of GERD and the potential for Barrett's esophagitis was first highlighted by Genco et al. in 2016 [2]. In his landmark paper, Genco reported that 5 years after SG, 68% of 110 patients presented with GERD versus 33% preoperatively and proton pump inhibitor (PPI) intake also increased to 57 from 19% preoperatively while 17.2% of patients developed Barrett's esophagitis[2]. Similarly, Mandeville et al. followed 100 patients after SG over 8.5 years and was able to show that 50% of patients developed severe reflux up from 17% preoperatively [6]. In this series, after conversion of SG to RYGB, 57% of patients converted had complete resolution of GERD symptoms [6]. There are other reasons to convert SG to RYGB. For example, a study by Landreneau et al. reported on patients converted for SG complications (47.2%), planned two-stage approach (40.5%) and weight regain (12.4%) [7]. Similarly, a multi-center study by Boru et al. revealed that 50% of patients converted were due to GERD, 40% IWL/WR and 10% GERD and IWL/WR and GERD resolution was 83% after conversion from SG to RYGB [8].

3   Pre-Operative Work-Up

Prior to converting SG patients to RYGB or other procedures, a thorough evaluation is required to evaluate the anatomy of SG, objective assessment for GERD, assessment of patient's compliance and nutritional status. To assess the anatomy of SG, an upper endoscopy (EGD) is often used to check the presence of a hiatal hernia, size of the SG pouch, presence of strictures or proximal migration of the Z line. In addition, an upper gastrointestinal (UGI) series is often used to estimate the function of the SG as well as the presence of any esophageal dilatation.

To objectively assess for the presence of GERD, one must not depend on symptoms as they are misleading. Objective assessment utilizing esophageal manometry and pH testing is necessary to document the presence or absence of GERD after SG. Finally, all patients considered for conversion of SG to RYGB or other procedures need assessment of their compliance to follow-up, behavioral and dietary recommendation of the dietitians and obesity medicine specialists as well a complete nutritional evaluation to assess for deficiencies can affect a patient's morbidity and quality of life.

4 Operative Technique for Conversion of SG to RYGB

The technical aspects of converting SG patients to RYGB involve important steps including always looking for a hiatal hernia (especially on the left side), using a higher surgical staplers height to compensate for thickness of the SG tissue as well as liberal over-sewing of the staple lines, utilizing the patients current BMI and prior weight loss success in deciding the length of the BP limb (100 cm up to a maximum of 1/3 of the small bowel up to 250–300 cm) [9]. For example, Nergaard et al. evaluated 187 primary RYGB patients randomized to a long BP limb (200 cm) versus a short BP limb (60 cm) over a median follow-up of 70.6 months[10]. Median pre-operation BMI was 44 kg/m^2. At 2-years post-RYGB, the long BP limb group had a higher mean EBMIL% of 88.5% compared to the short BP limb group at a mean EBMIL% of 77.7% [10]. A difference between groups was maintained throughout the study period and at 7 years post-surgery even in the superobese (BMI > 50 kg/m^2) [10]. However, nutritional deficiencies were more common in the long BP limb group (17–67%) compared to the short BP limb group (3.5–52%) [9]. In addition, others have shown that significant nutritional deficiencies (requiring hospital admission) can occur if the BP limb is made too long and studies have suggested that BP length over 200 cm may redispose patients to hospitalization [11].

5 How Common Do SG Patients Need Conversion to RYGB

It is difficult to council SG patients about the true incidence of conversion of SG to RYGB due to the lack of large series with long-term follow up. Nevertheless, Felsenreich et al. followed 96 patients for 10-years after SG and reported that 14% of SG patients were converted to RYGB due to GERD [12]. In addition, 38% of SG patients had symptomatic GERD but did not undergo revisional surgery [12]. The authors updated their study in 2018, and the conversion rate increased from 14 to 33% while the number of symptomatic patients who did not undergo revisional surgery increased from 38 to 57% [12]. Similary, Chang et al. reported on a series of SG patients with a 10-year follow-up. In this series 50% had de novo GERD symptoms and 21.5% needed revision to RYGB [13].

It appears that conversion of SG to RYGB leads to improvement in GERD symptoms, more weight loss and improvement of obesity related medical problems. For example, a Canadian study by Yorke et al. evaluated 273 SG for a mean of 41.8 months and 6.6% needing conversion to RYGB [14]. Reasons for conversion were inadequate weight loss (65.3%) and severe reflux (26.1%) [14]. The mean BMI after conversion was 36.4 kg.m^2, down from a mean BMI of 50.5 kg/m^2 preoperatively [14]. Similarly, Parmar et al. reported that conversion of SG to RYGB over a 3-year period with 16 month follow-up yields benefits for resolving GERD but not for further reducing weight [4]. Reasons for conversion were

GERD in 45.5% (pre-conversion BMI 30.5) and IWL/WR in 50% (pre-conversion BMI 43.3) [4]. All patients converted for GERD noted improvement in their symptoms, with 80% stopping their medications altogether [4]. In the IWL/WR group, the BMI drop was 2.5 point after 2 years similar to the BMI drop in the GERD group (2-point drop) [4].

6   Conversion of SG to RYGB Versus Other Procedures

In patients with weight regain post-SG, the BMI at the time of the conversion plays an important role in which procedure is recommended and patients with super obesity (BMI>50 kg/m^2) are not recommended to undergo conversion of SG to RYGB. This is particularly important since weight loss is lower in patients undergoing conversion of SG to RYGB and the rate of complications is higher than primary RYGB. For example, Malinka et al. compared outcomes of revisional RYGB vs primary RYGB [15]. The percent excess weight loss was higher in the primary group (74 ± 23%) versus the revisional group (52 ± 26%) at 3 years. With similar resolution of comorbidities such as diabetes and hypertension[15].

A study by Dijkorst et al. evaluated 140 patients after conversion of SG to RYGB or Single Anastomosis Duodenoileal Bypass (SADI) [5]. At 2 years, SG patients converted to SADI had 20% more total weight loss than those converted to RYGB [5]. The SADI group however also had more nutritional deficiencies than the RYGB group, 34 versus 26% [5]. Similarly, Homan et al. evaluated outcomes of SG patients converted to RYGB versus biliopancreatic diversion with duodenal switch (BPD/DS) [16]. The primary reasons for conversion were inadequate weight loss in 40% and weight regain in 19% [16]. After 34 months, median excess weight loss was 59% in BPD/DS and 23% in RYGB and nutritional deficiencies were more significant in patients converted to BPD/DS [16]. Likewise, Shimon et al. also studied the outcomes of SG patients converted to RYGB or BPD/DS for insufficient weight loss [17]. The mean follow-up was 49 months and conversion to RYGB led to lower BMI reduction of 8.5–31.9 kg/m^2 compared to SG conversion to BPD/DS BMI reduction of 12.8–31.9 kg/m^2 [17].

7   Conclusion

The data suggests that an important component in the decision making of converting SG patients to RYGB vs other procedures should be balancing the amount of weight loss desired with potential side effects such as diarrhea, steatorrhea and nutritional deficiencies that may lead to additional complications. Complications such as osteoporosis due to severe vitamin D deficiency or iron deficiency anemia. It appears that converting a SG patient to RYGB will have less weight loss than conversion of SG to SADI or BPD/DS but SG patients converted to RYGB tend to suffer fewer nutritional deficiencies compared to SG patients converted to BPD/DS.

Single Center retrospective cohort studies							
	SG to RYGB	Conv for GERD	Preop BMI Kg/m2	Post op BMI	FU Months	GERD resolution	BPL CC	Complications
Quezada et al SOARD 2016	50	32%	33.8	TWL 3 years 19.3%	36	90%		0%
Poghosyan et al SOARD 2016	34	8.8	44.7	40.9 TWL 23.8%	36	100%		11.7%
Casilas et al SOARD 2016	48	29%		TWL% 6.5%	36	96% 50% HH repair		31%
Iannelli et al SOARD 2016	40	27.5%	TWL% 34.7%		18.6	100%	50	16.7% Grade II 5 Grade IIIa 2 Clavein Dindo

Atrium Health

References

1. Rosenthal R, Szomstein S. Laparoscopic sleeve gastrectomy. UpToDate. 2020. www.upto-date.com/contents/laparoscopic-sleeve-gastrectomy.
2. Genco A, et al. Gastroesophageal reflux disease and Barrett's esophagus after laparoscopic sleeve gastrectomy: a possible, underestimated long-term complication. Surg Obes Relat Dis. 2017;13(4):568–74. https://doi.org/10.1016/j.soard.2016.11.029.
3. Iannelli A. Laparoscopic conversion of sleeve gastrectomy to Roux-en-Y gastric bypass: indications and preliminary results. Surg Obes Relat Dis. 2016;1533–8.
4. Parmar CD, et al. Conversion of sleeve gastrectomy to Roux-en-Y gastric bypass is effective for gastro-oesophageal reflux disease but not for further weight loss. Obes Surg. 2017;27(7):1651–8. https://doi.org/10.1007/s11695-017-2542-8.
5. Dijkhorst PJ, et al. Failed sleeve gastrectomy: single anastomosis Duodenoileal bypass or Roux-en-Y gastric bypass? A multicenter cohort study. Obes Surg. 2018;28(12):3834–42. https://doi.org/10.1007/s11695-018-3429-z.
6. Mandeville Y, et al. Moderating the enthusiasm of sleeve gastrectomy: up to fifty percent of reflux symptoms after ten years in a consecutive series of one hundred laparoscopic sleeve gastrectomies. Obes Surg. 2017;27(7):1797–803. https://doi.org/10.1007/s11695-017-2567-z.
7. Landreneau J. Conversion of sleeve gastrectomy to Roux-en-Y gastric bypass. Obes Surg. 2018;3843–50.
8. Boru CE, et al. Short-term outcomes of sleeve gastrectomy conversion to R-Y gastric bypass: multi-center retrospective study. Langenbeck's Arch Surg. 2018;403(4):473–9. https://doi.org/10.1007/s00423-018-1675-0.
9. Boerboom A, et al. A long Biliopancreatic and short alimentary limb results in more weight loss in revisional RYGB surgery. Outcomes of the randomized controlled ELEGANCE REDO Trial. Surg Obes Relat Dis. 2019;15(1):60–9. https://doi.org/10.1016/j.soard.2018.10.010.
10. Nergaard BJ, et al. Gastric bypass with long alimentary limb or long Pancreato-biliary limb—long-term results on weight loss, resolution of co-morbidities and metabolic parameters. Obes Surg. 2014;24(10):1595–602. https://doi.org/10.1007/s11695-014-1245-7.

11. Genser L, et al. Laparoscopic reversal of mini-gastric bypass to original anatomy for severe postoperative malnutrition. Langenbeck's Arch Surg. 2017;402(8):1263–70. https://doi.org/10.1007/s00423-017-1615-4.
12. Felsenreich DM, et al. Reflux, sleeve dilation, and Barrett's esophagus after laparoscopic sleeve gastrectomy: long-term follow-up. Obes Surg. 2017;27(12):3092–101. https://doi.org/10.1007/s11695-017-2748-9.
13. Chang D-M, et al. Thirteen-year experience of laparoscopic sleeve gastrectomy: surgical risk, weight loss, and revision procedures. Obes Surg. 2018;28(10):2991–7. https://doi.org/10.1007/s11695-018-3344-3.
14. Yorke E, Caroline S. Revision of sleeve gastrectomy to Roux-en-Y gastric bypass: a Canadian experience. The Am J Surg. 2017;970–4.
15. Malinka T, et al. Three-year outcomes of revisional laparoscopic gastric bypass after failed laparoscopic sleeve gastrectomy: a case-matched analysis. Obes Surg. 2017;27(9):2324–30. https://doi.org/10.1007/s11695-017-2631-8.
16. Homan J. Secondary surgery after sleeve gastrectomy: Roux-En-Y gastric bypass or biliopancreatic diversion with duodenal switch. Surg Obes Relat Dis. 2015;771–8.
17. Shimon O, et al. Long-term effectiveness of laparoscopic conversion of sleeve gastrectomy to a biliopancreatic diversion with a duodenal switch or a Roux-en-Y gastric bypass due to weight loss failure. Obes Surg. 2018;28(6):1724–30. https://doi.org/10.1007/s11695-017-3086-7.

Revisional Surgery: Second-Stage Duodenal Switch

Laurent Biertho, Simon Marceau, Stéfane Lebel, François Julien
and André Tchernof

1   Introduction

The prevalence of obesity has been increasing steadily over the last decades. It is predicted to reach 18% in men and 21% in women globally by 2025 [1]. For most individuals with severe obesity, lifestyle interventions, perhaps effective in inducing short-lived weight loss, are ineffective for long-term weight loss maintenance and durable metabolic recovery. For example, the vast majority (74%) of individuals with severe obesity undergoing intensive lifestyle intervention in the Look AHEAD trial did not maintain a weight loss greater or equal to 10% of initial body weight after 4 years [2]. Bariatric surgery represents the best option for these individuals, including patients with poorly controlled type 2 diabetes (T2D), with the demonstration that it is more effective than standard medical approaches, including use of medication and dietary counselling [3–6].

Among the weight-loss surgeries commonly performed around the world, a version of the biliopancreatic diversion with duodenal switch (DS, Fig. 1) was developed by our team in the early 90's [7, 8]. This modification was based on animal studies by DeMeester et al., who originally described duodenal switch procedure for the treatment of bile gastritis [4]. Our experience in a series of 2,615 consecutive DS patients followed up to 20 years (median follow-up of 8 years) has shown excellent results in terms of weight loss and metabolic recovery [9]. This operation offers one of the most pronounced and durable weight loss (71% excess

L. Biertho (✉) · S. Marceau · F. Julien · A. Tchernof
IUCPQ—Laval University, Quebec, QC, Canada
e-mail: laurentbiertho@gmail.com

S. Lebel
Laval University, Quebec, QC, Canada

BILIOPANCREATIC DIVERSION (Duodenal switch)

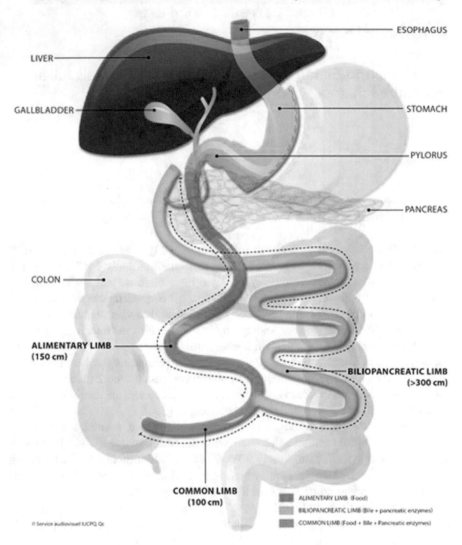

Fig. 1 Biliopancreatic diversion with duodenal switch (DS)

weight loss), and 80–90% remission rates for T2D [9, 10]. Yet, the technical complexity of this operation and the risk for long-term nutritional deficiencies has hindered its widespread use. According to the most recent data, DS represented 1.1% of the total number of surgeries worldwide and 5–6% of all bariatric operations in Canada [11, 12]. Conversely, **sleeve gastrectomy (SG)** now represents 46% and 58% of all surgeries in the world and North America, respectively [11].

It was initially offered as part of a staged-approach for standard DS, but has rapidly gained popularity as a stand-alone procedure [11, 13, 14]. SG is technically easier with less side-effects, but also has a much higher rate of weight regain and T2D relapse, especially in individuals with well-established disease [10]. Consequently, many bariatric centers are now faced with significant proportions of SG patients with insufficient weight loss and diabetes relapse. An increasing rate of revisional surgery has been witnessed in the US over the last few years [15]. This is where second-stage Duodenal Switch (DS) will play an increasing role as one of the most effective surgical options for patients with SG failure.

2   Preoperative Assessment

Classical indications for revisional surgery include patient that are (a) still meeting the initial criteria for obesity surgery, as defined in the 1991 NIH consensus guidelines [16]; (b) have insufficient weight loss, defined as an Excess Weight Loss (EWL) under 50%; (c) have experienced as significant weight regain of 25% EWL or more or d) for the management of a significant, potentially reversible comorbidity. In addition, revision to DS should not be considered before SG patients are weight stable with a minimal follow-up of 18 and 24 months.

Upper GI endoscopy is part of the routine evaluation to rule-out oesophageal or gastric pathology (ie Barrett's oesophagus) and to assess gastric volume. Other gastric volume assessment techniques, like CT-Scan volumetry or upper-GI swallow are done to rule-out technical errors, for example fundus enlargement, and assess the SG volume. Our preferred option however, to obtain significant long-term weight loss, is to convert patients to DS. Conversion to Roux-en-Y Gastric Bypass (RYGB) is considered for the management of refractory reflux, complications (i.e. stenosis or chronic fistula) or control of comorbidities, and not when significant weight loss is required. We only consider doing a re-sleeve in patients with significantly enlarged stomach who are not candidates or willing to undergo a DS.

Other pre-operative evaluation includes a standard multidisciplinary evaluation, with a bariatric surgeon, bariatric nurse, and a dietician. The dietician should be experienced with DS to educate patients on the recommended long-term post-operative diet (high-protein, >90gr per day with very low-fat diet). Before surgery, a low-calorie diet can also be used to decrease the size of the liver and the amount of intraperitoneal fat. A psychiatric or psychological evaluation is requested for patients with a history of mental health illnesses or when clinically indicated. Screening for diabetes, dyslipidemia and obstructive sleep apnea is performed and treatment is initiated.

Preoperative blood work consists of a complete blood cell count, ions, creatinine, liver enzymes, albumin, calcium, parathyroid hormone, vitamin D, vitamin A, vitamin B12, Thyroid Stimulating Hormone and iron panel. All patients receive a multivitamin complex with B1 supplement (ie Centrum Forte©) a few months *before surgery* and vitamin D3 (10,000U per day for 1 month followed by 1000

U per day until surgery). Other vitamins and minerals deficiencies are corrected before surgery.

3   Surgical Technique

The patient is positioned in a split leg position with both arms open. Thromboprophylaxis is given 2 hours prior to surgery and antibiotic-prophylaxis at induction (Heparin 5,000U s/c and Cefazolin 2 to 3 g for patients below and above 120 kg, respectively). Pneumatic compression devices are used during the procedure and until patients are walking. The surgeon stands between the patient's legs, with the assistant at the patient's left (Fig. 2).

A long Veress needle (15 cm) is first inserted in the left upper quadrant to create a 15 mmHg pneumoperitoneum. A 5-mm or 10-mm optical trocar is used to enter the abdominal cavity under direct vision, 2 handbreadths under the xyphoid. One 12-mm ports is placed at the same level in the left flank. A 5-mm port is placed in the right flank and at the epigastria for the liver retractor, in the left upper quadrant for the assistant, and in the left flank for the infra-mesocolic part of the procedure. Trocart position is described in Fig. 3.

The first step of the procedure is to release adhesions from the previous sleeve and confirm feasibility of the duodenal switch. Usually, when a patient has lost a significant amount of weight after the SG, the working space and length of the mesentery are sufficient to perform a DS. In rare occasions (ie extensive adhesions in the lower abdomen, chronic cholecystitis, significant weight regain after SG or

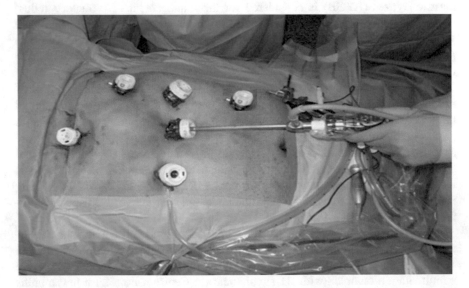

Fig. 2 Operative room setup

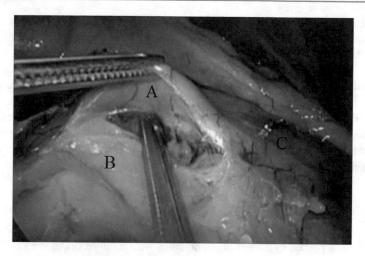

Fig. 3 Trocar position for second-stage duodenal switch

complex ventral hernia), the surgery may be postponed and weight loss obtained through medical/nutritional therapy before considering a second-stage surgery.

3.1 Duodenal Dissection

The relationships between the duodenum, pancreatic head, common bile duct and gastroduodenal artery should be familiar. A liver retractor is placed to retract segment IV and V of the liver and expose the first duodenum and pylorus. Mayo's vein, located at the inferior edge of the pylorus can be useful to identify the pylorus. The antrum is retracted to the patient's left to bring the first portion of the duodenum towards midline. The peritoneum is opened above and below the first duodenum. The common bile duct is often seen at the superior edge of the duodenum and represents a good landmark for dissection. Two different techniques can be used to mobilize the duodenum.

Gastro-duodenal approach: the dissection starts on the antrum and the gastrocolic ligament is released, past the pylorus. The pyloric artery can be controlled with clips. The posterior attachments of the duodenum are dissected to mobilize the first 3 to 4 cm of duodenum. The gastroduodenal artery, which lies at the posterior aspect of the first duodenum, marks the distal end of the dissection. A window is created at the upper aspect of the duodenum, just lateral and above the common bile duct. A 15-cm Penrose drain is then passed into that window to retract the duodenum. That window is slightly enlarged to accommodate the anvil of a linear stapler and an Echelon Flex with a blue cartridge or Endo-GIA tri-staple is passed through the 12-mm port in the left flank, to transect the duodenum.

Direct duodenal approach: This approach can be quicker, especially in second-stage surgery patients with significant weight loss. The duodenum is retracted medially by pulling the antrum to the left. The surgeon pulls the duodenum up and the peritoneum is opened 3–4 cm distal from the pylorus on the lower and the upper aspect of the duodenum. A window is created at the inferior part of the duodenum, 3 to 4 cm distal to the pylorus. Blunt dissection is used to identify the plane between the posterior duodenal wall and the pancreas (Fig. 4). A 15-cm Penrose drain is then passed into that window to retract the duodenum. The window is slightly enlarged to accommodate the anvil of the linear stapler and the duodenum is transected (Fig. 5).

3.2   Small Bowel Transection

The patient is placed in a head-down position with a slight tilt to the patient's left and the operating surgeon move to the patient's left. The 2 lower trocars in the left flank are used. The ileocecal junction is identified and adhesions between the ascending colon and the omentum are released. The ileum is measured from the ileo-caecal valve, using small bowel graspers (the length of our grasper's jaw is 5 cm). The small bowel is first marked at 100 cm from the ileocecal junction, using a large clip on each side of the mesentery to mark the location of the future ileo-ileostomy. The small bowel is then run another 150 cm and a Penrose drain is passed below the small bowel for retraction. The alimentary limb is identified directly using a metal clip on the mesentery to maintain orientation. The small bowel mesentery can be opened a few centimeters to decrease tension on the duodenal anastomosis.

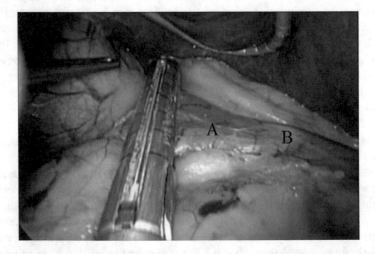

Fig. 4 The duodenum (**a**) is lifted up and the retro-duodenal window is created above the pancreatic head (**b**), 3-cm distal from the pylorus (**c**)

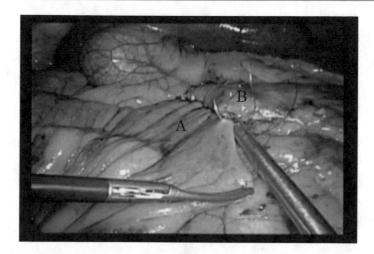

Fig. 5 The duodenum (**a**) is transected 3 cm distal from the pylorus (**b**)

3.3 Duodeno-Ileal Anastomosis

The patient is now placed in head-up position and the surgeon goes back between the patient's legs. The alimentary limb is brought to the right upper quadrant in an antecolic fashion and approximated to the transected duodenum. The Penrose drain is used for retraction and placed to the left of the anastomosis. A handsewn end-to-side anastomosis is then created with 23-cm 3–0 absorbable V-Loc sutures. The first posterior layer is created to approximate the antimesenteric side of the small bowel to the duodenum (Fig. 6). The intestinal lumens are opened and the back wall of the anastomosis is sewn using the same suture. The anterior layer of the anastomosis is then created, starting from the top of the anastomosis (Fig. 7). The 2 running sutures are crossed or tied together. The anastomosis can be tested by insufflating air through a nasogastric tube or with an endoscope. This also allows testing the patency of the anastomosis. The small bowel is then transected using a linear-stapler passed through the mesenteric window at the level of the Penrose.

3.4 Ileoileal Anastomosis

The patient is placed head-down and the surgeon goes to the patient's left. The ileoi-leal anastomosis is created 100 cm from the ileocecal valve. The biliary limb is attached to the ileon using a 2–0 Vicryl in an antiperistaltic technique (Fig. 8). The stitch is retracted to the patients' right and an enterotomy is made on the anti-mesenteric side of the marked ileon, at 100 cm, and the biliopancreatic limb. A 3 to 4 cm side-to-side anastomosis is created using another white load of a 60-mm linear stapler-cutter. The intestinal opening is closed using a single layer

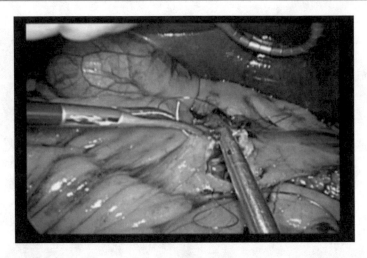

Fig. 6 The first posterior layer is created using 3–0 absorbable suture, to approximate the ileon (**a**) to the first duodenum (**b**)

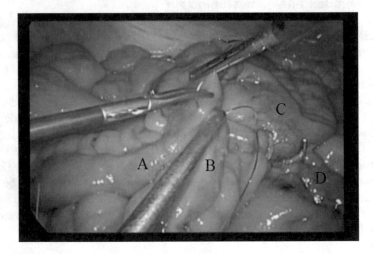

Fig. 7 Anterior layer of the anastomosis, starting from the top of the duodenum

of 3–0 V-Loc suture, starting from the mesenteric side (Fig. 9). The small bowel is then retracted to the right upper quadrant using the Vicryl stay suture. The mesenteric window is closed using a nonabsorbable 2–0 Prolene suture. The Petersen window is also closed using a 2–0 Prolene suture. The patient is placed head up and the assistant lift the transverse colon up. The alimentary limb is placed in the right flack to expose Petersen's defect. A routine cholecystectomy and liver biopsy are performed at the end of the surgery and the pneumoperitoneum is exsufflated under direct vision.

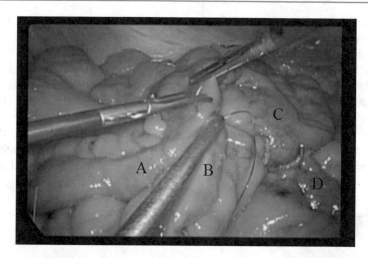

Fig. 8 A 2–0 Vicryl suture is placed to approximate **a** the common channel and **b** the biliary limp. **c** The alimentary limp is located in the patient's right flank and **d** proximal ileon

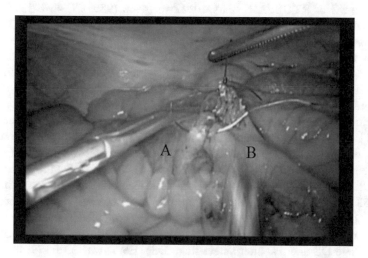

Fig. 9 The intestinal opening of the anastomosis is closed with a 3–0 absorbable suture. The common channel is on the left (**a**) and the biliary limb is on the right (**b**)

4 Post-Operative Care

Regular subcutaneous heparin is started 6 hours post surgery and patients are switched to a low-molecular-weight heparin on postoperative day 1. Pneumatic compression devices, incentive spirometry and non-invasive airway support are also used. Patients are started on water the day of surgery, and full liquids on postoperative day one. Typical discharge is on postoperative day three with a liquid diet for two weeks. The diet is progressed to pureed diet, minced diet and regular diet every 2 weeks. Patients who still have their gallbladder are placed on Ursodiol (Actigall, Ciba-Geigy, Summit, New Jersey), 250 mg PO twice a day for 6 months. Daily vitamins and mineral supplementations are started within the first month: ferrous sulfate, 300 mg; vitamin D3, 20,000 IU; vitamin A, 30,000 IU; calcium carbonate, 1000 mg and a multivitamin complex. Supplements are adjusted over time and education in consuming a high-protein diet is reinforced. Patients are followed with bloodwork (similar to pre-op) at 4, 8, 12, 18 and 24 months and annually thereafter. Fasting glucose, Haemoglobin A1C and lipid panel is done every year.

5   Surgical Outcomes

Five-year efficacy of SG has been confirmed in recent randomized controlled trials, however, 10-years good quality data is still missing. In the largest RCT trial, 240 patients (mean age of 48 [SD, 9] years and BMI of 46, [SD, 6]), were randomized to SG or RYGB. At 5 years, EWL was 49% (95% CI, 45%-52%), remission rate for T2D was 37%, dyslipidemia 47% and hypertension 29% [17]. These results are similar to other prospective trials [18–20] and illustrate the need for an effective revisional option for patients with suboptimal SG outcome. Second-stage DS offers such an option and has the advantage, compared to conversion to RYGB or re-sleeve, of a relatively simple procedure, avoiding scarred tissues at the level of the previous sleeve and approaching obesity in a stepwise approach.

A study recently reported on medium term outcomes with second-stage DS [21]. All patients who had a second stage DS with a minimal follow-up of 2 years were matched 1:1 for age, sex, BMI and year of surgery, with a group of patients who had a single-stage DS (Table 1). A total of 118 patients were included (59 in each group) and there was no significant difference in initial BMI (53.8 ± 9.7 vs. 52.7 ± 7.8 kg/m^2, P = 0.4), age and sex ratio between the 2 groups. Interestingly, the overall 90-days major complication rate of 2-stages DS was not significantly different from single-stage DS (2% after SG, 5% after second-stage DS and 5% after single-stage DS). EWL was 39 ± 17% at the time of conversion. After second-stage DS versus single-stage DS, EWL increased to 75 ± 18% versus 88 ± 18% at 1 year (p = 0.00021), 80.2 ± 17% versus 92.3 ± 14% at 2 years (p = 0.002), and 80.2 ± 18% versus 87.2 ± 16% at 3 years (p = 0.6) (Fig. 10). Remission rate for T2D increased from 59 to 94% after second-stage DS (p = 0.001), similar to the remission rate in the single-stage group, at 94%. Remission of hypertension increased from 42 to 77% after second-stage DS (p = 0.03), compared to 71% with single-stage DS (P = 0.8). In addition, second-stage DS was highly effective in controlling patients with T2D on insulin, with a remission rate of 80% (from 15% after SG).

Other series of staged DS have reported similar weight and metabolic benefits. Homan et al. [22] reported a retrospective series of SG patients converted to either

Table 1 Remission rate of obesity related comorbidities

Variable	SG	2nd Stage DS	1-stage DS (32)	p[a]/p[b]
T2D (n)	34	34	32	
Improved	41% [14]	6% [2]	6% [2]	0.001/1
Remission	59% [20]	94% (32)	94% (30)	0.001/1
T2D on insulin (n)	12	12	7	
Improved	83% [10]	17% [1]	29% [2]	0.04/0.6
Remission	17% [2]	83% [10]	71% [5]	0.04/0.6
Hypertension (n)	31	31	28	
Unchanged	9 (29%)	13% [4]	4% [1]	0.01/0.4
Improved	9 (29%)	10% [3]	25% [7]	0.7/0.8
Remission	13 (42%)	77% [24]	71% [20]	0.03/0.8
OSA (n)	39	39	41	
Unchanged	14 (36%)	2 (5%)	17% [7]	0.07/0.2
Improved	11 (28%)	7 (18%)	22% [9]	0.6/0.6
Remission	14 (36%)	14 (36%)	61% [25]	0.03/0.02

Data are reported as percentages (n). A Chi-square or Fischer exact test was used to compare SG to DS (a) and 2nd Stage to DS (b).

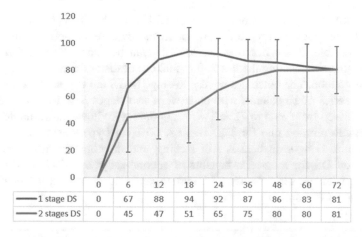

	0	6	12	18	24	36	48	60	72
1 stage DS	0	67	88	94	92	87	86	83	81
2 stages DS	0	45	47	51	65	75	80	80	81

Fig. 10 Percentage of excess weight loss (mean ± Standard Deviation) over time following one-stage and two-stage DS. Number of data available (1-stage/2-stages) at: T0 (59/59), 6 m (51/50), 12 m (56/54), 18 m (30/45), 24 m (45/54), 36 m (40/57), 48 m (30/45), 60 m (27/27), 72 m (17/17). Mean EWL at the time of conversion was 51%

RYGB (n = 18) or DS (n = 25). The additional median EWL was significantly greater for DS (59% [range 15–113]) compared to RYGB (23% [range −49–84], p = 0.008) at 34 months (range 14–79).

Iannelli et al. [23] also published a retrospective series of patients with an initial BMI≥ 50 kg/m^2 who underwent either single or 2-stage approach.

Second-stage DS was required in 39 patients and EWL reached 73% ± 14%, similar to patients who had a single-stage DS (73% ± 18%).

Overall, these results confirm the medium-term efficacy of a two-step approach, in terms of additional weight loss, remission rate of comorbidities and quality of life. The overall complication rate of the staged-approach, compared to single-stage DS, needs to be better defined but is likely inferior. The question of economic burden, loss of productivity, surgical costs and timing (early versus late revision) is still unanswered.

However, the problem with DS is not as much the efficacy than the risk of long-term nutritional deficiencies and side-effects. In our experience [21], the rate of moderate protein malnutrition was low, at 1.7%; and was not significantly different from that of patients undergoing a single-stage DS. The two-step approach could potentially improve the selection of patients who are compliant to follow-ups, blood work prescriptions and vitamin supplementations. When protein malnutrition occurs, it can usually be managed through nutritional consultation, protein supplements and pancreatic enzymes (ie Cotazyme 10000U, 2co with meals). When medical treatment is insufficient or for patients with some chronic medical conditions that are unlikely to improve (ie alcoholism, drug addiction, mental illness), surgical revision can be needed. In a series of 2615 primary DS with a mean follow-up 9.8 ± 4.8 years, readmission for protein malnutrition was needed in 8% of cases, including placement of feeding jejunostomy in 1.8% and lengthening of the common channel in 1.4% of cases.

The place of Single-Anastomosis Duodenal Switch (SADI) is beyond the scope of this chapter but could represent an option to decrease side-effects and protein malnutrition rate. It was described in 2011 by Sanchez-Pernaute and Torres [24], and consists in connecting the last 250 to 300 cm of distal ileon to the duodenum, as an omega loop. The outcomes of second-stage SADI are extremely scarce, however. In a series of 16 patients who underwent two-stages SADI-250 cm [25], the EWL increased from 39.5 to 72%. Two-years data were however available in only 5 patients. Remission rate for T2D was 88, 60% for hypertension, and 40% for dyslipidemia. Long-term data is still lacking and drawing conclusion from the literature on DS for long-term benefits of second-stage SADI is clearly biased. Prospective data on second-stage SADI are urgently needed to clarify the risk versus benefits of this option.

6   Conclusion

Second-stage DS represents an effective option for patients with SG failure, with an additional 41% EWL and 35% cure rate for T2D. Staged approaches could also improve selection of candidates for DS and simplify the surgical technique and early outcomes. The selection of patients that would benefit the most from a staged-approach is however not yet perfectly defined and single-stage DS remains a standard option for patients with severe obesity and long-lasting comorbidities.

Protein malnutrition remains a long-lasting risk and long-term follow-up is mandatory. Overall, the medium-term outcomes of a staged approach seem similar to single-stage DS and represent the most effective option for the management of obesity-related diseases and weight loss for patients with SG failure.

References

1. Trends in adult body-mass index in 200 countries from 1975 to 2014: a pooled analysis of 1698 population-based measurement studies with 19.2 million participants. Lancet. 2016;387(10026):1377–96.
2. Unick JL, Beavers D, Bond DS, Clark JM, Jakicic JM, Kitabchi AE, et al. The long-term effectiveness of a lifestyle intervention in severely obese individuals. the Am J Med. 2013;126(3):236–42.
3. Schauer PR, Kashyap SR, Wolski K, Brethauer SA, Kirwan JP, Pothier CE, et al. Bariatric surgery versus intensive medical therapy in obese patients with diabetes. the New Engl J Med. 2012;366(17):1567–76.
4. Schauer PR, Bhatt DL, Kirwan JP, Wolski K, Brethauer SA, Navaneethan SD, et al. Bariatric surgery versus intensive medical therapy for diabetes–3-year outcomes. the New Engl J Med. 2014;370(21):2002–13.
5. Mingrone G, Panunzi S, De Gaetano A, Guidone C, Iaconelli A, Leccesi L, et al. Bariatric surgery versus conventional medical therapy for type 2 diabetes. the New Engl Journal of Medicine. 2012;366(17):1577–85.
6. Gloy VL, Briel M, Bhatt DL, Kashyap SR, Schauer PR, Mingrone G, et al. Bariatric surgery versus non-surgical treatment for obesity: a systematic review and meta-analysis of randomised controlled trials. BMJ. 2013;347:f5934.
7. Marceau P, Biron S, Bourque RA, Potvin M, Hould FS, Simard S. Biliopancreatic diversion with a new type of gastrectomy. Obes Surg. 1993;3(1):29–35.
8. Biertho L, Marceau S, Biron S. A Canadian and historical perspective on bariatric surgery. Can J Diab. 2017;41(4):341–3.
9. Marceau P, Biron S, Marceau S, Hould FS, Lebel S, Lescelleur O, et al. Long-term metabolic outcomes 5 to 20 years after biliopancreatic diversion. Obes Surg. 2015.
10. Biertho L, Lebel S, Marceau S, Hould FS, Lescelleur O, Marceau P, et al. Laparoscopic sleeve gastrectomy: with or without duodenal switch? A consecutive series of 800 cases. Dig Surg. 2014;31(1):48–54.
11. Angrisani L, Santonicola A, Iovino P, Vitiello A, Zundel N, Buchwald H, et al. Bariatric Surgery and Endoluminal Procedures: IFSO Worldwide Survey 2014. Obes Surg. 2017.
12. Information CIfH. Bariatric surgery in Canada 2014.
13. Rosenthal RJ, Diaz AA, Arvidsson D, Baker RS, Basso N, Bellanger D, et al. International sleeve gastrectomy expert panel consensus statement: best practice guidelines based on experience of >12,000 cases. Surg Obes Relat Dis: Official J Am Soc Bariatric Surg. 2012;8(1):8–19.
14. Gagner M, Hutchinson C, Rosenthal R. Fifth international consensus conference: current status of sleeve gastrectomy. Surg Obes Relat Dis: Official J Am Soc Bariatric Surg. 2016;12(4):750–6.
15. English WJ, DeMaria EJ, Brethauer SA, Mattar SG, Rosenthal RJ, Morton JM. American society for metabolic and bariatric surgery estimation of metabolic and bariatric procedures performed in the United States in 2016. Surg Obes Relat Dis: Official J Am Soc Bariatric Surg. 2018;14(3):259–63.
16. NIH conference. Gastrointestinal surgery for severe obesity. Consensus Development Conference Panel. Ann Intern Med. 1991;115(12):956–61.

17. Salminen P, Helmio M, Ovaska J, Juuti A, Leivonen M, Peromaa-Haavisto P, et al. Effect of laparoscopic sleeve gastrectomy versus laparoscopic Roux-en-Y gastric bypass on weight loss at 5 years among patients with morbid obesity: the SLEEVEPASS randomized clinical trial. JAMA. 2018;319(3):241–54.
18. Peterli R, Wolnerhanssen BK, Peters T, Vetter D, Kroll D, Borbely Y, et al. Effect of laparoscopic sleeve gastrectomy vs laparoscopic Roux-en-Y gastric bypass on weight loss in patients with morbid obesity: the SM-BOSS randomized clinical trial. JAMA. 2018;319(3):255–65.
19. Schauer PR, Bhatt DL, Kirwan JP, Wolski K, Aminian A, Brethauer SA, et al. Bariatric surgery versus intensive medical therapy for diabetes—5-year outcomes. the New Engl J Med. 2017;376(7):641–51.
20. Mingrone G, Panunzi S, De Gaetano A, Guidone C, Iaconelli A, Nanni G, et al. Bariatric-metabolic surgery versus conventional medical treatment in obese patients with type 2 diabetes: 5 year follow-up of an open-label, single-centre, randomised controlled trial. Lancet. 2015;386(9997):964–73.
21. Biertho L, Theriault C, Bouvet L, Marceau S, Hould FS, Lebel S, et al. Second-stage duodenal switch for sleeve gastrectomy failure: A matched controlled trial. Surg Obes Relat Dis: Official J Am Soc Bariatric Surg. 2018;14(10):1570–9.
22. Homan J, Betzel B, Aarts EO, van Laarhoven KJ, Janssen IM, Berends FJ. Secondary surgery after sleeve gastrectomy: Roux-en-Y gastric bypass or biliopancreatic diversion with duodenal switch. Surg Obes Relat Dis: Official J Am Soc Bariatric Surg. 2015;11(4):771–7.
23. Iannelli A, Schneck AS, Topart P, Carles M, Hebuterne X, Gugenheim J. Laparoscopic sleeve gastrectomy followed by duodenal switch in selected patients versus single-stage duodenal switch for superobesity: case-control study. Surg Obes Relat Dis: Official J Am Soc Bariatric Surg. 2013;9(4):531–8.
24. Sanchez-Pernaute A, Rubio MA, Perez Aguirre E, Barabash A, Cabrerizo L, Torres A. Single-anastomosis duodenoileal bypass with sleeve gastrectomy: metabolic improvement and weight loss in first 100 patients. Surg Obes Relat Dis: Official J Am Soc Bariatric Surg. 2013;9(5):731–5.
25. Sanchez-Pernaute A, Rubio MA, Conde M, Arrue E, Perez-Aguirre E, Torres A. Single-anastomosis duodenoileal bypass as a second step after sleeve gastrectomy. Surg Obes Relat Dis: Official J Am Soc Bariatric Surg. 2015;11(2):351–5.

Revisional Surgery: Sleeve to Single Anastomosis Sleeve Ileal (SASI) Bypass

Tarek Mahdy and Waleed Gado

1   Introduction

Obesity and diabetes comprise a great health epidemic, involving millions of people. Morbid obesity, however, is a problem that cannot be prevented by a healthy diet and exercise alone [1]. Recently, Second Diabetes Surgery Summit (DSS-II), had recommended inclusion of bariatric/metabolic surgery among glucose-lowering interventions for select patients with type 2 diabetes mellitus (T2DM) and obesity [2]. The mechanism in which this weight loss and control of metabolic syndrome is attained involves a detailed understanding of the way the gut anatomy is modified, interconnected with the role of gut hormones and microbiota [3, 4]. Metabolic surgery represents the new hope to control both diseases in one shot. The concept of metabolic surgery involves operations and procedures to treat metabolic diseases, such as T2DM [5]. These procedures encompass operating on normal organs to procreate effects beneficial to treat medical health problems. Bariatric surgery now represents a developed form of metabolic surgery that is used on a large scale to fight obesity and metabolic syndrome through more than 50 implemented surgical operations [6–8]. However, recently it has been reported that up to 10–50% of inadequate weight loss or weight regain patients who underwent an initial restrictive bariatric procedure will require another secondary bariatric surgical rescue operation [9].

T. Mahdy (✉) · W. Gado
Mansoura Faculty of Medicine, Mansoura, Egypt
e-mail: tmahdy@yahoo.com

S. Al-Sabah et al. (eds.), *Laparoscopic Sleeve Gastrectomy*,
https://doi.org/10.1007/978-3-030-57373-7_56

579

2   Rationale for Another Bariatric Surgical Procedure Following Sleeve Gastrectomy

Sleeve gastrectomy (SG) is mainly a restrictive procedure that has become one of the most commonly performed stand-alone bariatric operations due to its efficacy in achieving weight loss and attractive improvement of comorbidities, easiness to perform, better quality of life, and absence of complications of other complex procedures like marginal ulceration, internal herniation, malabsorption and dumping syndrome [10]. However, with the higher number of SGs performed and availability of long term results, a higher appearance of post SG consequences will become present that raise alarm, like sleeve stenosis, intractable severe reflux, or suboptimal results such as weight loss failure (inadequate weight loss and weight regain especially in super obese) and inadequate remission or relapse of T2DM [11]. This leads predominately to revision of the gastric sleeve or a conversion to a diversion procedure such as Roux-en-Y Gastric Bypass (RYGB), Mini Gastric Bypass (MGB), Single-anastomosis Duodeno-Ileal Bypass with Sleeve (SADI-S), or Duodenal switch (DS). Some identified causes of weight regain following SG in patients at least 2 years post-surgery include: a large retained fundus, increased ghrelin levels, inadequate follow-up support, and maladaptive lifestyle behaviors [12].

3   Options of Secondary Bariatric Procedures Following Suboptimal Sleeve Gastrectomy Results: What is the Rightful Choice?

Although revisional bariatric surgery is usually complex, technically demanding and riskier in terms of postoperative complications than that of primary procedures, with a perioperative morbidity rate of 19–50% [13]; it can be done safely by well-trained experienced bariatric surgeons in special bariatric centers [14]. Revisional surgery rates following SG are variable worldwide; it accounts for about 1.1% of bariatric procedures over a 6 year follow-up as proven in a Swedish study, 1.7% over 6 years in a high volume center in the US, up to 4.2% in Norway over 5 years, 6.4% in a study from Turkey over 7 years, and 6.6% over 7 years in a Canada center [9, 10, 15–17]. Re-sleeve gastrectomy is suitable only for patients with large gastric pouch after the original sleeve. However, it has higher risk of complications such as gastric fistula formation compared to the primary sleeve procedure that may be difficult to manage, and is also of lower efficacy in comparison to other revisional procedures like DS [18, 19]. Reversal of SG to RYGB also carries problems, such as inability to monitor gastric residue by upper gastro-intestinal endoscopy keeping it under risk, lack of access to biliary tract, complete exclusion of the duodenum and proximal jejunum leading to calcium and iron deficiencies, complete bypassing of the pylorus leading to dumping syndrome, and increased risk of internal hernias due to mesenteric division [20, 21]. MGB has recently come into light, becoming a familiar competitive procedure in the last decade because of its effectiveness, however, has approximately the same limitations, in addition to alkaline reflux gastritis [22, 23].

Research recently shed light on the correlation between gastrointestinal physiology and the metabolic pathways in response to operative and anatomical changes of the classic restriction and/or malabsorption mechanisms [24]. Biliopancreatic diversion with duodenal switch (BPD-DS) effects can be explained by neurohormonal modulation and alterations of the microbiota and bile salt metabolism resulting from initial and strong distal intestinal stimulation, making malabsorption an unnecessary and avoidable side effect [25]. This understanding helped form the current surgical set up as well as create future possibilities for metabolic surgery [26].

Although classic malabsorptive operations such as the BPD-DS are the most effective surgery's known given that they promote the best weight loss [90% excess weight loss (EWL)], and glycemic control than other techniques [27], its greater technical complexity, gastrointestinal complications and long-term nutritional risks that requires long-life follow up have limited its use [28].

SADI-S is a loop modification of the BPD-DS [29]. Malabsorption is relatively lower compared to BPD-DS because the common channel length is between 200 to 250 cm, and has even been recently increased to 300 cm to lessen hypoalbuminemia and dramatic malabsorption effects, but it is still considered a procedure causing concern in several patients [30, 31]. Furthermore, access to the biliary tract is lost in the SADI-S procedure. These procedures that are dominantly diversion related may result in atrophy of the mucosa. This is proven histologically by the flattening of intestinal villi and an increase in mitotic frequency, which may be followed by bacterial translocation and hepatic decompensation of already altered hepatic function by nonalcoholic fatty liver disease in obese patients [32, 33]. Additionally, proximal intestinal exclusion will initiate increased secretion and unopposed incretin action that eventually leads to the risk of hypoglycemia. That, plus the continuing weight loss adds to the malabsorptive effect [34].

4   The Rising Concept of Bipartition in Bariatric Surgery

Santoro et al. [35] introduced new operative modifications to the BPD-DS in the year 2003 making it safer and easier to perform, with comparable dramatic weight loss and comorbidity resolution, while reducing its adverse effects. The procedure entails sleeve gastrectomy with transient intestinal bipartition (SG-TB), in which a gastro-ileal anastomosis in a Roux-en-Y fashion is done to the pre-pyloric region, at a point 250 cm from the ileocecal junction reconstruction. This technique differs from the classic BPD-DS given that there is no exclusion of intestinal segments. The purpose of this new surgical technique is to promote only a partial exclusion of the proximal bowel and to boost early distal intestinal stimulation [36]. In addition, the preservation of some duodenal food flow has many advantages like nutritional protection, ensuring full access to the digestive tract, maintaining proximal protective mechanisms against hypoglycemia and micronutrient absorption capacity [36, 37].

5   Single Anastomosis Sleeve Ileal (SASI) Bypass: Pathophysiological Merits and Role in Weight Reduction and T2DM Remission

SASI bypass was born as a loop modification of the SG-TB of Santoro rather than the Roux-en-Y double anastomosis (Fig. 1) [36]. It Gained its name and popularity by Mahdy et al. [33], and since, has erupted as a unique bariatric and metabolic model representing a bipartition technique to treat obesity, diabesity or weight regain after SG. It acts by decreasing ghrelin secretion through sleeve gastrectomy while increasing the flow of food majorly through the gastro-ileostomy instead of the pylorus, which is thought to intensify hindgut stimulation rather than the foregut that provides positive intervention with the neuroendocrine control of hunger and satiety and not causing harm to the important digestive processes unrelated to obesity. It only has one intestinal anastomosis which in turn is associated with less anastomotic complications and shorter operative time [33]. The perception of nutrients in the distal bowel makes SASI patients eat less food due to a hypothalamic-generated satiety sensation [39]. The profound distal bowel stimulation reduces proximal gastrointestinal activity through the distal gut hormones such as glucagon like peptide-1 (GLP-1), which has central satietogenic effects, and reduces gastric emptying by the ileal break mechanism [40–42].

Like the SG-TB, the SASI is described as safer and easier to perform than BPD-DS and carries similar weight-loss benefits without the nutrient deficiencies and protein caloric malnutrition seen with the latter. The duodenum and papilla

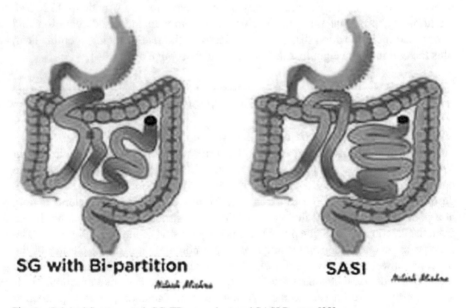

SG with Bi-partition   **SASI**

Fig. 1   Original Santoro et al. SG-TB procedure and SASI Bypass [38]

continue to be endoscopically accessible, with satisfactory short-term follow-up evidence now available for the SASI bypass [4].

6   SASI Bypass Technique

The operation is done as a two step procedure; SG followed by gastro-ileostomy, or a single complementary step added to the previously performed SG under general anesthesia. The latter is performed in the following steps:

The operating table is set in a horizontal position and the surgeon positioned on the left side of the patient. The procedure starts using 12-mm optical trocar to enter the abdomen under direct vision about 20 cm below the xiphoid process and 3 cm to the left side of the midline. Pneumo-peritoneum is achieved with carbon dioxide at 15 mmHg. Four additional ports are placed under direct vision, using the same sites as in SG. The ileocecal junction is identified and 250 cm is measured upwards. The selected loop is ascended without division of the greater omentum, and is stapled iso- peristaltic side-to-side to the anterior wall of the antrum of the stomach, just 3 cm away from the pylorus with a linear stapler charged with a green cartridge, the diameter of ileal antrum anastomosis should not exceed 3 cm in diameter. The anterior wall of the anastomosis is closed with a two-layer running 3/0 polydioxanone suture [33].

7   SASI Bypass Clinical Outcomes for Weight Regain and T2DM Remission

Mahdy et al.'s report was one of the initial studies that demonstrated the efficacy of the SASI bypass technique and included 50 patients [mean body mass index (BMI) 48.7 ± 7.6 kg/m^2]. The patients experienced significant (90%) excess weight loss (EWL) at 1 year. Also, serum glucose level was normalized in 100% of patients at 3 months, and all patients discontinued insulin and oral hypoglycemic medications [33]. In another study, Salama et al. reported on a 1-year follow-up of 45 patients (mean BMI 43.2 kg/m^2) BMI had decreased to 29.1 kg/m^2. Fasting plasma glucose (FPG), low-density lipoprotein (LDL), and insulin use were statistically significantly decreased, while high-density lipoprotein (HDL) was significantly increased [43]. In a multicenter study done also by Mahdy et al., fifty-eight patients underwent the SASI bypass after unsatisfactory SG outcomes. A significant decrease in weight and BMI from the mean preoperative weight at 12 months after SASI was recorded. The mean % total weight loss (TWL) at 12 months postoperatively was 17.3 ± 9.3 and the mean % EWL was 40.9 ± 22.1. Complete remission of T2DM was also documented, with complete remission of hypertension in 16.6%, while none of the patients with dyslipidemia or obstructive sleep apnea syndrome (OSAS) showed remission of their comorbidities [4].

The remarkable impact of the SASI bypass on glycemic control in diabetic patients is a major advantage of this procedure, with remission rates reaching

100%. This finding would suggest that the SASI bypassis an excellent option for patients with obesity and T2DM. As the procedure entails only a single gastroileal anastomosis, the risk of anastomotic complications may theoretically be less than other procedures that include more than one anastomosis [4]. In terms of comparison with SG-TB it is found to be more effective and simpler to perform, while also being an easily reversible technique.

Lower preoperative BMI and lower body weight were reported to predict higher %EWL after the SASI bypass. It should be emphasized that higher preoperative BMIs (>50 kg/m^2) scored poorer outcomes and lower % EWL after SG [44]. Performing the SASI to overcome sub-standard outcomes after SG was also associated with significantly lower % EWL (40.9 vs. 63.9%) compared with performing the SASI bypass as a primary bariatric procedure. Although weight regain was not observed in patients who underwent the SASI bypass compared with more than 5% of patients who underwent SG [12].

Furthermore, the SASI bypass was associated with significant improvement in other obesity-associated comorbidities, particularly gastroesophageal reflux disease (GERD) which is a considerable issue for the predominantly restrictive bariatric procedures such as SG. Moreover, research has proven that the leakage and GERD rates from SG was significantly decreased after performing gastrojejunostomy due to a decrease in the stomach tube pressure [45]. It is also worth mentioning that recent reports disclosed possible Barrett's esophagus risk following SG due to exposure of the distal esophagus to severe reflux, with de novo reflux seen in up to 23% of patients [46–48].

8   SASI Bypass Perioperative Morbidity, Reversal/ Revision

Salama et al. reported no mortalities in their study, with minimal postoperative nutritional complications in comparison to other procedures, reduced dumping syndrome and diarrhea [43]. Complications in the Mahdy et al. initial study included one complete obstruction at the gastroileal anastomosis, one post-operative internal hemorrhage, one pulmonary embolism, seven bilious vomiting and one leak in the biliary limb. At 6 months, one patient was diagnosed with a marginal ulcer; at 1 year, one patient was re-operated on to hault potential excessive weight loss, but no mortalities were seen [33]. From the multicenter study which included more than 600 patients, Mahdy et al. reported fifty-six (10.1%) complications after the SASI bypass, which is slightly higher than the mean overall complication rate after SG (8.7%) [4, 30]. Four (0.72%) patients required readmission within 30 days after surgery. However, the vast majority of morbidities after SASI bypass were minor, graded as grade I or II on the Clavien-Dindo scale. Complications included bilious vomiting, diarrhea, stomal ulcer, calcular obstructive jaundice, pulmonary embolism, intestinal obstruction, staple line bleeding, and ileal perforation (Table 1) [4].

Table 1 Grades of complications after SASI bypass [4]

Grade of complication	Type of complication	Number (%)
Grade I	Bilious vomiting	32 (5.8%)
	Diarrhea	15 (2.7%)
Grade II	Stoma ulcers	3 (0.54%)
Grade III	Staple line bleeding	1 (0.18%)
	Intestinal obstruction	1 (0.18%)
	Ileal perforation	1 (0.18%)
	Calcular obstructive jaundice	2 (0.36%)
Grade IV	Pulmonary embolism	1 (0.18%)

The most frequently reported complication after the SASI bypass was bilious vomiting. Bile reflux seems to be a common phenomenon in patients with a single gastroileal anastomosis, MGB and even RYGB [49] but even if dumping or biliary reflux is intractable, it can be simply reversed or revised to Braun's reconstruction [45]. In Mahdy et al.'s study, bilious vomiting and diarrhea were treated conservatively with fluids and medications. Stomal ulcers were managed with proton pump inhibitors, and calcular obstructive jaundice was treated with endoscopic retrograde cholangiopancreaticography (ERCP)and stone extraction, whereas a staple line bleeding, intestinal obstruction, and ileal perforation required surgical intervention. One patient who developed a pulmonary embolism was admitted to the ICU and was treated with intravenous fluids, anticoagulant medications, and thrombolytic therapy [4].

While most bariatric surgical procedures can be associated with nutritional deficiencies (as were reported for SG with median deficiency rates of iron, zinc, vitamin D, and vitamin B12 (9%, 20%, 35.5%, and 11.7%, respectively)) [50], SASI bypass has only a statistical decrease in serum albumen, which has proven to cause no clinical significance as serum albumin levels were still within the normal laboratory range so that none of the patients developed protein malabsorption after the SASI bypass [4, 43]. On the contrary, Salama et.al reported normal serum albumin and hemoglobin levels, with calcium deficiency in 2 cases of his study which improved with oral supplements [43]. On the other hand, Mahdy et al. demonstrated that vitamin D levels showed a significant increase at 1 year after the SASI bypass, which was explained by patients' compliance with systemic intake post operatively [33]. All options for weight regain after sleeve are associated with high failure and nutritional deficiency because they depend on malabsorption. SASI bypass, however, depends on modulation of gastrointestinal hormones without causing malabsorption, with easy conversion to the normal anatomy and a low morbidity rate.

9 Take Home Message

The ideal metabolic operation is one with high efficacy, cause resolution of comorbidities, easy to perform and have an easy exit strategy. The SASI bypass is an effective and safe bariatric procedure, with low and minor complication rate that can be added to suboptimal or failed SG to combat weight regain. It has also shown remarkable improvement in obesity-related comorbidities, namely T2DM and GERD.

References

1. Hall KD, Kahan S. Maintenance of lost weight and long-term management of obesity. Med Clin North Am. 2018;102:183–97.
2. Rubino F, Nathan DM, Eckel RH, Schauer PR, Alberti KG, Zimmet PZ, et al. Metabolic surgery in the treatment algorithm for type 2 diabetes: a joint statement by international diabetes organizations. Diab Care. 2016;39:861–77.
3. Cheng Y, Huang X, Wu D, Liu Q, Zhong M, Liu T, et al. Sleeve gastrectomy with bypass of proximal small intestine provides better diabetes control than sleeve gastrectomy alone under postoperative high-fat diet. Obes Surg. 2019;29:84–92.
4. Mahdy T, Emile SH, Madyan A, Schou C, Alwahidi A, Ribeiro R, et al. Evaluation of the efficacy of single anastomosis sleeve ileal (sasi) bypass for patients with morbid obesity: a multicenter study. Obes Surg. 2019. https://doi.org/10.1007/s11695-019-04296-3.
5. Buchwald H. The evolution of metabolic/bariatric surgery. Obes Surg. 2014;24:1126–35.
6. World Health Organization. Obesity and overweight key facts. Accessed July 2018. https://www.who.int/news-room/fact-sheets/detail/obesity-and-overweight. Accessed January 2020.
7. Dobbs R, Sawers C, Thompson F, Manyika J, Woetzel J, Child P, et al. Overcoming obesity: an initial economic analysis: McKinsey Global Institute; 2014.
8. Buchwald H, Buchwald JN. Review: metabolic (bariatric and non-bariatric) surgery for type 2 diabetes. Diab Care. 2019;42(2):331–40.
9. Almalki OM, Lee WJ, Chen JC, Ser KH, Lee YC, Chen SC. Revisional gastric bypass for failed restrictive procedures: comparison of single-anastomosis (mini-) and Roux-en-Y gastric bypass. Obes Surg. 2018;28(4):970–5.
10. Yilmaz H, Ece I, Sahin M. Revisional surgery after failed laparoscopic sleeve gastrectomy: retrospective analysis of causes, results, and technical considerations. Obes Surg. 2017;27(11):2855–60.
11. Biertho L, Thériault C, Bouvet L, Marceau S, Hould FS, Lebel S, et al. Second-stage duodenal switch for sleeve gastrectomy failure: a matched controlled trial. Surg Obes Relat Dis. 2018;14(10):1570–9.
12. Lauti M, Kularatna M, Hill AG, MacCormick AD. Weight regain following sleeve gastrectomy—a systematic review. Obes Surg. 2016;26(6):1326–34.
13. Spyropoulos C, Kehagias I, Panagiotopoulos S, Mead N, Kalfarentzos F. Revisional bariatric surgery: 13-year experience from a tertiary institution. Arch Surg. 2010;145(2):173–7.
14. Victorzon M. Revisional bariatric surgery by conversion to gastric bypass or sleeve–good short-term outcomes at higher risks. Obes Surg. 2012;22(1):29–33.
15. Yorke E, Sheppard C, Switzer NJ, Kim D, de Gara C, Karmali S, et al. Revision of sleeve gastrectomy to Roux-en-Y gastric bypass: a Canadian experience. Am J Surg. 2017;213(5):970–4.

16. Axer S, Szabo E, Naslund I. Weight loss and alterations in comorbidities after revisional gastric bypass: a case-matched study from the Scandinavian obesity surgery registry. Surg Obes Relat Dis. 2017;13(5):796–800.
17. Flolo TN, Andersen JR, Kolotkin RL, Aasprang A, Natvig GK, Hufthammer KO, et al. Five-year outcomes after vertical sleeve gastrectomy for severe obesity: a prospective cohort study. Obes Surg. 2017;27(8):1944–51.
18. Dapri G, Cadiere GB, Himpens J. Laparoscopic repeat sleeve gastrectomy versus duodenal switch after isolated sleeve gastrectomy for obesity. Surg Obes Relat Dis. 2011;7(1):38–43.
19. Cesana G, Uccelli M, Ciccarese F, Carrieri D, Castello G, Olmi S. Laparoscopic re-sleeve gastrectomy as a treatment of weight regain after sleeve gastrectomy. World J Gastrointest Surg. 2014;6(6):101–6.
20. Weng TC, Chang CH, Dong YH, Chang YC, Chuang LM. Anaemia and related nutrient deficiencies after Roux-en-Y gastric bypass surgery: a systematic review and meta-analysis. BMJ Open. 2015;5(7):e006964.
21. Higa KD, Ho T, Boone KB. Internal hernias after laparoscopic Roux-en-Y gastric bypass: incidence, treatment and prevention. Obes Surg. 2003;13:350–4.
22. Georgiadou D, Sergentanis TN, Nixon A, Diamantis T, Tsigris C, Psaltopoulou T. Efficacy and safety of laparoscopic mini gastric bypass. Surg Obes Relat Dis. 2014;10(5):984–91.
23. Mahawar KK, Kumar P, Carr WR, Jennings N, Schroeder N, Balupuri S. Current status of mini-gastric bypass. J Minim Access Surg. 2016;12(4):305–10.
24. Stefater MA, Wilson-Pérez HE, Chambers AP, Sandoval DA, Seeley RJ. All bariatric surgeries are not created equal: insights from mechanistic comparisons. Endocr Rev. 2012;33(4):595–622.
25. Celik A, Ugale S. Functional restriction and a new balance between proximal and distal gut: the tools of the real metabolic surgery. Obes Surg. 2014;24(10):1742–3.
26. Santoro S. From bariatric to pure metabolic surgery: new concepts on the rise. Ann Surg. 2015;2(2):e79-80.
27. Crea N, Pata G, Di Betta E, Greco F, Casella C, Vilardi A, et al. Long-term results of biliopancreatic diversion with or without gastric preservation for morbid obesity. Obes Surg. 2011;21(2):139–45.
28. Risstad H, Søvik TT, Engström M, Aasheim ET, Fagerland MW, Olsén MF, et al. Five-year outcomes after laparoscopic gastric bypass and laparoscopic duodenal switch in patients with body mass index of 50 to 60: a randomized clinical trial. JAMA Surg. 2015;150(4):352–61.
29. Sanchez-Pernaute A, Rubio MA, P´erez-Aguirre E, Barabash A, Cabrerizo L, Torres A. Single-anastomosis duodenoileal bypass with sleeve gastrectomy: metabolic improvement and weight loss in first 100 patients. Surg Obes Relat Dis. 2013;9:731–5.
30. Neichoy BT, Schniederjan B, Cottam DR, Surve AK, Zaveri HM, Cottam A, et al. Stomach intestinal pylorus-sparing surgery for morbid obesity. JSLS 2018;22(1):e2017.00063.
31. Mitzman B, Cottam D, Goriparthi R, Cottam S, Zaveri H, Surve A. Stomach intestinal pylorus sparing (SIPS) surgery for morbid obesity: retrospective analyses of our preliminary experience. Obes Surg. 2016;26:2098–104.
32. Spak E, Björklund P, Helander H, Vieth M, Olbers T, Casselbrant A, et al. Changes in the mucosa of the Roux-limb after gastric bypass surgery. Histopathology. 2010;57(5):680–8.
33. Mahdy T, Al Wahedi A, Schou C. Efficacy of single anastomosis sleeve ileal (SASI) bypass for type 2 diabetic morbid obese pa- tients: gastric bipartition, a novel metaboic surgery procedure: a retrospective cohort study. Int J Surg. 2016;34:28–34.
34. Dorman RB, Rasmus NF, al-Haddad BJ, Serrot FJ, Slusarek BM, Sampson BK, et al. Benefits and complications of the duodenal switch/biliopancreatic diversion compared to the Roux-en-Y gastric bypass. Surgery. 2012;152:758–65.
35. Santoro S, Malzoni CE, Velhote MC, Milleo FQ, Santo MA, Klajner S, et al. Digestive adaptation with intestinal reserve: a neuroendocrine- based operation for morbid obesity. Obes Surg. 2006;16(10):1371–9.

36. Santoro S, Castro LC, Velhote MC, Malzoni CE, Klajner S, Castro LP, et al. Sleeve gastrectomy with transit bipartition: a potent intervention for metabolic syndrome and obesity. Ann Surg. 2012;256(1):104–10.
37. Santoro S, Velhote MCP, Malzoni CE, Malzoni CE, Mechenas ASG, Damiani D, et al. Digestive adaptation with intestinal reserve: a new surgical proposal for morbid obesity. Rev Bras Videocir. 2004;2:130–8.
38. Bhandari M, Fobi MAL, Buchwald JN. Standardization of bariatric metabolic procedures: world consensus meeting statement. Obes Surg. 2019;29(4):S309–45.
39. Chambers AP, Sandoval DA, Seeley RJ. Integration of satiety signals by the central nervous system. Curr Biol. 2013;23(9):379–788.
40. Santoro S, Milleo FQ, Malzoni CE, Klajner S, Borges PC, Santo MA, et al. Entero hormonal changes after digestive adaptation five-year results of a surgical proposal to treat obesity and associated diseases. Obes Surg. 2008;18(1):17–26.
41. Carr RD, Larsen MO, Winzell MS, Jelic K, Lindgren O, Deacon CF, et al. Incretin and islet hormonal responses to fat and protein ingestion in healthy men. Am J Physiol Endocrinol Metab. 2008;295(4):779–84.
42. Lustig RH. The neuroendocrinology of obesity. Endocrinol Metab Clin North Am. 2001;30(3):765–85.
43. Salama TMS, Sabry K, Ghamrini YE. Single anastomosis sleeve ileal bypass: new step in the evolution of bariatric surgeries. J Invest Surg. 2017;30(5):291–6.
44. Elbanna H, Ghnnam W, Negm A, Youssef T, Emile S, El Metwally T, et al. Impact of preoperative body mass index on the final outcome after laparoscopic sleeve gastrectomy for morbid obesity. Ulus Cerrahi Derg. 2016;32(4):238–43.
45. Mui W, Lee D, Lam K. Laparoscopic sleeve gastrectomy with loop bipartition: a novel metabolic operation in treating obese type II diabetes mellitus. Int J Surg Case Rep. 2014;5(2):56–8.
46. Stenard F, Iannelli A. Laparoscopic sleeve gastrectomy and gastro- esophageal reflux. World J Gastroenterol. 2015;21(36):10348–57.
47. Emile SH. Gastroesophageal reflux disease after sleeve gastrectomy: the need to predict its onset and prevent its consequences. Obes Surg. 2019;29(8):2625–6.
48. Yeung KTD, Penney N, Ashrafian L, Darzi A, Ashrafian H. Does sleeve gastrectomy expose the distal esophagus to severe reflux? a systematic review and meta-analysis. Ann Surg. 2020;271(2):257–65.
49. Emile SH, Elfeki H, Elalfy K, Abdallah E. Laparoscopic sleeve gastrectomy then and now: an updated systematic review of the progress and short-term outcomes over the last 5 years. Surg Laparosc Endosc Percutan Tech. 2017;27(5):307–17.
50. Emile SH, Elfeki H. Nutritional deficiency after sleeve gastrectomy: a comprehensive literature review. EMJ Gastroenterol. 2017;6(1):99–105.

Revisional Surgery: Sleeve to Endosleeve

Aayed R. Alqahtani, Mohamed Elahmedi and
Abdullah Al-Darwish

1   Introduction

Teams treating patients who underwent LSG must be aware of evaluation and
management options for potential reasons behind poor weight loss and weight
regain. Interventional modalities that re-induce weight loss can be surgical,
endoscopic, medical, or combination therapy. A personalized management plan
must be established for each patient based on evaluation. Common reasons that
are associated with failure of LSG include poor compliance, baseline body mass
index (BMI) greater than 50 kg/m², retained antrum or fundus, use of an excessively large orogastric calibration tube, and gastric dilation. Volumetric analysis using computerized tomography following LSG has revealed that gastric
volume increases by about 60 ml on average during the first year, and that greater
increases in volume are associated with poor weight loss [1].

2   Patient Assessment

Weight loss trajectories after LSG vary between patients, and we recommend waiting 18 to 24 months after LSG before considering revision. Patients with poor
weight loss or weight regain (% excess weight loss <50%) should undergo evaluation for anatomical reasons for weight loss failure. The investigations assess the

A. R. Alqahtani (✉) · M. Elahmedi · A. Al-Darwish
New You Medical Center, Riyadh, Saudi Arabia
e-mail: qahtani@yahoo.com

M. Elahmedi
e-mail: elahmedi89@gmail.com

© The Editor(s) (if applicable) and The Author(s), under exclusive license to Springer   589
Nature Switzerland AG 2021
S. Al-Sabah et al. (eds.), *Laparoscopic Sleeve Gastrectomy*,
https://doi.org/10.1007/978-3-030-57373-7_57

presence and size of hiatal hernias, which could contribute to reflux symptoms and maladaptive eating. Segmental or generalized pouch dilations as well as the size of the antrum and fundus should be evaluated since these can limit the restrictive effect of the sleeve (Fig. 1). The rate of pouch emptying should be rapid without delays in any segment or significant reflux into the esophagus. It is important to recognize that weight regain can occur without pouch dilation or anatomic abnormality. Also, stable weight loss may exist with a very malformed or dilated pouch. Thus, it is important to fully evaluate each patient prior to embarking on any intervention to address failure.

3   Endoscopic Revision of LSG Using OverStitch

Given the evolving role of endoscopic suturing as a therapeutic bariatric intervention, there is growing interest in endoscopic revision of LSG as a minimally-invasive alternative to surgical revision for weight recidivism. Endoscopic sleeve gastroplasty (ESG) involves plication of the body of the stomach, reducing its lumen by approximately 70% [2]. The aim of the technique is to reduce the effective volume of the gastric lumen using lines of full-thickness sutures created along the greater curvature of the stomach. Current evidence Illustrates that ESG can safely induce 15–20% total body weight loss in 18–24 months [3, 4]. This approach has several advantages over traditional surgical revision options, including improved safety, technical ease, and the organ-sparing nature that allows for further revisional surgery.

After discussing all options, complete workup including evaluation with CT volumetry, upper gastrointestinal contrast study and/or EGD is performed. The choice of revision intervention is reached as an agreement between the surgeon/gastroenterologist and the patient considering the results of the workup and the expected weight loss with each option. Contraindications against performing revisional endoscopic gastroplasty (rEGP) include esophageal disorders, presence of a large hiatal hernia, and active peptic ulcer disease.

Fig. 1 Upper GI contrast study 6 years post LSG showing concentric dilatation

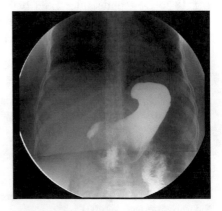

4 Technique

There are two aims from this procedure. The first is to reduce the capacity of the enlarged sleeve (Fig. 2), and the second is to shorten it. In general, the technique of rEGP post-LSG is the same for primary ESG [4] with two main exceptions: The surgeon must be wary of taking bites that traverse the diameter of the lumen as there is a risk of closing the lumen especially with the first suture. Secondly, the gastric caliber will be reduced resulting in poor visualization of the system's jaw. This raises the risk of damaging the gastric wall especially at the fundus. All sides of the gastric wall, including the greater curvature, are incorporated. The site of previous resection can be incorporated without major concerns. The gastric wall is expected to be thicker compared to patients who have not undergone sleeve gastrectomy, and the helix can safely have two or more full turns secure full thickness bites.

Under general anesthesia and with the patient in the left lateral position, a dual-channel gastroscope (Olympus, Tokyo, Japan) is inserted with an esophageal overtube placed over the scope. After reaching the stomach, the overtube is inserted using the scope as a guide. Surveillance gastroscopy is performed, delineating the exact anatomy of the sleeve, assessing for dilated or remnant areas in the antrum, body and fundus, and deciding on the suturing map. Suturing usually starts on the anterior wall at the level of incisura anteriorly. This point may be marked.

The gastroscope is withdrawn and an OverStitch system (Apollo Endosurgery, Austin, TX, USA) is mounted over the scope. The procedure commences at the referenced staring point. A helix is pushed, turning twice to thrice and grasping gastric tissue. The helix is pulled, presenting the gastric wall in a perpendicular position to the needle apparatus in the endcap (the jaw). A full-thickness bite is taken, exchanging the needle with the holder in the other channel. The tissue helix is then released. The process is repeated at the greater curvature and the posterior wall. The gastroscope is then repositioned proximally and a second bite line is performed. The needle is then released and the first cinch is deployed to secure the first knot of the procedure.

Fig. 2 EGD view showing dilated stomach after sleeve gastrectomy

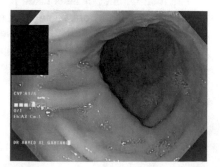

Fig. 3 Final look after
endoscopic revision of sleeve
gastrectomy using OverStitch

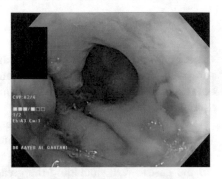

Fig. 4 Upper GI contrast
study after rEGP

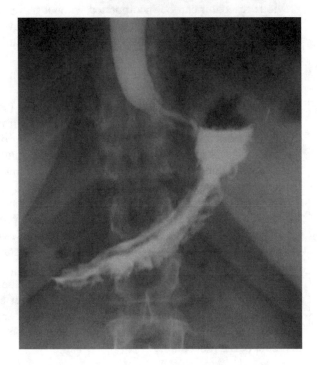

The total number of bites taken per suture is not fixed. This depends on tissue configuration and anatomy. Thorough plication leaving no pockets but a main, patent lumen is aimed for (Fig. 3). Additionally, the number of sutures depends on the gross volume of the gastric sleeve. Implanting of 2–4 sutures is expected considering the sleeve surface area. We believe that enlarged/retained fundus and antrum are major causes of weight regain, and we therefore focus on closing them during plication (Fig. 4).

5 Follow-Up

Postoperative visits are scheduled monthly for the first year and in 3–6 month intervals afterwards. At each visit, patients are counseled by multidisciplinary teams. Each team should include at least a clinical dietitian and a bariatric surgeon or a gastroenterologist.

6 Outcomes

The safety and efficacy of rEGP post-LSG were evaluated in two multicenter studies. The first was an international multicenter study that included 82 patients from Saudi Arabia, the United States, the UAE, and Brazil. More than 80% of patients lost at least 10% of their weight within one year, and mean weight loss was 16%. However, one patient experienced narrowing of the gastroesophageal junction that required endoscopic dilatation [5]. The second study included 34 patients primarily from Brazil. Patients lost 18% of their weight during the first year after revision, and similar to the international multicenter study, more than 80% lost at least 10% of their weight. No severe adverse events were recorded [6].

7 Conclusions

rEGP for patients with weight regain after LSG is feasible. The reversibility of the procedure, the fact that it induces weight loss without disruption of GI anatomy, and its day-case nature are important advantages that make it an intervention worth considering before revisional surgery.

References

1. Atkins ER, Preen DB, Jarman C, Cohen LD. Improved obesity reduction and co-morbidity resolution in patients treated with 40-French bougie versus 50-French bougie four years after laparoscopic sleeve gastrectomy. Analysis of 294 patients. Obes Surg. 2012;22(1):97–104.
2. Kumbhari V, Hill C, Sullivan S. Bariatric endoscopy: state-of-the-art. Curr Opin Gastroenterol. 2017;33(5):358–65.
3. Hedjoudje A, Dayyeh BA, Cheskin LJ, Adam A, Neto MG, Badurdeen D, et al. Efficacy and safety of endoscopic sleeve gastroplasty: a systematic review and meta-analysis. Clin Gastroenterol Hepatol. 2019.
4. Alqahtani A, Al-Darwish A, Mahmoud AE, Alqahtani YA, Elahmedi M. Short-term outcomes of endoscopic sleeve gastroplasty in 1000 consecutive patients. Gastrointest Endosc. 2019;89(6):1132–8.

5. de Moura DTH, Barrichello S Jr, de Moura EGH, et al. Endoscopic sleeve gastroplasty in the management of weight regain after sleeve gastrectomy. Endoscopy. 2020;52(3):202–10. https://doi.org/10.1055/a-1086-0627.
6. Daniel B. Maselli, Aayed R. Alqahtani, Barham K. Abu Dayyeh, et al. Revisional Endoscopic Sleeve Gastroplasty (R-ESG) of laparoscopic sleeve gastrectomy: an international, multi-center study. Gastrointest Endosc. 2020 (in-press).

Revisional Surgery: Sleeve to DJB

Hidenori Haruta, Kazunori Kasama, Yosuke Seki
and Alan Kawarai Lefor

1   Introduction

Sleeve gastrectomy (SG) was first described as a modification of the biliary-pancreatic diversion, then combined with the duodenal switch in 1998, and first performed laparoscopically in 1999 [1–3]. Having been shown to be safe and effective in the short term, SG subsequently became a standalone bariatric procedure [4].

According to recent data, SG has become the most commonly performed bariatric procedure around the world [5]. While short-term postoperative outcomes of SG are satisfactory, revision surgery is still unavoidable during mid to long-term follow up in some patients. In a recent systematic review and meta- analysis, the overall revision rate was 10.4%, but for patients with more than 10-years follow up, the rate was 22.6% [6]. During long-term follow-up, some patients may require revision due to insufficient weight loss, weight regain, intolerable gastroesophageal reflux disease (GERD) symptoms, or relapse of diabetes mellitus. Revision to a Roux-en-Y gastric bypass (RYGB) [6, 7] has been the most commonly performed procedure, but recently, revision to a duodeno-jejunal bypass (DJB) is also being performed. In this chapter, we report the significance of adding a DJB, surgical procedure and outcomes of revision surgery from SG to DJB.

H. Haruta (✉) · K. Kasama · Y. Seki
Weight Loss and Metabolic Surgery Center, Yotsuya Medical Cube, Tokyo, Japan
e-mail: haruta511@yahoo.co.jp

A. K. Lefor
Division of Gastroenterological, General and Transplant Surgery, Jichi Medical University, Tochigi, Japan

S. Al-Sabah et al. (eds.), *Laparoscopic Sleeve Gastrectomy*,
https://doi.org/10.1007/978-3-030-57373-7_58

2   Significance of Adding a DJB

It is known that biliopancreatic diversion with duodenal switch (BPD/DS) is the most effective bariatric procedure for weight loss and improvement of obesity-related complications [8]. But patients who undergo BPD/DS are susceptible to malabsorption of fat-soluble vitamins, calcium, zinc, iron, and protein, even when taking supplementation appropriately [9]. Above all protein intake varies from region to region. Amount of protein intake in the Asia Pacific population is much less than that of westerners due to the different dietary habits. However, there are few reports of malnutritional complications in long-term follow-up after RYGB. Therefore, the risk of nutritional deficiency after DJB (proximal intestinal bypass) is expected to be lower than that after DS [10].

The duodenal jejunum anastomosis in DJB is placed 1–2 cm distal to the pylorus, allowing a wider range of anastomosis than the RYGB anastomosis, and reducing the incidence of anastomotic stenosis. Pyloric preservation can reduce the rates of marginal ulcers, dumping syndrome, bile reflux and reactive hypoglycemia which are often problematic after RYGB [10, 11]. Also, unlike RYGB, there is no need to create an anastomotic stoma out of scarred or fibrotic tissues (the duodenum had not been dissected during the primary LSG).

Duodenal exclusion may have a significant role in the resolution of diabetes in addition to weight reduction. Several randomized trials have shown that procedures which include duodenal exclusion are associated with higher rates of diabetes remission or eliminating the need for medications than procedures without duodenal exclusion, especially in patients with diabetes and a lower body mass index [12, 13]. The mechanism of this effect is not fully elucidated. After the bypass procedure, there are changes in the secretion of intestinal hormones [14, 15], intestinal flora, and an elevation of serum bile acid concentration [13, 16, 17]. Investigators in the field of metabolic disorders are increasingly interested in the role of bile acids as a metabolic modulator [18]. Miyachi et al. reported that a long biliopancreatic limb contributes to metabolic improvement and elevation of serum bile acid concentration in a rat model [19]. These effects were negated after removing the biliopancreatic limb. Ise et al. reported that shortening the enterohepatic circulation by early reabsorption of conjugated bile acids in the biliopancreatic limb, not by the early influx of bile into the ileum, after DJB in a type 2 diabetes rat model [20]. The metabolic improvement effect and the increase in bile acid concentration after DJB may both depend on the length of the biliopancreatic limb.

3   Effects of DJB on Diabetes Mellitus

Patients who underwent bypass as the first operation serve as a reference for predicting the effect of revision surgery on the rate of relapse of diabetes mellitus. Raj et al. observed in a randomized controlled trial comparing laparoscopic RYGB and laparoscopic SG/DJB that the remission rate of diabetes mellitus (defined by achieving a HbA1c < 7.0% without the need for diabetes medication at 1 year) was similar (laparoscopic SG/DJB: 80%, laparoscopic RYGB: 81%) [21]. Lee et al. reported a retrospective matched case–control study comparing laparoscopic SG with single-anastomosis duodenal-jejunal bypass and laparoscopic SG alone. In their study, the length of the (loop) biliary limb was 150 to 250 cm based on the body mass index. The mean reduction in the HbA1c level in the laparoscopic SG/DJB group was also higher than that found for the laparoscopic SG group (2.8 versus 2.1%, p = 0.045) [22]. Naito et al. reported that laparoscopic SG/DJB is significantly more effective than laparoscopic SG alone for obese diabetic patients with a lower ABCD score [23] (patients with more severe type 2 diabetes mellitus) [24]. They also recommend that patients with type 2 diabetes mellitus who use insulin or whose ABCD score is ≤ 5 undergo laparoscopic SG/DJB.

Although the rate of diabetes remission after bariatric surgery may be strongly influenced by various factors such as patients' background especially in terms of diabetes severity, surgical technique, surgeon's preference, etc., it still seems to be safe to say that laparoscopic SG/DJB is superior to laparoscopic SG and at least equivalent to RYGB in terms of long-term glycemic control.

4   Reasons for Revising a SG to a DJB

Inadequate weight loss, weight regain, GERD and diabetes relapse are the most common reasons to revise a SG [25]. In patients with post-operative GERD, RYGB is considered as the first choice. If the sleeve pouch is dilated when considering revision from SG to DJB, a re-sleeve procedure needs to be added. Sleeve volume is an important determinant of weight loss/weight regain. Returning to a low volume restores satiety and appetite suppression [25–27]. In case of insufficient weight loss or weight regain without sleeve pouch dilatation, there are no definite recommendations for the choice of revision procedure. It is strongly recommended to add a DJB or bypass procedure (for example duodenal switch or single-anastomosis duodeno–ileal bypass with sleeve gastrectomy (SADI-S), as described in other chapters). If diabetes relapses, a bypass procedure should be added.

5   Surgical Procedure for Revising SG to DJB

5.1   Biliopancreatic Diversion/Duodenal Switch (Fig. 1)

As mentioned earlier, SG was originally developed as a first stage procedure for biliopancreatic diversion with duodenal switch (BPD/DS) [28]. In the original BPD/DS, the total alimentary limb, including the common limb, was 250 cm, the common channel was 50–100 cm from the ileocecal valve, and the rest was the biliopancreatic limb [28]. BPD/DS is the most effective bariatric procedure for weight loss and improvement of obesity-related complications [8], but is

Fig. 1 BPD/DS:
Biliopancreatic diversion with
duodenal switch

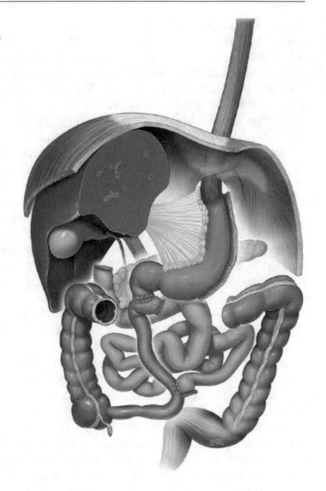

performed in only 1.1% of bariatric procedures worldwide [5]. The major obstacles to BPD/DS are the technical difficulties (two anastomoses and closure of two
mesenchymal defects: Petersen's defect and the mesenteric defect from the entero-
enterostomy) and the possibility of long-term nutritional problems [29]. Patients
who undergo BPD/DS are susceptible to malabsorption of fat-soluble vitamins,
calcium, zinc, iron, and protein, even when taking supplementation appropriately
[9]. Since BPD/DS results in malabsorption, it is important to evaluate long-term
nutritional changes.

6   Laparoscopic SG/DJB (Fig. 2)

A modified short duodenal switch has been proposed by Kasama et al. from Asia
with a procedure called laparoscopic SG with duodeno-jejunal bypass (laparoscopic SG/DJB) in 2009 [10]. Initially, SG and dissection of the posterior duodenal

Fig. 2 Laparoscopic SG with duodeno-jejunal bypass [10]

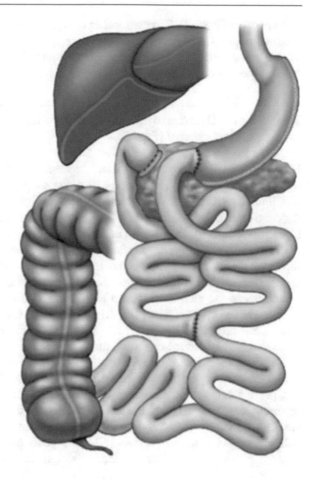

wall are carried out. Subsequently, DJB is added with 50–150 cm of biliopancreatic tract and 100–150 cm of alimentary tract resulting in a common channel length more than 300 cm. DJB consists of a jejuno-jejunostomy created using a linear stapler and hand sewn closure and duodeno-jejunostomy with a two layer hand-sewn closure. The duodeno-jejunostomy is placed 1–2 cm distal to the pylorus allowing a wide anastomosis compared to that in RYGB, which contributes to a lower rate of anastomotic stenosis. Pyloric preservation can reduce the rates of marginal ulcers, dumping syndrome and reactive hypoglycemia which are often problematic after RYGB. Bile reflux is not anatomically possible. The risk of nutritional deficiency after laparoscopic SG/DJB is expected to be lower than that after DS. Theoretically, the combination of SG and DJB (proximal intestinal bypass) is expected to have strong anti-diabetic effects. Seki reported the medium-term (up to 5 years) effects and outcomes after laparoscopic SG/DJB. Laparoscopic SG/DJB is effective for achieving significant weight loss and improvement of glycemic control, and the effects seem to be durable up to 5 years [30].

Laparoscopic SG/DJB is an ideal operation with no bile reflux into the stomach but requires advanced skill and more time (two anastomoses and closure of two mesenteric defects: Petersen's defect and the mesenteric defect from the entero-enterostomy).

7 Loop Duodenojejunal Bypass with Sleeve Gastrectomy (Fig. 3)

Huang CK et al. proposed the loop duodenojejunal bypass with sleeve gastrectomy in 2013 [11]. The concept of a one loop anastomosis is similar to the technique of SADI-S. SADI-S includes a sleeve gastrectomy followed by a loop duodeno-ileal anastomosis with a 200 cm efferent limb from the ileocecal valve (see other chapters). In the loop duodenojejunal bypass with sleeve gastrectomy, SG is initially carried out, the transection of the first part of the duodenum performed 2 cm from the pylorus, and an antecolic loop duodeno-jejunal anastomosis created 200 cm from the ligament of Treitz using a hand-sewn single-layer technique. In the anastomosis as a loop, there is only one anastomosis and one mesenteric defect (Petersen's defect) compared to the two anastomoses and two mesenteric defects in BPD/DS or laparoscopic SG/DJB. The elimination of one anastomosis may reduce operating time and needs no mesenteric opening, therefore decreasing the possibility of surgically related complication. Pyloric preservation can reduce the rates of marginal ulcer formation and dumping syndrome and prevent bile reflux. However, bile reflux is anatomically possible. Ser et al. reported long-term data after single-anastomosis duodenal-jejunal bypass with sleeve gastrectomy (logically the same operation as loop duodenojejunal bypass with sleeve gastrectomy) [33]. At 1, 2 and 5 years postoperatively, the mean percentage of total weight loss and excess weight loss in patients who underwent

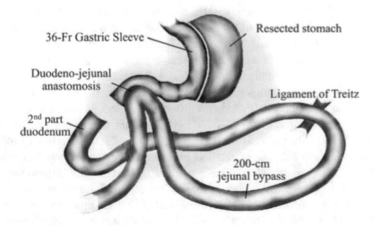

Fig. 3 Loop duodenojejunal bypass with sleeve gastrectomy [34]

single-anastomosis duodenal-jejunal bypass with sleeve gastrectomy were 25.5%, 22.8%, 22.5%, and 83.9%, 76.1%, 58.6%, respectively. Among 118 patients with type 2 diabetes mellitus, 62 (52.5%) achieved complete remission (HgbA1C<6.0%) at 1 year and 36.5% at 5 years after surgery. Their results showed that primary single-anastomosis duodenal-jejunal bypass with sleeve gastrectomy is a durable primary bariatric procedure with sustained weight loss and a high resolution of type 2 diabetes mellitus at 5 years.

8   Conclusions

There is no consensus on what operation should be carried out after failed SG [35]. Bariatric revision surgery is often technically challenging due to the altered anatomy and tissue fibrosis after the primary procedure [36]. Revision surgery has been associated with severe increases in the rate of surgical complications.

The need to revise a SG to a DJB is strongly influenced by a number of factors such as the patients' background, surgical technique, surgeon's preference, etc. Each procedure introduced in this chapter is effective for substantial weight loss and improvements in comorbidities which are maintained, but each has both advantages and disadvantages. It is important for surgeons to understand the characteristics of each procedure and to provide appropriate advice and treatment for patients.

References

1. Marceau P, Hould FS, Simard S, et al. Biliopancreatic diversion with duodenal switch. World J Surg. 1998;22:947–54.
2. Ren CJ, Patterson E, Gagner M. Early results of laparoscopic biliopancreatic diversion with duodenal switch: a case series of 40 consecutive patients. Obes Surg. 2000;10:514–23; discussion 524.
3. de Csepel J, Burpee S, Jossart G, et al. Laparoscopic biliopancreatic diversion with a duodenal switch for morbid obesity: a feasibility study in pigs. J Laparoendosc Adv Surg Tech A. 2001;11:79–83.
4. Gagner M, Deitel M, Kalberer TL, et al. The second international consensus summit for sleeve gastrectomy, Surg Obes Relat Dis. 2009;5(4):476–85.
5. Angrisani L, Santonicola A, Iovino P, et al. Bariatric surgery and endoluminal procedures: IFSO worldwide survey 2014. Obes Surg. 2017;27(9):2279–89.
6. Guan B, Chong TH, Peng J, et al. Mid-long-term revisional surgery after sleeve gastrectomy: a systematic review and meta-analysis. Obes Surg. 2019;29(6):1965–75.
7. Weiner RA, Theodoridou S, Weiner S. Failure of laparoscopic sleeve gastrectomy--further procedure? Obes Facts. 2011;4(Suppl 1):42–6. https://doi.org/10.1159/000327343. Epub 2011 Apr 4.
8. Buchwald H, Avidor Y, Braunwald E, et al. Bariatric surgery: a systematic review and meta-analysis. JAMA. 2004;292:1724–37.
9. Strain GW, Torghabeh MH, Gagner M, et al. Nutrient status 9 years after Biliopancreatic Diversion with Duodenal Switch (BPD/DS): an observational study. Obes Surg. 2017;27(7):1709–18.

10. Kasama K, Tagaya N, Kanehira E, et al. Laparoscopic sleeve gastrectomy with duodenojejunal bypass: technique and preliminary results. Obes Surg. 2009;19(10):1341–5.
11. Huang CK, Goel R, Tai CM, et al. Novel metabolic surgery for type II diabetes mellitus: loop duodenojejunal bypass with sleeve gastrectomy. Surg Laparosc Endosc Percutan Tech. 2013;23(6):481–5.
12. Gerhard GS, Styer AM, Wood GC, et al. A role for fibroblast growth factor 19 and bile acids in diabetes remission after Roux-en-Y gastric bypass. Diabetes Care. 2013a;36(7):1859–64.
13. Liou AP, Paziuk M, Luevano Jr JM, et al. Conserved shifts in the gut microbiota due to gastric bypass reduce host weight and adiposity. Sci Transl Med. 2013;5(178):178ra41.
14. Ionut V, Bergman RN. Mechanisms responsible for excess weight loss after bariatric surgery. J Diab Sci Technol. 2011;5(5):1263–82.
15. Meryn S, Stein D, Straus EW. Pancreatic polypeptide, pancreatic glucagon and enteroglucagon in morbid obesity and following gastric bypass operation. Int J Obes. 1986;10(1):37–42.
16. Batterham RL, Cummings DE. Mechanisms of diabetes improvement following bariatric/metabolic surgery. Diab Care. 2016;39(6):893–901.
17. Gerhard GS, Styer AM, Wood GC, et al. A role for fibroblast growth factor 19 and bile acids in diabetes remission after Roux-en-Y gastric bypass. Diab Care. 2013b;36(7):1859–64.
18. Ryan KK, Tremaroli V, Clemmensen C, et al. FXR is a molecular target for the effects of vertical sleeve gastrectomy. Nature. 2014;509(7499):183–8.
19. Miyachi T, Nagao M, Shibata C, et al. Biliopancreatic limb plays an important role in metabolic improvement after duodenal-jejunal bypass in a rat model of diabetes. Surgery. 2016;159(5):1360–71.
20. Ise I, Tanaka N, Imoto H, et al. Changes in enterohepatic circulation after duodenal-jejunal bypass and reabsorption of bile acids in the bilio-pancreatic limb. Obes Surg. 2019;29(6):1901–10.
21. Praveen Raj P, Kumaravel R, Chandramaliteeswaran C, et al. Is laparoscopic duodenojejunal bypass with sleeve an effective alternative to Roux en Y gastric bypass in morbidly obese patients: preliminary results of a randomized trial. Obes Surg. 2012;22(3):422–6.
22. Lee WJ, Almulaifi AM, Tsou JJ, et al. Duodenal-jejunal bypass with sleeve gastrectomy versus the sleeve gastrectomy procedure alone: the role of duodenal exclusion. Surg Obes Relat Dis. 2015;11(4):765–70.
23. Lee MH, Lee WJ, Chong K, et al. Predictors of long-term diabetes remission after metabolic surgery. J Gastrointest Surg. 2015;19(6):1015–21.
24. Naitoh T, Kasama K, Seki Y, et al. Efficacy of sleeve gastrectomy with duodenal-jejunal bypass for the treatment of obese severe diabetes patients in Japan: a retrospective multicenter study. Obes Surg. 2018;28(2):497–505.
25. Yilmaz H, Ece I, Sahin M. Revisional surgery after failed laparoscopic sleeve gastrectomy: retrospective analysis of causes, results, and technical considerations. Obes Surg. 2017;27(11):2855–60.
26. Iannelli A, Schneck AS, Noel P, et al. Re-sleeve gastrectomy for failed laparoscopic sleeve gastrectomy: a feasibility study. Obes Surg. 2011;21(7):832–5.
27. Saliba C, El Rayes J, Diab S, et al. Weight regain after sleeve gastrectomy: a look at the benefits of re-sleeve. Cureus. 2018;10(10):e3450.
28. Hess DS, Hess DW. Biliopancreatic diversion with a duodenal switch. Obes Surg. 1998;8(3):267–82.
29. Aasheim ET, Björkman S, Søvik TT, et al. Vitamin status after bariatric surgery: a randomized study of gastric bypass and duodenal switch. Am J Clin Nutr. 2009;90(1):15–22.
30. Seki Y, Kasama K, Umezawa A, et al. Laparoscopic sleeve gastrectomy with duodenojejunal bypass for type 2 diabetes mellitus. Obes Surg. 2016;26(9):2035–44.
31. Sanchez-Pernaute A, Herrera AR, Perez-Aguirre MEP, et al. Proximal duodenal-ileal end-to-side bypass with sleeve gastrectomy: proposed technique. Obes Surg. 2007;17:1611–8.

32. Sanchez-Pernaute A, Herrera AR, Perez-Aguirre MEP, et al. Single anastomosis duodeno-ileal bypass with sleeve gastrectomy (SADI-S). One- to three-year follow-up. Obes Surg. 2010;20:1720–6.
33. Ser KH, Lee WJ, Chen JC, et al. Laparoscopic single-anastomosis duodenal-jejunal bypass with sleeve gastrectomy (SADJB-SG): surgical risk and long-term results. Surg Obes Relat Dis. 2019;15(2):236–43.
34. Huang CK, Tai CM, Chang PC, et al. Loop duodenojejunal bypass with sleeve gastrectomy: comparative study with Roux-en-Y gastric bypass in type 2 diabetic patients with a BMI <35 kg/m(2), first year results. Obes Surg. 2016;26(10):2291–301. https://doi.org/10.1007/s11695-016-2118-z.
35. Langer FB, Shakeri-Leidenmühler S, Bohdjalian A, et al. Strategies for weight regain after sleeve gastrectomy. Surg Laparosc Endosc Percutan Tech. 2010;20:159–61.
36. Barrett AM, Vu KT, Sandhu KK, et al. Primary sleeve gastrectomy compared to sleeve gastrectomy as revisional surgery: weight loss and complications at intermediate follow-up. J Gastrointest Surg. 2014;18(10):1737–43.

How to Manage Sleeve Complications: The Unresponsive Sleeve

Rudolf Weiner and Sylvia Weiner

1   Introduction

Currently, the sleeve gastrectomy (SG) is the leading procedure for the treatment of obesity, and associated diseases worldwide. The procedure is standardized in many surgical involvements, but not performed identically in general. Consensus Conferences on SG organized by M. Gagner [5] and R. Rosenthal [8]had a pivotal role in establishing the fundamental standards of the procedure There is notable evidence that weight loss, after SG, has a wide range, especially in the mid- and long-term periods. Per definition inadequate weight loss is an excess weight loss of less than 50% in the post-operative period. The view of each obese patient can differ, and any EWL less than 70 or 100% can be considered as failure by the individual patient. This is the result of unrealistic expectations and anticipations by the obese patient.

The EWL is highly dependent on the amount that the individual patient is overweight (BMI classes). Higher initial weight, higher BMI-classes would ultimately achieve lower rates of EWL. While there is no scientific basis for the limit of exact 50% EWL, excessive weight loss (also inadequate) is defined as EWL of more than 100%. The inadequate (poor) weight loss can be due to several factors, such as insufficient gastric volume reduction for nutritional uptake (restriction) and/or incorrect habits in daily nutrition.

R. Weiner (✉)
Sana-Klinikum Offenbach, Frankfurt, Germany
e-mail: profweiner@gmail.com

S. Weiner
Krankenhaus Norwest, Steinbacher Hohl, Frankfurt am Main, Germany
e-mail: sylvia.weiner@gmx.de

S. Al-Sabah et al. (eds.), *Laparoscopic Sleeve Gastrectomy*,
https://doi.org/10.1007/978-3-030-57373-7_59

The "normal" range of EWL after SG in BMI-classes between 35 and 50 kg/m^2 were reported in literature with large series to be between 75 and 90% EWL [9].

2   Diagnosis

The diagnostic algorithm normally begins with non-invasive tools.

(A) An evaluation of nutritional behaviors that include eating disorders is fundamental.
(B) A 3-D CT-volume measurement of the sleeve after ingestion of gas-forming agents is an important next step. The gastric volume should not exceed 180 ml. If this technical tool is not available, then an experienced physician in bariatric surgery should follow up with an upper endoscopy procedure.
(C) The exploration by upper endoscopy should be readily available. The highest diagnostic value can be reached if the endoscopy is performed by a "bariatric" surgeon. That is due to the fact that they will have a better ability to determine:
     a. Persistent gastric volume,
     b. Herniation of the sleeve into the mediastinum,
     c. Non-resected fundus
     d. Pylorus function. If the pylorus is always open, then the duodenum would become a new reservoir and weight loss would be poor.

3   Treatment

The treatment of the unresponsive sleeve is mostly based on the diagnostic findings of the aforementioned tests. The most common cause for ineffective weight loss has been found to be the lack of restriction. In contrast to primary BPD-DS, the volume of the gastric sleeve should be smaller after a stand-alone procedure than that preceding a double stage procedure such as the BPD-DS. DS surgeons using larger bougie sizes (e.g.. 50–56) than what is commonly used in single-stage sleeve gastrectomy, or performing the part of SG during BPD-DS "free-handedly" without calibration tend to result in less restriction.. Thus, the reduction of gastric volume is not sufficient.

Studies from the last decade have shown that a resected gastric volume of less than 500 cc is associated with poor weight loss and therefore, with failure in treatment [10]. Early weight loss results were not considerably different between SG using a 32 French and a 44 French tube for calibration, but after 2 years follow-up, the more restrictive LSG results were significantly better in patients without calibration. A removed gastric volume of <500 cc appears to be a predictor of failure in treatment or in early weight regain.

4 Laparoscopic Redo Sleeve Gastrectomy (LRSG) in Short and Midterm Follow-Up

Laparoscopic redo sleeve gastrectomy (LRSG) has been shown to be an efficient revisional surgery option for insufficient weight loss after primary gastric sleeve in short and medium term follow-up [4]. This study from Rumania was able to prove that the initial weight reduction was effective. Mean BMI before LRSG was 35.69 kg/m^2 (range 28,58–52) and follow-up results at 6 months after re-sleeve revealed a mean BMI of 28.39+ −5.32 kg/m^2 corresponding to an EWL of 83.88%, while at 1 year mean BMI reached 27.23+ −5.23 kg/m^2 with EWL of 94.45% and at 3 years BMI reached 27.65+ −5.13 kg/m^2 with EWL of 85.41%. There are statistically significant differences (p 0.01), between BMI before LRSG and BMI for all other periods of measurement at 6 months, 1 year and 3 years after LRSG.

Similar results were reported by Mehmet [7]. He concluded that LRSG is an available and efficient method to correct the weight regain or inadequate weight loss following SG.

A total of 21 patients underwent LRSG after SG, due to inadequate weight loss. This study revealed that, 7 (33.3%) of them were males, and 14 (66.7%) were females. The mean body weight index (BMI) before primary LSG was 52.3±4.7 kg/m^2 and EWL% was 32.7±4.6. After an average follow-up of 24 months. BMI of patients before LRSG was 46.1±4.3 kg/m^2. Following a 1-year observation period, there was a substantial (p<0.001) improvement in BMI (21.6±3.1 kg/m^2) and excess weight loss percentage (86.82% EWL).

Al Sabah et al. [1] reported about the outcome of 1300 SG in the period of 2009 to 2012. A total number of 36 patients needed a conversion due to insufficient weight loss and weight regain. 24 underwent a LRSG and 12 were converted to RYGB. The mean BMI prior to LSG for the LRYGB and LRSG patients were 52 kg/m^2, and 50 kg/m^2, respectively. The EWL after the initial LSG was 37.9 and 43%, for LRYGB and LRSG.. Results of conversion of LSG to LRYGB involved a mean EWL of 61.3% after 1 year (p value 0.009). Results of LRSG involved a mean EWL of 57% after an interval of 1 year (p value 0.05). Comparison of the EWL% of LRYGB and LRSG for failed primary LSG was not significant (p value 0.097).

5 Laparoscopic Redo Sleeve Gastrectomy (LRSG) in Long-Term Follow-Up

The long-term results have proven to be different and non sufficient. De Angelis et al. [3] presented the outcomes of a cohort of LRSG at 52 months. Around 40% of the patients complained of GERD symptoms after 36 months and finally were converted to RYGB. Based on our disappointing results, De Angelis et al. [3] concluded that LRSG should not currently be offered as a revisional procedure any longer.

In the case of a proper sleeve, the conversion to a malabsorptive procedure is the solution for long-term success in weight loss. Beside the classic BPD-DS, SADI, MGB/OAGB, SASI, many other variations can be offered. The BPD-DS has proven to be very effective after failed sleeve [3]. While the technique of duodenoileostomy has no influence [11], the RYGB has been shown to be the best solution for gastroesophageal reflux symptom. If further weight loss is indicated, then the biliopancreatic limb should be extended (100–150 cm). The correct sleeve is a *conditio sine qua non*, if a BPD-DS or SADI will be added. Lebel et al. [6] has shown, that after SG, the biliopancreatic diversion with a common channel (CC), of 100 cm and 200 cm do not result in considerable differences in weight loss (EWL $61 \pm 22\%$ versus $68 \pm 18\%$) ($P = 0.18$).

Patients with 200 cm CC showed a lower incidence of severe protein deficiency (11% versus 19%, $p = 0.3$) and hyperparathyroidism (17.1% versus 35.3%, $p = 0$ 0.17); require a lower amount of vitamins A and D ($P < 0.05$); and had a decreased number of daily bowel movements (2.0 versus 2.9, $p = 0$ .03). In this population, BPD-DS with a 200-cm common channel offered similar remission rate of co-morbidities compared to standard BPD-DS. It was associated with similar weight loss at nadir, followed by a more significant weight regain, while yielding a lower rate of nutritional complications [9]. Long-term randomized data are needed to detect other potential advantages.

6   Conclusion

The proper and perfect gastric sleeve is the basis for success in weight loss and treatment of obesity-related diseases.

References

1. Al Sabah S, Alsharqawi N, Almulla A, Akrof S, Alenezi K, Buhaimed W, Al-Subaie S, Al Haddad M. Approach to poor weight loss after laparoscopic sleeve gastrectomy: re-sleeve versus gastric bypass. Obes Surg. 2016;26(10):2302–7
2. Biertho L, Thériault C, Bouvet L, Marceau S, Hould FS, Lebel S, Julien F, Tchernof A. Second-stage duodenal switch for sleeve gastrectomy failure: a matched controlled trial. Surg Obes Relat Dis. 2018;14(10):1570–9.
3. De Angelis F, Avallone M, Albanese A, Foletto M, Silecchia G. Re-sleeve gastrectomy 4 years later: is it still an effective revisional option? Obes Surg. 2018;28(11):3714–6.
4. Filip S, Hutopila I, Coapescu C. Re-sleeve Gastrectomy—an efficient revisional bariatric procedure—3 years results. Chirurgia (Bucur). 2019;114(6):809–23.
5. Gagner M, Hutchinson C, Rosenthal R. Fifth international consensus conference: current status of sleeve gastrectomy. Surg Obes Relat Dis. (2016).

6. Lebel S, Dion G, Marceau S, Biron S, Robert M, Biertho L. Clinical outcomes of duodenal switch with a 200-cm common channel: a matched, controlled trial. Surg Obes Relat Dis. 2016;12(5):1014–20.
7. Mehmet B. Re-sleeve gastrectomy for failed primary laparoscopic sleeve gastrectomy. J Coll Physicians Surg Pak. 2019;29(1):62–5.
8. Rosenthal RJ; Diaz AA, Arvidsson D, Baker RS, Basso N, Bellanger D, Boza C, El Mourad H, France M, Gagner M, Galvao-Neto M, Higa KD, Himpens J, Hutchinson CM, Jacobs M, Jorgensen JO, Jossart G, Lakdawala M, Nguyen NT, Nocca D, Prager G, Pomp A, Ramos AC, Rosenthal RJ, Shah S, Vix M, Wittgrove A, Zundel N. International sleeve gastrectomy expert panel consensus statement: best practice guidelines based on experience of >12,000 cases. Surg Obes Relat Dis. (2012).
9. Strain GW, Gagner M, Pomp A, Dakin G, Inabnet WB, Hsieh J, Heacock L, Christos P. Comparison of weight loss and body composition changes with four surgical procedures. Surg Obes Relat Dis. 2009;5(5):582–7.
10. Weiner RA, Weiner S, Pomhoff I, Jacobi C, Makarewicz W, Weigand G. Laparoscopic sleeve gastrectomy–influence of sleeve size and resected gastric volume. Obes Surg. 2007;17(10):1297–305.
11. Weiner RA, Blanco-Engert R, Weiner S, Pomhoff I, Schramm M. Laparoscopic biliopancreatic diversion with duodenal switch: three different duodeno-ileal anastomotic techniques and initial experience. Obes Surg. 2004;14(3):334-40.

Nutritional Considerations

Nutritional Status of Sleeve Patients, Micronutrients and Vitamins: Pre-op

Eliana Al Haddad

1 Introduction

1.1 Problem Statement

The LSG procedure involves major gastric resection as 60–80% of the stomach capacity is removed including the ghrelin producing fundus [28]. Accordingly, weight loss occurs through a combination of food restriction and a hormonal mechanism [19]. The consequences of the limited oral intake, food intolerance, and malabsorption following LSG are a major nutritional concern in the short and long term. Studies have shown that micronutrients including iron, thiamin, folate, vitamin B_{12}, and vitamin D are the most affected post LSG procedure [6, 10, 31]. Worth noting is the fact that obesity is associated with nutritional deficiencies [7, 26, 27, 35]. These deficiencies might be further exacerbated post LSG procedure. Severe nutritional deficiencies after bariatric surgeries may lead to anemia Brolin et al. [9, 8], bone mass loss [12], protein malnutrition [16], peripheral neuropathies [18], visual impairment [24], Wernicke encephalopathy Aasheim et al. [2, 3], and fetal malformations [21]. Beside the nutritional deficiencies, it is also important to mention that some studies reported undesirably high micronutrients levels post LSG surgery [1, 31]. Excess level may progress into toxicity which is also associated with devastating conditions.

E. Al Haddad (✉)
Columbia University Medical Center, New York, NY, USA
e-mail: Eliana.h91@gmail.com

Amiri Hospital, Kuwait City, Kuwait

© The Editor(s) (if applicable) and The Author(s), under exclusive license to Springer Nature Switzerland AG 2021
S. Al-Sabah et al. (eds.), *Laparoscopic Sleeve Gastrectomy*,
https://doi.org/10.1007/978-3-030-57373-7_60

2   Literature Review

2.1   Nutritional Concerns Pre Bariatric Surgeries

Obesity is associated with low micronutrient levels. Although, obese individuals have excess energy stores, they are quite often not well nourished (Fig. 1). Many obese subjects have already existing nutritional deficiencies before bariatric procedures. These deficiencies commonly include iron, vitamin B_{12}, thiamin, folate, and vitamin D [7, 27, 35]. Screening and correction of micronutrient deficiencies

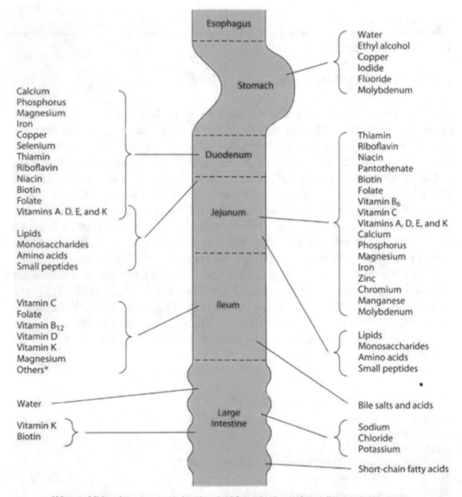

*Many additional nutrients may be absorbed from the ileum depending on transit time.

Fig. 1   Sites of nutrients absorption in gastrointestinal tract

preoperatively are crucial, as these deficiencies may be more exacerbated post bariatric procedures.

Several studies have examined nutritional deficiencies among morbidly obese patients prior to bariatric procedures. An overview of selected studies representing nutrients status pre bariatric procedures is shown in Table 1. Schweiger et al. [26] studied nutritional deficiencies in 114 bariatric candidates who underwent surgery between 2006 and 2008. The prevalence of pre-operative nutritional deficiencies was: 35% for iron, 24% for folate, 24% for ferritin, 3.6% for vitamin B_{12}, 2% for phosphorous, and 0.9% for calcium. Hemoglobin and Mean Corpuscular Volume (MCV) levels were low in 19% of the patients. High levels of Parathyroid Hormone (PTH) were found among 39% of the patients. No hypoalbuminemia was encountered. Low iron and ferritin were more common in females than males (40.8% vs.14.3%) and (31.8% vs. 0%), respectively. Similarly, another study conducted in Saudi Arabia by Al-Mulhim [4] evaluated nutritional status in 112 patients prospectively. Pre-operatively, 64% of the patients had one deficiency and 11% had more than one. Deficiencies rates were reported as follows: hemoglobin 24%, iron 11.6%, vitamin D 60%, vitamin B_{12} 1.8%, and folate 0.9%.

3 Discussion

3.1 Nutritional Status Pre LSG Surgery

3.1.1 Nutritional Deficiencies Pre LSG

Nutritional deficiencies among LSG candidates are commonly attributed to unhealthy dietary and lifestyle habits (Moizé et al. [23]; Aasheim et al. [2, 3]. Obese individuals often displace nutritious foods with high calorie foods that are rich in refined carbohydrates and fat. Moreover, chronic dieting, which is common among obese individuals, might further deteriorate their nutritional status as a result of food restrictions. Besides diet and lifestyle, a further explanation includes the volumetric dilution factor. Obese individuals have relatively high amounts of total body water, and their extracellular compartment appeared to be more expanded than the intracellular compartment [33]. Aasheim et al. [2, 3] suggested that the low micronutrient levels might be related to the dilution effect of the extracellular fluid on micronutrient concentrations. The following sections will address pre-operative status for each nutrient parameter studied.

3.1.2 Protein Deficiency Pre LSG: Albumin and Transferrin

Reports of albumin status vary widely in literature as percentage of low albumin ranged from 0–27% before LSG [31, 10, 22, 25, 26]. Since obesity is associated with chronic low grade inflammation, acute phase protein levels, including albumin and transferrin, might be altered [34].

Table 1 Selected studies of nutrients status pre bariatric surgeries

Percentage of patients with low nutrients level

Study	Design	n	B_1	B_6	B_9	B_{12}	A	D	Hgb	Ferritin	Fe	Mg	Phos	Ca	Zinc	Albumin
Ben-Porat et al. [6]	Prospective	192			32	13		99	15	7	47					
van Rutte et al. [31]	Prospective	200	6 / 3↑	3 / 21↑	24	12 / 1↑	0 / 72↑	81	5	7	38	2	14	1	0	0
Coupaye et al. [10]	Prospective	43	37	19	7	2	16	91	2					5		7
Gjessing et al. [15]	Retrospective	150			23	16 / 2↑		47 / 1↑	1 / 1↑					5 / 3↑		1 / 21↑
Moizé et al. [22]	Prospective	61	0	75		3		90	10	8	31	38		3	8	5
Saif et al. [25]	Retrospective	82	9					75	21	0	7	18	5	10		27
Damms-Machado et al. [11]	Prospective	54		11	6	9	0	83			29			0		
Moizé et al. [23]	Prospective	231	7		16	2		68	22	10	26	29		5	32	1
Al-Mulhim [4]	Prospective	112			1	2		60	24		12	6	5	0		
Toh et al. [29]	Retrospective	232			0	2		57	6	1	16					1
Schweiger et al. [26]	Retrospective	114			24	4			18	24	35		2	1		0
Gehrer et al. [14]	Prospective	136	0	0	3	3		23			3			0	14	6

↑ High; excess nutrient level, Hgb = Hemoglobin, Fe = Iron, Mg = Magnesium, Phos = Phosphorous, Ca = Cal

3.2 Vitamins Deficiencies Pre LSG

3.2.1 B Vitamins Deficiencies Pre LSG

Vitamin B_{12} was the only B vitamin that showed considerable deficiency prevalence prior to LSG (13–16%) [16, 15, 31]. However, several studies had also reported significant deficiencies in vitamin B_1, B_6, and folate [6, 31, 10, 22, 26]. These variations in B vitamins status may be partially explained by the differences in the extent of food fortifications between countries. It can also be related to food and supplement intake. Chronic alcoholism can be a contributing factor to vitamin B_1 deficiency as alcohol interferes with the active transport of vitamin B_1 across the intestinal wall and hastens its excretion in urine [13, 20].

3.2.2 Vitamin D Deficiency Pre LSG

A prevalence of vitamin D deficiency can be seen in previously reported studies, falling in the range of 60–91% [4, 10, 31, 22, 25].

Several reasons can be attributed to vitamin D deficiency in current LSG candidates. One reason is the decreased dietary consumption of vitamin D rich sources including fortified dairy products. A second reason is the reduced exposure to sunlight. The psychological status of the obese individual and the cultural and lifestyle factors of the population might further explain the limited sun exposure. A third possible reason of vitamin D deficiency is the sequestration of vitamin D in adipose tissues. The degree of adiposity appears to be inversely correlated with vitamin D levels. Correspondingly, several studies reported that obese individuals tend to have lower levels of vitamin D due to its increased uptake in adipose tissue [17, 30, 32]. A fourth reason for deficiency might be related to the decreased synthesis of vitamin D by the liver as a result of impaired liver function due to fatty liver disease, which is common among obese individuals [5]. Lastly, regarding the variation in vitamin D deficiency prevalence in the literature, it can also be related to the geographical, seasonal, and fortification policy differences.

3.2.3 Anemia and Iron Deficiency Pre LSG

Based on low hemoglobin levels as an indicator for anemia, anemia was observed in 18–24% in previously reported literature [4, 23, 25, 26]. However, anemia is variably reported in the literature, as others observed a much lower prevalence (1–5%) [10, 15, 31]. Iron biochemical parameters such as ferritin, serum iron, and transferrin saturation indicated poor iron status pr-eoperatively. Low ferritin was found in 24% of patients as reported by Schweiger et al. [26]. Low serum iron was observed in half of the patients before surgery according to Ben-Porat et al. [6] data (47%). On the contrary other previous studies reported a much lower prevalence in term of low ferritin (1–10%) [6, 23, 29, 31] and serum iron levels (7–29%) [4, 11, 25, 29].

The high percentages of pre-operative anemia and iron deficiency may be attributed to the inadequate iron intake due to poor dietary choices. It can also be attributed to the dominance of female gender (75%) in the reproductive age in

LSG candidates. Women in the reproductive age are at increased risk of iron deficiency anemia due to blood loss through menstruation. Furthermore, blood investigation of ferritin, serum iron, and transferrin saturation were not part of the routine preoperative assessment, hence, these tests might only be requested when deficiencies were suspected.

4   Excess Micronutrient Level Pre LSG

Some patients were found to have excess micronutrient levels which are consistent with data reported by van Rutte et al. [31]. This excess level might be due to consuming large doses of over the counter supplements by the patient's own initiative or by intense preoperative nutritional optimization from healthcare providers.

5   Conclusions and Recommendations

The rising prevalence of obesity is causing a parallel increase in the use of bariatric surgery. LSG is an effective procedure for morbid obesity management. Nutritional status is one of the main concerns in bariatric field. However, little is known about the nutritional status as well as the optimal nutritional care plan post LSG at longer term. Nutritional deficiencies were already present in LSG candidates as seen in multiple previous studies. Vitamin D, vitamin B_{12}, and iron deficiencies were the most commonly observed before surgery.

The current data emphasize the importance of pre and post-operative nutritional assessment. Since nutritional deficiencies are common among obese individual, optimizing LSG candidates before surgery is crucial to avoid further deterioration. Routine screening and adequate supplementation are vital post LSG to prevent and correct nutritional problems at an early stage. Data on iron, vitamin B_{12} and folate prove that these parameters deserve more attention particularly in females in the childbearing age. However, it is important to note that supplementation should be tailored to patient laboratory test to prevent excessive rise towards toxic level. Health care providers should be aware of vitamins toxicity risks, particularly vitamin B_6 and its adverse effect leading to neuropathy.

References

1. Aarts E, Janssen I, Berends F. The gastric sleeve: losing weight as fast as micronutrients? Obes Surg. 2011;21(2):207–11. https://doi.org/10.1007/s11695-010-0316-7.
2. Aasheim E, Hofsø D, Hjelmesæth J, Birkeland KI, Bøhmer T. Vitamin status in morbidly obese patients: a cross-sectional study. Am J Clin Nutr. 2008;87(2):362–9.
3. Aasheim E, Hofsø D, Hjelmesæth J, Sandbu R. Peripheral neuropathy and severe malnutrition following duodenal switch. Obes Surg. 2008;18(12):1640–3. https://doi.org/10.1007/s11695-008-9539-2.
4. Al-Mulhim A. Laparoscopic sleeve gastrectomy and nutrient deficiencies. Surg Laparosc Endosc Percutaneous Techn. 2016;26(3):208–11. https://doi.org/10.1097/sle.0000000000000270.

5. Bell N, Epstein S, Greene A, Shary J, Oexmann M, Shaw S. Evidence for alteration of the vitamin D-endocrine system in obese subjects. J Clin Investig 1985;76(1):370–3. https://doi.org/10.1172/jci111971.

6. Ben-Porat T, Elazary R, Yuval J, Wieder A, Khalaileh A, Weiss R. Nutritional deficiencies after sleeve gastrectomy: can they be predicted preoperatively? Surg Obes Relat Diseas. 2015;11(5):1029–36. https://doi.org/10.1016/j.soard.2015.02.018.

7. Bordalo L, Sales Teixeira T, Bressan J, Mourão D. Bariatric surgery: how and why to supplement. Revista Da Associação Médica Brasileira. 2011;57(1):111–8. https://doi.org/10.1016/s2255-4823(11)70025-x.

8. Brolin R, Gorman J, Gorman R, Petschenik A, Bradley L, Kenler H, Cody R. Are vitamin B12 and folate deficiency clinically important after Roux-en-Y gastric bypass? J Gastrointestinal Surg. 1998;2(5):436–42. https://doi.org/10.1016/s1091-255x(98)80034-6.

9. Brolin R, Gorman J, Gorman R, Petschenik A, Bradley L, Kenler H, Cody R. Prophylactic iron supplementation after Roux-en-Y gastric bypass. Arch Surg. 1998;133(7). https://doi.org/10.1001/archsurg.133.7.740

10. Coupaye M, Rivière P, Breuil M, Castel B, Bogard C, Dupré T, et al. Comparison of nutritional status during the first year after sleeve gastrectomy and Roux-en-Y gastric bypass. Obes Surg. 2014;24(2):276–83. https://doi.org/10.1007/s11695-013-1089-6.

11. Damms-Machado A, Friedrich A, Kramer K, Stingel K, Meile T, Küper M, et al. Pre- and postoperative nutritional deficiencies in obese patients undergoing laparoscopic sleeve gastrectomy. Obes Surg. 2012;22(6):881–9. https://doi.org/10.1007/s11695-012-0609-0.

12. Fleischer J, Stein E, Bessler M, Badia M, Restuccia N, Olivero-Rivera L, et al. The decline in hip bone density after gastric bypass surgery is associated with extent of weight loss. J Clin Endocrinol Metab. 2008;93(10):3735–40. https://doi.org/10.1210/jc.2008-0481.

13. Gastaldi G, Casirola D, Ferrari G, Rindi G. Effect of chronic ethanol administration on thiamine transport in microvillous vesicles of rat small intestine. Alcohol Alcohol. 1989;24(2):83–9.

14. Gehrer S, Kern B, Peters T, Christoffel-Courtin C, Peterli R. Fewer nutrient deficiencies after laparoscopic sleeve gastrectomy (LSG XE "laparoscopic sleeve Gastrectomy (LSG)") than after laparoscopic Roux-Y-Gastric bypass (LRYGB)—a prospective study. Obes Surg. 2010;20(4):447–53. https://doi.org/10.1007/s11695-009-0068-4.

15. Gjessing H, Nielsen H, Mellgren G, Gudbrandsen O. Energy intake, nutritional status and weight reduction in patients one year after laparoscopic sleeve gastrectomy. Springerplus. 2013;2(1):352. https://doi.org/10.1186/2193-1801-2-352.

16. Hamoui N, Chock B, Anthone G, Crookes P. Revision of the duodenal switch: indications, technique, and outcomes. J Am Coll Surg. 2007;204(4):603–8. https://doi.org/10.1016/j.jamcollsurg.2007.01.011.

17. Holick MF. Vitamin D deficiency. N Engl J Med. 2007;357(3):266–81.

18. Juhasz-Pocsine K, Rudnicki S, Archer R, Harik S. Neurologic complications of gastric bypass surgery for morbid obesity. Neurology. 2007;68(21):1843–50. https://doi.org/10.1212/01.wnl.0000262768.40174.33.

19. Karamanakos S, Vagenas K, Kalfarentzos F, Alexandrides T. Weight loss, appetite suppression, and changes in fasting and postprandial ghrelin and peptide-YY levels after Roux-en-Y gastric bypass and sleeve gastrectomy. Ann Surg. 2008;247(3):401–7. https://doi.org/10.1097/sla.0b013e318156f012.

20. Mahan L, Escott-Stump S. Krause's food & nutrition therapy, 12th ed. vol. 1229. St. Louis, Mo: Saunders/Elsevier;2008. pp. 84–85.

21. Martin L, Chavez G, Adams M, Mason E, Hanson J, Haddow J, Currier R. Gastric bypass surgery as maternal risk factor for neural tube defects. The Lancet. 1988;331(8586):640–1. https://doi.org/10.1016/s0140-6736(88)91430-4.

22. Moizé V, Andreu A, Flores L, Torres F, Ibarzabal A, Delgado S, et al. Long-term dietary intake and nutritional deficiencies following sleeve gastrectomy or Roux-En-Y gastric bypass in a mediterranean population. J Acad Nutr Dietetics. 2013;113(3):400–10. https://doi.org/10.1016/j.jand.2012.11.013.

23. Moizé V, Deulofeu R, Torres F, de Osaba J, Vidal J. Nutritional intake and prevalence of nutritional deficiencies prior to surgery in a spanish morbidly obese population. Obes Surg. 2011;21(9):1382–8. https://doi.org/10.1007/s11695-011-0360-y.
24. Moschos M, Droutsas D. A man who lost weight and his sight. The Lancet. 1998;351(9110):1174. https://doi.org/10.1016/s0140-6736(97)11074-1.
25. Saif T, Strain G, Dakin G, Gagner M, Costa R, Pomp A. Evaluation of nutrient status after laparoscopic sleeve gastrectomy 1, 3, and 5 years after surgery. Surg Obes Relat Diseas. 2012;8(5):542–7. https://doi.org/10.1016/j.soard.2012.01.013.
26. Schweiger C, Weiss R, Berry E, Keidar A. Nutritional deficiencies in bariatric surgery candidates. Obes Surg. 2009;20(2):193–7. https://doi.org/10.1007/s11695-009-0008-3.
27. Shankar P, Boylan M, Sriram K. Micronutrient deficiencies after bariatric surgery. Nutrition. 2010;26(11–12):1031–7. https://doi.org/10.1016/j.nut.2009.12.003.
28. Snyder-Marlow G, Taylor D, Lenhard M. Nutrition care for patients undergoing laparoscopic sleeve gastrectomy for weight loss. J Am Diet Assoc. 2010;110(4):600–7. https://doi.org/10.1016/j.jada.2009.12.022.
29. Toh S, Zarshenas N, Jorgensen J. Prevalence of nutrient deficiencies in bariatric patients. Nutrition. 2009;25(11–12):1150–6. https://doi.org/10.1016/j.nut.2009.03.012.
30. Tsiaras W, Weinstock M. Factors influencing vitamin D status. Acta Derm Venereol. 2011;91(2):115–24. https://doi.org/10.2340/00015555-0980.
31. van Rutte P, Aarts E, Smulders J, Nienhuijs S. Nutrient deficiencies before and after sleeve gastrectomy. Obes Surg. 2014;24(10):1639–46. https://doi.org/10.1007/s11695-014-1225-y.
32. Vanlint S. Vitamin D and obesity. Nutrients. 2013;5(3):949–56. https://doi.org/10.3390/nu5030949.
33. Waki M, Kral JG, Mazariegos M, Wang J, Pierson RN, Heymsfield SB. Relative expansion of extracellular fluid in obese vs. nonobese women. Am J Physiol Endocrinol Metab. 1991;261(2):E199–E203.
34. Wellen KE, Hotamisligil GS. Inflammation, stress, and diabetes. J Clin Investig. 2005;115(5):1111–9.
35. Ziegler O, Sirveaux M, Brunaud L, Reibel N, Quilliot D. Medical follow up after bariatric surgery: nutritional and drug issues General recommendations for the prevention and treatment of nutritional deficiencies. Diabetes Metab. 2009;35(6):544–57. https://doi.org/10.1016/s1262-3636(09)73464-0.

Nutritional Status of Sleeve Patients, Micronutrients and Vitamins: Post-op

Christine Stier

1 Introduction

The preoperative nutritional status of patients undergoing sleeve gastrectomy (SG) has already been discussed in the previous chapter and represents at least one precondition for the postoperative nutritional status.

In addition, postoperative specific changes such as the limited oral intake, emerging food intolerances, and possible malabsorption in the short and long term have further impact on the postoperative nutritional status. Studies have shown that the most affected micronutrients after SG are **iron, thiamine, folate, vitamin B12,** and **vitamin D** [1]. It seems that the nutritional consequences of SG are fundamentally different from that of bypass surgery. Bypass surgery excludes the duodenum from food passage, which is the major absorption site for minerals, with resulting respective resorption limitations.

SG differs fundamentally. This procedure exclusively modifies the anatomy of the stomach by reducing its extensible volume along the "Magenstrasse" by about 90%. Thus, the cause of possible postoperative deficiency symptoms may be explained with anatomical and physiological alterations of the stomach.

C. Stier (✉)

Sana Obesity Center Northrhine Westphalia, Krankenhausstrasse 42, Hürth, Germany

e-mail: christine.stier@sana.de

S. Al-Sabah et al. (eds.), *Laparoscopic Sleeve Gastrectomy*,

https://doi.org/10.1007/978-3-030-57373-7_61

2 Effect on Vitamin B12

SG involves, in particular, the resection of the fundus and the largest part of the corpus, while the volume of the antrum is only marginally diminished [2]. Thus, the parietal cells that produce acid and **intrinsic factor** are drastically reduced in number (Fig. 1), while the number of gastrin-producing antral G cells remains only slightly reduced.

The intrinsic factor forms a complex with **vitamin B12** (cobalamin) ingested from food, thus enabling its absorption. Subsequently this certainly plays an influential part after SG on the absorption of vitamin B12. Vitamin B12 cannot be synthesized by the body itself and must therefore be gained through food. As it is sensitive to acids, it is first attached to haptocorrin secreted by the parotid glands and thus protected from the acidic pH of the stomach. Haptocorrin is then split off from vitamin B12 in the alkaline milieu of the duodenum by pancreatic proteases and further linked to intrinsic factor. This complex formation between vitamin B12 and the intrinsic factor is essential for its absorption which is mediated by the cubam receptor complex in the terminal ileum [3–6].

3 Effect on Iron

Furthermore, volume reduction can interfere with **iron** absorption. The human organism utilizes both bivalent (Fe2+) and trivalent (Fe3+) iron ions, only divalent iron is able to be absorbed directly, whereas trivalent iron needs to be converted into bivalent ions. A distinction is made between heme–iron, which is

Parietal cells are located in the fundus and the corpus. They produce hydrochloric acid and intrinsic factor.
Acid plays a crucial role in the brake down of iron. Haptocorrin is bond to the acid-sensitive vitamin B12. This bond is spit by pancreatic proteases in the duodenum. Then vitamin B12 is linked to intrinsic factor. Intrinsic factor is the protective binding-protein of vitamin B12 throughout the small intestine until it reaches the cubam receptor complex for absorption in the terminal ileum.

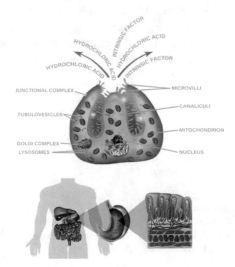

Fig. 1 Parietal cell of the stomach

present as bivalent iron protoporphyrin, and non-heme iron, which is present as free ionized iron bivalent or trivalent iron. Since Fe^{3+} and Fe^{2+} are basically firmly bound to food proteins, the breakdown of the proteins by special digestive enzymes such as pepsin is a prerequisite for the absorption of iron. If there is sufficient gastric acid (HCl) production in the stomach, this breakdown is ensured. The amount of gastric acid production is modified after SG, as well. Thus, another influence of the remaining petite gastric volume with thereby reduced acid and pepsin production on the absorption behavior of iron can be supposed. However, usually SG only marginally affected the antrum with its gastrin-producing G-cells. Gastrin is a peptide hormone and is the strongest stimulus for the production of gastric acid, but the interaction between the surgical significantly increased numbers of parietal cells at almost the same number of G-cells in SG still remains unclear [4, 7, 8].

4   Effect of Volume Reduction on Vitamin Status

A further anatomical influence can be derived from the quantity of volume reduction and the resulting shape of SG. In adults the average stomach volume is about 1.5–2 L. SG reduces stomach volume down to 75–150 ml [2]. There is very little literature available that describes objectively the volume determination with SG, and only one paper dealt specifically with the preoperative stomach volume, the achieved SG volume, and the volume of the obtained specimen and its correlation to weight (Fig. 2a, b) [9]. Hence, it does not seem to be clear at what extent the quantity of volume change itself exactly influences weight loss, nor are there many facts available regarding the influence of the extend of gastric volume change on possible postoperative nutritional deficiencies, especially on vitamin B 12 and iron. However, it appears that the rhythm and speed of gastric emptying has a significant influence on many aspects of the effects and side effects of bariatric interventions. In the physiological stomach the exact tuned regulation of gastric emptying speed of the chyme into the duodenum is crucial for further digestion processes and subsequently provides feedback from the intestine via a variety of gastrointestinal hormones [10, 11]. However, it seems to be clear that a too rapid gastric emptying of the physiological stomach alters the secretion of intestinal hormones and thus has complex effects not only on carbohydrate metabolism. A surgical induced accelerated gastric emptying has been reliably proven for SG, even if only few data are available due to rare publications on basic physiology of bariatrical procedures [12]. In addition, it has not yet been demonstrated to what extent and how pronounced the influence of the reduced volume leads to this acceleration of gastric emptying [13–15]. It is conceivable whether this will lead to a shorter enterocyte contact time with subsequently reduced absorption rates of vitamins and minerals, but this has not yet been investigated. In the case of **folic acid**, this could be an aspect for the, albeit low, rates of folic acid deficiencies observed following SG [16]. Folic acid must be broken down enzymatically in the duodenum and proximal jejunum, but is subsequently absorbed in the entire small

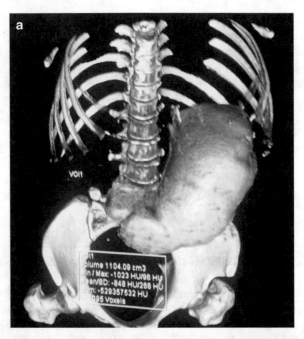

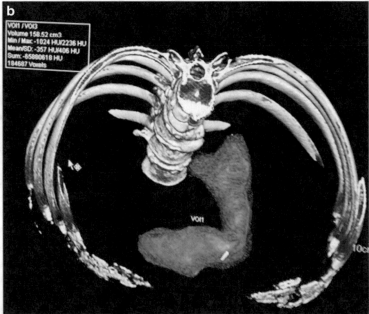

Fig. 2 a Volume-rendered 3D image of the distended stomach with multi-detector CT (preoperative) (volume 1108 ml). b Volume-rendered 3D image of the gastric sleeve 3 months postoperatively (volume 158 ml)

intestine. The ubiquitous nutritional undersupply with folic acid can be another aspect of the observed deficiencies [4].

5   Effect on Thiamine

Thiamine (Vitamin B1) is also absorbed throughout the entire small intestine. The enteral uptake of thiamine is subject to a dose-dependent dual mechanism. Physiological amounts of thiamine below a concentration of 2 µmol/l are absorbed by an energy-dependent sodium-mediated carrier mechanism, above a concentration of 2 µmol/l, vitamin B1 is absorbed by passive diffusion. The comparison of biopsies of the intestinal mucosa of patients with and without thiamine deficiency revealed a significantly higher intestinal vitamin B1 intake in subjects with poor thiamine status. The increased absorption of thiamine in the deficient state results from the upregulation of apical thiamine transporters in the intestinal mucosa cells [17–19].The biological **half-life of thiamine is relatively short** and is reported to be 9.5–18.5 days in humans. The maximal limited storage capacity and high conversion rate of thiamine make a daily supply of sufficient quantities necessary to meet demand [19]. These facts may lead to special nutritional problems with thiamine, which must be kept in mind after bariatric surgery, and especially after SG, as postoperative nausea and vomiting (PONV) may be considered the most common adverse effect of LSG. Without prophylaxis the incidence can be as high as 80% [20]. Another and even more important and longer lasting reason for chronic vomiting after SG is due to functional gastric stenosis at the angulus fold [21–24]. The incidence can be as high as 4%, but with that incidence only proven and treated cases are represented [21–24]. In fact, more patients suffer from chronic vomiting after SG. Further reasons for this issue can be the presence of a hiatal hernia or emerging food intolerances. Important in this context is the fact that chronic vomiting easily leads to a **thiamine deficiency** based on its short half-life and its absolute limited storage capacity. Another contributing aspect is the fact that these patients often almost stop eating due persistent nausea.

This can lead to two clinical pictures with a pronounced thiamine deficiency, both of which can take a dramatic course. Acute thiamine deficiency occurs when patients in an already catabolic state (e.g. like after bariatric surgery) additionally fast for some time, (e.g. due to chronic vomiting) and then resume eating.

5.1   Refeeding Syndrome

The initial phase of starvation (e.g. low food intake after bariatric surgery plus nausea) leads to a high consumption of the total concentration of essential electrolytes within the extracellular space. During such a period carbohydrate metabolism is minimized, and thus insulin release is suppressed, whereas gluconeogenesis, lipolysis and proteolysis are increased, the substrates of which are fatty acids, glycerol, ketones and amino acids. At the same time intracellular electrolyte concentration is still high. Subsequently, along this concentration gradient magnesium, phosphate and potassium shift to the extracellular space. "Starvation seizes the cellular level" is probably the best way to describe convincingly this state. In this phase of starvation, when electrolytes already have been shifted from intra- to extracellular, resumption of food results in a massive insulin release, which immediately leads to increased glycogeno-, proteino- and lipogenesis. Henceforth, massive amounts of thiamine are consumed by acting as cofactor for the glucose transport into the intracellular space. Simultaneously, with indication of this metabolic process, phosphate, potassium and magnesium massively flux back into the cell. This results in an engraving and persisting deficiency of potassium, phosphate, magnesium and thiamine in the extra cellular space followed by all its clinical consequences. This phenomenon is known as **refeeding syndrome** (Fig. 3a–c) that has so far been recognized mainly in the context with anorexia [25–28]. The hallmark biochemical feature of this phenomenon is **hypophosphatemia**. Regardless of the serious symptoms of that malignant electrolyte imbalance, additionally, the acute thiamine deficiency may result in symptoms of an acute dry and/or wet **Beriberi** syndrome with severe cordial and neurological impairments (Table 1). This situation mostly represents a life-threatening condition. Milder forms of electrolyte shifts have been frequently observed as moderate hypophosphatemia in the post-bariatric phase, characterized by the significant reduction of

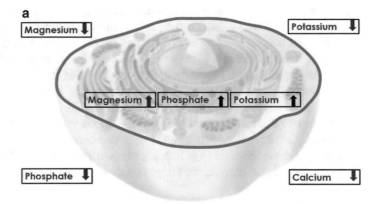

Fig. 3 **a** Starvation leads to a consumption of extracellular electrolytes. Carbohydrate metabolism is minimized, gluconeogenesis, lipolysis, and proteolysis is increased. This results in a concentration gradient of electrolytes from intracellular to extracellular. **b** "Starvation seizes the cellular level". This results in a shift of intracellular phosphate, magnesium and potassium into the extracellular space. **c** Refeeding Syndrome. Resumption of food in the state of starvation results in a massive insulin release, which simultaneously leads to increased glycogeno-, proteino- and lipogenesis. Thiamine is consumed as cofactor for the transport of glucose, phosphate, potassium and magnesium back into the intracellular space. The hallmark biochemical feature of refeeding syndrome is **hpophosphatemia and thus phosphate is the indicator electrolyte**

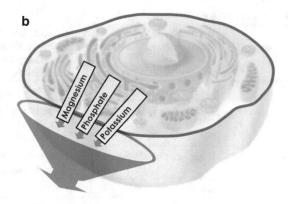

Fig. 3 (continued)

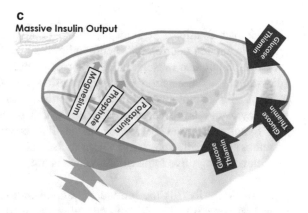

Fig. 3 (continued)

food intake over weeks. Some published cases of patients with "bariatrical refeeding syndrome" demonstrated impressively that this clinical picture can occur independently of body weight, but is solely induced by prolonged starvation with a subsequent electrolyte shift [28].

Emergency intensive care therapy of the refeeding syndrome includes a reduced and controlled protocol of nutrient supply under monitoring and ad hoc substitution of electrolytes and thiamine, potassium and magnesium according to the NICE guidelines [25]. Often the adequate therapy necessitates very high doses especially of phosphate and thiamine for several days,

The Refeeding Syndrome leads to an excessive lack of thiamine by shifting the vitamin between the different spaces of the body. If the deficiency is due to an insufficient extrinsic supply or waste through vomiting, Beriberi syndrome can develop without further phosphate imbalance. The Beriberi syndrome shows

Table 1 Classification and symptoms of beriberi syndrome

Dry Beriberi More frequent than wet Beriberi	Wet Beriberi Cardio-vascular manifestation	Cerebral Beriberi Wernicke-Korsakoff syndrome Complete remission is rare Mortality rate: 10–20%
Neuritis	Cardiac insufficiency	Encephalopathy
Neuropathy, esp. of the lower limbs with loss of tendon reflexes	Tachycardia	Omphtalmoplegia, with nystagmus and impairment of eye movements
Muscle atrophy with muscle pain	Right heart insufficiency	Hemorrhagic lesions of the 3.and 4. Ventricle
General weakness	Edema	Ataxia
	Respiratory symptoms	Korsakoff pychosis
	Hypertension	Coma

three different clinical manifestations, with dry Beriberi being the most common of all. Its symptoms include neuritis and neuropathy that manifests particularly at the lower extremity, but also muscle pain and atrophy with loss of tendon reflexes. The cardio-vascular manifestation with hypertension, formation of edemas and possible respiratory symptoms is called wet beriberi. An acute severe thiamine deficiency may even lead to cerebral Beriberi, which is also known as Wernicke-Korsakoff Syndrome. If the disease occurs in this severe form, complete remission is rare and mortality rate ranges high as between 10–20%. Even early therapy cannot cure the cognitive impairment, which is not reversible in most cases [29].

Therapy of symptomatic Beriberi is the immediate administration of thiamine (up to 400 mg parenteral per day) [29, 30], directly after the blood sample has been taken for current vitamin level determination. In suspected cases, there is no need to wait for the result and an initial dose of 100 mg is administered ex juvantibus. In such situations, however, it is always worth controlling the indicator electrolyte phosphate to differentiate suspected Beriberi from refeeding syndrome.

6   Effect on Vitamin D

Vitamin D deficiency is not specific.

Although only parts of the stomach are removed in SG, the resulting reduction in gastric acid and intrinsic factor and the rapid emptying of the stomach can have effects on the vitamin and mineral balance. Other influencing factors are the drastically reduced postoperative food and vitamin intake or recurrent vomiting after SG. Additionally, proton pump inhibitor (PPI) intake, which is frequently after SG, has a considerable effect on iron, and vitamin B12 levels, as well as it

Table 2 Nutrient supplementation for patients with weight loss surgery according to the guidelines of American Society for Metabolic and Bariatric Surgery integrated health nutritional guidelines for the surgical weight loss patient 2016 update: micronutrients [35]

	Patients after sleeve gastrectomy
Vit B1	At least 12 mg/d At risk patients: at least 50–100 mg/d
Vit B12	350–500 ug/d oral, disintegrating tablet, sublingual or liquid or nasal—as directed or 1000mcg/mo IM
Folate	400–800 mcg oral 800–1000 mcg F childbearing ages
Calcium	1200–1500 mg/d1800
Vit A	5000 IU/d
Vit E	15 mg/d
Vit K	90–120ug/d
Vit D	At least 3000 IU/d to maintain D,25(OH) levels > 30 ng/mL
Iron	At least 18 mg/d from multivitamin At least45–60 mg/d in F with menses and/patients with history of anemia
Zinc	8–11 mg/d
Copper	1 mg/d

interferes with the calcium and bone metabolism [31–34]. Besides that, PPI retard the clinical response to iron supplementation [34].

A **vitamin D** deficiency is not specific after SG, but is generally widespread in obese patients. Indeed, deficiencies of fat-soluble vitamins are more likely after bypass procedures due to the duodenal exclusion.

7   Conclusion

In summary of all these influences on the absorption of vitamins and minerals following SG, the lifelong supplementation is obligatory according to the guidelines (Table 2). Standardized follow up examinations and lab tests are necessary to monitor the vitamin and mineral status in bariatric patients after SG, to conclude, according to the current state of knowledge, postoperative supplementation after SG should be recommended life-long, since anatomical and physiological changes provide at least deficiencies in **iron, thiamine, folate, vitamin B12,** and **vitamin D.**

References

1. Al-Mutawa A, Al-Sabah S, Anderson AK, Al-Mutawa M. Evaluation of nutritional status post laparoscopic sleeve—5 years outcome. Obes Surg. 2018;28:1473–83.

2. Bhandari M, Fobi Mal, Buchwald JN, Bariatric Metabolic Surgery Standardisation (BMSS Working Group). Standardization of bariatric metabolic procedures: world consensus meeting statement. Obes Surg. 2019;29(Suppl 4):309–45.

3. Shane B. Folate and vitmin B12 metabolism: overview and interaction with riboflavin, vitamin B6, and polymorphisms. Food Nutr Bull. 2008;29(2 Suppl):5–16.

4. Gu L, Fu R, Chen P, et al. In terms of nutrition, the most suitable method for bariatric surgery:laparoscopic sleeve gastrectomy or Roux-en-Y gastric bypass? A systematic review and meta-analysis. Obes Surg. 2020. https://doi.org/10.1007/s11695-020-04488-2. [Epub ahead of print].

5. Herrmann W, Obeid R. Cobalamin deficiency. Subcell Biochem. 2012;56(3):01–22.

6. Herrmann W, Obeid R, Schorr H, Geisel J. Functional vitamin B12 deficiency and determination of holotranscobalamin in populations at risk. Clin Chem Lab Med. 2003;41(11):1478–88.

7. German Society for Nutrition, Austrian Society for Nutrition, Swiss Society for Nutrition Research, Swiss Association for Nutrition: reference values for nutrient intake. 5 Edn. In: DGE/ÖGE/SGE/SVE. Umschau- Braus-Verlag, Frankfurt/Main (2013).

8. Camaschella C, Nai A, Silvestri L. Iron metabolism and iron disorders revisited in the hepcidin era. Haematologica. 2020;105(2):260–72.

9. Pawanindra L, Vidal A, Migha M, et al. Early post-operative weight loss after laparoscopic sleeve gastrectomy correlates with the volume of the excised stomach and not with that of the sleeve! Preliminary data from a multi-detector computed tomography-based study. Surg Endosc. 2015;29(10):2921–7.

10. Goyal RK, Guo Y, Mashimo H. Advances in the physiology of gastric emptying. Neurogastroenterol Motil. 2019;31(4):e13546.

11. Khiyani N, Tulchinsky M, Hava S, et al. Gastric emptying results may influence the selection of the type of bariatric surgery. Medicine (Baltimore). 2019;98(41):e17205.

12. Vargas EJ, Bazerbachi F, Calderon G, et al. Changes in time of gastric emptying after surgical and endoscopic bariatrics and weight loss: A systematic review and meta-analysis. Clin Gastroenterol Hepatol. 2020;18:57–68.

13. Coupaye M, Rivière P, Breuil M, et al. Comparison of nutritional status during the first year after sleeve gastrectomy and roux-en-Y gastric bypass. Obes Surg. 2014;24(2):276–83.

14. Ben-Porat T, Elazary R, Yuval J, et al. Nutritional deficiencies after sleeve gastrectomy: can they be predicted preoperatively? Surg Obes Relat Dis. 2015;11(5):1029–36.

15. van Rutte P, Aarts E, Smulders J, et al. Nutrient deficiencies before and after sleeve gastrectomy. Obes Surg. 2014;24(10):1639–46.

16. Campos AJ, Risch L, Nydegger U, et al. Diagnostic accuracy of holotranscobalamin, Vitamin B12, Methylmalonic acid, and Homocysteine in detecting B12 deficiency in a large, mixed patient population. Dis Markers. 2020;2020:7468506.

17. Singleton CK, Martin PR. Molecular effects of thiamine deficiency. Curr Mol Med. 2001;1(2):197–207.

18. Song Q, Singleton CK. Mitochondria from cultured cells derived from normal and thiamine-responsive megaloblastic anemia individuals efficiently import thiamine diphosphate. BMC Biochem. 2002;25(3):8.

19. Pan X, Nan X, Yang L, et al. Thiamine status, metabolism and application in dairy cows: a review. Br J Nutr. 2018;120(5):491–9.

20. Chandrakumar A, Bhardwaj A, Jong GW. Review of thiamine deficiency disorders: Wernicke encephalopathy and Korsakoff psychosis. J Basic Clin Physiol Pharmacol. 2018;30(2):153–62.

21. Fathy M, Abdel-Razik MA, Ayman. Impact of Pyloric Injection of Magnesium Sulfate-Lidocaine Mixture on Postoperative Nausea and Vomiting After Laparoscopic Sleeve Gastrectomy: a Randomized-Controlled Trial Obesity Surgery 2019; 29:1614–1623

22. Parikh A, Alley JB, Peterson RM, et al. Management options for symptomatic stenosis after laparoscopic vertical sleeve gastrectomy in the morbidly obese. Surg Endosc. 2012;26:738–46.
23. Yu JX, Baker JR, Watts et al. Functional lumen imaging probe is useful for the quantification of gastric sleeve stenosis and prediction of response to endoscopic dilation: a pilot study. Obes Surg. 2020;30(2):786–9.
24. Turcu F, Balahura C, Doras I, et al. Symptomatic stenosis after laparoscopic sleeve gastrectomy—incidence and management in a high-volume bariatric surgery. Chirurgia. 2018;113:826–36.
25. National Institute for Health and Clinical Excellence. Nutrition support in adults. Clinical guideline CG32;2006. www.nice.org.uk/page.aspx?o=cg032.
26. Mehanna HM, Moledina J, Travis J. Refeeding syndrome: what it is, and how to prevent and treat it. BMJ. 2008;336:1495–8.
27. Pacei F, Iaccarino L, Bugiardini E, et al. Wernicke's encephalopathy, refeeding syndrome and wet beriberi after laparoscopic sleeve gastrectomy: the importance of thiamine evaluation. Eur J Clin Nutr. 2020. https://doi.org/10.1038/s41430-020-0583-x. [Epub ahead of print].
28. Chiappetta S, Stein J. Refeeding syndrome: an important complication following obesity surgery. Obes Facts. 2016;9(1):12–6.
29. Stroh C, Meyer F, Manger T. Beriberi, a severe complication after metabolic surgery - review of the literature. Obes Facts. 2014;7(4):246–52.
30. Alves LF, Gonçalves RM, Cordeiro GV, et al. Beriberi after bariatric surgery: not an unusual complication. Report of Two Cases and Literature ReviewArq Bras Endocrinol Metabol. 2006;50(3):564–8.
31. Qorraj-Bytyqi H, Hoxha R, Sadiku S, et al. Proton pump inhibitors intake and iron and vitamin B12 status: a prospective comparative study with a follow up of 12 months. Maced J Med Sci. 2018;6(3):442–6.
32. Johnson DA. Nutritional consequences of long-term acid suppression; are they clinically important? Curr Opin Gastroenterol. 2016;32(2):136–40.
33. Schubert ML. Functional anatomy and physiology of gastric secretion. Curr Opin Gastroenterol. 2015;31(6):479–85.
34. McColl KE. Effect of proton pump inhibitors on vitamins and iron. Am J Gastroenterol. 2009;104(Suppl 2):S5–9.
35. Parrott J, Fran L, Rabena R, et al. American society for metabolic and bariatric surgery integrated health nutritional guidelines for the surgical weight loss patient 2016 update: Micronutrients SOARD. 2017.

Long-Term Consequences of Nutritional Deficiencies

Samantha Stavola

1   Pre-operative Deficiencies

The World Health Organization (WHO) estimates 13% of the world's adult population were obese in 2016 [1]. The sleeve gastrectomy (SG) can be argued as the fastest growing weight loss surgical procedure since 2003, resulting in excess weight loss percentages of 33–90% [2, 3]. From 2003 to 2013, the percentage of sleeve gastrectomy procedures performed in North America increased by 244%, in Europe there was an increase of 48%, South America experienced a 14% increase, and Asia/Pacific countries reported a 75% increase in procedure volume; this details only about 0.01% of the world's population having bariatric surgery [2].

Although there are many health advantages and resolutions of co-morbidities, many micronutrient deficiencies can result from metabolic changes associated with the sleeve gastrectomy [4]. Patients undergoing a sleeve gastrectomy procedure are at risk for nutrient deficiencies due to: limited food intake, increased risk of postoperative nausea and vomiting, food intolerances which may be newly developed since surgery, and reduced amounts of hydrochloric acid and intrinsic factor secretions within the stomach [4]. Nutritional deficiencies can be common in pre-operative patients and should be addressed and treated prior to surgery, to avoid postoperative complications [4, 5].

S. Stavola (✉)
Nutrition for Celebrate Nutritional Supplements, Wadsworth, OH, USA
e-mail: sam@celebratevitamins.com

S. Al-Sabah et al. (eds.), *Laparoscopic Sleeve Gastrectomy*,
https://doi.org/10.1007/978-3-030-57373-7_62

2   Post-operative Deficiencies

Weight loss surgery procedures can decrease nutrient intake, specifically in patients undergoing a sleeve gastrectomy procedure, due to the restrictive nature of the procedure [6]. The current and updated 2019 ASMBS(American Society for Metabolic and Bariatric Surgery) Guidelines provide the following early postoperative care and immediate follow up period checklist for monitoring during the first year after a sleeve gastrectomy procedure [7].

Early care related to vitamin supplementation for sleeve gastrectomy:

- Multivitamin plus minerals in 2 tablets to supply minimum requirements
- Elemental calcium in citrate form 1,200–1,500 mg/d
- 3,000 IU/d vitamin D
- Vitamin B12 at dose to maintain normal levels
- Oral hydration of minimum 1.5 L/d.

Immediate follow up care related to vitamin supplementation for sleeve gastrectomy:

- Office visits at one, three, six, twelve months and then annually thereafter
- Comprehensive metabolic panel (CMP) at each visit
- Complete blood count with platelet testing at each visit
- Iron studies test for baseline and as needed thereafter
- Bone density scan at 2 years
- Vitamin B-12 performed annually and every 3–6 months if needing supplementation (methymalonic acid-MMA test- and homocysteine test as preferred)
- Thiamine evaluation as needed.

Postoperative micronutrient deficiencies, specifically in thiamine and vitamin D and calcium, can cause serious complications. Thiamine plays a role in major metabolic pathways within the body by creating many precursors for brain metabolism, separating ATP (adenosine triphosphate) molecules from glucose, and providing the core function in initiating many biochemical reactions in the central and peripheral nervous system [6, 8].

Deficiency in thiamine can lead to Wernicke-encephalopathy, wet Beriberi, and ultimately death, if left untreated. Wernicke-encephalopathy is diagnosed by a change in mental status, ocular movement abnormalities, and ataxia. Early onset symptoms of thiamine deficiency are non-specific and can include: fatigue, lethargy, uneasiness, and headaches [8]. If left untreated, symptoms can progress to congestive heart failure or wet beriberi, peripheral neuropathy, dysphagia, depression, or Korsakoff syndrome [8]. Kröll et al. developed an overview of Wernicke-Encephalopathy after sleeve gastrectomy (Table 1) [8].

Weight loss surgery procedures can increase the risk of developing thiamine deficiency due to nausea and vomiting, rapid weight loss, and excessive alcohol

Table 1 Progression of wernicke-encephalopathy after sleeve gastrectomy

Risk factors	– Recurrent emesis – Non-compliance and inadequate vitamin supplementation – Preoperative vitamin B deficiencies – Surgical complications (stenosis) – Parenteral feedings, caloric carbohydrate diet – Co-morbidities: alcohol consumption, type 2 diabetes, hepatic stenosis, non-alcoholic fatty liver disease, delayed gastric emptying
Time of neurological symptoms	Early: within 2–6 weeks (stores can be depleted) Late: within 7 months with variability, usually 3–5 months
Clinical manifestations	– Wernicke encephalopathy (ocular dysfunction, gait ataxia, encephalopathy) classic triad often not seen – Altered mental status changes – Korsakoff syndrome (amnestic-confabulatory syndrome) – Peripheral neuropathy and polyradiculopathy – Nonspecific symptoms: fatigue, lethargy, restlessness – Atypical symptoms: vestibular dysfunction without hearing loss, dysphagia, depression
Diagnostic tools	– Clinical diagnosis Laboratory examination may not be specific, serum thiamine levels may be reduced MRI may show increased T2 signals in periventricular regions
Differential diagnosis	Other nutrient deficiencies: vitamin B-12, copper, folate, niacin, vitamin E
Treatment	500 mg thiamine IV TID for 2 days, followed by 500 mg/d IV or IM for 5 days with magnesium and other B vitamins, followed by long-term oral supplementation of 50 or 100 mg/d
Outcome	Complete recovery is rare

Adapted from Kröll et al. [8]

intake [8]. Since thiamine is a water-soluble vitamin, daily intake is needed to maintain normal serum levels, in fact, Sechi et al. found that lack of thiamine intake can lead to a deficiency in as few as 20 days without appropriate thiamine supplementation [9]. Angelou et al. found Wernicke encephalopathy onset occurred as early as 2 weeks and as late as 60 weeks after sleeve gastrectomy [10].

Postoperative thiamine deficiency was found to be as great as 25% in patients up to 2 years, and ranged from 0–30.8% by the 5-year mark regardless of supplementation [6]. A study conducted by Johns Hopkins University, found that out of 105 patients status post sleeve gastrectomy, patients with a higher BMI that were also of a minority ethnicity, or whom were of a minor ethnicity, independently, had a higher risk of developing thiamine deficiency: 20% at 3 months, 17% at 6 months, and 20% at 12 months post-surgery, even while taking recommended 3 mg thiamine supplementation daily [6].

There is evidence that suggests that weight loss procedures can cause a negative effect on bone mineral density, accelerate bone loss, and increase bone fragility [11]. However, these negative effects can mostly be reversed with adequate supplementation after surgery [12]. Serum calcium levels often remain within normal limits in post-operative patients due to the regulatory pathways within the body. Unfortunately, obese individuals typically have abnormal 25(OH)D levels due to sequestration of vitamin D within adipose tissue and due to a sedentary lifestyle with reduced sunlight exposure [12]. It is believed that changes in gut hormone concentrations after the sleeve gastrectomy can cause vitamin D deficiency in post-operative patients [13].

Lu et al. conducted a twelve-year study to observe fracture risk in weight loss surgery patients. Their results showed that out of the total 1,775 patients that had a restrictive procedure, 154 (8.7%) patients had fractures. The fracture rate for the surgical group were: 1.6% for 1 year, 2.37% for 2 years, 1.69% for 5 years, and 2.06% greater than 5 years, with most fractures occurring in the extremities [11].

Likewise, Mihmanli et al. studied 119 post sleeve gastrectomy patients and their vitamin D levels during the first year after surgery. At 12 months after surgery, 32.7% of patients needed high-dose vitamin D supplementation to combat deficiency [13].

Carrasco et al. noted vitamin D deficiency in sleeve gastrectomy patients in 31.6% preop, 5.6% 6 months, and 15.8% 12 months after surgery. Coincidentally, hyperparathyroidism was observed in 57.9% preop, 31.6% 6 months, and 5.3% 12 months after surgery. Patients who achieved higher vitamin D and calcium intake via diet and supplementation had reduced parathyroid hormone levels. Calcium intake of patients, closer to ASMBS recommendations, showed an association with less bone loss in the lumbar region of the spinal cords of sleeve gastrectomy patients [14].

Pluskiewicz et al. noted bone mineral density reductions of 1.2% in the spine, 7% in femoral neck, and 5.3% in total hip in sleeve gastrectomy patients that were 6 months post-surgery [15]. A review of evaluation and management of bone health in the surgical patient (Table 2) and recommendations for calcium and vitamin D supplementation (Table 3) are described below [16].

Although the causes for micronutrient deficiencies is multifactorial, resecting the gastric fundus in the sleeve gastrectomy procedure thus leading to reduced dietary intake, reduced hydrochloric acid and intrinsic factor, and a hypo acidic environment, can lead to micronutrient deficiencies such as iron, folic acid, vitamin B-12, thiamine, vitamin B-6, and copper [17].

In a literature review conducted by Emile and Elfeki, several studies were reviewed to compare nutritional deficiencies after sleeve gastrectomy (Table 4).

Table 2 Evaluation and management of bone health in surgical patients

Parameter	Pre op management	Post-op management	Treatment
Calcium	Serum parathyroid hormone, serum calcium, 25(OH)D, DXA of spine and hip for women aged ≥65, men aged ≥70, patients with conditions associated with bone loss or low bone mass	1200–1500 mg/d. Monitor serum parathyroid hormone, calcium, and 25(OH)D every 6–12 months and then annually. DXA at spine and hip 2 years post op, then every 2–5 years	Evualate secondary causes, if low bone mass in pre op phase. Consider bisphosphonates when bone density T score is <2.5
Vitamin D	25 (OH)D, serum parathyroid hormone	3000 IU/d or dose needed to reach 25(OH)D>30 ng/ml. Monitor serum parathyroid hormone and 25(OH)D every 6–12 months, then annually. 24-h urinary calcium at 6 months, then annually	For rapid correction of vitamin D deficiency ≥3,000 IU and ≤6,000 IU vitamin D_3/d or 50,000 Iu vitamin D_2 1–3 times/ week. Severe malabsorption may require higher dosing of ≤50,000 IU D_2 or D_3 1–3 times/week to once daily. High vitamin D dosing should be administered over a limited period of time and should be monitored by medical professionals
Protein	Serum albumin; can also measure serum protein, pre-albumin, DXA of fat-free mass	60–80 g/d or 1.1–1.5 g/kg ideal body weight. Monitor serum albumin 6–12 months and then annually	Oral protein supplementation or enteral/ parenteral nutrition as needed
Physical activity	N/A	Moderate aerobic physical activity at minimum 150 min/wk with a goal of 300 min/ wk. Strength training 2–3 times/wk	N/A

Adapted from Ben-Porat et al. [16]

Table 3 Recommendations for calcium and vitamin D supplementation

	Calcium	Vitamin D
Threshold values	Serum calcium (without renal disease) 9–10.5 mg/dl Serum parathyroid hormone: hyperparathyroidism > 65 pg/ml	25(OH)D: reference range 30–100 ng/ml; preferred range: 30–50 ng/ml; insufficiency: 20–30 ng/ml, deficiency < 20 ng/ml
Routine preventative supplementation	1200–1500 mg/d	3000 IU/d
Supplemental source	Calcium citrate is preferred over calcium carbonate due to it being independent of stomach acidity absorption	D_3 is more potent that D_2, but both can be effective and dose dependent
Additional considerations	Divided doses no greater than 600 mg; separate by at least 2 hours from iron containing products; calcium carbonate should be taken with meals, calcium citrate can be taken with or without meals	Vitamin D should be taken with meals containing a fat source for best absorption
Tolerable daily upper intake level	19–50 yrs: 1500 mg/d, > 51 yrs: 2000 mg/d, pregnancy/lactation: 2500 mg/d	> 9 yrs: 4000 IU/d
Safety and risk assessment	Potential adverse effects of excess intake include increased risk of kidney stones, constipation, hypercalciuria, hypercalcemia, vascular and soft tissue calcification, renal insufficiency, and interference with another mineral's absorption	Contraindications for vitamin D supplementation include patients with hypercalcemia or metastatic calcification Serum 25OHD chronically > 50 ng/mL may be related to potential adverse effects. Levels of 25(OH)D > 100 ng/mL reflect excess of vitamin D, levels of 25(OH)D > 150 ng/mL indicating intoxication. Vitamin D doses < 10,000 IU/d are unlikely to cause toxicity in adults Excessive vitamin D intake is associated with clinical adverse effects including hypercalcemia, hypercalciuria, and renal stones (when taken together with excess calcium supplementation) In sensitive subpopulations (granuloma-forming disorders, chronic fungal infections, lymphoma, thiazide diuretics treatment) 25(OH)D and calcium levels should be monitored carefully Serum calcium levels should be monitored 1 mo after completing the loading regimen of high-dose vitamin D supplements to treat deficiency. If calcium levels are elevated, any calcium-containing vitamin D supplements should be stopped and further vitamin D loading should be delayed. Elevated calcium despite stopping calcium and vitamin D supplements requires PTH monitoring and referring to endocrinologist

Adapted from Ben-Porat et al. [16]

Table 4 Micronutrient deficiencies after sleeve gastrectomy

Study	Type[a]	# of patients	Iron	Anemia	Calcium	Zinc	Magnesium	B1	B6	B12	Vit D	Folic Acid	Hypoalbuinaemia	Follow-Up
			Deficiency percentage (%)											
Hakeam et al. (2009)	P	61	4.9	4.9	NA	NA	NA	NA	NA	26.2	NA	9.8	NA	12
Salle et al. (2010)	P	33	25	NA	NA	18.8	NA	NA	NA	NA	NA	NA	0	12
Aarts et al. (2011)	P	60	43	26	0	NA	NA	11	0	9	39	15	15	12
Ruiz-Tovar et al. (2012)	R	30	3.3	NA	NA	NA	NA	NA	NA	NA	3.3	NA	NA	24
Moore and Sherman (2014)	P	60	N/A	NA	NA	NA	NA	NA	NA	NA	27.3	NA	NA	3
Damms-Machado et al. 2012	P	54	4.3	NA	4.3	NA	NA	NA	17.2	17.2	70.4	13.8	NA	12
Van Rutte et al. (2014)	P	200	18.5	6.5	2	5	3	9	4	11.5	36	12.5	0.5	12
Ben-Porat et al. 2015	R	77	27.7	20	NA	NA	NA	NA	NA	16.7	93.6	21.4	NA	12
Belfiore et al. (2015)	R	47	8.8	NA	NA	32.4	NA	17.7	NA	6	11.8	11.8	NA	6
Al-Mulhim (2016)	P	112	7.1	6.25	9.8	NA	2.7	NA	NA	14.3	8.9	6.25	NA	12
Saif et al. [18]	R	30	0	28.6	0	14.3	0	30.8	NA	0	42	0	5.5	60
Pellitero et al. (2017)	P	51	NA	4	NA	NA	NA	0	0.2	0	35	0	NA	60
Gehrer et al. (2010)	P	50	18	NA	0	34	NA	0	0	18	56.3	22	4	36
Alexandrou et at (2014)	P	40	30	54.2	NI	NA	NA	NA	NA	5	NA	20	NA	48
Kheniser et al. (2017)	R	50	6	49	NI	NA	NA	NA	NA	12	35.5	NA	NA	48
Median	–	907	8.8	20	1	18.8	2.7	10	0.2	11.7	35.5	12.5	4	12

[a]P = prospective, R = retrospective. Adapted from Emile and Elfeki [17]

Table 5 2019 ASMBS guidelines for vitamin/mineral supplementation post weight loss surgery

Vitamin/mineral	Prevalence of deficiency	Recommended supplementation	Repletion for deficiency	Screening
Thiamin (B1)	<1–49% depending on procedure and post surgery time frame	≥ 2 mg thiamine daily; preferably a 50–100 mg daily dose of thiamine from a B-complex supplement or high-potency multivitamin	Bariatric patients with suspected thiamine deficiency should be treated before or in the absence of laboratory confirmation and monitored/evaluated for resolution of signs and symptoms Repletion dose for thiamine deficiency varies based on route of administration and severity of symptoms: Oral therapy: 100 mg 2–3 times daily until symptoms resolve IV therapy: 200 mg 3 times daily to 500 mg once or twice daily for 3–5 d, followed by 250 mg/d for 3–5 d or until symptoms resolve, then consider treatment with 100 mg/d orally, indefinitely, or until risk factors have been resolved IM therapy: 250 mg once daily for 3–5 d or 100–250 mg monthly Magnesium, potassium, and phosphorus should be given simultaneously to patients at risk for refeeding syndrome	Recommended for high-risk groups: Females, African Americans, Patients with lack of nutritional care post-surgery, Patients experiencing symptoms such as intractable nausea and vomiting, poor appetite, or constipation, Patients with comorbidities that are taking medications, Excessive alcohol use, Malnutrition, Extreme weight loss Post-WLS patients with signs and symptoms or risk factors should be assessed for thiamin deficiency at least during the first 6 months and then every 3–6 months until symptoms resolve
Cobalamin (B12)	4–20% at 2–5 years post SG	Supplement dose varies based on route of administration. Orally by disintegrating tablet, sublingual, or liquid: 350–1,000 mcg daily Nasal spray as directed by manufacturer Parenteral (IM or SQ): 1,000 mcg monthly	1,000 mcg/d to achieve normal levels and then resume dosages recommended to maintain normal levels	Recommended for patients who have undergone SG More frequent screening (every 3 months) recommended in the first-year post-surgery, and then at least annually or as clinically indicated for patients who chronically use medications that exacerbate risk of B_{12} deficiency, such as nitrous oxide, neomycin, metformin, colchicine, proton-pump inhibitors, and seizure medications Screening should include serum MMA with or without homocysteine to identify metabolic deficiency of B_{12} in symptomatic and asymptomatic patients and in patients with history of B_{12} deficiency or preexisting neuropathy Vitamin B_{12} deficiencies can occur due to food intolerances or restricted intake of protein and vitamin B_{12}-containing foods

(continued)

Table 5 (continued)

Vitamin/mineral	Prevalence of deficiency	Recommended supplementation	Repletion for deficiency	Screening
Folic Acid	Up to 65% of patients	400–80 mcg oral folate daily from their multivitamin 800–1,000 mcg oral folate daily in women of child-bearing age	Oral dose of 1000 μg of folate daily to achieve normal levels and then resume recommended dosage to maintain normal levels >1 mg/d supplementation is not recommended because of the potential masking of vitamin B12 deficiency	Screening recommended for all patients, females of childbearing age, noncompliance with vitamin supplementation, and poor dietary intake of folate-containing foods
Iron	<18% SG 3 months–10 years post surgery	Males and patients without a history of anemia: 18 mg of iron from multivitamin Menstruating females and patients who have undergone RYGB, SG, or BPD/DS: 45–60 mg of elemental iron daily (cumulatively, including iron from all vitamin and mineral supplements) Oral supplementation should be taken in divided doses separately from calcium supplements, acid-reducing medications, and foods high in phytates or polyphenols	Oral supplementation should be increased to provide 150–200 mg of elemental iron daily to amounts as high as 300 mg 2–3 times daily Oral supplementation should be taken in divided doses separately from calcium supplements, acid-reducing medications, and foods high in phytates or polyphenols Vitamin C supplementation may be added to increase iron absorption and decrease risk of iron overload IV iron infusion should be administered if iron deficiency does not respond to oral therapy	Iron deficiency can occur after any bariatric procedure, despite routing supplementation Routine post-bariatric screening is recommended within 3 months after surgery, and then every 3 to 6 months until 12 months, and annually thereafter for all patients Iron status should be monitored in post-bariatric patients at regular intervals using an iron panel, complete blood count, total iron-binding capacity, ferritin, and soluble transferrin receptor (if available), along with clinical signs and symptoms Additional screening should be performed based on clinical signs and symptoms and/or laboratory findings or in cases where deficiency is suspected

(continued)

Table 5 (continued)

Vitamin/ mineral	Prevalence of deficiency	Recommended supplementation	Repletion for deficiency	Screening
Vitamin D	UP to 100% of patients post-surgery depending on procedure and timeframe post-op	Appropriate dose of daily calcium from all sources varies by surgical procedure SG: 1,200–1,500 mg/d To enhance calcium absorption in post WLS patients Calcium should be given in divided doses Calcium carbonate should be taken with meals Calcium citrate may be taken with or without meals Recommended preventative dose of vitamin D should be based on serum vitamin D levels Recommended vitamin D3 dose is 3,000 IU daily, until blood levels of 25(OH)D are greater than sufficient (30 ng/mL) 7–90% lower vitamin D3 bolus is needed (compared to vitamin D2) to achieve the same effects as those produced in healthy nonbariatric surgical patients	All bariatric patients with vitamin D deficiency or insufficiency should be repleted as follows: Vitamin D3 at least 3,000 IU/d and as high as 6,000 IU/d, or 50,000 IU vitamin D2 1–3 times weekly Vitamin D3 is recommended over vitamin D2 as a more potent treatment when comparing frequency and amount needed for repletion Repletion of calcium deficiency varies by surgical procedure: SG: 1,200–1,500 mg/d	Routine screening is recommending for all patients. 25(OH)D is the preferred biochemical assay Elevated PTH levels and increased bone formation/resorption markers may also be considered
Vitamin A	Up to 70% of patients within 4 years post-surgery depending on procedure	Dosage is based on type of procedure: SG: 5,000–10,000 IU/d Higher maintenance doses of fat-soluble vitamins may be required for bariatric patients with a previous history of vitamin A deficiency Water-miscible forms of fat-soluble vitamins are also available to improve absorption Special attention should be paid to post-bariatric supplementation of vitamin A in pregnant women	For bariatric patients with vitamin A deficiency without corneal changes, a dose of 10,000–25,000 IU/d of vitamin A should be given orally until clinical improvement is evident For bariatric patients with vitamin A deficiency with corneal changes, a dose of 50,000–100,000 IU of vitamin A should be administered IM for 3 d, followed by 50,000 IU/d IM for 2 weeks Bariatric patients with vitamin A deficiency should also be evaluated for concurrent iron and/or copper deficiencies because these can impair resolution of vitamin A deficiency	Screening is recommended within the first postoperative year, especially for those with symptoms of protein-calorie malnutrition

(continued)

Table 5 (continued)

Vitamin/mineral	Prevalence of deficiency	Recommended supplementation	Repletion for deficiency	Screening
Vitamin E	Uncommon	15 mg/d Higher maintenance doses of fat-soluble vitamins may be required for post-bariatric patients with a previous history of vitamin E deficiency Water-miscible forms of fat-soluble vitamins are also available to improve absorption	Optimal therapeutic dose for bariatric patients is not defined Potential antioxidant benefits can be achieved with supplements of 100–400 IU/d, which is higher than the amount found in multivitamins. Additional supplementation may be required for repletion	Screening is recommended in patients who are symptomatic
Vitamin K	Uncommon	SG: 90–120 mcg/day Higher maintenance doses of fat-soluble vitamins may be required for post-WLS patients with a previous history of vitamin K deficiency Water-miscible forms of fat-soluble vitamins are also available to improve absorption Special attention should be paid to post-WLS supplementation of vitamin K in pregnant women	A parenteral dose of 10 mg is recommended for bariatric patients with acute malabsorption A dose of either 1–2 mg/d orally or 1–2 mg/week parenterally is recommended for post-WLS patients with chronic malabsorption	Screening is recommended in patients who are symptomatic
Zinc	UP to 19% post SG	All post-WLS patients should take 4 RDA zinc, with dosage based on type of procedure SG: Multivitamin with minerals containing 100% of the RDA (8–11 mg/d) The supplementation protocol should contain a ratio of 8–15 mg of supplemental zinc per 1 mg of copper to minimize the risk of copper deficiency The formulation and composition of zinc supplements should be considered in post-WLS patients to calculated accurate levels of elemental zinc provided by the supplement	A dose-related recommendation for repletion cannot be made due to insufficient evidence Repletion doses should be chosen carefully to avoid inducing a copper deficiency Zinc status should be routinely monitored using consistent parameters throughout treatment	Zinc deficiency is possible, even during zinc supplementation Serum and plasma zinc are the preferred biomarkers for screening in post-bariatric patients

(continued)

Table 5 (continued)

Vitamin/ mineral	Prevalence of deficiency	Recommended supplementation	Repletion for deficiency	Screening
Copper	Uncommon	All post-WLS patients should take 4 RDA copper as part of routine multivitamin and mineral supplementation, with dosage based on type of procedure: SG: 100% of the RDA (1 mg/d) Supplementation with 1 mg copper is recommended for every 8–15 mg of elemental zinc to prevent copper deficiency in all post-WLS patients Copper gluconate or sulfate is the recommended source of copper for supplementation	Recommended repletion regimen varies with severity of deficiency: Mild to moderate (including low hematologic indices): 3–8 mg/d oral copper gluconate or sulfate until indices return to normal Severe: 2–4 mg/d intravenous copper can be initiated for 6 d or until serum levels return to normal and neurologic symptoms resolve Copper levels should be monitored every 3 months after they return to normal	Serum copper and ceruloplasmin are recommended biomarkers for copper status

SG Sleeve gastrectomy

The studies ranged in dates from 2009 through to 2017 to provide a comprehensive review of micronutrient deficiencies ranging from 3 months to 5 years after surgery [17].

Obesity related, low grade inflammation caused by obesity can lead to anemia. For the correct diagnosis of anemia after surgery, it is important to conduct a broad assessment of not only iron levels, but also vitamin B-6, B-12, folic acid, copper, selenium and zinc because deficiencies of these vitamins and minerals can lead to iron deficiency anemia [19].

A hypo acidic environment and over supplementation of zinc can lead to copper deficiency, which is a nutrient needed for iron mobilization, and thus will cause a reduction in numbers of red blood cells. Copper deficiencies are often mistaken for iron or vitamin B-12 deficiency, and usually are not diagnosed until advanced neurologic conditions such as unstable gait, numbness in the extremities, or damage to peripheral nerves [19].

The ASMBS released updated 2019 clinical practice guidelines for care and management of patients undergoing weight loss surgery procedures. Table 5 provides a comprehensive review of the vitamin and mineral recommendations for supplementation and repletion of deficiencies.

Saif et al. monitored blood levels of major vitamins and minerals of 82 patients who underwent a sleeve gastrectomy over the course of 5 years. In this study, 20% of the population had low hemoglobin and hematocrit values, however, these values normalized up to year 3. By year 5, levels had returned to preoperative deficiency levels. There was an increase in low levels for thiamine, however, enough values were not collected. Vitamin D status improved by year 1 for those that were deficiency pre-op, but by year 5 parathyroid hormone levels began to rise [18].

Likewise, Ben-Porat et al. observed long term results of 27 patients who underwent a sleeve gastrectomy procedure, below are their findings in Table 6 [20].

Similarly, Moizé et al. conducted a 5 year study to review micronutrient deficiencies in malabsorptive versus restrictive procedures. Of 355 patients, 61 underwent a sleeve gastrectomy with their laboratory findings detailed in Table 7 [21].

Although the sleeve gastrectomy is a restrictive procedure, patients are still at a nutritional risk for developing deficiencies of major micronutrients due to an array of clinical reasons. The research studies reviewed in this chapter, prove

Table 6 Nutrient deficiencies at baseline, 1 year, and 4 years after sleeve gastrectomy

Micronutrient	Baseline deficiency (%)	1 year deficiency (%)	4 year deficiency (%)
Hemoglobin	11.5	20	18.5
Iron	44	41.2	28.6
Vitamin B-12	7.7	13.6	15.4
Folate	46	14.3	12.5
Vitamin D	96.2	89	86.4
Hyperparathyroidism	52	15.4	60

Ben-Porat et al. [20]

Table 7 Percentage of deficiencies of patients post sleeve gastrectomy

Nutrient	Baseline	6 months	12 months	24 months	48 months	60 months
Total protein	5.4	0	3.4	0	4.5	0
Albumin	5.4	4.3	0	0	4.8	0
Prealbumin	11.8	8.7	14.3	3.1	0	0
Hemoglobin	10	12.1	11.5	11.5	15.8	14.3
Ferritin	8.3	0	6.5	20.6	23.8	0
Transferrin	2.8	0	7.1	9.4	0	0
Iron	30.8	4.3	10.3	9.4	9.5	12.5
Folic acid	0	13.6	20.7	6.1	0	12.5
Zinc	8.1	31.8	39.3	25	47.6	12.5
Calcium	2.9	0	3.6	3.1	4.8	12.5
Magnesium	37.8	12.5	10.3	6.3	4.8	12.5
Thiamine	0	4.8	9.1	25	0	0
B-6	75	26.3	11.1	0	16.7	0
B-12	2.7	3.7	3.2	5.9	0	12.5
Vit D sufficiency > 30 ng/ml	6.7	22.7	22.2	13.3	33.3	0
Vit D Insufficiency > 10–<30 ng/ml	3.3	54.5	40.7	20	22.2	100
VIt D Deficiency <10 ng/ml	90	22.7	37	66.7	44.4	0
Parathyroid hormone	62.5	40.9	37	40.6	57.1	87.5

Moize et al. [21]

the importance of, and need for, long-term supplementation for vitamins and minerals after weight loss surgery. There is limited research that has been done on patients greater than 2 years post-surgery. However, the research that has been conducted, shows a trend towards reappearance of deficiencies that were noted in the pre-operative phase for surgery.

References

1. World health Organization. Obesity and overweight fact sheet. 2018. https://Who.int/en/news-room/fact-sheets/detail/obesity-and-overweight.
2. Angrisani L, Santonicola A, Iovino P, Formisano G, Buchwald H, Scopinaro N. Bariatric surgery worldwide 2013. Obes Surg. 2015;25(10):1822–32. https://doi.org/10.1007/s11695-015-1657-z.
3. Damms-Machado, A., Friedrich, A., Kramer, K. M., et al. (2012). Pre-and postoperative nutritional deficiencies in obese patients undergoing laparoscopic sleeve gastrectomy. *Obesity Surgery, 22*(6), 881–889. https://doi.org/10.1007/s11695-012-0609-0.

4. Ben-Porat T, Weiss R, Sherf-Dagan S, Nabulsi N, Maayani A, Khalaileh A, Abed S, Brodie R, Harari R, Mintz Y, Pikarsky A, Elazary R. Nutritional deficiencies in patients with severe obesity before bariatric surgery: what should be the focus during the preoperative assessment?. J Acad Nutr Dietetics. 2019;120. https://doi.org/10.1016/j.jand.2019.10.017.

5. Flancbaum L, Belsley S, Drake V, et al. Preoperative nutritional status of patients undergoing Roux-en-Y gastric bypass for morbid obesity. J Gastrointest Surg. 2006;10:1033–7. https://doi.org/10.1016/j.gassur.2006.03.004.

6. Tang L, Alsulaim HA, Canner JK, Prokopowicz GP, Steele KE. Prevalence and predictors of postoperative thiamine deficiency after vertical sleeve gastrectomy. Surg Obes Relat Dis. 2018;14(7):943–50. https://doi.org/10.1016/j.soard.2018.03.024.

7. Mechanick JI, et al. Clinical practice guidelines for the perioperative nutrition, metabolic, and nonsurgical support of patients undergoing bariatric procedures—2019 update: cosponsored by American association of clinical endocrinologists/American college of endocrinology, the obesity society, American society for metabolic & bariatric surgery, obesity medicine association, and American society of anesthesiologists—executive summary. Endocrine Pract. 2019;25(12):1346–59.

8. Kröll D, Laimer M, Borbély YM, et al. Wernicke encephalopathy: a future problem even after sleeve gastrectomy? a Systematic Literature Review. Obes Surg. 2016;26:205–12. https://doi.org/10.1007/s11695-015-1927-9.

9. Sechi G, Serra A. Wernicke's encephalopathy: new clinical settings and recent advances in diagnosis and management. Lancet Neurol. 2007;6(5):442–55. https://doi.org/10.1016/S1474-4422(07)70104-7.

10. Athanasiou A, Angelou A, Diamantis T. Wernicke's encephalopathy after sleeve gastrectomy. Where do we stand today? A reappraisal. Surg Obes Relat Dis. 2014;10(3):563. https://doi.org/10.1016/j.soard.2014.01.028.

11. Lu CW, Chang YK, Chang HH, et al. Fracture risk after bariatric surgery: a 12-year nationwide cohort study. Medicine (Baltimore). 2015;94(48):e2087. https://doi.org/10.1097/MD.0000000000002087.

12. Folli F, Sabowitz BN, Schwesinger W, Fanti P, Guardado-Mendoza R, Muscogiuri G. Bariatric surgery and bone disease: from clinical perspective to molecular insights. Int J Obes (Lond). 2012;36(11):1373–79.https://doi.org/10.1038/ijo.2012.115.

13. Mihmanli M, Isil RG, Isil CT, et al. Effects of laparoscopic sleeve gastrectomy on parathyroid hormone, vitamin d, calcium, phosphorus, and albumin levels. Obes Surg. 2017;27(12):3149–55. https://doi.org/10.1007/s11695-017-2747-x.

14. Carrasco F, Basfi-Fer K, Rojas P, et al. Changes in bone mineral density after sleeve gastrectomy or gastric bypass: relationships with variations in vitamin D, ghrelin, and adiponectin levels. Obes Surg. 2014;24(6):877–84. https://doi.org/10.1007/s11695-014-1179-0.

15. Pluskiewicz W, Buzga M, Holeczy P, Bortlik L, Smajstrla V, Adamczyk P. Bone mineral changes in spine and proximal femur in individual obese women after laparoscopic sleeve gastrectomy: a short-term study. Obes Surg. 2012;22(7):1068–76.

16. Ben-Porat T, Elazary R, Sherf-Dagan S, et al. Bone health following bariatric surgery: implications for management strategies to attenuate bone loss. Adv Nutr. 2018;9(2):114–27.https://doi.org/10.1093/advances/nmx024.

17. Emile SH, Elfeki H. Nutritional deficiency after sleeve gastrectomy: a comprehensive literature review. EMJ Gastroenterol. 2017;6(1):99–105.

18. Saif T, Strain GW, Dakin G, Gagner M, Costa R, Pomp A. Evaluation of nutrient status after laparoscopic sleeve gastrectomy 1, 3, and 5 years after surgery. Surg Obes Relat Dis. 2012;8(5):542–7. https://doi.org/10.1016/j.soard.2012.01.013.

19. Gletsu-Miller N, Wright BN. Mineral malnutrition following bariatric surgery. Adv Nutr. 2013;4(5):506–17. https://doi.org/10.3945/an.113.004341.

20. Ben-Porat T, Elazary R, Goldenshluger A, Sherf-Dagan S, Mintz Y, Weiss, R. Nutritional deficiencies four years after laparoscopic sleeve gastrectomy-are supplements required for a lifetime?. Surg Obes Relat Diseas. 2017;13.https://doi.org/10.1016/j.soard.2017.02.021.

21. Moize V, Andreu A, Flores L, Torres F, Ibarzabal A, Delgado S, Lacy A, Rodriguez L, Vidal J. Long-term dietary intake and nutritional deficiencies following sleeve gastrectomy or Roux-En-Y gastric bypass in a mediterranean population. J Acad Nutr Dietetics. 2013;113:400–10. https://doi.org/10.1016/j.jand.2012.11.013.

The Sleeve Diet and Exercise programs

Laparoscopic Sleeve Gastrectomy: Beyond the 10 years

Ashraf Haddad

1   Introduction

The laparoscopic sleeve gastrectomy (LSG) was introduced initially as the first step of a staged procedure for high risk super-obese patients to be later followed by Roux-en-Y gastric bypass (RYGB) or duodenal switch (DS) [1]. The initial experiences and results with the LSG at that time suggested that it has the potential to be considered as a stand-alone single stage bariatric operation [2].

The LSG became extremely popular over the following years. Initially it constituted 5% of all bariatric procedures , as reported by the 2008 IFSO survey (International Federation for the Surgery of Obesity and related disorders), afterwards, the LSG dominated the bariatric field in 2016 and constituted 50% of all primary bariatric procedures [3] Fig. 1.

This trend can be explained by the fact that the LSG is seemingly easy and likey has a lower learning curve compared to the other procedures, especially that it was reported to have a slightly lower 30 days adverse outcome rate compared to the RYGB [4].

The safety profile and good short term outcomes are not enough. The lack of longterm data, particularly 10 years follow up, became an area of crticisim and debate. Longterm weight loss outcomes, the rate of weight regain, resolution of comorbidities, the risk of gastroesophageal reflux disease, and the need for reoperation became the pilars of this ongoing debate.

In this chapter we will examine the available longterm outcomes (beyond the 10 years) of the LSG.

A. Haddad (✉)
Minimally Invasive, Advanced GI and Bariatric surgery, GBMC-Jordan Hospital, Amman, Jordan
e-mail: drajhaddad@gmail.com

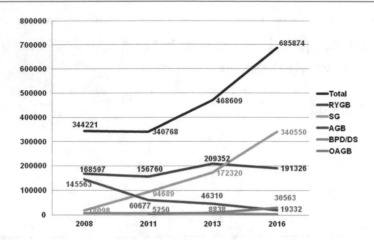

Fig. 1 Number of the main primary bariatric/metabolic surgical procedures from 2008 to 2016. AGB adjustable gastric banding, RYGB Roux-en-Y gastric bypass, SG sleeve gastrectomy, BPD-DS biliopancreatic diversionduodenal switch, OAGB oneanastomosis gastric bypass Angrisani et al. [3].

Table 1 Summary of 10 years weight loss outcomes after LSG

Study	Number of patients	% EBWL
Arman et al. [7]	47	62.5
Rodriguez et al. [8]	40	53.8
Gissey et al. [9]	114	52.5
Chang et al. [5]	65	70.5
Felsenreich et al. [6]	65	50

2   Weight Loss Outcomes

Despite the LSG's impressive short term and midterm weight loss outcomes, longterm weight loss outcomes beyond the 10 years mark are minimal, consisiting of few series and small amounts of patients.

Chang et al. reported on 65 post LSG patients with more than 10 years follow up. The perentage of excess body weight loss (%EBWL) was 70.5% [5]. A second study by Felsenreich et al. descibed the outcomes of another 65 patients who reached 10 years follow-up with only 50% EBWL [6]. Arman et al. similarly reported on 47 patients that were not converted who sustained 62.5% EBWL at 10 years [7]. Rodriguez et al. and Gissey et al. both reported on EBWL at 10 years being 53.8% in 40 patients and 52.5% in 114 patients respectively [8, 9]. To summarize, data is only available on the outcomes of 331 patients beyond 10 years with EBWL ranging between 50 and 70.5% Table 1.

3   Weight Regain

Weight regain has been descibed in 10.4% of LSG patients at 10 years [8]. The overall revision rate post LSG for all reasons was reported to be 21.5 to 33% [5–8]. Revisions for weight regain constitutes 27.5 to 81% of all revisions, with the RYGB being the most commonly performed revisional procedure post LSG for all purposes [5, 7, 8].

4   Gastroesphageal Reflux Disease Post Sleeve Gastrectomy

Gastroesophageal reflux disease (GERD) is one of the other major longterm concerns after LSG. These concerns sharply increased with the longterm de-novo GERD rate being reported between 21.4 and 58.4% at 10 years [5, 7, 8]. This significant rise in GERD, erosive esophagitis, and Barrets esophagus with no resolution of preoperative GERD at 10 years follow up led to substantially more people taking proton pump inhibitors (PPI) late after the procedure [7, 8].

With almost half of the patients (50%) consuming PPI regularly at 10 years, together with longterm GERD constituting 19–65.2% of all indications for post LSG revisions, this translated into a 16.9% conversion rate to RYGB, further highlighting GERD as a major pitfall of the LSG at 10 years [5–7] Table 2.

It is important to highlight that patients with GERD symptoms report significantly lower quality of life scores at 10 years [6].

5   Barretts Esophagus Post LSG

It is known that morbidly obese patients are more affected by GERD than lean patients. Furthermore; the duration and severity of GERD symptoms has a direct relationship to Barretts esophagus (BE). Although there is no longterm data on BE after LSG we felt it is important to disccuss the short and midterm outcome of LSG and BE in this chapter.

Table 2 Summary of all studies reporting GERD outcomes at 10 years post LSG

Study	Denovo GERD rate (%)	Coversion rate due to GERD
Arman et al. [7]	21.4	19% of all conversions
Gissey et al. [9]	42.9	1.8% of the total cohort of patients
Chang et al. [5]	58.4	65.2% of all conversions
Felsenreich et al. [6]	57	34% of all conversions

Although the diagnosis of GERD post LSG has been based on symptoms and PPI use, in 2017 Genco et al. reported on 110 post LSG patients that underwent both pre and post operative endoscopy and biopsies with a 58 months follow up. They reported 68.1% GERD symptoms and 57.2% PPI intake. This translated into a significant increase in erosive esophagitis leading to upward migration of the "Z" line in 73.6% of patients and a new diagnosis of non dysplastic BE in 17.2% of patients [10].

A follow up study by the same group with 144 patient and a mean follow up of 66 months showed an increase in GERD and PPI rate to 70.2% and 63.9% respectively. 72.9% had pathological endoscopic findings with 13.1% documentd BE [11]. This is similar to the BE rate of 14% documented by Felsenreich et al. [6].

This worrisome issue of GERD leading to the early development of BE in a young population led the International Federation for the Surgery of Obesity and related disorders (IFSO) to release a position statement on endoscopy and bariatric surgery in July 2020 stating:

> EGD should be undertaken routinely for all patients after bariatric surgery at 1 year and then every 2–3 years for patients who have undergone LSG or OAGB to enable early detection of Barrett's esophagus or upper GI malignancy until more data is available to confirm the incidence of these cancers in practice [12].

6   Comorbidities Beyond the 10 years

Comorbidities resolution should constitute the main long-term interest in bariatric surgery. Although long-term outcomes of comorbidity resolution are available for the RYGB, outcomes beyond the 10 years for LSG are minimal. We will summarize the data available on comorbidities and LSG beyond the 10 years.

The LSG showed resolution of comorbidities at 1 year with some persistence in the results at 10 years. Chang et al. reported type II diabetes (DM) remission of 60% at 1 year that drops to 39.6% at 10 years [5]. Felsenreich reported 71.4% 10 years DM resolution in 5 patients only [6]. Arman et al. reported on 3 patients with DM in their series. All 3 required revisional surgery during the follow up period (2 converted to RYGB, 1 to DS) [7]. Rodriguez reported a 54.9% improvement rate in his 40 patient's cohort. However; 33.3% required DM medications again [9]. Gissey et al. followed 17 diabetic post LSG patients and reported 64.7% DM resolution rate at 10 years.

As for Hypertension (HTN), resolution rates between 28.6 and 78.4% in very small numbers of patients have been reported [5–9]. However; 31.1% of patients had to restart HTN medications during follow up [9]. Resolution of comorbidities at 10 years after LSG is summarized in Table 3.

Table 3 Resolution rate of comorbidities at 10 years after LSG

Study	Type II DM (Remission/ Improvement at 10 years)	Hypertension (Remission/ Improvement at 10 years)	Hyperlipidemia (Remission/ Improvement at 10 years)	Obstructive sleep apnea (Remission/ Improvement at 10 years)
Chang et al.	39.6%	78.4%	51.3%	–
Felsenreich et al.	71.4% (5 patients)	36.1% (13 patients)	–	–
Arman et al.	All patients with DM required revision prior to 10 years. 1 denovo case recorded	28.6% either remission or improvement	10 patients: 2 remission 2 improvement 6 did not improve	66%
Gissey et al.	64.7%/23.5%(17 patients)	44.2%/36.5%	36.4%/45.5%	72.2%/27.8%
Rodriguez et al.	–/54.9% 33.3% of patient required medications again	–/48.2% 31.1% restarted HTN medication	–	–

7   Conclusion

The LSG has become one of the most commonly performed bariatric procedures worldwide. It has good short to mid term outcomes. Longterm results beyond the 10 years are lacking and is constituted of small series of patients. Weight regain, relapse of comorbidities that initially resloved, GERD, and Barretts esophagus are longterm concers that need to be closely observed and followed in larger series of patients to document the long term efficacy and safety of the LSG.

References

1. Regan JP, Inabnet WB, Gagner M, Pomp A. Early experience with two-stage laparoscopic Roux-en-Y gastric bypass as an alternative in the super-super obese patient. Obes Surg. 2003;13(6):861–4. https://doi.org/10.1381/096089203322618669.
2. Mognol P, Chosidow D, Marmuse JP. Laparoscopic sleeve gastrectomy as an initial bariatric operation for high-risk patients: initial results in 10 patients. Obes Surg. 2005;15(7):1030–3. https://doi.org/10.1381/0960892054621242.

3. Angrisani L, Santonicola A, Iovino P, et al. IFSO worldwide survey 2016: primary, endoluminal, and revisional procedures. Obes Surg. 2018;28(12):3783–94. https://doi.org/10.1007/s11695-018-3450-2.

4. Guerrier JB, Dietch ZC, Schirmer BD, Hallowell PT. Laparoscopic sleeve gastrectomy is associated with lower 30-day morbidity versus laparoscopic gastric bypass: an analysis of the american college of surgeons NSQIP. Obes Surg. 2018;28(11):3567–72. https://doi.org/10.1007/s11695-018-3396-4.

5. Chang DM, Lee WJ, Chen JC, Ser KH, Tsai PL, Lee YC. Thirteen-year experience of laparoscopic sleeve gastrectomy: surgical risk, weight loss, and revision procedures. Obes Surg. 2018;28(10):2991–7. https://doi.org/10.1007/s11695-018-3344-3.

6. Felsenreich DM, Ladinig LM, Beckerhinn P, et al. Update: 10 years of sleeve gastrectomy-the first 103 patients. Obes Surg. 2018;28(11):3586–94. https://doi.org/10.1007/s11695-018-3399-1.

7. Arman GA, Himpens J, Dhaenens J, Ballet T, Vilallonga R, Leman G. Long-term (11+years) outcomes in weight, patient satisfaction, comorbidities, and gastroesophageal reflux treatment after laparoscopic sleeve gastrectomy. Surg Obes Relat Dis. 2016;12(10):1778–86. https://doi.org/10.1016/j.soard.2016.01.013.

8. Rodriguez J, Zerrweck C, Inzunza E, et al. Laparoscopic sleeve gastrectomy: results at 10 years oral presentations. Surg Obes Relat Dis. 2016;12:S1–32.

9. Gissey LC, Casella Mariolo JR, Genco A, Troisi A, Basso N, Casella G. 10-year follow-up after laparoscopic sleeve gastrectomy: outcomes in a monocentric series. Surg Obes Relat Dis. 2018;14(10):1480–1487. https://doi.org/10.1016/j.soard.2018.06.021.

10. Genco A, Soricelli E, Casella G, et al. Gastroesophageal reflux disease and Barrett's esophagus after laparoscopic sleeve gastrectomy: a possible, underestimated long-term complication. Surg Obes Relat Dis. 2017;13(4):568–74. https://doi.org/10.1016/j.soard.2016.11.029.

11. Soricelli E, Casella G, Baglio G, Maselli R, Ernesti I, Genco A. Lack of correlation between gastroesophageal reflux disease symptoms and esophageal lesions after sleeve gastrectomy. Surg Obes Relat Dis. 2018;14(6):751–6. https://doi.org/10.1016/j.soard.2018.02.008.

12. Brown WA, Johari Halim Shah Y, Balalis G, et al. IFSO position statement on the role of esophago-gastro-duodenal endoscopy prior to and after bariatric and metabolic surgery procedures [published online ahead of print, 2020 May 29]. Obes Surg. 2020. https://doi.org/10.1007/s11695-020-04720-z.

Suggested Reading

Clapp B, Wynn M, Martyn C, Foster C, O'Dell M, Tyroch A. Long term (7 or more years) outcomes of the sleeve gastrectomy: a meta-analysis. *Surg Obes Relat Dis*. 2018;14(6):741–47. 10.1016/j.soard.2018.02.027.

The Sleeve Diet and Exercise Programs

Samantha Stavola

1 Recommended Diet Post Sleeve

Prior to sleeve gastrectomy, all patients should be counseled on the importance of making dietary changes that focus on lean protein intake to preserve fat free mass, while promoting the loss of fat tissue following weight loss surgery [1]. Fat free tissue within the body is responsible for resting metabolic rate and normal body functioning, making it crucial to promote high protein, well-balanced, well-hydrated dietary intake that increases lean tissue mass and prevents any stalling of weight loss due to dehydration [1, 2]. Table 1 provides recommendations for macronutrient and fluid intake and behavior changes for long-term success after surgery [2].

2 Types of Exercises: Recommended Exercise Programs

Physical activity and exercise are important components of comprehensive care and long-term weight loss success following bariatric surgery. Thus, it is important to provide individualized exercise recommendations to patients, that are within their specific capabilities, to promote long-term compliance [3]. Increased exercise after bariatric surgery contributes not only to supporting weight loss, but also improving quality of life [4]. Practice guidelines from The American Association of Clinical Endocrinologists/American College of Endocrinology and The American College of Cardiology, The American Heart Association, and

S. Stavola (✉)
Nutrition for Celebrate Nutritional Supplements, Wadsworth, OH, USA
e-mail: sam@celebratevitamins.com

© The Editor(s) (if applicable) and The Author(s), under exclusive license to Springer Nature Switzerland AG 2021
S. Al-Sabah et al. (eds.), *Laparoscopic Sleeve Gastrectomy*,
https://doi.org/10.1007/978-3-030-57373-7_64

Table 1 Recommendations following bariatric procedures

Recommendations	UpToDate: postoperative nutritional management	2008 ASMBS allied health nutritional guidelines	Guidelines for perioperative care in bariatric Surgery: ERAS society recommendations	Academy of nutrition and dietetics pocket guide to bariatric surgery, 2nd ed
Intake	Surgeon or institution specific Long-term diet: Sleeve Gastrectomy/Roux-en-Y gastric bypass – well balanced diet containing all the essential nutrients; possible postoperative diets may include • My Plate • DASH Diet The Vegetarian Resource Group Sleeve gastrectomy – same advancement and recommendations post-SG as for post- RYGB	Diet Stage: Regular textured (6–8 weeks after surgery and forward) * Purpose of nutrition care after surgical weight loss procedures: Adequate energy and nutrients to support tissue healing after surgery and support preservation of lean body mass during extreme weight loss Foods and beverages must minimize reflux, early satiety, and dumping syndrome while maximizing weight loss and weight maintenance	Balanced meal plan to include: >5 servings of fruit and vegetables daily for optimal fiber consumption, colonic function, and phytochemical intake Avoid concentrated sweets to reduce caloric intake and to minimize symptoms of dumping (gastric bypass)	Postoperative nutrition care of the bariatric patient has 2 distinct stages during the first year, then advance to: Diet Stage 4: Regular Solid Food Diet
Fluids	Throughout all the diet stages, patients should be counseled to consume adequate fluid to prevent dehydration	N/A	>1.5 L daily	Women: 48 oz/d Men: 64 oz/d 50% goal should be met with clear liquids
Protein	46 g/day–women 56 g/day–men Protein needs: Should constitute 10–35% of daily caloric intake Weight maintenance: 0.8–1.2 g/kg body weight per day Active weight loss: 1.2 g/kg body weight	Exact needs have yet to be defined	Should average 60–20 g daily	Guidelines for protein consumption not defined

(continued)

Table 1 (continued)

Recommendations	UpToDate: postoperative nutritional management	2008 ASMBS allied health nutritional guidelines	Guidelines for perioperative care in bariatric Surgery: ERAS society recommendations	Academy of nutrition and dietetics pocket guide to bariatric surgery, 2nd ed
Carbohydrates	Early postop–50 g/day As diet intake increases–130 g/day	N/A	N/A	N/A
Fat	20–35% of the daily caloric intake; bulk of the fat intake should be unsaturated fat	N/A	N/A	N/A
Behavior	Eat slowly Chew food extensively Stop eating as soon as reach satiety Avoid taking food and beverages at the same time Simple sugars should be limited to less than 10% of daily caloric intake	Avoid/Delay Concentrated sweets Carbonated beverages Fruit juice High-saturated fat, fried foods Soft doughy bread, pasta, rice Tough, dry, red meat Nuts, popcorn, other fibrous foods Caffeine and alcohol	Multiple small meals each day Chewing food thoroughly without drinking beverages at the same time Consume fluids slowly	Practice mindful eating Chew all food until it is smooth Make sure food is soft and moist enough to swallow without sticking Do not drink liquids during meals Wait 30 min after eating before resuming fluid intake Avoid bread, rice and pasta until able to comfortably consume adequate protein, vegetables and fruits

(continued)

Table 1 (continued)

Recommendations	UpToDate: postoperative nutritional management	2008 ASMBS allied health nutritional guidelines	Guidelines for perioperative care in bariatric Surgery: ERAS society recommendations	Academy of nutrition and dietetics pocket guide to bariatric surgery, 2nd ed
Other	Close monitoring with a registered dietitian	Dietitian's role is a vital component of the bariatric surgery process, follow up with registered dietitian	Nutritional and meal planning guidance should be provided to patient and family before bariatric surgery and during the postoperative hospital course and reinforced at subsequent outpatient visits Consultation should be provided with a dietitian and a protocol-derived staged meal progression, based on the type of surgical procedure, should be adhered to	RD responsible for the nutrition care of the post-surgery patient and plays an important role in every aspect of care, from pre-operative assessment of the patient to long-term follow-up, evaluation, and monitoring

Adopted and Modified from Mechanick et al. [2]

the Obesity Society Task Force recommend daily physical activity consisting of moderate aerobic activity equaling a minimum of 150 min per week, spanning a range of 3–5 days, in addition to dietary changes to promote weight loss, with the need of higher levels of activity, near 300 min weekly, to prevent weight gain [3, 5]. Jointly, the American College of Sports Medicine and American Diabetes Association recommend resistance training 2 to 3 times weekly to reduce visceral fat mass and improve body composition [3, 6]. There are two main areas of focus for exercise after weight loss surgery: aerobic activity and muscle strengthening/resistance exercise to preserve lean muscle mass [7].

Obesity is associated with a high energy expenditure needed to move a greater physical mass, this causes a compressed capacity to exercise and shorter duration periods of activity [8–10]. Promoting a negative energy balance of 500 cal per day promotes a net weight loss of one pound each week [11]. A thirty-minute period of moderate exercise can utilize up to 300 kilocalories of energy and represent approximately 20% of total energy intake for the day [12, 13]. Individuals attempting to maintain their weight status and prevent weight regain, may have to increase their weekly exercise routine to 300 minutes of moderate-intensity exercise to maintain weight loss [7]. Further, long term maintenance of weekly energy expenditures of 1,500–2,000 kilocalories have been proven to prevent weight regain [14]. Exercise after surgery should focus on key areas that include: cardiovascular health, strength training, and flexibility.

There are three main aerobic activities that should be promoted after surgery due to their ease and accessibility to improve cardiac health:

- Walking/Treadmill-simplest and most available form of exercise
- Cycling/Elliptical-low impact that is less stressful on knees, hips, and back
- Swimming-moderate activity that provides full body range of motion [6, 7].

A detailed beginner's exercise program is outlined in Table 2 to help patients begin a structured walking program.

A study conducted by de Souza et al. monitored 65 patients' ability to walk on a treadmill pre-operatively, six months, and twelve months post bariatric surgery. In the pre-operative period, patients were able to walk a distance of 401 meters in 5.37 minutes. At their first visit at six months post-op, patients averaged 513 meters in 6.42 minutes. At their final visit at twelve months, patients were able to cover a distance of 690 meters in 8.81 minutes. These results showed a 27.8% increase in distance from pre-op to six months; 34.5% increase from six to twelve months; and 71.9% increase from pre-op to twelve months post-op [15]. A study conducted by Shah et al. followed 33 post-surgical patients through a twelve-week high volume exercise program and compared them to a control group that did not endure high volume activities. 80% of the group assigned to the exercise program depleted at minimum 1,500 kilocalories each week, spanning five days, on aerobic activities that consisted of treadmill, elliptical, or rowing machines and increased their daily step count from 4,500 to 10,000 steps daily

Table 2 Six-week beginner walking plan

	Monday	Tuesday	Wednesday	Thursday	Friday	Weekend (Optional)
Week 1	Easy walk: 5–10 minutes Stretch: 2 minutes Easy walk: 5–10 minutes	Easy walk: 10–15 minutes NOTE: always rest when necessary!	Easy walk: 5–10 minutes Stretch: 2 minutes Easy walk: 5–10 minutes	Easy walk: 10–15 minutes	Rest	Easy walk: 15–20 minutes
Week 2	Easy walk: 10–15 minutes Stretch: 2 minutes Brisk walk: 5–10 minutes	Easy walk: 10–15 minutes	Easy walk: 10–15 minutes Stretch: 2 minutes Brisk walk: 5–10 minutes	Easy walk: 10–15 minutes Remember: rest when necessary!	Rest	Easy walk: 15–20 minutes
Week 3	Easy walk: 10–15 minutes Stretch: 2 minutes Brisk walk: 5–10 minutes	Easy walk: 15–20 minutes Stretch: 2 minutes	Easy walk: 10–15 minutes Stretch: 2 minutes Brisk walk: 5–10 minutes	Easy walk: 15–20 minutes Stretch: 2 minutes	Rest	Easy walk: 15–20 minutes
Week 4	Easy walk: 10–15 minutes Brisk walk: 5–10 minutes Stretch: 2 minutes	Easy walk: 15–20 minutes Stretch: 2 minutes	Easy walk: 10–15 minutes Brisk walk: 5–10 minutes Stretch: 2 minutes	Easy walk: 15–20 minutes Stretch: 2 minutes	Rest	Brisk walk: 20–25 minutes

(continued)

Table 2 (continued)

	Monday	Tuesday	Wednesday	Thursday	Friday	Weekend (Optional)
Week 5	Easy walk: 10–15 minutes Brisk walk: 10–15 minutes Stretch: 2 minutes	Easy walk: 25–30 minutes Stretch: 2 minutes	Easy walk: 10–15 minutes Brisk walk: 10–15 minutes Stretch: 2 minutes	Easy walk: 25–30 minutes Stretch: 2 minutes	Alternate activity of your choice: Go dancing, rake leaves for 20+ minutes	Easy walk: 25–30 minutes
Week 6	Total time: 24–34 minutes Easy walk: 15–20 minutes Power intervals: Power walk: 30 seconds Easy walk: 1 minutes Repeat 4–6 times Easy walk: 3–5 minutes	Alternate activity of your choice for 20–30 minutes	Easy walk: 30–35 minutes Stretch: 2 minutes	Easy walk: 25–30 minutes Stretch: 2 minutes	Rest	Easy walk: 25–35 minutes

Adopted from American Heart Association in collaboration with American Council on Exercise 2011. [24]

[16]. These studies clearly demonstrate a positive correlation between continued exercise post bariatric surgery and improved activity tolerance.

Strength training should consist of 12–15 repetitions of low to moderate free weights to maintain lean muscle mass while losing weight [17]. Herring et al. examined 24 sedentary patients 12–24 months after surgery. The patients were enrolled in an exercise program of 3- sixty-minute gym sessions per week of moderate aerobic activity and resistance training for a twelve-week period. Those in the exercise program lost, on average, 5.6 kg body weight more than those in the control group [18]. Huck et al. enrolled 15 patients in a twelve-week resistance training program to monitor physical fitness and functionality of individuals. At the conclusion of the program, there was significant improvement in functional strength and flexibility in the group that underwent resistance training [19].

However, when evaluating a patient for exercise programs, it is important to first gather an understanding of their current exercise routine and any concerns or fears they may have regarding an increase in their aerobic activity or transitioning from a sedentary lifestyle to a more active lifestyle [20].

3 Long-Term Outcomes-What to Expect

Since the late 1990s, weight loss surgery has been the most effective long-term treatment for weight loss for obese patients. Weight loss after surgery is primarily affected by a reduction in the secretion of the hormone ghrelin, which stimulates appetite. A study conducted by BuŽga et al. followed 37 patients for 3, 6, and 12 months after laparoscopic sleeve gastrectomy to monitor biochemical, physical and dietary changes after surgery. Prior to surgery, 5.4% patients reported low appetites, whereas 27% reported low appetites and 48.6% noticed a decrease in overall appetite in the first year after surgery due to reductions in ghrelin secretion.

However, at twelve months post sleeve gastrectomy, it was noticed that ghrelin hormone levels began to trend upwards near pre-operative levels.

It is known that with the removal of the large portion of the gastric fundus with the sleeve gastrectomy, there is a change in ghrelin production. However, Meier et al. was able to show that negative energy balance can increase ghrelin production [21].

At six months post surgery, patients reported statistically significant reductions of fatty foods and simple carbohydrates in their diets, with increased intake of fish. At twelve months, patients reported statistically significant reductions in intake of fatty foods, however, there was a lack of statistical significance in the reported reduced intake of simple carbohydrates such as rice and baked goods [22]. Another study conducted by Odom et al. showed that 79% of patients included in the study experienced weight regain, with 15% regaining greater than or equal to 15% of their total amount of weight loss. However, it is important to note that there was an inverse association of weight regain and attendance of post-operative appointment visits by patients [23].

4 Ways to Prevent Weight Regain

- Stay connected with clinical team to monitor bloodwork and anthropometric changes
- Stay engaged through a supportive environment whether through patient focused support groups or behavioral therapy appointments with a specialist
- Continue to eat a balanced diet focusing on higher protein intake of 0.8–1.2 g/kg body weight
- Long term maintenance of weekly energy expenditures of 1,500–2,000 kilocalories
- Continue to celebrate non-scale victories to promote positive mind-set.

Many study outcomes show it is beneficial for patients to stay engaged with clinical appointments with their registered dietitians and behavioral support clinicians to monitor dietary intake and lifestyle changes to prevent weight regain after sleeve gastrectomy.

References

1. Andrue A, Moize V, et al. Protein intake, body composition, and protein status following bariatric surgery. Obes Surg. 2010;20:1509–15. https://doi.org/10.1007/s11695-010-0268-y.
2. -Mechanick JI, et al. Clinical practice guidelines for the perioperative nutrition, metabolic, and nonsurgical support of patients undergoing bariatric procedures—2019 update: cosponsored by american association of clinical endocrinologists/american college of endocrinology, the obesity society, american society for metabolic & bariatric surgery, obesity medicine association, and american society of anesthesiologists—executive summary. Endocrine Pract. 2019;25(12):1346–59.
3. Garvey WT, Mechanick JI, Brett EM, Garber AJ, Hurley DL, Jastreboff AM, Nadolsky K, Pessah-Pollack R, Plodkowski R, Reviewers of the AACE/ACE Obesity Clinical Practice Guidelines. American association of clinical endocrinologists and american college of endocrinology comprehensive clinical practice guidelines for medical care of patients with obesity. Endocrine Pract. 2016;22(Supplement 3):1–203. https://doi.org/10.4158/EP161365.GL.
4. Wouters E, Larsen J, Zijlstra H, et al. Physical activity after surgery for severe obesity: the role of exercise cognitions. Obes Surg. 2011;21:1894–9. https://doi.org/10.1007/s11695-010-0276-y.
5. - Jensen MD, Ryan DH, Apovian CM, et al. 2013 AHA/ACC/TOS guideline for the management of overweight and obesity in adults: a report of the American College of Cardiology/American Heart Association Task Force on Practice Guidelines and The Obesity Society. J Am Coll Cardiol. 2014;63(25 Pt B):2985–3023.
6. Colberg SR, Sigal RJ, Fernhall B, et al. Exercise and type 2 diabetes: the American College of Sports Medicine and the American Diabetes Association: joint position statement executive summary. Diabetes Care. 2010;33(12):2692–6.
7. Physical Activity Guidelines for Americans 2nd Edition. U.S. Department of Health and Human Services. 2018. https://Health.gov/sites/default/files/2019-09/Physical_Activity_Guidelines_2nd_edition.pdf.
8. Vanhecke TE, Franklin BA, Miller WM, et al. Cardiorespiratory fitness and sedentary lifestyle in the morbidly obese. Clin Cardiol. 2009;32(3):121–4.

9. Barlow CE, Kohl HW III, Gibbons LW, et al. Physical fitness, mortality and obesity. Int J Obes Relat Metab Disord. 1995;19:41–4.
10. Cristofaro PD, Pietrobelli A, Dragani B, et al. Total energy expenditure in morbidly obese subjects: a new device validation. Obes Res. 2005;13:A175.
11. Noel PH, Pugh JA. Management of overweight and obese adults. BMJ. 2002;325:757–61.
12. Jakicic JM, Clark K, Coleman E, et al. American College of Sports Medicine position stand. Appropriate intervention strategies for weight loss and prevention of weight regain for adults. Med Sci Sports Exerc. 2001;33(12):2145–56.
13. Colles SL, Dixon JB, O'Brien PE. Hunger control and regular physical activity facilitate weight loss after laparoscopic adjustable gastric banding. Obes Surg. 2008;18(7):833–40.
14. Fogelholm M, Kukkonen-Harjula K. Does physical activity prevent weight gain–a systematic review. Obes Rev. 2000;1:95–111.
15. de Souza SAF, Faintuch J, Sant'Anna AF. Effect of weight loss on aerobic capacity in patients with severe obesity before and after bariatric surgery. Obes Surg. 2010;20:871–75. https://doi.org/10.1007/s11695-010-0109-z.
16. Shah M, Snell PG, Rao S, Adams-Huet B, Quittner C, Livingston EH, Garg A. High-volume exercise program in obese bariatric surgery patients: a randomized, controlled trial. Obesity. 2011;19:1826–34. https://doi.org/10.1038/oby.2011.172.
17. Karlstad J. Weight loss surgery and fitness. The Do's and Don'ts for a successful exercise program. Obesity Action Coalition. Accessed Dec 2019. https://4617c1smqldcqsat27z78x17-wpengine.netdna-ssl.com/wp-content/uploads/WLS-and-Fitness-Dos-Donts.pdf.
18. Herring L, Stevinson C, Carter P, et al. The effects of supervised exercise training 12–24 months after bariatric surgery on physical function and body composition: a randomised controlled trial. Int J Obes. 2017;41:909–16. https://doi.org/10.1038/ijo.2017.60.
19. Huck CJ. Effects of supervised resistance training on fitness and functional strength in patients succeeding bariatric surgery. J Strength Cond Res. 2015;29(3):589–95.
20. Livhits M, Mercado C, Yermilov I, et al. Exercise following bariatric surgery: systematic review. Obes Surg. 2010;20:657–65. https://doi.org/10.1007/s11695-010-0096-0.
21. Meier U, Gressner AM. Endocrine regulation of energy metabolism:review of pathobiochemical and clinical chemical aspects of leptin, ghrelin, adiponectin, and resistin. Clin Chem. 2004;50:1511–25.
22. BuŽga M, Zavadilová V, et al. Dietary intake and ghrelin and leptin changes after sleeve Gastrectomy. Videosurgery Miniinv. 2014;9(4):554–61. https://doi.org/10.5114/wiitm.2014.45437.
23. Odom J, Zalesin K, et al. Behavioral predictors of weight regain after bariatric surgery. Obes Surg. 2010;20:349–56. https://doi.org/10.1007/s11695-009-9895-6.
24. American Heart Association. Six-week beginner walking program. walking program developed by american council on exercise in collaboration with the AHA. 2011. American Council on Exercise. Accessed Jan 2020. https://www.heart.org/idc/groups/heart-public/@WCM/@fc/documents/downloadable/UCM_449261.pdf.

Types of Exercises: Recommended Exercise Programs

Naji Alamuddin

1 Introduction

The prevalence of obesity has increased dramatically in the United States and around the world over the last several decades. Several factors have been implicated in the rise of this epidemic including dietary and lifestyle factors. Expert panels sponsored by the World Health Organization, the National Institutes of Health, and several professional societies have recommended that obese individuals lose approximately 5–10% of initial body weight to improve their health and quality of life [1–3]. This can be achieved through behavioral weight loss programs, which consist of three components: dietary modification, physical activity, and behavioral modification strategies. This chapter provides an overview of physical activity recommendations for weight management and reviews the literature for physical activity post-bariatric surgery.

2 Overview of Physical Activity

Physical activity plays a key role in obesity management. It also reduces the risk of cancer incidence, cancer recurrence, and helps reduce risk of co-morbidities such as type 2 diabetes and hypertension [4–6]. Despite all this evidence, the vast majority of adults in the United States continue to not meet physical activity recommendations. In fact, only 23.0% of U.S. adults meet the aerobic physical activity and

N. Alamuddin (✉)
Royal College of Surgeons in Ireland—Medical University of Bahrain, Busaiteen, Bahrain
e-mail: naalamuddin@rcsi.com

King Hamad University Hospital, Al Sayh, Bahrain

Perelman School of Medicine at the University of Pennsylvania, Philadelphi, Pennsylvania, US

© The Editor(s) (if applicable) and The Author(s), under exclusive license to Springer Nature Switzerland AG 2021
S. Al-Sabah et al. (eds.), *Laparoscopic Sleeve Gastrectomy*,
https://doi.org/10.1007/978-3-030-57373-7_65

muscle-strengthening guidelines [7]. The guidelines from the American College of Sports Medicine recommend 150 minutes per week of moderate physical activity or 75–150 minutes of vigorous physical activity for health benefits, but also recognize that higher amounts are needed for prevention of weight gain, to promote weight loss, in combination with reduction in energy intake [8].

Physical activity is an important component of a comprehensive lifestyle intervention, in which participants are typically instructed to increase their physical activity gradually to approximately 150–180 minutes/week over the first 6 months. This goal can be achieved by engaging in moderate physical activity (e.g., brisk walking) for 30 minutes on 5 days per week [3, 9]. Physical activity can be increased by incorporating short bouts of activity into individual's daily routines, such as increasing the amount of daily walking or using the stairs when possible, or by longer bouts of structured physical activity (e.g., at the gym). Individuals should be encouraged to engage in physical activities that they enjoy rather than be prescribed a particular activity. The effects of physical activity on weight loss, the maintenance of weight loss, and CVD risk factors have been investigated extensively and will be discussed next.

3   Physical Activity and Weight Loss

The role of physical activity in weight loss remains debatable. While exercise is recommended by all public health organizations for weight loss and prevention of weight gain, the evidence has been conflicting. A review by Wing et al. revealed that exercise alone results in a minimal weight loss of 2 kg compared to control conditions [10]. This data predominantly comes from multiple short-term behavioral weight loss studies which demonstrated that physical activity has a minimal impact on weight loss when compared with the effect of caloric restriction [11]. For example, in a 12-week study, participants lost 0.3–0.6% (male vs female) of initial weight with physical activity alone, compared to 5.5–8.4% (female vs male) and 7.5–11.4% (female vs male) losses for participants who reduced their calorie intake and those who changed both diet and physical activity, respectively [12]. The exercise performed in this study consisted of 30 minutes/day on 5 days per week. Similarly, Wing et al. [13] reported weight losses of 2.1, 9.1, and 10.3 kg after 6 months in participants assigned to physical activity alone, diet alone, and diet plus physical activity groups, respectively, all of whom were provided behavioral intervention. These short term studies suggest that exercise administered alone is not generally viewed to cause substantial weight loss.

However, longer term efficacy studies have demonstrated an opposing conclusion, in which exercise alone can result in clinically significant weight loss, independent of any dietary changes. The Midwest Diet and Exercise Trial (MET) was a long-term (16 months) efficacy trial aimed to evaluate the benefits of exercise on its own; subjects were randomized into an intervention group and a control group. The study consisted of supervised exercise 5 days/week (225 minutes per week of moderate physical activity) with an ad libitum diet for the intervention group [14]. Men in the exercise group lost 5.2 kg compared to control whereas women maintained baseline weight despite performing the same physical activity. This discrepancy in weight loss between men and women may be explained by significant differences in energy balance between women and men, where women were expending approximately 400 kcal/session compared to 700 kcal/session in men.

These findings led to a second trial designed to evaluate if there are differences in weight loss between men and women prescribed the same level of energy expenditure of exercise (EEEx) (either 400 or 600 kcal/session) without diet restriction [15]. Subjects in the 400 and 600 kcal/session lost 4.3 and 5.7% weight, respectively, which was not significantly different. This is important because it highlights that physical activity can lead to clinical meaningful weight losses. Furthermore, 44.5% of men and 47.4% of women lost>5% of their weight in the 400 kcal/session group compared to 68.4% and 55.6%, respectively in the 600 kcal/session group. Most of the weight loss was fat mass. These studies illustrate that unlike the short-term studies described earlier, exercise can lead to clinically meaningful weight loss when it is supervised and EEEx is of a sufficient magnitude. Supervision is critical since compliance decreases as physical activity prescription increases, leading to less weight loss compared to unsupervised exercise. This is evident in an 18-months behavioral weight loss program, where participants who were achieving 300 minutes/week of exercise under supervision in the first 6 months; Once the exercise became unsupervised, only a third of subjects maintained the 300 minutes/week at 18 months, and over 40% did not even achieve the minimal guidelines for health benefits [16].

The amount of physical activity needed to induce weight loss are very high for most individuals who are obese and sedentary, especially in a non-supervised setting. Alternatively, they can lose 1 lb./wk by only reducing their food intake by 500 kcal/d (the equivalent of eliminating 2 20 oz sugared sodas per day). This is likely the reason most the studies indicate that exercise alone, without caloric restriction, is insufficient to produce significant weight loss.

Regarding type of physical activity, minute by minute, aerobic training generally burns more calories than resistance training, and works best for reducing fat mass and body mass [17, 18]. However, resistance training can lead to favorable changes in body composition, physical function, markers of metabolic health and muscle efficiency [19]. Resistance training may be easier and more enjoyable for some individuals with overweight and obesity [20].

Current, generic approaches to increasing physical activity within a behavioral weight loss intervention work well for some, but not others. The best approach to increasing physical activity may depend on the characteristics of the person. Understanding the phenotypes that contribute to differences in physical activity adoption and maintenance could inform novel targets for personalized physical activity interventions. Research identifying phenotypes relevant top physical activity, particularly as it relates to weight management is limited [21].

Adaptive interventions are a promising area where the type and dose of interventions are altered based on personal characteristics and adjusted over time, typically using a series of a priori decision rules about when and how to modify and intervention [22–24]. One example of this is a study in 20 adults with overweight and obesity who were randomized to a 6 months physical activity intervention: an adaptive intervention group, where the daily step goal was adjusted based on a algorithm that responded to the individual's performance compared to a static intervention of 10,000 steps/day. The idea in the adaptive intervention group is to keep the activity challenging yet attainable. The results showed that the adaptive intervention group increased their steps by 1,130 more than the static intervention group [25]. This study shows the promise of how personalizing the physical activity goals can enhance activity adherence. Simply monitoring physical activity does not seem to increase physical activity adherence or weight loss. Closing the loop with personalized feedback and support shows promise.

4   Physical Activity and Weight Maintenance

Exercise plays an important role in weight loss maintenance. Several studies have shown that the more physical activity the patient engages in, the better the maintenance of lost weight [26, 27]. Jeffery et al., for example, randomly assigned patients enrolled in a comprehensive lifestyle modification program to expend either 1000 kcal/week or 2500 kcal/week (principally through walking) [28]. There were no significant differences in weight loss between the two groups at month 6 (8.1 and 9.0 kg, respectively), consistent with the previous discussion of the limited effects of exercise on short-term weight loss. However, at month 18, patients in the high activity group maintained a loss of 6.7 kg, compared with a significantly smaller 4.1 kg for the low-activity group. Jakicic et al. [27] similarly demonstrated in a secondary analysis of a randomized controlled trial, that women who exercised more than 200 minutes/week maintained greater weight losses than those who exercised 150–199 minutes/week or < 150 minutes/week. Data from the National Weight Control Registry have also provided evidence that high levels of physical activity are characteristic of individuals who report for long-term, sustained weight loss [29]. The Registry follows patients who have lost a minimum of 13.6 kg (i.e., 30 lb) in six months and maintained this loss for at least one year. Of these successful weight loss maintainers, 91% reported that they were exercising consistently, with women expending 2,545 kcal/week and men 3,293 kcal/week [30]. Based on these findings and other evidence, the current recommendation by the American College of Sports Medicine is that, for weight maintenance, individuals should exercise at a minimum level equivalent to an hour of brisk walking per day [11].

Practitioners should emphasize that, for weight control, this activity can be performed at a moderate intensity and in short bouts, as brief as 10 minutes. When included as part of a comprehensive weight loss program, multiple short bouts of activity (throughout the day) are as effective as one long bout (>40 minutes) in achieving weight control [31, 32]. Additional studies have shown that lifestyle activity, which involves increasing energy expenditure throughout the course of the day, without concern for the intensity or duration of the activity, is as effective for weight control as more traditional programmed activity (such as jogging, swimming, or biking) [33, 34]. Furthermore, short-term studies comparing high-intensity interval training with moderate-intensity continuous training result in similar adherence, enjoyment and body composition changes in individuals with obesity [35]. Pedometers and activity trackers (e.g., Fitbit, Jawbone, smart phones) provide some of the most convenient methods of monitoring lifestyle activity [36]. The ultimate goal is to walk approximately 10,000 steps daily, the equivalent of 4 to 5 miles, as practiced by members of the National Weight Control Registry. When prescribing exercise and trying to personalize exercise recommendations for patients, it is important to consider factors such as patient preference, time constraints, fitness level, and risk for musculoskeletal injury.

5   Physical Activity and Cardiovascular Health

Physical activity is crucial for improving cardiovascular health for both average-weight and obese individuals. In the absence of significant weight loss, regular bouts of aerobic activity have been found to reduce blood pressure [5], lipids [37], and visceral fat [38], the latter which is associated with improved glucose tolerance and insulin sensitivity (in non-diabetic individuals) and glycemic control (in patients with type 2 diabetes) [39, 40]. Several authors have evaluated the independent effects of cardiorespiratory fitness and adiposity on subsequent CVD mortality, and have suggested that high levels of cardiorespiratory fitness significantly decrease the CVD mortality risk in overweight and obese individuals, regardless of adiposity. Barry et al. [41] performed a meta-analysis of 10 studies and concluded that, compared to individuals who were normal weight and fit, unfit individuals had twice the risk of all-cause mortality regardless of their BMI, whereas individuals who were obese and fit had similar mortality risks as normal-weight, fit individuals. Similarly, in a longitudinal study of 25,000 men, Lee et al. [42] found that those who were lean but unfit had double the mortality of fit, lean men. Even in the absence of weight loss, regular aerobic activity reduces blood pressure, lipid concentrations, and visceral fat, while also ameliorating glucose intolerance and insulin resistance in non-diabetic individuals, and improving glycemic control in persons with type 2 diabetes [43]. These findings indicate that obese individuals should increase their physical activity to improve their health, regardless of its impact on their weight.

6   Physical Activity and Bariatric Surgery

While there is extensive evidence to the benefits of physical activity in obesity, the same does not apply to patients who have had bariatric surgery. There are relatively few studies of physical activity in bariatric surgery patients to date, and those available are limited by small sample size, short interventions, and inability to assess adherence to intervention. Consequently, it is not known what the optimal physical activity prescription is for patients [44, 45]. The few studies available mainly target the first few months after surgery, and lack longer term follow up and intervention. For example, a post hoc analysis of patients who underwent a RYGB who were randomized into either a 6-month structured exercise program or a health education control demonstrated that those who exercised heavily (i.e., 286 ± 40 minutes per week) lost a significantly greater amount of body weight, total fat mass, and abdominal subcutaneous abdominal fat compared with the health education control group. These studies only focused on exercise interventions and short-term outcomes [9, 10]. In a small randomized controlled trial of twenty-four inactive adult bariatric surgery patients whose BMI remained ≥30 kg/m^2 12 to 24 months post-surgery were randomized to an exercise intervention $(n = 12)$ or control group $(n = 12)$ [46]. Supervised exercise consisted of three 60-minutes gym sessions per week of moderate intensity aerobic and resistance training for 12 weeks. Control participants received usual care. The results revealed a 5.6 kg difference between groups in body mass change from baseline to 24 weeks favoring the exercise group. The majority of reports demonstrate a positive effect of exercise on body composition, blood pressure control, insulin sensitivity, and inflammatory markers [47]. A metanalysis demonstrated the benefits of exercise after bariatric surgery on weight loss with a mean of 3.62 kg (CI = 1.28, 5.96) greater weight loss compared to the minimal exercise groups [45]. However, a recent metanalysis on the effects of a physical activity program after bariatric surgery demonstrated no significant weight loss with exercise when compared to usual postoperative care [48].

Expert panels from The American Society of Metabolic and Bariatric Surgery (ASMBS), the American Association of Clinical Endocrinologists (AACE), and the National Institute for Health and Care Excellence (NICE) recommend multi-component perioperative care that includes increased physical activity for patients undergoing bariatric procedures. Patients should be advised to incorporate moderate aerobic physical activity to include a minimum of 150 minutes per week and goal of 300 minutes per week, including strength training 2 to 3 times per week. However, other expert groups from the Institute of Medicine and American College of Sports Medicine all agree that 150 minutes/week is insufficient for the prevention of weight regain. More recently, the ASMBS/ACSM have assembled an expert panel to develop specific pre- and post-operative recommendations.

7 Summary

Obese individuals should be counseled on the importance of physical activity on their health and on the recommendations from the American College of Sports Medicine consisting of 150 minutes per week of moderate physical activity or 75–150 minutes of vigorous physical activity for health benefits. Current generic approaches to increasing physical activity within a behavioral weight loss intervention work well for some, but not others. Physical activity can promote weight loss, especially when enrolled in supervised programs, as supervised exercise generally results in greater weight loss compared to unsupervised exercise. However, long term adherence to physical activity is challenging in weight loss interventions. There is a lack of data and number of unanswered questions regarding the role of exercising following bariatric surgery, especially regarding weight loss. Further robust research is needed to study the health benefits of physical activity and its effect on weight after bariatric surgery in order to provide guidance to patients.

References

1. Obesity: preventing and managing the global epidemic. Report of a WHO consultation. World Health Organ Tech Rep Ser. 2000;894:i–xii, 1–253.
2. Clinical Guidelines on the Identification. Evaluation, and treatment of overweight and obesity in adults-the evidence report National Institutes of Health. Obes Res. 1998;6(Suppl 2):51s–209s.
3. Jensen MD, et al. 2013 AHA/ACC/TOS guideline for the management of overweight and obesity in adults: a report of the American College of Cardiology/American Heart Association Task Force on Practice Guidelines and The Obesity Society. Circulation. 2014;129(25 Suppl 2):S102–38.
4. Knowler WC, et al. Reduction in the incidence of type 2 diabetes with lifestyle intervention or metformin. N Engl J Med. 2002;346(6):393–403.
5. Whelton SP, et al. Effect of aerobic exercise on blood pressure: a meta-analysis of randomized, controlled trials. Ann Intern Med. 2002;136(7):493–503.
6. Kyu HH, et al. Physical activity and risk of breast cancer, colon cancer, diabetes, ischemic heart disease, and ischemic stroke events: systematic review and dose-response meta-analysis for the Global Burden of Disease Study 2013. BMJ. 2016;354:i3857.
7. Katzmarzyk PT, et al. Epidemiology of physical activity and exercise training in the united states. Prog Cardiovasc Dis. 2017;60(1):3–10.
8. Services, U.S.D.o.H.a.H., Physical Activity Guidelines for Americans, U.S.D.o.H.a.H. Services, Editor. Washington, DC;2018.
9. Wing RR, et al. Cardiovascular effects of intensive lifestyle intervention in type 2 diabetes. N Engl J Med. 2013;369(2):145–54.
10. Wing RR. Physical activity in the treatment of the adulthood overweight and obesity: current evidence and research issues. Med Sci Sports Exerc. 1999;31(11 Suppl):S547–52.
11. Donnelly JE, et al. American College of Sports Medicine Position Stand. Appropriate physical activity intervention strategies for weight loss and prevention of weight regain for adults. Med Sci Sports Exerc. 2009;41(2):459–71.
12. Hagan RD, et al. The effects of aerobic conditioning and/or caloric restriction in overweight men and women. Med Sci Sports Exerc. 1986;18(1):87–94.
13. Wing RR, et al. Lifestyle intervention in overweight individuals with a family history of diabetes. Diabetes Care. 1998;21(3):350–9.
14. Donnelly JE, et al. Effects of a 16-month randomized controlled exercise trial on body weight and composition in young, overweight men and women: the Midwest Exercise Trial. Arch Intern Med. 2003;163(11):1343–50.
15. Donnelly JE, et al. Aerobic exercise alone results in clinically significant weight loss for men and women: midwest exercise trial 2. Obesity (Silver Spring). 2013;21(3):E219–28.
16. Catenacci VA, et al. The impact of timing of exercise initiation on weight loss: an 18-month randomized clinical trial. Obesity (Silver Spring). 2019;27(11):1828–38.
17. Swift DL, et al. The effects of exercise and physical activity on weight loss and maintenance. Prog Cardiovasc Dis. 2018;61(2):206–13.
18. Willis LH, et al. Effects of aerobic and/or resistance training on body mass and fat mass in overweight or obese adults. J Appl Physiol. 2012;113(12):1831–7.

19. Rosenbaum M, et al. Resistance training reduces skeletal muscle work efficiency in weight-reduced and non-weight-reduced subjects. Obesity (Silver Spring). 2018;26(10):1576–83.
20. Ten Hoor GA, et al. A benefit of being heavier is being strong: a cross-sectional study in young adults. Sports Med Open. 2018;4(1):12.
21. Bryan AD, et al. Behavioral and psychological phenotyping of physical activity and sedentary behavior: implications for weight management. Obesity (Silver Spring). 2017;25(10):1653–9.
22. Lai TL, Lavori PW, Shih MC. Adaptive trial designs. Annu Rev Pharmacol Toxicol. 2012;52:101–10.
23. Murphy SA, Collins LM, Rush AJ. Customizing treatment to the patient: adaptive treatment strategies. Drug Alcohol Depend. 2007;88(Suppl 2):S1-3.
24. Lei H, et al. A "SMART" design for building individualized treatment sequences. Annu Rev Clin Psychol. 2012;8:21–48.
25. Adams MA, et al. An adaptive physical activity intervention for overweight adults: a randomized controlled trial. PLoS ONE. 2013;8(12):e82901.
26. Fogelholm M, Kukkonen-Harjula K. Does physical activity prevent weight gain–a systematic review. Obes Rev. 2000;1(2):95–111.
27. Jakicic JM, et al. Effect of exercise duration and intensity on weight loss in overweight, sedentary women: a randomized trial. JAMA. 2003;290(10):1323–30.
28. Jeffery RW, et al. Physical activity and weight loss: does prescribing higher physical activity goals improve outcome? Am J Clin Nutr. 2003;78(4):684–9.
29. Thomas JG, et al. Weight-loss maintenance for 10 years in the national weight control registry. Am J Prev Med. 2014;46(1):17–23.
30. Klem ML, et al. A descriptive study of individuals successful at long-term maintenance of substantial weight loss. Am J Clin Nutr. 1997;66(2):239–46.
31. Murphy MH, Blair SN, Murtagh EM. Accumulated versus continuous exercise for health benefit: a review of empirical studies. Sports Med. 2009;39(1):29–43.
32. Jakicic JM, et al. Prescription of exercise intensity for the obese patient: the relationship between heart rate, VO2 and perceived exertion. Int J Obes Relat Metab Disord. 1995;19(6):382–7.
33. Epstein LH, et al. Ten-year outcomes of behavioral family-based treatment for childhood obesity. Health Psychol. 1994;13(5):373–83.
34. Andersen RE, et al. Effects of lifestyle activity vs structured aerobic exercise in obese women: a randomized trial. JAMA. 1999;281(4):335–40.
35. Vella CA, Taylor K, Drummer D. High-intensity interval and moderate-intensity continuous training elicit similar enjoyment and adherence levels in overweight and obese adults. Eur J Sport Sci. 2017;17(9):1203–11.
36. Bravata DM, et al. Using pedometers to increase physical activity and improve health: a systematic review. JAMA. 2007;298(19):2296–304.
37. Kraus WE, et al. Effects of the amount and intensity of exercise on plasma lipoproteins. N Engl J Med. 2002;347(19):1483–92.
38. Ross R, et al. Reduction in obesity and related comorbid conditions after diet-induced weight loss or exercise-induced weight loss in men. A randomized, controlled trial. Ann Intern Med. 2000;133(2):92–103.
39. Hayes C, Kriska A. Role of physical activity in diabetes management and prevention. J Am Diet Assoc. 2008;108(4 Suppl 1):S19-23.
40. Sigal RJ, et al. Physical activity/exercise and type 2 diabetes: a consensus statement from the American diabetes association. Diabetes Care. 2006;29(6):1433–8.
41. Barry VW, et al. Fitness vs. fatness on all-cause mortality: a meta-analysis. Prog Cardiovasc Dis. 2014;56(4):382–90.
42. Lee CD, Blair SN, Jackson AS. Cardiorespiratory fitness, body composition, and all-cause and cardiovascular disease mortality in men. Am J Clin Nutr. 1999;69(3):373–80.

43. Gaesser GA, Angadi SS, Sawyer BJ. Exercise and diet, independent of weight loss, improve cardiometabolic risk profile in overweight and obese individuals. Phys Sportsmed. 2011;39(2):87–97.
44. King WC, Bond DS. The importance of preoperative and postoperative physical activity counseling in bariatric surgery. Exerc Sport Sci Rev. 2013;41(1):26–35.
45. Egberts K, et al. Does exercise improve weight loss after bariatric surgery? a systematic review. Obes Surg. 2012;22(2):335–41.
46. Herring LY, et al. The effects of supervised exercise training 12–24 months after bariatric surgery on physical function and body composition: a randomised controlled trial. Int J Obes (Lond). 2017;41(6):909–16.
47. Ahmadi N, et al. Effects of intense exercise and moderate caloric restriction on cardiovascular risk factors and inflammation. Am J Med. 2011;124(10):978–82.
48. Carretero-Ruiz A, et al. Effects of exercise training on weight loss in patients who have undergone bariatric surgery: a systematic review and meta-analysis of controlled trials. Obes Surg. 2019;29(10):3371–84.

Completing the Weight Loss Journey for Laparoscopic Sleeve Gastrectomy Patients: The Role of Body Contouring Surgery

Sarah Al Youha, Osama Samargandi and Jason G. Williams

1   Introduction

The American Society of Plastic Surgery declared 2018 as, 'The Year of the Body' [1], as global statistics showed a rise in the number of body contouring procedures performed around the world [2]. The psychological and functional benefits of body contouring procedures after bariatric surgery are well documented in the literature and are an essential component of providing comprehensive care for these patients, after the dramatic changes their bodies undergo [3, 4]. In addition to the psychosocial benefits that body contouring surgeries offer these patients, evidence has recently emerged that bariatric patients who have undergone body contouring procedures undergo greater weight loss than those that have not and are able to sustain those weight losses for longer [3, 5–10]. Despite the numerous advantages that body contouring surgery offers and the high desire for it by patients who have undergone laparoscopic sleeve gastrectomies (LSG) [11], (around 60% of bariatric patients reported interest in body contouring surgery one year after their bariatric surgery [12]), a relatively low proportion, around 5–7% of bariatric patients end up actually having body contouring procedures [11]. Some have attributed this low uptake to the high out-of-pocket costs for patients who must personally fund

S. Al Youha (✉)
Jaber Al Ahmad Al Sabah Hospital, Kuwait City, Kuwait
e-mail: sarahalyouha@gmail.com

O. Samargandi · J. G. Williams
Division of Plastic Surgery, Dalhousie University, Nova Scotia, Canada
e-mail: osamargandi@gmail.com

J. G. Williams
e-mail: drjwilliams@gmail.com

S. Al-Sabah et al. (eds.), *Laparoscopic Sleeve Gastrectomy*,
https://doi.org/10.1007/978-3-030-57373-7_66

these operations, as they are often not covered by insurance providers. The lack of access to plastic surgeons in the public hospital system is another factor that may be contributing to the discrepancy in the number of patients who desire body contouring surgery and those who end up getting it [13].

Another reason for the lack of access to body contouring procedures is the low prevalence of plastic surgeons on multi-disciplinary bariatric teams. The UK's National Institute for Health and Care Excellence (NICE) guidelines explicitly state in their recommendations that, 'bariatric surgery should be undertaken by a multi-disciplinary team (MDT) that can provide information on access to plastic surgery (such as apronectomy), where appropriate' [14]. Despite this, a recent survey, completed by over 70% of bariatric surgeons that are members of the British Obesity and Metabolic Surgery Society, reported that only 1 out of 61 respondents involved a plastic surgeon in their bariatric MDTs on a regular basis [15]. A prime example of how both bariatric and plastic surgery groups can be integrated to provide ongoing support for patients during all phases of weight loss, is the 'Life After Weight Loss' Program, which is a joint venture between the Department of Plastic Surgery and Bariatric Surgery Division at the University of Pittsburgh Medical Center (UPMC). Patients are prescribed personalized exercise and nutrition programs as well as behavioral seminars and are continuously assessed by both surgical teams to ensure that patients are optimized for the multiple procedures they require [15]. Adequate counselling regarding the deleterious impact of the excess amount of skin that is left behind after massive weight loss has been shown to improve patient satisfaction with their overall treatment, as their expectations are managed [16]. In addition, inter-disciplinary care can improve patient selection for body contouring surgery, reducing unnecessary referrals for patients who are unsuitable candidates [17].

2   Importance of Patient Selection and Timing for Body Contouring Surgery Safety and Optimized Outcomes

Several factors need to be considered prior to referring patients for body contouring surgery after LSG. It is advisable that patients wait around 12–18 months after bariatric surgery, until their weight stays constant for 2 months, to ensure that their weight loss and nutritional status are stable[18]. This allows time for protein, micronutrients, and vitamin deficiencies to be corrected. In bariatric patients seeking body contouring procedures, 40% of patients were found to have iron deficiency anemia, despite 50% of those patients reporting that were taking iron supplements. The next most common vitamin deficiency in the same group patients was reported to be vitamin B12 deficiency (14.5%) [19]. Hypoalbuminemia was also found to be present in 14% of post-bariatric patients seeking body contouring surgery[19]. Although the impact of low albumin levels on wound complications is unclear [20], there is some evidence that pre-operative consumption of over-the-counter protein supplements prior to abdominoplasty in massive weight loss patients reduces post-operative wound complications (0.0% in protein supplement group versus 21.8% in the non-supplemented group).

To optimize patients prior to body contouring surgery, the following blood work can be ordered to identify potential nutrient deficiencies so that they can corrected via pre-operative supplementation: full blood work, electrolytes, albumin and pre-albumin levels, iron, ferritin, total iron binding capacity, vitamin B12 levels, folate and glucose levels [21].

Another safety consideration is adequate risk stratification for thromboembolic episodes and appropriate administration of thromboprophylaxis. Although uncommon, thromboembolic episodes are a serious, preventable complication, whose occurrence can be minimized through careful patient selection and by taking adequate precautions [22]. Older age (>65 years old), BMI at the time of surgery (>30 kg/m^2) and multiple combined body contouring procedures (>2 at the same time), have shown to be significantly associated with thromboembolic episodes in bariatric patients undergoing body contouring procedures [23]. Anti-coagulation has been demonstrated to safely decrease that risk, whilst not being shown to increase the hematoma rates after surgery [24, 25].

In addition to medical optimization, psychological counseling and assessment is important to adequately manage patient expectations and to prepare them for the upcoming changes in their body after body contouring surgeries. Adequate informed consent and a detailed explanation of what to expect has been shown to improve patient satisfaction [16]. Minimally invasive procedures are rarely an option for these patients, as the large amount of skin redundancy that must be managed and the poor skin quality can often only be addressed through direct excision [26]. These patients are trading scars for a more aesthetic body contour, as their skin is essentially being tailored to fit their bony framework again, after undergoing years of expansion. Patients need to be informed about this tradeoff and the potential impact of their scars' visibility on their psychological well-being. The potential need for multiple staged procedures also needs to be discussed, to prepare patients psychologically [27].

3   Overview of Body Contouring Procedures and Staging

As already stated, most body contouring procedures for massive weight loss patients, such as those who have undergone LSG, tend to rely on direct excision of excess skin and subcutaneous tissue. Considerations for scar placement include: placing the scars in the least visible area, avoiding distortion to adjacent tissues through appropriate scar placement (e.g. placing the incision far away enough from the labia in an abdominoplasty incision to avoid labial distortion) and ensuring that the scar length and vector is able to correct the majority of the skin redundancy that is concerning the patient (Figs. 1 and 2). Multiple areas of the body tend to be concurrently affected in these patients, including the trunk, arms, thighs, and face, and may all need to be addressed in the same patient. The types of surgeries that are available to massive weight loss patients are summarized in Table 1. Whether the procedures are staged and how they are staged depends on what surgeries the patient desires and whether the grouping of those procedures can be performed safely [27].

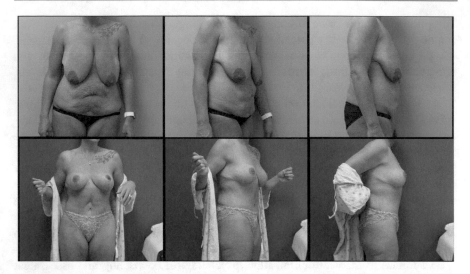

Fig. 1 'Before' and 'after' pictures for a massive weight loss patient. Significant breast and abdominal deformities can be seen in the 'before' pictures (top). For example, massive deflation of the breasts, asymmetry, loss of definition of the lateral breast borders and prominent lipodystrophy of the abdomen. Significant improvement of the breast deformity (bottom) can be seen after breast reduction surgery using an inverted T-scar and auto-augmentation. The abdominal contour has also significantly improved after a traditional abdominoplasty and liposuction of the flanks (photos courtsey of Dr John Stein, Dalhousie University)

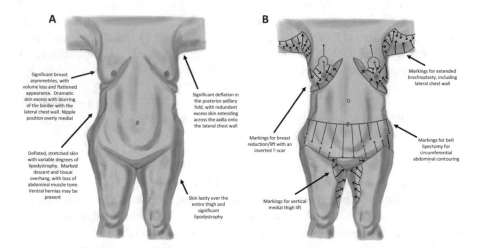

Fig. 2 Illustrations demonstrating the classical deformities that occur after massive weight loss (**a**) and the surgical markings for the body contouring procedures required to improve those deformities (**b**)

Table 1 Summary of commonly performed body contouring procedures in laparoscopic sleeve gastrectomy patients ([27] adapted from Almutairi et al.)

Procedure	Type of Procedure	Description
Brachioplasty (arm lift)	Upper extremity contouring	• In mild deformities, liposuction or a short axillary scar technique might be adequate. More commonly a posteromedial long scar extending from the elbow to the axilla, and sometimes the chest, is required to address the deformity in most MWL[a] patients
Breast procedures	Upper trunk contouring	• Breast reshaping can be a challenge in these patients as the breasts are often severely deflated and their associated supporting structures are very lax. Volume replacement via an implant, fat grafting or tissue redistribution is often required along with skin tightening procedure
Bra-line back lift or other upper body lifts to address upper body rolls	Upper trunk contouring	• A transverse scar at the back or bilateral vertical scars on the lateral chest can be used to excise upper back rolls. These procedures are often combined with other upper trunk contouring procedures
Panniculectomy	Abdominal contouring	• For patients who are unsuitable candidates for an abdominoplasty, this is a functional operation, where the undesirable lower abdominal excess tissue is directly excised without undermining or rectus plication
Abdominoplasty • Traditional • High Lateral Tension • Mini abdominoplasty • Umbilical float abdominoplasty • Lipo-abdominoplasty • Vertical or Fleur-de-lis or Gauthier abdominoplasty • Reverse abdominoplasty	Abdominal contouring	• The type of abdominoplasty that is carried out should be tailored to the amount of excess skin that the patient has and where it is located • A mini abdominoplasty or an umbilical float abdominoplasty is an option for minor skin excess, where the umbilicus is placed high in the abdomen • Traditional abdominoplasties involve a horizontal incision that is strategically placed, some undermining of the abdominal flap and plication of the rectus abdominis muscle. A high lateral tension abdominoplasty is a refinement, where most of the skin that is excised, is excised laterally, where it is predominantly present • A vertical abdominoplasty includes a vertical midline scar, in addition to a horizontal scar to correct skin excess in both dimensions • A reverse abdominoplasty involves a scar that is placed in the lower part of the chest, often below the breast in women, to address epigastric laxity

(continued)

Table 1 (continued)

Procedure	Type of Procedure	Description
Monsplasty	Lower trunk contouring	• A ptotic mons can be distressing to MWL patients and suspension techniques can help improve function and aesthetics for those patients
Lower body lift and belt lipectomy	Lower body contouring	• These circumferential procedures can be powerful in addressing skin excess in massive weight loss patients. Body lifts differ from belt lipectomies in that their scar placement are located differently. Auto-augmentation of the buttock and reshaping can also be incorporated in combination with these procedures
Thigh lift	Lower trunk contouring	• Medial and vertical incisions can be used to correct thigh laxity. Body lifts do address some of the lateral thigh laxity. Combining them with a medial vertical thigh lift is a common way of addressing lower extremity skin deformities in MWL patients
Facelift	Facial volumization and contouring	• MWL patients faces can also be severely affected after MWL. Skin excision through facelifts and volume replacement via fat grafting can help rejuvenate this area if it is a cause of distress for patients

ªMWL = massive weight loss

Most patients prefer not to stage their procedures and to have all their areas of concern addressed in a single operation. Several safety concerns must be considered, as the complication rate and the overall recovery time for patients increases significantly when multiple procedures are grouped together [28]. These complications often include an increase in the rate of thromboembolic episodes, wound healing complications, unnecessary blood transfusions and infections [22]. For example, combining surgeries with opposing vectors of tension, such as an upper body lift with a lower body lift can be associated with a much longer recovery and wound healing complications. Ultimately, a frank discussion regarding the risks/benefits is an important component of the informed consent process. Safety must never be compromised for convenience or patient preference, especially these elective procedures [27].

4 Future Trends in Body Contouring Surgery

Body contouring techniques are becoming more sophisticated. Reshaping and re-sculpting the body to achieve a more aesthetically desirable contour has become the focus of most plastic surgeons, rather than just skin and fat reduction in massive weight loss patients. An appreciation for the influence of light and shadows on the perception for contour, has resulted in an increased uptake of additive surgical procedures, such as those that utilize fat grafting and auto-augmentation techniques to reshape anatomical regions [29]. The use of liposuction as an adjunct to body contouring surgeries is becoming more popular as a result. Liposuction can also be combined with reductive procedures to help preserve key anatomical structures, reducing the risk of injuring critical lympho-vascular and neural structures [30].

Lastly, ambulatory surgical care and enhanced recovery after surgery (ERAS) protocols are becoming an essential component of modern care for body contouring patients, minimizing the discomfort and certain risks associated with these surgeries [31, 32]. As a result, drainless procedures are becoming more common, as well as measures to minimize seroma formation, which can be time-consuming to manage in the outpatient setting [33]. Future studies should be directed towards confirming the benefits and safety of these protocols need to be conducted, to ensure that these measures are more widely adopted [31].

References

1. ASPS. ASPS Statistics Suggest Surge in Body Sculpting Procedures—Plastic Surgery Practice. https://www.plasticsurgerypractice.com/client-objectives/aesthetics/body-make-over/sculpting/asps-statistics-suggest-surge-body-sculpting-procedures/. Accessed 25 May 2020.
2. ISAPS. ISAPS International Survey on Aesthetic/Cosmetic Procedures performed in 2018. www.isaps.org. Accessed 25 May 2020.
3. Toma T, Harling L, Athanasiou T, Darzi A, Ashrafian H. Does body contouring after bariatric weight loss enhance quality of life? a systematic review of QOL studies. Obes Surg. 2018. https://doi.org/10.1007/s11695-018-3323-8.
4. Marek RJ, Steffen KJ, Flum DR, et al. Psychosocial functioning and quality of life in patients with loose redundant skin 4 to 5 years after bariatric surgery. Surg Obes Relat Dis. 2018. https://doi.org/10.1016/j.soard.2018.07.025.
5. Balagué N, Combescure C, Huber O, Pittet-Cuénod B, Modarressi A. Plastic surgery improves long-term weight control after bariatric surgery. Plastic and Reconstructive Surgery. 2013;826–33.
6. Wiser I, Avinoah E, Ziv O, et al. Body contouring surgery decreases long-term weight regain following laparoscopic adjustable gastric banding: A matched retrospective cohort study. J Plast Reconstr Aesthetic Surg. 2016. https://doi.org/10.1016/j.bjps.2016.08.012.
7. Wiser I, Heller L, Spector C, Fliss E, Friedman T. Body contouring procedures in three or more anatomical areas are associated with long-term body mass index decrease in massive weight loss patients: a retrospective cohort study. J Plast Reconstr Aesthetic Surg. 2017. https://doi.org/10.1016/j.bjps.2017.05.055.
8. Paul MA, Opyrchał J, Knakiewicz M, et al. The long-term effect of body contouring procedures on the quality of life in morbidly obese patients after bariatric surgery. PLoS ONE. 2020;15:e0229138.
9. Agarwal S, Shenaq D, Teven CM, Prachand V, Roughton M, Zachary L. Body contouring after obesity surgery is associated with a weight loss benefit among patients. J Plast Reconstr Aesthetic Surg. 2017;70:1186–90.
10. Froylich D, Corcelles R, Daigle CR, et al. Weight loss is higher among patients who undergo body contouring procedures after bariatric surgery. Surg Obes Relat Dis. 2016. https://doi.org/10.1016/j.soard.2015.09.009.

11. Altieri MS, Yang J, Park J, et al. Utilization of body contouring procedures following weight loss surgery: a study of 37,806 patients. Obes Surg. 2017. https://doi.org/10.1007/s11695-017-2732-4.

12. Giordano S, Victorzon M, Stormi T, Suominen E. Desire for body contouring surgery after bariatric surgery: do body mass index and weight loss matter? Aesthetic Surg J. 2014. https://doi.org/10.1177/1090820X13515701.

13. Aldaqal SM, Samargandi OA, El-Deek BS, Awan BA, Ashy AA, Kensarah AA. Prevalence and desire for body contouring surgery in postbariatric patients in Saudi Arabia. N Am J Med Sci. 2012. https://doi.org/10.4103/1947-2714.93386.

14. NICE. 1 Recommendations | Obesity: identification, assessment and management | Guidance | NICE. https://www.nice.org.uk/guidance/cg189/chapter/1-recommendations. Accessed 25 May 2020.

15. Highton L, Ekwobi C, Rose V. Post-bariatric surgery body contouring in the NHS: a survey of UK Bariatric Surgeons. J Plast Reconstr Aesthetic Surg. 2012. https://doi.org/10.1016/j.bjps.2011.09.047.

16. Sarwer DB, Thompson JK, Mitchell JE, Rubin JP. Psychological considerations of the bariatric surgery patient undergoing body contouring surgery. Plast Reconstr Surg. 2008. https://doi.org/10.1097/PRS.0b013e3181772aa8.

17. Warner JP, Stacey DH, Sillah NM, Gould JC, Garren MJ, Gutowski KA. National bariatric surgery and massive weight loss body contouring survey. Plast Reconstr Surg. 2009. https://doi.org/10.1097/PRS.0b013e3181b03880.

18. Peter Rubin J, Nguyen V, Schwentker A. Perioperative management of the post-gastric-bypass patient presenting for body contour surgery. Clin Plast Surg. 2004. https://doi.org/10.1016/j.cps.2004.03.017.

19. Naghshineh N, O'Brien Coon D, McTigue K, Courcoulas AP, Fernstrom M, Rubin JP. Nutritional assessment of bariatric surgery patients presenting for plastic surgery: a prospective analysis. Plast Reconstr Surg. 2010. https://doi.org/10.1097/PRS.0b013e3181de2473.

20. Karamanos E, Kandagatla P, Wang H, Gupta AH, Siddiqui A. Challenging the surgical axiom: albumin level does not reliably predict development of wound complications in patients undergoing body contouring. Perm J. 2020. https://doi.org/10.7812/TPP/18.206.

21. Davison SP, Clemens MW. Safety first: precautions for the massive weight loss patient. Clin Plast Surg. 2008. https://doi.org/10.1016/j.cps.2007.08.002.

22. Michaels J, Coon D, Rubin JP. Complications in postbariatric body contouring: strategies for assessment and prevention. Plast Reconstr Surg. 2011. https://doi.org/10.1097/PRS.0b013e3182063144.

23. Wes AM, Wink JD, Kovach SJ, Fischer JP. Venous thromboembolism in body contouring: an analysis of 17,774 patients from the national surgical quality improvement databases. Plast Reconstr Surg. 2015. https://doi.org/10.1097/PRS.0000000000001251.

24. Morales R, et al. Safety and efficacy of novel oral anticoagulants vs low molecular weight heparin for thromboprophylaxis in large-volume liposuction and body contouring procedures. Aesthetic Surg J. 2016;36. https://doi.org/10.1093/ASJ/SJV243.

25. Sarhaddi D, et al. Fondaparinux significantly reduces postoperative venous thromboembolism after body contouring procedures without an increase in bleeding complications. Aesthetic Surg J. 2019;39. https://doi.org/10.1093/ASJ/SJZ184.

26. Afrooz PN, Pozner JN, DiBernardo BE. Noninvasive and minimally invasive techniques in body contouring. Clin Plast Surg. 2014. https://doi.org/10.1016/j.cps.2014.07.006.

27. Almutairi K, Gusenoff JA, Rubin JP. Body contouring. Plast Reconstr Surg. 2016. https://doi.org/10.1097/PRS.0000000000002140.

28. Coon D, Michaels J, Gusenoff JA, Purnell C, Friedman T, Rubin JP. Multiple procedures and staging in the massive weight loss population. Plast Reconstr Surg. 2010. https://doi.org/10.1097/PRS.0b013e3181c87b3c.

29. Hoyos AE, Perez ME, Castillo L. Dynamic definition mini-lipoabdominoplasty combining multilayer liposculpture, fat grafting, and muscular plication. Aesthetic Surg J. 2013. https://doi.org/10.1177/1090820X13484493.
30. Chia CT, Neinstein RM, Theodorou SJ. Evidence-based medicine: liposuction. Plast Reconstr Surg. 2017. https://doi.org/10.1097/PRS.0000000000002859.
31. Nuveen EJ, Matthesen J, Cox K, Caplin CJ. An enhanced recovery after surgery (ERAS) protocol for outpatient bodylift surgery. Am J Cosmet Surg. 2020. https://doi.org/10.1177/0748806819898990.
32. Egrari S. Outpatient-based massive weight loss body contouring: a review of 260 consecutive cases. Aesthetic Surg J. 2012. https://doi.org/10.1177/1090820X12441618.
33. Isaac KV, et al. Drainless abdominoplasty using barbed progressive tension sutures. Aesthetic Surg J. 2017. https://doi.org/10.1093/asj/sjw241.

Index

Printed in the United States
by Baker & Taylor Publisher Services